Five Element Constitutional Acupuncture

For Churchill Livingstone

Commissioning Editors: *Karen Morley, Claire Wilson*
Project Development Editors: *Natalie Meylan, Louisa Welch*
Project Manager: *Alan Nicholson*
Designer: *Stewart Larking*

Five Element Constitutional Acupuncture

SECOND EDITION

Angela Hicks MAc, DIP CHM, MBAcC, MRCHM
Joint Principal of the College of Integrated Chinese Medicine, Reading, Berkshire, UK

John Hicks PhD, DR Ac DIP CHM, MBAcC, MRCHM
Joint Principal of the College of Integrated Chinese Medicine, Reading, Berkshire, UK

Peter Mole MA (OXON), MAc, MBAcC
Dean, College of Integrated Chinese Medicine, Reading, Berkshire, UK

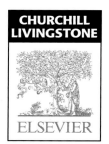

CHURCHILL LIVINGSTONE

ELSEVIER

Edinburgh   London   New York   Oxford   Philadelphia   St Louis   Sydney   Toronto   2011

CHURCHILL
LIVINGSTONE
ELSEVIER

First edition 2004
Second edition 2011

ISBN 978-0-7020-3175-5

British Library Cataloguing in Publication Data
A catalogue record for this book is available from the British Library

Library of Congress Cataloging in Publication Data
A catalog record for this book is available from the Library of Congress

Notices
Knowledge and best practice in this field are constantly changing. As new research and experience broaden our understanding, changes in research methods, professional practices, or medical treatment may become necessary.

Practitioners and researchers must always rely on their own experience and knowledge in evaluating and using any information, methods, compounds, or experiments described herein. In using such information or methods they should be mindful of their own safety and the safety of others, including parties for whom they have a professional responsibility.

With respect to any drug or pharmaceutical products identified, readers are advised to check the most current information provided (i) on procedures featured or (ii) by the manufacturer of each product to be administered, to verify the recommended dose or formula, the method and duration of administration, and contraindications. It is the responsibility of practitioners, relying on their own experience and knowledge of their patients, to make diagnoses, to determine dosages and the best treatment for each individual patient, and to take all appropriate safety precautions.

To the fullest extent of the law, neither the Publisher nor the authors, contributors, or editors, assume any liability for any injury and/or damage to persons or property as a matter of products liability, negligence or otherwise, or from any use or operation of any methods, products, instructions, or ideas contained in the material herein.

ELSEVIER   your source for books, journals and multimedia in the health sciences

www.elsevierhealth.com

Working together to grow
libraries in developing countries
www.elsevier.com | www.bookaid.org | www.sabre.org

ELSEVIER   BOOK AID International   Sabre Foundation

The Publisher's policy is to use **paper manufactured from sustainable forests**

Printed in China

Contents

Section 1   The Foundations

Contents

Section 4   Blocks to Treatment

Section 5   Treatment Techniques

Section 6   The Use of Points

Appendices

Introduction

Recent history

The practice of Five Element Constitutional Acupuncture in the form described in this book is of relatively recent origin. It is based on the style developed some time in the late 1960s and 1970s by J. R. Worsley (1923–2003), an Englishman. He drew on passages in the *Nei Jing* and *Nan Jing*, as well as what he learnt from a number of teachers in the East and West in the 1960s (Eckman, 1996). J. R. Worsley and some of his students have subsequently taught this style of treatment to thousands of acupuncture students and practitioners in the UK and the USA, and to a lesser extent in other countries such as Norway, Holland, Canada, Switzerland and Germany. A survey carried out in 1995 of members of the British Acupuncture Council in the UK showed that 38% of practitioners were using this style 'regularly' compared with 66% using Traditional Chinese Medicine (TCM) and 8% using Japanese Meridian Therapy (Dale, 1996). (Note that throughout this book the abbreviation TCM is used to describe that style of Chinese medicine currently practised in China.)

Diversity in Chinese medicine

The history of Chinese medicine has been characterised by diversity and innovation. Its principles were laid down in antiquity and its style of practice has varied according to where and when it has been used. Recent scholarship has given us some glimpse of just how varied and innovative the practice of acupuncture has been (see Unschuld, 1992; Hsu, 2001; and Scheid, 2002).

It is inevitable that Western practitioners, steeped in the philosophical and intellectual traditions of the West, will continue to evolve new ways of practising acupuncture that honour traditional Chinese concepts and introduce ideas and practices from Western traditions.

There are currently a number of styles of acupuncture being practised in Western countries. Some have little or no basis in the classics of Chinese medicine. All were essentially formulated in the late twentieth century. Some were developed in countries with long traditions of traditional acupuncture; some arose in the West. Styles that draw on traditional concepts include TCM (China; the countries in brackets indicate the country of origin), Tong family style (Taiwan), Eight Constitutions (Korea), Meridian Therapy (Japan), Six Energetic levels (France), Stems and Branches (China), and Five Element Constitutional Acupuncture (UK). Even within these styles, individual practitioners and teachers practise in quite different ways from each other.

There is as yet no adequate research that establishes the relative efficacy of these various styles of diagnosis and treatment. TCM, with the backing of the Chinese government, is currently the style practised by the majority of practitioners. It has contributed greatly to the spread and acceptance of acupuncture throughout the world. The other styles, however, with their emphasis on other traditional concepts, have much to offer both patients and practitioners.

Chinese medicine has always had a 'continuous tendency toward a syncretism of all ideas that exist (within accepted limits). Somehow a way was always found in China to reconcile opposing views and to build bridges' (Unschuld, 1992, p. 51). It is to be hoped that colleges of acupuncture, professional associations and statutory bodies will continue to respect the diversity of traditional acupuncture and these styles will continue to flourish.

The recent history of Five Element Acupuncture in the UK

In the 1960s there was a loose grouping of practitioners of various forms of medicine who showed a keen interest in acupuncture. J. R. Worsley, who was previously trained as a physiotherapist and naturopath, was a member of this group and attended seminars in the UK given by various teachers of acupuncture (Worsley, 1987). In the absence of teachers from China, due to the political situation at the time, he and others learnt from practitioners from Japan, Korea, Taiwan, Vietnam, Hong Kong and Singapore, as well as Europe. J. R. Worsley also visited the Far East several times.

At this time Five Element theory was the major philosophical influence on the group. This is because at that time Japan and Taiwan were the main sources of inspiration. Three of the group members subsequently wrote books primarily focused on the Five Elements (Austin, 1983, and Lawson-Wood and Lawson-Wood, 1965).

In Japan, the Five Elements has always been the dominant underlying principle, and the *Nan Jing* the main classic of Chinese medicine. The *Nan Jing* is based almost exclusively on Five Element theory. Taiwan, which J. R. Worsley visited, had been ruled by Japan for much of the twentieth century and its style of acupuncture was heavily influenced by Japanese-inspired Five Element thinking. In Japan it was customary for acupuncture to be used alongside massage, often by blind practitioners, rather than with herbal medicine as was customary in China. (One of J. R. Worsley's main teachers, Bunkei Ono, had himself received his initial training in one of the schools of acupuncture for the blind, which naturally stressed the importance of touch in diagnosis.) Japanese practitioners also had not embraced the changes in emphasis that had taken place in China in the Qing dynasty (1644–1911).[1]

It is also important to remember that it was virtually impossible to enter China until some time after President Nixon's visit in 1972. What few books were available from China did not explain TCM in any coherent form. For example, *The Academy of Traditional Chinese Medicine* (1975) was the only official Chinese text available in English. It had virtually no theoretical discussion in it and concentrated on point location, practical techniques and purely symptomatic treatments for various ailments. The slightly enhanced *Essentials of Chinese Acupuncture* from the same publisher in 1980 included exactly the same material with the addition of an extremely brief outline of the theoretical basis of TCM.

It was not until 1979 that Ted Kaptchuk gave a series of lectures on TCM in London, based on instruction he had received in Macao. This was the first introduction most British practitioners had to this style. Knowledge of TCM was available in the USA at approximately the same time. Practitioners from the British Acupuncture Association and Register visited China in 1976 and came back with some grasp of the style being practised there. Mann (1963) included a translation of *A General Survey of Common Diseases and their Treatment by Acupuncture* compiled by The Beijing School of Chinese Medicine in 1960. This laid out a simple version of TCM differentiation of disease, but had no discussion of theory at all. It is striking how little effect it had on the general development of acupuncture in the UK.

In the late 1960s J. R. Worsley broke from most of his peers and started to teach his vision of Five Element acupuncture in Leamington Spa, in the Midlands of England. He stopped teaching for a time, but was persuaded to start again to teach a class of Americans in 1972. In subsequent years he taught several classes of Americans, with a few British students, at the Buddhist Centre at Farmoor near Oxford.

From 1972 until 1993 he was the Principal of the College of Traditional Chinese Acupuncture in Leamington Spa and taught hundreds of students. Looking at the notes of students who trained in 1972, it is striking that his teaching was fundamentally identical then to what he was teaching at the end of the century.[2] For a time in the 1980s this style was probably the most widely practised style in the UK. Its emphasis on the diagnosis of an individual's constitutional imbalance means that practitioners must rely largely on their sensory and intuitive skills. After TCM was

---

[1] Although the concepts had been laid down in the early Classics, this era saw the development of the Eight Principles (*ba gang bian zheng*), the syndromes of the *zang-fu* and tongue diagnosis elevated to their current level of importance in contemporary Chinese acupuncture.

[2] Connelly (1994) gives an exposition of J. R. Worsley's teaching in the early 1970s. There is, however, only one reference to what rapidly became a salient feature of Five Element Classical Acupuncture, which is the constitutional imbalance or CF. His students from the 1960s were not familiar with the concept. There were some small differences from the mid-1970s to the present day, so students of the style from different eras are inclined to have somewhat differing emphases in their work.

introduced to the UK, some practitioners abandoned the more esoteric Five Element style in favour of TCM's understanding of the body's energetic physiology and its more analytical diagnostic approach. Other practitioners incorporated TCM into their practice and evolved an integration of the two styles. Some chose to continue practising Five Element Acupuncture on its own.

Bob Duggan and Dianne Connelly, along with other American students of J. R. Worsley, left the UK in 1974 to form the Traditional Acupuncture Institute in Columbia, Maryland, USA. At the time of writing there are several colleges in the USA and UK that teach Five Element Constitutional Acupuncture as their dominant model, and there are several more which incorporate it into their curriculum. For example, at the College of Integrated Chinese Medicine, in Reading, UK, where the authors teach, it is taught with TCM to provide an integrated style of practice.

What is Five Element Constitutional Acupuncture?

J. R. Worsley did not coin the phrase Five Element Constitutional Acupuncture, which we use in this book. He mainly used the term Five Element Classical Acupuncture, There are many styles of acupuncture that use the Five Elements as their principal basis. The style that he pioneered is different from these other styles in several ways, but especially in regard to his emphasis on the diagnosis and treatment of a primary imbalance. Practitioners using this style of treatment strive to diagnose and treat each individual's fundamental Five Element constitutional imbalance. Chapter 64 of the *Ling Shu* set out the concept of the Five Element types, including the concept of each Element having each of the Five Elements represented within it. It was therefore possible to diagnose 25 constitutional types. The Five Element associations laid down in the *Nei Jing* and *Nan Jing* formed the crux of his diagnostic method. From the early 1970s onwards J. R. Worsley's concept of the 'Causative Factor' (CF) or constitutional imbalance became the dominant focus of his method of working.

This style of treatment is remarkable in several ways. Diagnosis of the CF is based entirely on the sensory acuity of the practitioner. It places particular priority on the health of the person's body, mind and spirit. It recognises four particular 'blocks' to treatment and it also stresses preventive treatment.

Five Element Constitutional Acupuncture is a style of acupuncture developed by Westerners and is a part of the overall process of adapting and transforming Chinese medicine to make it more appropriate for Western patients and practitioners. In China acupuncture is often practised in out-patient hospital clinics and emphasis is placed on acute and short-term health problems. In the West we have a high proportion of patients with longer-term chronic problems with a mixture of physical and psychological issues. In the clinic at the College of Integrated Chinese Medicine (CICM), which has a relatively youthful patient base, over 50% of the patients had been suffering from their main complaint for over 5 years. This means that Western practitioners need to look for diagnoses and treatment protocols different from those currently used in China. As Ted Kaptchuk wrote,

> As Western practitioners, we must have access to accurate information from first-hand sources. Concomitantly we need to become poignantly aware of how culture and history demand from us different answers from those presently fixed in the tradition as it is variously understood in different Asian countries.
>
> (Introduction to Wiseman *et al.*, 1985)

It has been rightly said that, 'to justify and legitimise ourselves we perpetually invent a history of Chinese medicine' (V. Scheid, Rothenberg Congress, 2001), and this is true of the authors as much or as little as anybody else. Although there are a couple of significant innovations, we intend to show that Five Element Constitutional Acupuncture is firmly rooted in the Han dynasty (−202 to +220) classics of Chinese medicine. In fact it is the acupuncture style that in some ways most closely adheres to many of the values expressed in the *Nei Jing* and other classics. It has adopted nothing of the tendency to diagnose by bio-medical disease labels (*bianbing*). It has also remained loyal to the traditional values of focusing treatment on the patient's 'spirit' (*shen*), illnesses frequently being caused by the seven emotions (*qi qing zhi bing*), and the need for preventive treatment and minimum therapeutic intervention.

About this book and its authors

This is the first comprehensive textbook that explains the concepts of Five Element Constitutional Acupuncture and how to use it in diagnosis and treatment. There are several influences on the material that we present in this book. The first is what we learned from J. R. Worsley as students and then as teachers in his college. This includes working with him over a long period of time supervising student clinical training. The other main source is our experience of using Five Element Constitutional Acupuncture in our own practices since the early 1970s. In this book we attempt to be true to both what we learned from J. R. Worsley and our own experiences. Other areas that influenced us include reading the classics of Chinese medicine as well as the accumulated insights of various writers and colleagues. At the time of writing the authors have each been practising this style for 30–35 years and have each been teaching it for over 25 years.

This book is different from other books written about this style of acupuncture. The emphasis is on enabling the practitioner to recognise how people reveal their constitutional imbalance. It also concentrates on clinical practice.

For those who are practitioners or students of TCM, or any of the other styles of acupuncture, we believe that this style of treatment offers a huge amount. Just as all systems of medicine have their strengths and weaknesses, so each style of acupuncture has its strengths and weaknesses. The strengths of Five Element Constitutional Acupuncture complement the weaknesses of TCM, and the strengths of TCM complement the weaknesses of Five Element Constitutional Acupuncture. They go together so elegantly that we believe an integration of the two styles offers an excellent paradigm for practitioners. It is effective for the treatment of physical illnesses and also enables practitioners to practise a person-centred style of acupuncture, which holds that the health of the spirit is essential to a person's well-being.

Notes to the edition

The authors assume that the readers of this book are familiar with the basic concepts of Chinese medicine, such as *qi*, *yin/yang*, Five Elements, *jing*, *xue*, *shen*, etc. In our opinion, *The Foundations of Chinese Medicine* by Giovanni Maciocia (2005) is a lucid and thorough exposition of these concepts and is recommended to any reader unfamiliar with them. In addition, we do not cover point location in this text. For point location *A Manual of Acupuncture* by Peter Deadman, Mazin Al-Khafaji and Kevin Baker (1998) is an outstanding work and can hardly be bettered.

The authors have used *pinyin* throughout the text except in certain specific cases. For example, references for the *Chinese* characters from the book *Chinese Characters* by L. Weiger (1965) are written in Wade–Giles. As well as this, terms such as Confucius and the *I Ching*, are also in Wade–Giles. These transliterations are so well known as to make rendering them into *pinyin* confusing. Chinese words have generally been put into italics.

Where an organ is described as one of the *zang fu* they are started with a capital letter. When they are used with a small letter in front it denotes that the word is being used in the context of Western medicine.

Acknowledgements

This book is respectfully dedicated to J. R. Worsley. We would also like to thank all the friends and colleagues we worked with at the Oxford Acupuncture Clinic in Farmoor including Judy Becker-Worsley, Meriel Darby, Julia Measures and Allegra Wint. We learned so much with you over those years! We have also been inspired by the extraordinary scholarship of Claude Larre and Elisabeth Rochat de la Vallée. The authors would like to wholeheartedly thank the following for their assistance in the publication of this book.

Firstly, we would like to thank Allegra Wint, Peter Eckman, Ben Wint, Carey Morgan and Rebecca Avern, who read and made so many valuable comments about the book at various stages. We are also grateful to those who provided copy for the pictures and diagrams: Eric Goodchild, who provided all of the diagrams; Liong Sen Liew, who gave so much time and advice and who provided us with the Chinese characters in the book; David Hatfull, for patiently taking the photographs; and Sharon Ashton, for having her photograph taken in so many facial expressions.

We are also indebted to James Rodriguez for finding Weiger references and for assisting us with Wade–Giles versus *pinyin* translations. Also thank you to Viv Lo for her help with quotations and Sara Hicks for providing the translations of point names.

Thanks also go to Giovanni Maciocia for all of his support, to Inta Ozols for commissioning the first edition of this book, and to Karen Morley and Kerry McGechie for their work on the first edition. We also extend our thanks to the staff at Elsevier for their work on this new edition.

Finally, we'd like to thank all the patients and practitioners who so kindly offered their insights, experiences and case histories to this book: Rebecca Avern, Gill Black, Sally Blades, Janice Booth, Charlotte Bryden-Smith, Sarah Collison, Di Cook, Ian Dixon, Clare Dobie, Susan East, Janice Falinska, Janet Hargreaves, Gaby Hock, Mary Kaspar, Chris Kear, Sandra King, Magda Koc, Sylvie Martin, Carey Morgan, Keith Murray, Barbara Pickett, Jo Rochford, Marcus Senior, James Unsworth, Julie Wisbey and Helen Vlasto.

Alas, medicine is so subtle that no one seems able to know its complete secrets. The way of medicine is so wide that its scope is as immeasurable as the Heaven and the Earth, and its depth is as immeasurable as the four seas.

Su Wen, Chapter 78; Lu, 1972

Who is to speak for Five Element Acupuncture? While J. R. Worsley was alive, he was universally acknowledged as its living Master. With his passing however, the next generation has a chance to demonstrate how well they have absorbed his teachings – not just the formal system he promulgated, but also the methods by which he got there: intensive study with anyone who might contribute ideas and practices conducive to healing, a propensity for integrating diverse traditions, a commitment to maintaining the vision of the ancients that the spirit is the fundamental determinant of health, and years of clinical experience with acupuncture – keeping what works and discarding what doesn't.

Over the years I have followed the authors' careers as they grappled with the challenges inherent in practicing Five Element Constitutional Acupuncture. This text presents the fruit of their endeavours. In principle, such practice is wondrously simple: just notice a colour, a sound, an odour, an emotion! Of course, then we usually need to spend years trying to develop our sensory faculties so as to do this accurately. The authors have devised a series of exercises to help speed this process of self-development, which are introduced in Chapter 25. In Chapter 24 we are introduced to the technique of "matching" in order to facilitate rapport. Chapter 26 provides an Elemental analysis of body language (postures and gestures) that can help pin down the diagnosis. In short, the learning process is greatly facilitated. The text is peppered with citations from the Classics, some of which will be new to even the most scholarly reader, documenting once again that the fundamental teachings of Five Element Constitutional Acupuncture are as authentic as any other style of practice. Finally, the authors have shown how their approach can even integrate with TCM findings to treat patients more completely and rapidly. As the case histories illustrate, Five Element Constitutional Acupuncture is a style of practice that is second to none, and this innovative text is an excellent resource for learning it.

Peter Eckman, MD, PhD, MAc (UK)
San Francisco

Section 1

The Foundations

The philosophical foundations of Five Element Constitutional Acupuncture

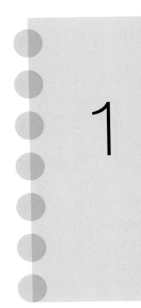

1

CHAPTER CONTENTS

Introduction

The foundations of Five Element Constitutional Acupuncture were laid down over 2000 years ago. The values and beliefs of the physicians of the time continue to shape the practice of the system of medicine today.

Two major texts constitute the main theoretical foundations of Five Element Constitutional Acupuncture. The first is the *Nei Jing* (approximately −200), which comprises *Su Wen* (Simple Questions) and the *Ling Shu* (Spiritual Pivot). This applies the concepts of *yin/yang* and the Five Elements to medicine. The second text is the *Nan Jing* (Classic of Difficulties, approximately +200). This further develops the application of ideas put forward in the *Nei Jing*.

The era in which these texts were written was the Han dynasty (−202 to +220). During this time a complex system of medicine was developed from a diverse range of ideas concerning health, illness, treatment and the causes of disease (see Unschuld, 1992, for a discussion of the transformation in Chinese medicine during the Han dynasty). At that time, little distinction was made between religion, philosophy, science and medicine, and the classics of Chinese medicine are permeated with ideas arising from Daoism, Naturalism, Confucianism and other branches of religious and philosophical thought (a good introduction to these ideas and their influence on Chinese science can be found in Ronan and Needham, 1993, pp. 78–84, 85–113 and 127–190).

Naturalism and Daoism

Naturalism and Daoism maintain that humans are an integral part of Nature and the *Dao*, not the creation of a divine supernatural being. Both schools of thought emphasise the unity of all phenomena in the universe. What unites everything is *qi*. *Qi* is the insubstantial matter that underlies everything that is manifest.

The character for *qi* (Weiger, 1965, lesson 98A) shows the 'vapour' or 'gas' given off during the cooking of rice. It defies adequate translation into English, but is usually translated as 'energy' (for example, Porkert, 1982), 'influences' (Unschuld, 1992) or 'breaths' (Larre and Rochat de la Vallée, 1995). In Chinese and Daoist thinking, *qi* has many contexts and meanings. Ever present, however, is the idea that, in any situation, what is ultimately significant is the nature of the *qi* present. For example, an illness may manifest, but the way to understand and transform it is to understand the underlying imbalance in the *qi*.

Qi pervades the entire universe. Naturalists and Daoists thought that all phenomena in nature were 'immersed' in *qi*, whether they were inanimate objects or whether they were alive and more obviously full of life-force. In approximately −400 Wen Tian Xiang sang:

> Heaven and Earth have correct *qi*. Its form is flexible and fluid. In the lower parts, it is in earth's rivers and mountains. In the upper parts, it is in the heaven's sun and stars. In it human beings are said to be overwhelmingly and universally immersed.
>
> (Manaka *et al.*, 1995, p. 5)

Nature as inspiration

Daoism and Naturalism were concerned with how humans can best conform to the laws of nature. In fact, nature provided the root metaphors for the most fundamental concepts of Chinese philosophy. *Dao* (the way), *de* (virtue), *wu wei* (non-action), *xin* (mind/heart), *qi*, *yin/yang*, *wu xing* (Five Elements) and other ideas were all described by referring to different aspects of the natural world (Allan, 1977). The *Dao* was seen as being the 'the way the universe works' (Waley, 1965, p. 30) or 'the Order of Nature' (Ronan and Needham, 1993, p. 85). Han dynasty Daoists drew on their observations of nature in order to further understand the *Dao*. Lao Tse stated that, 'the *Dao* follows the way of nature' (Zhang and Rose, 2000, Chapter 25).

As Joseph Needham, the historian of Chinese science, put it:

> If there was one idea the Daoists stressed more than any other, it was the unity of Nature and the uncreated and eternal nature of the *Dao*. The sage embraces the Oneness (of the Universe), making it his testing-instrument for everything under Heaven.
>
> (Ronan and Needham, 1993)

But *Su Wen* states: 'The Supreme *Dao* is imperceptible; its changes and transformations are endless' (Larre *et al.*, 1986). The study of those 'changes and transformations' led to the realisation that the unity of the *Dao* was divided into *yin/yang* (duality) and the Five Elements. The *Huainanzi*, a Han dynasty Daoist text written at approximately the same time as the *Nei Jing*, describes the relationship between the *Dao*, *yin/yang* and the Five Elements:

> It [the *Dao*] softens Heaven and Earth and harmonises *yin* and *yang*. It regulates the four seasons and harmonises the Five Elements.
>
> (Chan, 1963)

This emphasis on the observation of nature led to an extraordinary growth in intellectual and scientific curiosity during the Han and succeeding dynasties. This curiosity led to rapid developments in all branches of science and technology, including medicine. (Many of these developments, for example, smelting of cast-iron, the invention of paper, developments in porcelain, working with brass, were not emulated in Western civilisation until many centuries later.)

The *Dao*, as revealed through the patterns of nature, also sets out the 'path' or 'way' by which humanity should live. Water, for example, symbolises the characteristics of stillness, power and adaptability that humans should seek to emulate. Trees that bend in the wind and therefore do not break were proposed as models for how people should respond to the varying changes of fortune in life (for example, *Dao de Jing*, Chapters 8 and 22).

> The sage infers the far from the near, and concludes that the myriad things are based upon a single principle.
>
> (*Huainanzi*; Needham, 1956, p. 66)

The unity of the microcosm of human life and the macrocosm of nature was a guiding principle for Daoist thinkers in their efforts to understand how people should conduct their lives. The Daoist classic, the *Huainanzi*, put it like this:

> I have gazed upwards to study Heaven and examined the Earth below me and about me, and sought understanding of the principles of humanity.
>
> (De Bary *et al.*, 1960, p. 185)

Humans stand between Heaven and Earth

> Heaven arose out of the accumulation of *yang qi*, the Earth arose out of the accumulation of *yin qi*.
>
> (*Taisu*; Unschuld, 1992, p. 283)

Humanity was regarded as forming a bridge between Heaven and Earth. This is usually expressed in the phrase 'Heaven (*tian*), Earth (*di*) and Man (*ren*)'. The same immutable laws were seen to unite everything in nature, from the movement of the stars to small cyclical changes in the plant and animal world. Each person was regarded as a microcosm of the universe, their *qi* resonating with the *qi* of Heaven and Earth (Chapter 71 of the *Ling Shu* is largely devoted to this theme). Needham (1956, p. 300) quotes Wang Kubei as saying: 'The human body imitates Heaven and Earth very distinctly and exactly.'

Chuang Tse, the great Daoist sage, also stressed the resonance between humanity and the world outside. Changes in the season or climate were bound to induce changes in the *qi* of the person: 'Heaven exists inside, Man exists outside' (Merton, 1970, Chapter 17). This micro/macrocosm concept is also to be found in the *Huainanzi*, Chapter 7. A person's place in the natural order, therefore, is to form the bridge between the *yang* of Heaven and the *yin* of Earth. As it says in the *Huainanzi*:

> The vital spirit belongs to Heaven, the physical body belongs to Earth: when the vital spirit goes home and the physical body returns to its origin, where then is the self?
>
> (Cleary, 2000, p. 29)

The Three Treasures

Humanity was regarded as having a special place amongst all living creatures. Only humans are endowed with the 'Three Treasures' (*san bao*), *jing*, *qi* and *shen* (see the Glossary for a description of these terms). This is a very old concept in Chinese thought, the first written reference being in the *Guanzi*, an early Daoist classic that predates the *Nei Jing*. The condition of these 'treasures' determines the individual's health.

Jing, or Essence – our constitutional and 'physical' energy – is what we inherit from our parents. We now know that we share 99.4% of our genes with our closest relatives, the higher primates. Even in antiquity the Chinese were well aware that our links to animals are extremely close. (It is perhaps striking that one of the most popular Chinese stories, *Wu Ch'eng-en* (Monkey), has a monkey not only as its main character but also as the most intelligent of the characters.) The *jing* carries our biological link with the animal world. Much behaviour in all animals, humans included, is driven by basic biological instincts. The drive for survival, the need to bond with others, aggression and lust are common to humanity and all of the higher primates. These primal instincts are largely carried in our *jing*. They play an important role in how we live our lives. A substantial amount of human suffering and illness results from imbalances in these drives.

Qi we share with all matter in the universe or the 'ten thousand things' (*wan wu*). *Qi* literally gives us our life and our vitality.

Shen, or spirit, is the treasure we do not share with animals. Animals possess *jing* and *qi*, but they do not possess *shen*. *Shen* is bestowed on us from Heaven and gives humanity its glory and human consciousness. That is why humanity is 'the most precious thing in the universe' (*Xunzi*, Larre *et al.*, 1986, p. 59).

In the *Huainanzi* it says that: 'The gross *qi* becomes animals, the subtle *qi* becomes Man' (Major, 1993). The Three Treasures therefore reflect the Heaven, Humanity and Earth concept. *Jing*, which gives us our biological link with the other animals, is linked with Earth. *Qi* is what we share with all the 'ten thousand things', and *shen* is humanity's unique gift from Heaven. The relationship between these 'treasures' and *yin* and *yang* is shown in Table 1.1.

The great physician Zhang Jiebin succinctly expressed the relationship between the *Dao*, nature and humanity.

> The *dao* produces and completes the 10,000 beings. It is nothing but the exchange between the *yin* and *yang* and then the luminous radiance of the spirits (*shen ming*). In order to be alive, mankind needs the combination of *yin* and *yang qi*, the union of the essences (*jing*) of the father and mother. Two essences combine, the physical form and the spirits are then completed, uniting the *qi* of heaven and earth, and giving mankind.
>
> (Larre and Rochat de la Vallée, 1995)

On the one hand, people have a physical body that needs to be fed from the fruits of the Earth, just as all animals and living things do. On the other hand, people possess a connection to Heaven, which requires a different type of nourishment. This gives them the wonder of human consciousness and the human spirit. As well as taking care of the body, the writers of the *Nei Jing* emphasised the idea that the health of the human spirit is central to people's passage through life. They must strive to cultivate their connection with Heaven in order to fulfil their destiny (*ming*). The *Huainanzi* sums up the Han dynasty Daoist view:

Table 1.1 The Three Treasures in relation to Heaven, Earth and Humanity

Heaven	*yang*	*shen*
Humanity	*yin/yang*	*qi*
Earth	*yin*	*jing*

Heaven is calm and clear, Earth is stable and peaceful. Beings who lose these qualities die, while those who emulate them live.

(Cleary, 2000, p. 24)

Summary

1 In the Han dynasty (−202 to +220) Chinese medicine came to be based on a study of the processes of nature and how they are manifested in human beings.

2 *Qi* is the insubstantial matter that underlies everything that is manifest.

3 For the early Daoists, little distinction was made between the *qi* of Heaven and Earth and of Humanity.

4 Humanity forms a bridge between Heaven and Earth.

5 Humanity alone possesses the 'Three Treasures'. Animals possess *jing* and *qi*, but only humans have the gift of Heaven, *shen*.

Five Element theory

The Five Elements

The idea that all of nature is governed by *yin/yang* and the Five Elements (Figure 2.1) lies at the heart of Chinese medicine. Zhu Yen (some time between −350 and −270) wrote extensively on the subject and the Five Elements are mentioned in both the *Book of History* and the *Book of Rites* (the dates for these are uncertain). The *Ling Shu* states that: 'Nothing on earth or within the universe is unrelated to the Five Elements and Man is no exception' (*Ling Shu* Chapter 64; quoted in Liu, 1988, p. 48).

The Five Elements, which are Wood, Fire, Earth, Metal and Water, represent the fundamental qualities of all matter in the universe. The Chinese term for Element is *xing*. *Xing* means to walk or to move, and therefore the word 'Element' is somewhat misleading because it implies something more akin to a basic constituent of matter. For this reason, the translation 'The Five Phases' is often used. However, because the term 'Element' is so established, we continue to use it here, but the reader should be clear that an Element is a process, movement or quality of *qi*, not a fixed 'building block' (Rochat, 2009, p. 13; Kaptchuk, 2000, p. 437; Maciocia, 1989, p. 15; Needham, 1956, p. 244).

Each Element has its own particular quality of *qi*: 'As soon as the Five Elements are formed, they have each their specific nature' (Chou Tun-I; quoted in Needham, 1956, p. 461). One of the earliest texts describing the Five Elements outlined this emphasis on the different qualities of the Elements.

> Water is that quality in Nature which we describe as soaking and descending. Fire which we describe as blazing and uprising. Wood which permits of curved surfaces or straight edges. Metal which can follow the form of a mould and then becomes hard. Earth which permits of sowing, growth and reaping.
>
> (Shu Ching, −4th century; quoted in Needham, 1956, p. 243)

Above all, the Five Elements serve as a model for understanding the inexorable succession of the seasons. For many Daoists and Naturalists virtually no distinction was made between the nature of the seasons, the climate resonant with each season and the cyclical changes taking place in the human, animal and vegetable worlds. In plants the never-ending cycle of growth, flowering, harvest, decline and storing informed them of the differing qualities of each season. The behaviour of animals and humans in each season was also seen to be governed by the same laws.

> Men have no choice but to go by this succession; officials have no choice but to operate according to these powers. For such are the calculations of heaven.
>
> (Tung Chung-shu, −135; quoted in Needham, 1956, p. 249)

Over the course of history there have been several different models of Five Element theory, some coming from its application to agriculture or politics (see,

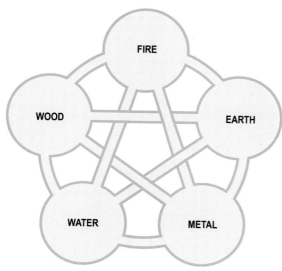

Figure 2.1 • The Five Elements

for example, Cheng, 1987, pp. 18–22; Maciocia, 1989, pp. 15–35; Matsumoto and Birch, 1983, pp. 1–8). Five Element Constitutional Acupuncture is based on the model of the Five Elements set out in the *Nei Jing* and *Nan Jing*. This model, which envisages the Five Elements in a cyclical creative cycle, has always been the dominant one used by acupuncture practitioners.

Chinese medicine, like any system of medicine, is predominantly concerned with understanding and alleviating physical and psychological suffering. The writers of the medical classics strove to understand how the Five Elements affected people and how physicians could observe this. The 'resonances' associated with each Element are how the condition of the Elements inside the person is revealed to the practitioner. 'Associations' or 'correspondences' are the usual words used in this context, but these words imply a relationship between separate entities. We have chosen to use the word 'resonances' as it implies an underlying sameness.

The Five Element resonances

When people's *qi* becomes either deficient (*xu*) or full (*shi*) within an Element, changes start to take place in various aspects of the physical body as well as in the mind and spirit. (This idea is present in both the *Nei Jing* and the *Nan Jing*, but is put most succinctly in *Nan Jing*, Chapter 16.)

The practitioner diagnoses the dysfunction by perceiving disharmony in patients' odour, voice tone, facial colour and in the external expression of their inner state. It is not that the imbalanced *qi* 'causes' the changes to happen, but that the odour, colour, tone and emotion 'resonate' (*ying*) in harmony with the condition of the *qi* of the Element (see Birch and Felt, 1998, p. 93, for a description of how 'resonance' is a more understandable concept to the Chinese than to Westerners).

The *Ling Shu* states: 'Between Heaven and Earth, the number five is indispensable. Man also resonates with it' (Yang and Chace, 1994, p. 54). This concept of 'resonance', exemplified by sympathetic vibrations in gongs across a temple hall, was vital to early Chinese ideas concerning science and medicine (Needham, 1956, pp. 282–283). Indeed, 'The fundamental idea of the *Book of Changes* (*I Jing*) can be expressed in one word – resonance' (Shih Shuo Hsu Yu; quoted in Needham, 1956, p. 304).

The quality of *qi* resonant with the Wood Element in Heaven manifests as the season of spring, the climatic *qi* of wind and in a person as the emotion of anger. Humanity stands between Heaven and Earth and the Five Elements are present within us just as they are present throughout all the manifestations of the *Dao*.

> According to *Su Wen* there are Five Elements in the sky and Five Elements on the earth. The *qi* of earth, when in the sky, is moisture. ... the *qi* of wood, when in the sky, is wind.
>
> (Shen Kua; quoted in Needham, 1956, p. 267)

There have been many resonances attributed to the Elements over the centuries, many not in a medical context. Table 2.1 sets out the resonances commonly used by practitioners of Five Element Constitutional Acupuncture (these resonances are often referred to in the classics, but *Nan Jing* Chapter 34 is devoted to this topic). They are the resonances that most clearly give us an understanding of how the Five Elements manifest in people. It is easy to say that the Wood Element plays the same role in people's character as the spring plays in the annual cycle of the seasons. It requires considerable experience and depth of understanding, however, to be able to make an accurate diagnosis based on observation of how these resonances manifest in people. For example, when the Water Element is out of balance then a putrid odour, an imbalance in the person's ability to deal effectively with fear, a groan in the voice tone and a blue facial colour also arise.

Table 2.1 Five Element resonances

	Wood	Fire	Earth	Metal	Water
Colour	green	red	yellow	white	blue
Sound	shouting	laughing	singing	weeping	groaning
Emotion	anger	joy	sympathy/worry	grief	fear
Odour	rancid	scorched	fragrant	rotten	putrid
Season	spring	summer	late summer	autumn/fall	winter
Climate	wind	heat	humidity	dryness	cold
Taste	sour	bitter	sweet	pungent	salty
Power	growth	maturity	harvest	decrease	storage

Cultivating the ability to diagnose from such signs is one of the main challenges for the Five Element Constitutional Acupuncturist.

Human emotions in particular are seen as being equivalent to the different forms of *qi* present throughout Nature. Often they are the most overt manifestations of the Element that can be discerned in the person.

> Just as there are wind and rain in Heaven, so there are joy and anger in man.
>
> *(Ling Shu, Chapter 71; Lu, 1972)*

Heaven has four seasons and five Elements or phases to engender (*sheng*), make grow (*zhang*), gather (*shou*) and store (*cang*), to produce cold, heat, dryness, dampness and wind. Man has five *zang* (Organs) and, through transformation, five *qi* to produce elation (*xi*), anger (*nu*), sadness (*bei*), grief (*you*) and fear (*kong*).

> *(Su Wen, Chapter 5; Larre and Rochat de la Vallée, 1996, p. 27)*

If practitioners understand, for example, how winter is the period of storing (*cang*) and of holding reserves during a phase of little discernible activity, they can gain a great deal of understanding into the role the Water Element plays in a person. Observing and understanding the different qualities of *qi* in each season enables the practitioner to diagnose patients according to the balance of the Five Elements within them. Understanding the difference between the *qi* of spring and the *qi* of summer or how the *qi* of dampness is different from the *qi* of cold, informs the practitioner of the difference between the Elements in a person.

Five Element interrelationships

The other key concept in Five Element theory and the practice of Five Element Constitutional Acupuncture is the interrelationships between the Elements, a concept that featured particularly in the *Nan Jing*. This great classic of Chinese medicine has been the most influential text in the development of Japanese and Five Element acupuncture (see Unschuld, 1986, p. 3). Focusing on issues of interrelationships and interdependence is a typically Oriental way of looking at things. Many Western students and practitioners of acupuncture find this less easy. They are more inclined to focus on the 'things' relating rather than on the relationships themselves. The translation of 'Element' rather than 'phase' or 'process' colludes with this way of thinking.

Oriental concepts of gardening, *feng shui*, cuisine, and many other aspects of life place much of their focus on the relationships *between* objects rather than on the object itself. Confucianism stresses the importance of maintaining a 'proper' relationship between the individuals in a family or society. It regards these relationships as crucial to the proper functioning of society and to the person's own well-being. In Chinese communities an individual's psychological problems are usually seen as being problems *in relation* to other individuals, especially other family members. The concepts of *yin/yang* and the Five Elements are based on an exploration and an understanding of relationships.

This emphasis on relationships means that establishing balance and harmony between the Five

Elements is crucially important in this style of acupuncture. The goal of the practitioner is to achieve equilibrium between all the Elements. In the *Ling Shu* it says: 'The principles of needling dictate that needling should stop as soon as *qi* is brought into harmony' (Lu, 1972, Chapter 9).

It is important to reinforce or reduce the *qi* of an Element if it leads to greater harmony between that Element and other Elements. If a person is deficient in *qi* but the Elements are in relative harmony, then this may lead to a lack of well-being but it is unlikely to cause a serious disorder. If, on the other hand, there is a large discrepancy between the *qi* of different Elements, then this can cause more severe physical or psychological symptoms. This view is summed up in the *Nei Jing*.

> It is necessary to promote the flow of qi and blood according to the laws of mutual victories among the Five Elements in order to strike a balance among them and bring about peace.
>
> (*Su Wen*, Chapter 74; Lu, 1972)

The most important relationships between the Five Elements are those controlled by the *sheng* and *ke* cycles.

The *sheng* cycle

The transition of the seasons provides the most obvious model for this cycle of the Elements. Just as summer follows spring and winter follows autumn, so the seasons 'generate' each other according to the *sheng* cycle, as illustrated in Figure 2.2. The character for *sheng* (Weiger, 1965, lesson 79F) is shown below.

The Daoist Liu I Ming described the *sheng* cycle like this:

> When *yin* and *yang* divide, the Five Elements become disordered (*luan*). The Five Elements, Metal, Water, Wood, Fire, and Earth, represent the five *qi*. The Five Elements of early heaven create each other following the *sheng* cycle. These Five Elements fuse to form a unified *qi*.
>
> (translation by Jarret, 1998; based on Cleary, 1986b, p. 66)

Just as the *qi* of Heaven in the form of the seasons are seen to follow each other, the *qi* of Earth is also seen

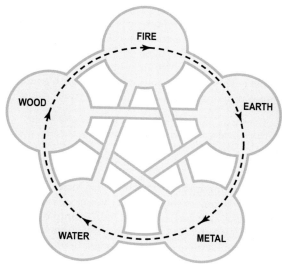

Figure 2.2 • The *sheng* cycle

to follow the same cycle. This is described by practitioners of Chinese medicine in the following way:

- Wood creates Fire by burning.
- Fire creates Earth from ashes.
- Earth creates Metal by hardening. (Metal in this context is synonymous with rock or ore found within the Earth.)
- Metal creates Water by containment.[1]
- Water creates Wood by nourishment.

Mother–child relationship

The *sheng* cycle is of the utmost importance in Five Element Constitutional Acupuncture as it is fundamental to the idea that a practitioner can generate change in the organs of one Element by treating another Element. Chapter 69 of the *Nan Jing* discusses the *sheng* cycle in terms of the relationship between a mother and child. If the 'child' Element is deficient, then it may be because it is not receiving sufficient *qi* from its 'mother'. It may be more effective to treat the 'mother' to engender more *qi* in the

---

[1] Joseph Needham cites the ritual use of metal mirrors as receptacles to gather water through condensation as the likely model for 'Metal creates Water'. It seems far more likely to us that the connection is the presence of impermeable rock in the ground without which all water would soak away into the earth. Elisabeth Hsu recounts a story of hearing a Daoist monk using the phrase while entering a granite cave on Mount Hua and seeing water droplets sitting on the rock (Hsu, 1999, p. 211).

'child' Element than treating the child itself. For example, if the Fire Element is deficient the practitioner may reinforce the Wood Element in order to provide *qi* for the Fire Element (by analogy, throwing more wood on the fire in order to generate more flames). This kind of connection fitted into contemporary thinking during the Han dynasty.

> There is an unvarying dependence of the sons on the fathers and a direction from the fathers to the sons. Such is the *Dao* of Heaven.
>
> (Tung Chung-shu, −135; quoted in Needham, 1956, p. 249)

Five Element theory also mentions that if a 'child' Element becomes too full (*shi*) it can deleteriously affect the 'mother' Element. For example, if the Wood Element is too full then it may have 'robbed' the Water Element, which becomes depleted. This relationship is known as '*zi dao mu qi*' or 'the son steals the mother's *qi*'.

The *ke* cycle

The Chinese character for *ke* shown here is taken from Weiger (1965), lessons 29A and 75K. The *ke*, or 'control', cycle describes a relationship between the Elements which is less apparent from nature than the *sheng* cycle. Focusing on interrelationships, the writers of the *Nei Jing* and *Nan Jing* observed pathological effects on the Element two stages along the *sheng* cycle.

> In the mystery of nature, neither promotion of growth (*sheng*) nor control (*ke*) is dispensable. Without promotion of growth, there would be no development; without control, excessive growth would result in harm.
>
> (*Ling Shu*; Liu, 1988, p. 53)

The *ke* cycle is illustrated in Figure 2.3. It is described in the following way:

- Fire controls Metal by melting.
- Metal controls Wood by cutting.
- Wood controls Earth by covering.[2]

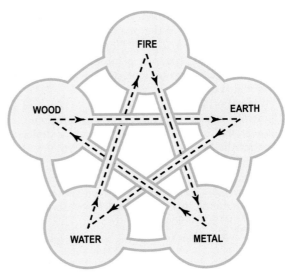

Figure 2.3 • The *ke* cycle

- Earth controls Water by damming.[3]
- Water controls Fire by extinguishing.

The cycle of control maintains unity within the Five Elements. As the *Ling Shu* says, 'Without control, excessive growth would result in harm.' If an Element starts to become dysfunctional, however, it may easily lose 'control' or it may 'over-act' on the Element it controls across the *ke* cycle. (When the *ke* cycle becomes pathological, it is called the 'contempt' cycle.) For example, if the Organs of the Wood Element struggle, the Organs of the Earth Element will often start to show signs of distress.

The elements 'insulting' each other

The *sheng* cycle is the most important relationship of the Elements in that deficiency in one Element easily leads to a secondary deficiency or excess in the 'child' Element. The *ke* cycle, however, tends to produce more complex interrelationships.

> Being excessive, *qi* not only acts on what it should, but also counteracts on what it should not. Being insufficient, *qi* is not only overacted on by what acts upon it, but is also counteracted upon by what it should act upon.
>
> (Treatise on the Five Circuit Phases in *Su Wen*; Liu, 1988, p. 56)

This means that if the organs of an Element are out of balance they may 'insult' the organs of the Element

---

[2]The Earth may become rapidly eroded when it no longer has vegetation in order to bind it together, for example, the dust bowls of the American Midwest.

[3]An analogy that came easily to the Chinese with their extensive use of flooded paddy-fields for the cultivation of rice.

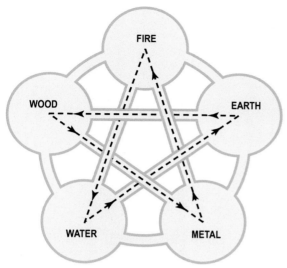

Figure 2.4 • The Elements insulting each other

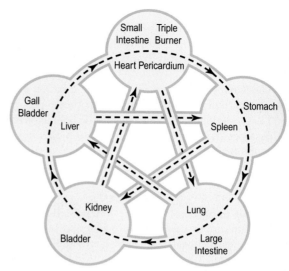

Figure 2.5 • The Five Elements with their associated Organs

that should be controlling it (see Figure 2.4). For example, if the Liver suffers it may produce imbalance in the Lungs.

Treating the constitutional imbalance

Any Element can be adversely affected along the *sheng* and/or *ke* cycles by imbalance in any other Element (see Scheid, 1988, for a discussion of these relationships). In clinical practice practitioners see complex pictures of imbalance that make it hard to be sure by which route one Element has been affected by another. The key lies in understanding which Element was the first to become imbalanced. The practitioner focuses much of the treatment on this Element and thereby affects other Elements that have become imbalanced. This enables the practitioner to generate improvement in the person's *qi* by treating at the root of the person's disharmony.

The Organs or 'Officials'

The twelve organs have been associated with particular Elements from the time of the *Nei Jing* (see Figure 2.5). As well as teaching the more commonly accepted functions of the Organs, Five Element Constitutional Acupuncture places particular emphasis on Chapter 8 of *Su Wen* (see Larre and Rochat de la Vallée, 1992, for a detailed and thought-provoking commentary on *Su Wen* Chapter 8). This chapter

describes the twelve organs as though they were 'officials' in a court, each with a particular ministry or role. This way of thinking about the Organs is similar to a Daoist concept, prevalent at that time, that people are composed of several different 'deities' who reside within them. For example, the *Ling Hsien*, written by Chang Heng (+7 to +139), describes the various gods sitting around in heaven, each of them occupying the position of an official in a court.

Su Wen, Chapter 8, portrays the Organs more in terms of their functions in a person's mind and spirit than of their functions in the physiology of the body.

The Officials and their 'ministries' are as follows (Larre and Rochat de la Vallée, 1992, pp. 151–152):

- *The Heart* holds the office of lord and sovereign. The radiance of the spirit stems from it.
- *The Lung* holds the office of minister and chancellor. The regulation of the life-giving network stems from it.
- *The Liver* holds the office of general of the armed forces. Assessment of circumstances and conception of plans stem from it.
- *The Gall Bladder* is responsible for what is just and exact. Determination and decision stem from it.
- *Tan zhong* (an early name for the *Pericardium*) has the charge of resident as well as envoy. Elation and joy stem from it.
- *The Stomach and Spleen* are responsible for storehouses and granaries. The five tastes stem from them.

11

- *The Large Intestine* is responsible for transit. The residue from transformation stems from it.
- *The Small Intestine* is responsible for receiving and making things thrive. Transformed substances stem from it.
- *The Kidneys* are responsible for the creation of power. Skill and ability stem from them.
- *The Triple Burner* is responsible for opening up passages and irrigation. The regulation of fluids stems from it.
- *The Bladder* is responsible for regions and cities. It stores the body fluids. The transformations of the *qi* then give out their power.

Placing importance on these functions diagnostically is unique in contemporary practice (as far as the authors are aware) to Five Element Constitutional Acupuncture. Awareness of the 'Officials' leads to a practitioner emphasising modes of behaviour and ways of thinking when diagnosing patients. This focus supersedes any indications arising from the physical symptoms (see Chapters 3, 4 and the chapters on the Elements, this volume, for discussion of the priority given to diagnosis based on the person's psychological characteristics).

The Law of Midday–Midnight

Each Official has a 2-hour period in the day when its *qi* is stronger (Figure 2.6). This concept is an ancient one. It comes from the school of biorhythmic methodology known as *zi wu liu zhu fa* and goes back to at least the Tang dynasty (+618 to +906) (Soulié de Morant, 1994, p. 121, claims it goes back to −104 in the Han dynasty but gives no reference). There is also a period of time (roughly 12 hours from the strongest time) when the Organ is at its weakest.

In practice it can give useful diagnostic information about the condition of an Organ. Patients, for example, often report that they find it hard to sleep during the strongest time of day for the Liver (1–3 a.m.) and then find it especially hard to stay awake after lunch (1–3 p.m.).

In treatment, the horary points can be used to tonify an Organ at its strongest time (see Section 6,

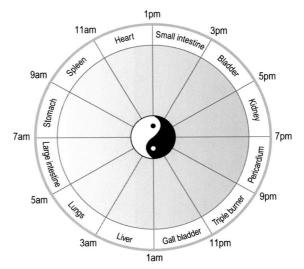

Figure 2.6 • The Chinese Clock

this volume). The relevance of the time of day and how this is used diagnostically is discussed for each Organ in Section 2.

Summary

1 The *qi* of each Element is different in its nature. Season, climatic factors and human emotions are all variations of the Elements.

2 When one of a person's Five Elements becomes out of balance, the 'resonances' of that Element manifest themselves.

3 Diagnostically the most important resonances are the facial colour, voice tone, emotion and odour.

4 The Five Elements are bound by a complex system of interrelationships. This means that each Element is affected by changes taking place in another Element.

5 Balance and harmony between the Elements is of prime importance.

6 Emphasis is placed on the descriptions of the Organs as 'Officials' given in *Su Wen*, Chapter 8.

7 Each Official has a 2-hour period in the day when its *qi* is stronger.

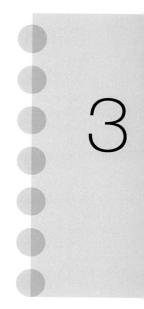

The importance of the spirit

3

CHAPTER CONTENTS

The primacy of the spirit

Five Element Constitutional Acupuncture is a very 'person-centred' style of treatment. When a patient comes for treatment, a Five Element Constitutional Acupuncturist is more likely to consider, 'how can this *person* be treated?' rather than 'how can this person's *symptom* be treated?' This is because one of the practitioner's core values is that diagnosis and treatment should be focused on the health of the individual, rather than on the physical symptoms presented.

Chronic physical symptoms are seen as being the manifestation of the illness (*biao*), which stems from the root (*ben*). The root usually lies in the mind or spirit. This is not true for all symptoms, of course. For example, symptoms caused by physical trauma or acute infections are likely to have their *ben* arising from an external cause rather than from a deeper internal one.

Although a person's most underlying imbalance can arise from body, mind or spirit, the majority of patients coming for treatment in the West are suffering primarily from an imbalance of the spirit. Around a quarter of all drugs prescribed by the National Health Service in the UK are for mental health problems (The Stationery Office, 1996). There are also huge numbers of patients who present with symptoms that have a psychosomatic component. In addition, there are a large number of substances taken for their symptom-relieving effects, such as coffee, alcohol and 'recreational' drugs. Stress-related absence accounts for half of all sickness from work (Patel and Knapp, 1998). A recent study of 22,000 people in the UK found that:

- 58% of people suffer from mood swings
- 52% feel apathetic and unmotivated
- 50% suffer from anxiety
- 47% have difficulty sleeping
- 43% have poor memories or difficulty concentrating
- 42% suffer from depression (Holford, 2003, pp. 2–3)

As Cicero observed long before the advent of modern lifestyles and contemporary neuroses, 'Diseases of the soul are more dangerous and more numerous than those of the body.' It is fair to say that today many Westerners are suffering from what seems to be spiritual malaise with much accompanying mental dysfunction.

Diagnosing and treating the whole person

A practitioner of Five Element Constitutional Acupuncture diagnoses patients by assessing which is the primary Element in distress. This diagnosis is based on various sensory signs, especially the patient's emotional balance, facial colour, odour and voice tone. The patient's personality is also of utmost importance. The focus is on diagnosing the balance of the Five Elements within the person rather than making a differential diagnosis of the symptoms presented by the person. As the great physician Xu Dachun described it, 'Illnesses may be identical but the persons suffering from them are different' (Unschuld, 1990, p. 17). This idea is also reflected in the Chinese phrase *yin ren zhi yi*, which translates as 'different patients require different treatment'.

Treatment is only perceived as fully successful if patients report improvement in how they 'feel in themselves', as well as in their signs and symptoms. Sometimes patients are surprised to notice positive differences in how they feel even if they did not perceive anything to be 'wrong' with them in the first place. Five Element Constitutional Acupuncture has the ability to direct treatment to any level of the patient's mind and spirit if that is what is required to help the patient to return to good health.

The meaning of mind and spirit

What do we mean by 'spirit'?

Many people already have a view, albeit indistinct, of what the word 'spirit' means. Others do not accept that human beings have a spirit at all. The word 'spirit' also has many different meanings in the English language. For these reasons this topic can be difficult to discuss.

The Oxford English Dictionary lists 34 separate meanings for 'spirit'. The one that is closest to its meaning in Chinese medicine is 'the animating or vital principle in man'. Cicero called it 'the true self, not that physical figure which can be pointed out by your finger'. In the Chinese language the words *shen* and *jing-shen* most closely describe the spirit, although it also encompasses some aspects of the mind. The sinologist Claude Larre described *shen* like this:

> The *shen* are that by which a given being is unlike any other; that which makes an individual an individual and more than a person.
>
> (Larre et al., 1986, p. 164)

People often equate 'spirit' with the spiritual and religious sides of the person. The word 'spirit', however, encompasses many other aspects of being. Religion, mysticism and spiritual awareness emanate from the human spirit, but so also does the desire to look at a radiant sunset, to listen to beautiful music or to achieve one's potential as a human being. When people wake up and experience the joy of seeing a beautiful day dawning, it is their spirit that is touched by that experience. Love and compassion are expressions of the spirit.

People who have problems in their spirit struggle when under stress and have difficulties coping with their lives. This may manifest in areas such as their relationships, communication, posture, use of language or the look in their eyes (for more on this, see Chapter 27, this volume). Resignation, anguish, despair, depression, disappointment, sadness, anxiety and many other states are present to some extent in almost all of our patients. As Thoreau said in *Walden*, 'the mass of men lead lives of quiet desperation'.

What do we mean by mind?

The mind is the cognitive faculty and gives people the ability to think. This includes being able to concentrate, remember, plan and make decisions. The phrase 'mentally ill' is legitimately used in Western medicine to describe problems in sense perception, personality, emotions or behaviour. This use of the word goes far beyond the core meaning of the word 'mental'. Many people in psychiatric hospitals have extremely astute and able minds. It is their spirits that are in distress.

In the context of Chinese medicine, symptoms on the mental level include being obsessed, forgetful, indecisive, unable to concentrate, disorganised, muddled, vague, inarticulate, dyslexic, etc. In Chinese medicine the mind and spirit are considered to be an aspect of the person's *qi*. Just as *qi* is present in every cell in the body, so also is the person's mind and spirit (see Pert, 1999).

The *shen* in Chinese medicine

Several different words are used in Chinese medical texts to describe the mind and spirit. *Shen* is most commonly used and it has different meanings according to the context in which it is used. Some writers translate it as 'mind' (see Maciocia, 2005, p. 109), some as 'spirit' (see Kaptchuk, 2000, p. 58) and some as 'spirits' (see Larre and Rochat de la Vallée, 1995, p. 4). Spirits is used to emphasise that the *shen* is more than just the spirit of the Heart (see below) but also describes the 'whole sphere of emotional, mental and spiritual aspects of a human being' (see Maciocia, 2005, p. 109). In this sense of the word *shen* includes the mental and spiritual aspects of all the Organs.

It is the *shen* that gives people their human consciousness, as the following two quotations illustrate.

> To have the spirits (*de shen*) is the splendour of life. To lose the spirits (*shi shen*) is annihilation.
>
> (*Su Wen*, Chapter 13; Larre and Rochat de la Vallée, 1995)

> Let me discuss *shen*, the spirit. What is the spirit? The spirit cannot be heard with the ear. The eye must be brilliant of perception and the heart must be open and attentive, and then the spirit is suddenly revealed through one's own consciousness. It cannot be expressed through the mouth; only the heart can express all that can be looked upon. If one pays close attention one may suddenly know it but one can just as suddenly lose this knowledge. But *shen*, the spirit, becomes clear to man as though the wind has blown away the cloud. Therefore one speaks of it as the spirit.
>
> (*Su Wen*, Chapter 26; Veith, 1972)

The ability to perceive the nature of the imbalances in a person's mind and spirit is important and is one of the crucial skills the practitioner of Five Element Constitutional Acupuncture strives to develop.

Chinese medicine's approach to the spirit and health

The emphasis on enhancing the health of the person's spirit above all else is consistently referred to in the early classics. For example:

> When the Spirits are overwhelmed, they leave; when left in peace they remain. Thus the most important thing in the conduct and treatment of a being is maintenance of the Spirits, and then comes maintenance of the body.
>
> (Zhang Jiebin; quoted in Larre and Rochat de la Vallée, 1995)

> When the spirit is master, the body follows and a man prospers. When the body is master, the spirit follows and man is degraded.
>
> (*Huainanzi*, Chapter 1; Larre et al., 1986)

These passages emphasise that the health of the spirit and mind is regarded as being of ultimate importance. Most people face a struggle with illness at some time in their lives. Their prognosis is often dependent on the condition of their will and spirit.

It is well known that when a person gives up and 'turns his face to the wall' the end is not far away.[1]

> The essential point in the treatment of an illness is to root oneself in the five spirits of the person: to know whether they dwell or have been lost, whether one possesses or loses them, to know if the intent is for death or life.
>
> (*Taisu*; Larre and Rochat de la Vallée, 1995)

> How can a disease be cured if there is no spiritual energy left in the body?
>
> (*Su Wen*, Chapter 14; Veith, 1972)

> When one applies medical treatment, one must keep in mind first of all, the patient's spirit
>
> (*Ling Shu*, Chapter 8; Sunu, 1985)

> In order to make all acupuncture thorough and effective one must first cure the spirit
>
> (*Su Wen*, Chapter 25; Veith, 1972)

Using acupuncture to treat the spirit

At the time of the *Nei Jing* and *Nan Jing*, the period when Daoism's influence on Chinese medicine was at its height, acupuncture was the form of therapy most discussed. The *Ling Shu* is solely concerned with acupuncture. With its ability to influence the person's *qi* in the channels acupuncture was regarded as the primary therapeutic modality for initiating change in a person's spirit and mind.

> If the body is healthy and the *xin* (Heart-Mind housing the Spirit) suffers, illnesses arise in the meridians (channels). Moxa and needles are the proper treatment.
>
> (*Su Wen*, Chapter 24; Unschuld, 1992, p. 293; additional translation of *xin* by Claude Larre)

Five Element Constitutional Acupuncture continues the tradition of regarding the health of the mind and spirit as being of prime importance. Acupuncture and moxibustion are profoundly effective therapies for treating these levels in a person.

The five *shen*

The word *shen* is used in two ways. As discussed in the section above, one use encompasses the 'whole sphere of emotional, mental and spiritual aspects

---

[1]Many modern Chinese textbooks of Chinese medicine make no reference to the spirit and often do not stress that it is the underlying cause of many physical illnesses. This is in stark contrast to the *Nei Jing*'s priorities.

of a human being'. Although a person's spirit is ultimately indivisible, the Chinese also discussed it in terms of five different 'spirits' which interact together. Each of the spirits is responsible for a different aspect of the person and is also associated with one of the *yin* Organs. In this context *shen* describes the 'spirit' of the Heart specifically. This is used alongside the *hun, po, zhi* and *yi*, which are the spirits of the other *yin* organs (see Table 3.1).

In many ways the five *shen* are closely linked to the 'Officials' described in *Su Wen*, Chapter 8 (see Chapter 2, this volume). Both describe important aspects of the spirit. Some of the *shen*, especially the *hun* and the *po*, also describe the spirit in relation to life and death. This is of interest, although of less use diagnostically, to a practitioner.

An overview of the five *shen*

The following is an overview of each of the five *shen*. They are described in more detail in Section 2 of this volume.

Hun

The *hun* of the Liver or Ethereal Soul is most closely linked to what in the West is called a person's 'soul'. The *hun* is said to enter the body at birth and to leave the body and continue on when a person dies. When people relate that they have separated from the body, for example, during 'out of body experiences' or 'near death experiences' (Moody, 1973) or if people sleepwalk or are in a trance, these experiences involve the *hun*. Strengthening the spirit of the Liver can help to keep the *hun* in the body if this is pathological. In less extreme cases people can become rather vague and day-dreamy.

Also useful diagnostically is the fact that the *hun* is associated with people's ability to fulfil their life plan

as well as their ability to have spiritual vision or insight. If a person constantly has dreams, either in the form of dreams during the night or daydreams or just being rather vague or 'spacey', this may be due to an imbalance in the Liver that affects the *hun*. This is often noticeable in people who have taken significant amounts of recreational drugs.

Po

The *po* of the Lung or 'corporeal soul' is an exclusively Chinese concept. It is an aspect of the spirit associated with the physical body and it dies when the body ceases to function. The *po* allows people to have instinctive reactions, for example, the ability to put out a hand to catch something while in flight. It also enables people to become animated. For example, when a person becomes 'spirited' or excited, the Chinese use the term '*po li*'. This describes someone who is vigorously involved in an activity (see Yang, 1997, p. 293).

The *po* is closely aligned to a person's breathing, which is called 'the pulsation' of the *po*. Good breathing roots the *po* into the body and allows people to feel more animated or alive. The *po* also gives people the ability to feel bodily sensation. Weak Lungs cause them to be less able to register physical sensations arising from such things as feeling, seeing and hearing. In consequence people may start to become distanced, inert or cut off from others when the Lungs are out of balance.

Shen

The *shen* of the Heart or the mind/spirit aligns a person's consciousness to the world and allows her or him to communicate with others. It is the most visible of the spirits as it allows people to think clearly and act appropriately in social relationships as well as be settled and calm in order to relax and sleep. The state of a person's spirit generally and especially of the Heart itself is reflected in the brightness of the eyes and a person's ability to make eye contact with others.

Zhi

The *zhi* of the Kidney is often translated as the will or drive. It has been called the 'will that can't be willed' because it allows people to move forward in their lives without consciously pushing or driving themselves. A person with strong Kidneys will reflect a strong Kidney spirit by having a 'drive to be alive'. Conversely people with less strong Kidneys may have

Table 3.1 The five *shen*

Organ	Spirit	Translation
Heart	*shen*	mind/spirit
Spleen	*yi*	intellect/intention
Lungs	*po*	corporeal soul
Kidneys	*zhi*	will/drive
Liver	*hun*	ethereal soul

a lack of drive or may overcompensate for their lack by pushing themselves overly hard and appearing to have extreme drive or strong willpower.

Yi

Finally, the *yi* of the Spleen is sometimes translated as the intellect or 'intention'. The *yi* allows us to bring our thoughts and ideas to fruition and make ideas manifest in the world. When the Spleen is weak a person is unable to accomplish things and may feel unfulfilled by what they do. The inability to bring things to fruition has been termed being 'unable to reap a harvest'. This is a term often used by J. R. Worsley when diagnosing Earth CF patients.

The spirit and the emotions

The spirit is affected by a person's intense and long-standing emotions. Although the effect is on the patient's *shen*, *hun*, *po*, *zhi* or *yi*, the practitioner will often state this in terms of needing to treat the 'spirit level' of the Element. For example, a practitioner who thinks that the patient's spirit has been damaged by intense grief, will focus attention on the spirit level of the Metal Element. The practitioner is always striving to bring about balance between the emotions resonant with each of the Elements. The Han dynasty text, the *Zhong Yang*, describes this:

> The state when the emotions are aroused and relaxed, each attaining its appropriate measure, limit and articulation, is called harmony.
>
> (Davis, 1996)

Summary

1 Focusing diagnosis and treatment on the health of the mind and spirit is a core principle of Five Element Constitutional Acupuncture.

2 The Chinese word *shen* describes both the mind and spirit of a person. It gives people their human consciousness.

3 Each Organ has a spiritual aspect. The names of these are the *shen* (mind/spirit), *hun* (ethereal soul), *po* (corporeal soul), *zhi* (will/drive) and the *yi* (thought/intention).

The Constitutional Factor

4

CHAPTER CONTENTS

The concept of the constitutional imbalance in Chinese medicine

The notion that people have a particular constitutional imbalance is very old and widespread in Chinese medicine. *Ling Shu* Chapter 64 is devoted to an exploration of Five Element constitutional types, based mainly on physical shape and aspects of a person's character. Another system given in *Ling Shu* Chapter 72 outlines a four-fold *yin/yang* system that divides people into *taiyang, shaoyang, taiyin* and *shaoyin* types (see Flaws and Lake, 2000, p. 27). In Japan there is a strong tradition of treating people according to constitutional type. For example, there is a style based upon the six-fold system outlined in the late Han dynasty classic, the *Shang-han Lun*. Using somewhat different criteria it divides people into six types, *taiyang, shaoyang, taiyin, shaoyin, yangmimg* and *jueyin* (Schmidt, 1990). Master practitioners such as Fukushima

and Honma (Eckman, 1996) have also developed styles that diagnose and treat constitutional types. In Korea, Kuon Dowon teaches yet another constitutional style (see Eckman, 1996, p. 209).

The phrase that is currently used in Chinese medicine today to describe a person's constitution is *chang ti*, which means 'bodily type'. This is an appropriate phrase to describe diagnosis that is primarily based upon the physical shape of the person's body (see Maciocia, 2005, pp. 292–298, or Requena, 1989, pp. 81–93, for discussion of these systems). J. R. Worsley, however, developed his style based upon completely different diagnostic criteria, which are set out in the *Nei Jing* and *Nan Jing*. The practitioner's focus is on certain signs that arise as a patient's *qi* goes out of balance.

What do we mean by the Constitutional Factor?

The Constitutional Factor, known as the CF, is one of the most important concepts in Five Element Constitutional Acupuncture. J. R. Worsley used the phrase 'Causative Factor' because, as it is the primary imbalance, it 'causes' other Elements to become imbalanced. Although this is true there are also other causes. Along with many other practitioners of this style we prefer, for clarity, the term 'Constitutional Factor'. The word factor is used, partly because it is the word used by J. R. Worsley and partly because it is commonly used in Chinese medicine, as in 'pathogenic factor'. It is the main focus of the practitioner's diagnosis and much of the patient's treatment is centred on it. Because it is the patient's most underlying imbalance it creates much of the imbalance that can be detected in other Elements. For this reason, as it returns to a better state of health through treatment, it in turn enables many other imbalances to respond and improve. Many of the most dramatic and profound changes that patients can experience from acupuncture treatment are achieved by focusing treatment on it.

The word constitution is defined in the Oxford English Dictionary as: 'The character of the body as regards health, strength, vitality, etc. Condition of mind; disposition; temperament.' The concept of a person's constitution covers both the physical body and the mind and temperament. The word gives a sense of a person's constitution having lifelong characteristics that may manifest in their physical health or psychological make-up.

There is some debate amongst practitioners of Five Element Constitutional Acupuncture about whether the CF is always inherited or whether it can be acquired in early childhood. Examining the occurrence of the same CF in several members of different generations in a family suggests that many constitutional imbalances are carried in the genes. The person's responses to subsequent traumatic life situations further imbalance that Element. Other Elements are also affected over time but the CF is the person's Achilles heel and is the most vulnerable.

Just as people can inherit diseases or weaknesses in particular Organs, people can also inherit imbalances in their temperament or disposition depending on the balance of the Five Elements. The 'nature versus nurture' debate is probably irresolvable and will continue wherever people study humanity, whether they are psychologists, educationalists, acupuncturists or anyone interested in the formation of character. The key task of the acupuncture practitioner is to diagnose the pattern of the person's imbalances and to assist them to achieve a better state of health.

According to Chinese medicine theory the *jing* is the main vehicle by which imbalances are handed down from generation to generation. *Jing* is governed by the Kidneys and determines people's constitutional strength or weakness. This is different from the CF. It is obvious that not all congenital imbalances are found in people's Kidneys. Just as, for example, heart problems or skin problems can be inherited, so also are imbalances in any of the Elements or Organs.

How does a practitioner diagnose the CF?

The four diagnostic signs

The four diagnostic signs are:

- the *emotion* that has the most inappropriate expression in the person
- the *colour* can be observed on the face, particularly on the lower temples beside the eye
- the *odour* that is emitted by the body
- the *sound* present in the voice, particularly a tone that is not congruent with the emotion being expressed.

As well as focusing on these four signs, a practitioner also concentrates on assessing the nature of the person's character in the light of the Five Elements and twelve Officials (see Chapters 8–22, this volume, for a discussion of the Elements). The idea that imbalance of an Organ or Element produces these energetic signs comes from both the *Nei Jing* and the *Nan Jing*. Chapter 34 of the *Nan Jing*, *Su Wen* Chapters 4 and 5 and *Ling Shu* Chapter 49, amongst others, outline the emotion, colour, sound and odour that 'resonate' with each Organ. The odour, colour, season and climate are also given in the *Huainanzi*, a non-medical Han dynasty text.

Chapter 16 of the *Nan Jing* says that when a person's Organ becomes distressed the emotion and colour associated with that Element will manifest themselves. The *Ling Shu* laid down the basic idea by stating, 'Examine the external resonances of the body to know the body's inner viscera' (Wu, 1993, Chapter 47). These four signs enable practitioners to use their senses and intuition to discern which Elements have become dysfunctional.

The importance of diagnosing by signs

This emphasis on diagnosing purely by signs is a distinctive feature of this style. (The use of pulse diagnosis and palpation of the body to reveal signs is discussed in Chapter 28, this volume.) Chronic physical symptoms are usually regarded as merely a manifestation (*biao*) of the primary underlying imbalance (*ben*), and should not distract the practitioner. Even if a patient has obvious signs or symptoms of a congenital or constitutional imbalance in a particular Organ, for example, a heart abnormality or being born with only one kidney, this offers no clue to the person's CF. Diagnosis by signs always takes precedence over physical symptoms when diagnosing the CF. In practice, a significant physical dysfunction is often in the CF Element, but it *cannot* be relied on diagnostically.

Su Wen Chapter 54 and *Ling Shu* Chapter 3 both stress that the practitioner should not rely only on symptoms for making a diagnosis. In fact, hoping to reach a diagnosis of the person's CF by questioning patients about their physical symptoms or even their own perception of their emotional tendencies is regarded as missing the point. As it says in *Nan Jing* Chapter 61:

> To be able to make a diagnosis by observation alone is to possess divine power. To be able to make a diagnosis by hearing alone is to be a sage. To be able to make a diagnosis by questioning alone is to be skilled physician.
>
> (Lu, 1972)

That said, there is no doubt that basing nearly all of the diagnosis on signs and virtually none on symptoms is an extremely difficult path to follow. Practitioners who practise Five Element Constitutional Acupuncture without integrating it with another style pay little attention to the information that can be gained from questioning the patient. This places huge demands on the practitioner. Depending on their inclination, this style suits some practitioners more than others.

Practitioners of Five Element Constitutional Acupuncture need to hone their senses in order to become adept at diagnosis using only signs. Liu I Ming writes of the 'encrustation of the senses' (Cleary, 2001, p. 66). It is this numbing of our sensory perception that has to be transcended. Much of an acupuncturist's training, both while a student and throughout their career as a practitioner, is devoted to refining sensory and intuitive faculties.

Diagnosis by assessing the emotion

Of the four diagnostic signs the emotion is probably the most reliable indicator of the CF. The ability to use the intuition (*zhiguan*) to gain insight into the patient's emotional life is therefore one of the most important skills that the practitioner needs to develop. As the *Huainanzi* stated, 'The external is manifest, the internal is concealed' (Major, 1993, Chapter 7).

Practitioners need to develop the ability to understand the balance of the *qi* of the Five Elements. To do this they interact with the emotions of the patient. As emotions arise, they create movements in the patient's *qi* (see Chapter 5, this volume). Patients will often attempt to hide their emotions, especially when they are intense or painful. In Britain, for example, mastery of the 'stiff upper lip' is much admired. The art of the practitioner lies in discerning these movements of *qi*, however well the person tries to hide them. The movements that arise in the *qi* inevitably also produce subtle changes in the person's voice tone, eyes, face and body language (see also Chapter 26, this volume). This enables the practitioner to decide which emotions are producing the greatest disturbance in the person's *qi* and how appropriately or inappropriately these emotions are being expressed.

The concept of 'inappropriate' emotions

> The sage is joyous because according to the nature of things before him he should be joyous, and he is angry because according to the nature of things before him he should be angry.
>
> (Ch'eng Hao; quoted in Chan, 1963, p. 526)

When a loving relationship is abruptly ended, the practitioner expects a patient to feel sad and hurt. It is 'inappropriate' if another emotion, such as anger, the need for sympathy or fear is the *most* powerful or prolonged emotion exhibited. It probably means that either:

1 The person finds it difficult to experience feelings of hurt and rejection and finds it easier to express another emotion instead. It is, for example, sometimes less painful for people to express their anger than to fully experience their profound sense of abandonment. This means that the person's Fire Element is not healthy and may be the CF.

   or

2 Fire is not the CF and the inappropriate emotion gives a valuable diagnostic clue to the CF.

In this situation, it is relatively straightforward for the practitioner to determine the range of emotional response a person might exhibit. In many situations, it is far less clear and there may be a range of emotions that must be regarded as appropriate. Being aware of the 'structure' of emotions makes it easier for the practitioner to assess the appropriateness of an emotion (see Chapter 25, this volume, for further details). There are no easy objective criteria in this form of diagnosis, however.

It is essential that the practitioner respects the individuality of the patient at the same time as drawing conclusions concerning which emotions are being inappropriately expressed. Which emotions weaken the person and which help them to express themselves in the world? For one person, getting irritable and impatient one more time is another step away from good health. For another, becoming able to assert and stand up for her or himself against a tyrannical boss or partner strengthens the person significantly. Are the tears the patient is shedding a mark of strength or weakness? Does the expression of an emotion enhance or diminish the person's vitality and life?

The answer also partly lies in the practitioner evolving an idea of how a person would be if they returned to a state closer to their 'true nature'. Many people, for example, fearful of the consequences of their fiery temper in childhood, repress their anger to such an extent that they become diminished and excessively inhibited in themselves. Much as being more hot-tempered might make their life difficult in many ways, it is only by returning to something closer to their 'true nature' that they can hope to recover their inner vibrancy and strength.

Diagnosing only by signs is not always difficult, however. Once a practitioner, or even a student, becomes familiar with the key resonances, it is possible to diagnose some people almost immediately. Some patients wear their CFs on their sleeves. When they have voices that laugh, and they easily bring joy and warmth to a room, their CF is very likely to be in the Fire Element. For practitioners to be sure of their diagnosis they also need to ascertain the odour and the colour, but having two of the four diagnostic criteria is sufficient to make a tentative diagnosis.

Confirming the diagnosis of the CF

A practitioner of Five Element Constitutional Acupuncture confirms the diagnosis through treatment. This is done in two main ways:

- by observing improvement in the patient's signs
- by an improvement occurring in the patient's overall health and well-being.

Improvement in the patient's signs

During the course of treatment emphasis is placed on detecting changes in the patient's signs. For example, the practitioner looks for a lessening in intensity in the patient's colour, sound, emotion and odour during the treatment session. If this occurs it is an excellent indication that the treatment is on the CF. Over the course of treatment the practitioner constantly monitors these key signs. Pulse changes are also extremely important and overall improvement in the quality of the person's pulses is an indication that the Element treated is probably the CF.

Improvement in the patient's overall health and well-being

Over the course of treatment amelioration of symptoms is obviously vital. When confirming the CF it is especially significant when the symptoms are linked with Organs not associated with the CF. For example, initiating improvement in the Lungs while treating the patient on the Fire Element.

A positive change in how patients feel 'in themselves' may manifest as improved vitality, greater *joie de vivre*, feeling more relaxed, more tolerant, more self-assured, more emotionally resilient or in other ways that are difficult to describe, but are none the less very real for the patient. Changes in how people feel in themselves are often crucial to their ability to heal their chronic symptoms. Emotions primarily affect the spirit. Illnesses produced by stress and unresolved emotions cannot be cured without a change in the person at this level (see Chapter 5 for a discussion of the causes of disease).

A positive change in a person's sense of well-being is therefore not just a bonus on top of the alleviation of symptoms, but an essential part of their return to a long-term better state of health.

Elements within Elements

Once the patient's CF has been diagnosed, practitioners may attempt to refine their diagnosis so that they can more accurately discern the nature of the imbalance. One way of doing this is by diagnosing the Element within the Element. The *Ling Shu* Chapter 64 also sets out the idea that each Element is represented within each Element. Qi Bo says:

> First establish the five appearances of Metal, Wood, Water, Fire and Earth. Separate them into the five colours. Differentiate them into the five body types of man, and then the twenty-five types of men as a whole.
>
> (Lu, 1972)

This is reflected in the attribution of a point on each channel that corresponds to each Element. The

Earth point on the Heart channel, for example, is *shen men* or Heart 7; the Water point is *shao hai* or Heart 3, etc.

An Earth CF, for example, may be deficient in Water within the Earth. This could lead to the body fluids drying up and a more agitated and insecure personality. Patients can also have excess Water within Earth. In this case they might exhibit an excess of body fluids and perhaps a stodgy mind and character. This diagnosis can only be made by perceiving, for example, that the yellow on the face is a bluish kind of yellow, that the singing tone of voice is a groaning kind of singing, that the odour is a putrid kind of fragrant and a fearful craving for sympathy. This is obviously a very hard diagnosis to make. It is extremely difficult to differentiate between someone whose CF is Earth and whose Water within the Earth is also imbalanced compared with someone whose CF is Earth, but the Water Element itself is imbalanced.[1]

The diagnosis and treatment of patients at this level requires considerable experience and aptitude and is necessarily beyond the scope of this book. However we give a brief introduction in Appendix H.

This difficulty in diagnosing and treating the Element within the Element was even noted by Po-Kao when talking to the Yellow Emperor.

Yellow Emperor '. . . . I wish to hear about the physical shapes of the twenty-five categories of people, how their *qi* and blood are governed, how to distinguish them from their appearances, how to infer their internal conditions from their external outlooks; could you tell me about such things?'

Po-Kao replied, 'That is indeed a complete question. But it is the secret of the ancient teachers, and even I am unable to understand it.'

(*Ling Shu*, Chapter 64; Lu, 1972)

How does our Constitutional Factor affect us?

The effect of the CF on the emotions

The CF inevitably shapes a patient's responses to the circumstances of their life. It may affect their physical shape or function, the way their mind works

and the nature of their character. By definition the emotion that resonates with the Element of the CF is also out of balance.

Situations are bound to arise that provoke emotional responses. How these manifest are affected by a person's CF. Certain situations are obviously inclined to provoke certain emotions. For example, if somebody one loves dies, it is normal to experience grief. Metal CFs are likely to have more dysfunctional reactions to this particular situation than other people. They may be flooded with feelings of loss to such an extent that their spirit never fully recovers. They may generate physical symptoms and they may be unable to return to their previous state of relative balance. Some Metal CFs go to the other extreme and are unable to fully access the feelings of loss. This may also have a lasting impact on the state of health of the person's Metal Element. As Proust said: 'We are healed of our suffering only by experiencing it to the full' (*A la Recherche du Temps Perdu*).

A profound grief can obviously seriously affect people who are not Metal CFs. How much their Metal Element is affected depends on the state of their Metal Element and the state of their *qi* in general. Metal CFs, however, are particularly inclined to find grief difficult to deal with.

It is also often the case that a particular situation evokes a complex mixture of emotions in a person. For example, very different emotions may be felt when people lose their jobs. Anger directed towards the company, a sense of loss, anxiety about the future, a need for support and sympathy or a sense of emotional flatness may all be felt. Which feelings predominate is partially determined by the specific nature of the situation, but most crucially they are shaped by the temperament of the person. For example, a Wood CF whose tendency is to be excessively angry will be inclined to struggle most with the feelings of anger that arise from the redundancy. A Water CF who is inclined to be fearful may well be most affected by the anxiety inherent in the situation. The person's CF, as well as the state of the *qi* of the other Elements, accounts for why different people respond differently to the same event.

Positive characteristics arising from the CF

Practitioners understandably usually concentrate on how the CF makes it difficult for patients to lead spontaneous, happy and fulfilled lives. People's

---

[1]Practitioners of TCM may recognise a correlation to a person suffering from Spleen *qi* deficiency with damp. Whichever viewpoint you come from, Spl 9, the Water point on the Spleen channel, is a point that jumps to mind.

CFs also give them strengths, however. Practitioners may diagnose the excess joy in a Fire CF as a pathological sign. This excess joy may, however, also mean that the person has an extraordinary ability to bring joy into other people's lives. The 'tears of the clown' may be excruciating to the clown, but he or she comes to life once the band strikes up and the spotlight picks out the figure. Only certain people have this ability to bring joy to a crowd of people (the strengths that the different CFs can manifest are discussed in more detail in Chapters 8–22, this volume).

Treating the CF

Nourishing the root (yangben)

One of the strengths of Chinese medicine is its understanding of how imbalances in a person's *qi* manifest in signs, such as the pulse, the colour on the face, voice tone, odour, etc. This enables the practitioner to concentrate treatment on the Elements emanating such signs, sometimes before symptoms have arisen. This initiates change at the root of the patient's disharmony. *Su Wen* Chapter 77 outlined the emphasis many great practitioners of antiquity placed on tracing illnesses back to their origin: 'The sages..., knew the root and the beginning of the illness' (*Su Wen*, Chapter 77; Unschuld, 1992).

The following quotation also recognises this:

> The foundation for the treatment of illness is that one must seek out the root ... if one does not know how to seek out its root, then one's treatments are as vague as if one was gazing at the wide sea and would not know how to ask for water.
>
> (Yu Chang)

Each Element is in relationship with the other Elements through the *sheng* and *ke* cycles. This is crucial to the practitioner's understanding that change is created in any Element by treating the CF. As discussed in Chapter 2, the Elements are not discrete entities but phases in a cycle. Any change in the condition of an Element inevitably has an effect on the other Elements to some degree. One of the key aspects of treatment focused on the CF, the weakest link in the chain, is the extent of changes evoked in other Elements. The pulses normally become more balanced and stronger.

When a patient is in a life-endangering situation, concentrating treatment exclusively on the root is not appropriate. There are also some situations when a practitioner might find that treating the underlying constitution is inappropriate, for example, when treating some musculo-skeletal disorders or acute infections.

Chronic diseases, however, form a large percentage of conditions presented to practitioners in the West. It is these chronic conditions that respond so well to treatment on the CF.

The importance of minimum intervention

One of the advantages of focusing treatment on the CF is that the practitioner needs to use only a small number of points when treating. Some patients require treatment on several different channels in order to respond satisfactorily. Many patients, however, even those with severe and complex conditions, improve hugely with the use of only a few points.

The ethos of minimum intervention has been much prized by many acupuncture practitioners over the course of history. The great physician Hua To (+110 to +207), for example, was admired for only using one or two points in his treatments.

> As for moxa, he applied it to no more than two places and not more than seven or eight times in one place. In needling two places were sufficient and often only one.
>
> (Li Chan: Soulié de Morant, 1994, p. 10)

A thirteenth century ode, describing some of the great practitioners of the past, asserted:

> What these doctors (who used what is known as spiritual healing) in all sincerity thought most highly of was a single needle inserted into a hole, the disease responding to the hand and it lifting. In recent times, this class of doctors has nearly broken from tradition.
>
> (*Da Cheng*; Bertschinger, 1991, p. 17)

This kind of 'spiritual healing' is only possible because changes in the *qi* of one Element affect the *qi* of other Elements through the complex relationships of the *sheng* and *ke* cycles. Practitioners who do not give these processes a chance to operate lose the chance to discover whether the patient can get better by nourishing just the root.

Preventive treatment

Practitioners of Five Element Constitutional Acupuncture place a high value on preventive treatment. Once the Five Elements have returned to a state of greater balance between themselves, patients can expect to enjoy better physical and psychological health. They may then wish to continue treatment in order to stay healthy. The idea of the physician using treatment in order to help patients to avoid illness is often referred to in the classics of Chinese medicine. However, the story that in antiquity patients paid their physician when they were well and not when they were ill, touching tale that it is, appears to have no basis in fact.

> When medicinal therapy is initiated only after someone has fallen ill, when there is an attempt to restore order only after unrest has broken out, it is as though someone has waited to dig a well until he is already weak from thirst, or as if someone begins to forge a spear when the battle is already underway. Is this not too late?
>
> (Su Wen, Chapter 1; Unschuld, 1992, p. 283)

> The really excellent physician controls disease before any illness has declared itself, the man of middling art practises acupuncture before the disease has come to a crisis, and the inferior practitioner does it when the patient is declining and dying.
>
> (Nan Jing, Chapter 61; quoted in Yang and Chace, 1994)

Focusing treatment on symptoms does not ultimately prevent disease from occurring. This is because preventing disease involves harmonising the underlying imbalance that occurred before symptoms arose. The emphasis on diagnosis using signs enables the practitioner to diagnose before symptoms develop. Treatment focused on the CF, or root, lessens patients' predisposition to suffer future problems. This concept of the 'Achilles heel', which may lead to physical and/or psychological illness, is fundamental to the concept of the CF.

In +500, T'ao Hung-Ching wrote in the herbal classic Shen Nong Ben Cao:

> Who, except a brilliant physician, can recognise a disease which is not yet a disease by listening to the tones of the patient's voice, examining the colours of the face, or feeling the pulse?
>
> (Chung, 1982)

Fulfilling our potential

Some people may think that the goal of diagnosis is to fit people into one of five boxes, but this is to seriously misunderstand the approach of practitioners of this style of acupuncture. Everybody is unique. The responsibility of the practitioner is to honour that uniqueness. One of the goals of treatment is to assist

people to fulfil their potential, to achieve their 'contract with heaven', or their destiny.[2] It is not that practitioners desire patients to be 'balanced' in a way that robs them of their individuality. On the contrary, it is disharmony of qi (sometimes in the body, but more commonly in the mind and spirit) that holds people back from achieving their potential. The spirit of writers, artists or musicians often shines through more fully in the creativity of their work if they are strengthened through effective acupuncture treatment. (The authors have treated a number of artists and writers who have attributed the end of a fallow period to acupuncture treatment.) To see people change because the depth of their spirit has been touched by treatment, is one of the greatest joys of practice.

Harmonising our qi

In the Han dynasty the goal of acupuncture treatment was to harmonise the patient's qi with that of Heaven and Earth: 'Unite these two to make a whole person. When they are in harmony there is vitality. When they are not in harmony there is no vitality' (Nei Yeh; Roth, 1986, p. 619).

Practitioners of Five Element Constitutional Acupuncture also strive for this and the method for doing this is to concentrate on enhancing and harmonising the Five Elements. This is largely achieved through treatment of the CF. As the patient's Five Elements become more balanced the mind and spirit become more settled and the emotions become less inappropriate. Patients frequently report feeling as well as they did earlier in their lives. The goal is balanced Elements and therefore appropriate emotions. The Han dynasty text, the Zhong Yang, describes this as: 'The state when the emotions are aroused and relaxed, each attaining its appropriate measure, limit and articulation, is called harmony' (Davis, 1996).

Confucius described it in another way:

> Before the feelings of pleasure, anger, sorrow and joy are aroused it is called equilibrium (chung). When these feelings are aroused and each and all attain due measure and degree, it is called harmony. Equilibrium is the great

[2]See Jarret (1998), for example, pp. 28–32, for discussion of the Chinese concept of each person having a 'contract with heaven' ming, an individual obligation to achieve one's own destiny. Confucians were inclined to see this as being achieved by fulfilling one's duty to society and the family and cultivating the classic Confucian virtues. Daoists typically were inclined to have a much less structured and more mystical vision of how best to 'nourish their destiny'.

foundation of the world, and harmony its universal path. When equilibrium and harmony are realised to the highest degree, heaven and earth will attain their proper order and all things will flourish.

(Chan, 1963, p. 98)

Summary

1 The Constitutional Factor (CF) is the primary imbalance in the person's *qi*. It is usually present at birth, certainly by the end of infancy, and remains constant throughout a person's life.

2 Diagnosis is mainly by signs rather than symptoms. These are predominantly the inappropriate emotion, the colour on the face, the sound of the voice and the odour.

3 Emphasis is placed on improvement in the signs and the person's feeling of well-being rather than on the alleviation of symptoms.

4 The CF has a profound effect on how people respond, either positively or negatively, to different life situations.

5 A high value is placed on the practitioner needling as few points as possible.

6 Using acupuncture to treat patients preventively in order to enhance their state of health and reduce the likelihood of future illness is regarded as important.

The causes of disease

5

CHAPTER CONTENTS

History of the causes of disease

The Daoists, who were the main creators of Chinese science, were fascinated with nature. Their influence and that of the Naturalists during the Han dynasty ensured that Chinese medicine started to evolve a systematic view of aetiology based on a study of nature. In fact 'find the causes' became the watchword of Daoist scientists (Ronan and Needham, 1993, p. 93) For example, in −239, Shi Chun Jiu wrote:

> All phenomena have their causes. If one does not know these causes, although one may happen to be right about the facts, it is as if one knew nothing, and in the end one will be bewildered.
>
> (Needham, 1956, p. 55)

Before this time practitioners of Chinese medicine viewed disease as a hostile entity which was external to the body. From the Han dynasty onwards the emphasis moved away from this and towards viewing disease as the 'breakdown of a state of harmony within the body' (Lo, 2000). The *Nei Jing* described the emotions, invasion by climatic

factors and poor lifestyle as the main causes of disease. The *San-yin Fang*, written by Chen Yen in +1174, is the great classic on the causes of disease and it was in this book that the categories were laid down as they are still taught in China today. Chen divided the causes into internal (*nei yin*), external (*wai yin*) and 'miscellaneous' (*bu wai bu nei yin* – neither internal nor external) causes.

The causes of disease

Practitioners of Five Element Constitutional Acupuncture place most emphasis on the internal causes of disease. These arise from inside people and directly affect the Organs and Elements. They are anger, joy, sadness, over-thinking, grief, fear and shock. The external causes of disease are due to climatic conditions. They are wind, cold, damp, dryness, summer heat and fire. The miscellaneous causes are predominantly linked with a person's lifestyle. They are poor constitution, overwork and fatigue, too much or too little exercise, diet, sex (too much or too little), trauma, parasites and poisons and incorrect treatment. The external and miscellaneous causes are discussed in Appendix B. The internal causes of disease are discussed in greater depth in this chapter and also in the chapters on the Elements (Section 2, this volume).

The internal causes of disease

The *San-yin Fang* and *Su Wen* are emphatic that people's spirits are primarily affected by the internal rather than the external or miscellaneous causes. The *San-yin Fang* states:

> In the interior (of the body) reside the *jing* and the *shen*, the *hun* and the *po*, the mind (*chih*) and the sentiments (*I*), mourning (*yu*) and thoughts. They tend to be harmed by the seven emotions.
>
> (Unschuld, 1988, p. 102)

Su Wen Chapter 5 is equally clear on the role of the emotions:

> The emotions of joy and anger are injurious to the spirit (*shen*). Cold and heat are injurious to the body.
>
> (Veith, 1972)

Although excessive emotions were perceived as being injurious to the spirit in the first place, there was never any doubt that once a person's spirit became disturbed, illness was likely to follow.

> The *shen* is the ruler of the whole body. It controls the seven affects. Harming the *shen* will result in illness.
>
> (Dong Yi Bao Jian)

> Apprehension and anxiety, worries and pre-occupations injure the *shen* ... the spirits injured under the effect of fear, one loses possession of oneself, well-rounded forms become emaciated and the mass of flesh is ravaged.
>
> (*Ling Shu*, Chapter 8; Larre and Rochat de la Vallée, 1995)

Given Five Element Constitutional Acupuncture's emphasis on the health of the spirit, it is natural that it places more emphasis on the internal causes than on the external and miscellaneous causes. In relatively affluent Western cultures it is distress in people's spirits that is the cause of so much illness and suffering. This was true amongst the affluent even in ancient China.

> The reason that nobility get illness is that they do not harmonise their joys and passions ... The reason that lowly people become ill is exhaustion from their labour, hunger and thirst.
>
> (*Yinshu*; Lo, 2003)

Traditional Chinese Medicine, in contrast, is inclined to focus more of its attention on the external and miscellaneous causes. It does, however, recognise the importance of internal causes but to a lesser degree (see Mole, 1998, for a discussion of changes in attitudes to the internal causes in recent Chinese history).

Emotions as a cause of disease

It is normal for people to experience a variety of emotions in different circumstances. For example, it is normal for people to feel grief when they have lost someone or something. Anger helps people to assert their rights and fear protects them from danger. Appropriate emotional response is the goal. It is when emotions are prolonged, intense, repressed or not acknowledged that they can become a cause of imbalance in a person's *qi*. Prolonged or intense emotion creates excessive or disharmonious movement of the *qi*. Emotions that are consistently suppressed tend to inhibit the normal movement of the *qi*. In the Han dynasty text, the *Li Ji*, it says: 'The movements of the Heart are brought about by things; things affect it, thus there is motion' (Davis, 1996).

In the Qing dynasty, Shen Jin-ao made clear that it was excessive emotion that was deleterious: 'Due to having great fear, great joy, great anxiety, great fright, the result is suffering loss of spirit' (quoted in Flaws and Lake, 2000, p. 18). This is a typically Confucian view, advocating the need to avoid intense emotional states.

Many patients have experienced traumas and situations that have evoked intense emotions. When talking about aspects of their past the practitioner can detect movement in the patient's face, changes in their body language or a different tone to the voice. Their *qi* has been unable to return to its previous level of balance. The emotions that arise pervade their spirit and body. Their emotional life and physical function are inevitably affected.

A young child is perhaps the best model of emotional balance and health. Although sadly some babies are born with severe problems, most are born with only slight imbalances in their *qi*. One of the striking and endearing aspects of young children is their extraordinary vitality in body, mind and spirit and the spontaneity and fluency of their emotions. Often when small children hurt themselves, they go to their mothers for sympathy, but only for the time required to get their needs met. Then suddenly they are off, running and shouting again. A temper tantrum may be all-consuming, but rarely lasts more than a few minutes. The emotion, though it can be passionate, does not become stuck. Anger, joy, fear and sorrow may all be felt intensely by an infant, but only rarely do they become prolonged or habitual.

This emotional balance regrettably does not last. As Wordsworth says in his ode, *Intimations of Immortality*,

Heaven lies about us in our infancy!

Shades of the prison-house begin to close around the growing boy.

As children become older they begin to lose that wonderful sense of freedom and happiness, that state when all the emotions are available and none has become habitual or entrenched. Even in a young child one can usually perceive that certain emotions are more powerful and intense than others. There may be many reasons for this, but life events and the emotional and mental idiosyncrasies of other family members usually start to take their toll. For example, Ernest Becker has proposed that children never fully recover from the discovery in early childhood that their lives, and those of the people they love and depend upon, will inevitably end in death (see Becker, 1975). Where once the *qi* of the Five Elements flowed freely, the *sheng* and *ke* cycles were in harmony, now the balance of the Elements in the cycle becomes disturbed.

> When the Five Elements are united, the five virtues are present and *yin* and *yang* form a chaotic unity. Once the Five Elements divide, the distinguishing spirit (*shishen*) gradually arises, and the encrustation of the senses gradually takes place; truth flees and the false becomes established. Now, even the state of the child is lost.
>
> (Liu I Ming; quoted in Cleary, 2005, p. 66)

In time the effects on the body and spirit can become chronic. Physical illness develops and the spirit is diminished. Patients all have their own personal history, which has formed their unique personality and created imbalances in the Five Elements.

The movement of emotions

The English word 'emotion' has the idea of movement inherent in its composition. The Chinese also understood that the emotions create movement and disturbance in a person's *qi*. The Chinese character for emotion is *qing* (Weiger, 1965, lesson 79F). Elisabeth Rochat de la Vallée describes the character:

It is made with two parts, the heart on the left side and the greeny blue colour of life on the right. The right hand side expresses the deep power of life, the richness of the sap flowing or circulating within vegetation. It is made

with the character for life (*sheng*) itself, which is the image of a plant growing up from the earth, and with cinnabar (*dan*). The first impression of this character is that there is a kind of manifestation of the power of life at the level of the heart.

(Larre and Rochat de la Vallée, 1996, p. 21)

Su Wen describes how the different emotions affect a person's *qi*. More *yang* emotions of joy and anger create upward and expansive movement. More *yin* emotions, such as sadness and anxiety, generate downward and contracting movement. This can be clearly seen in an acute situation. Shock or fright affects the Heart and Kidneys intensely. Its effects are both *yin* and *yang* in nature. If, for example, people become intensely frightened or shocked, their bodies immediately produce a huge surge of adrenaline. The effects of increased adrenaline production have been extensively studied by physiologists. There is an increase in perspiration, heart rate, urination, circulation of blood to the muscles, etc. In short, it prepares the body for physical action. The downward moving aspects of the *qi* may affect the bladder and bowel. The more upward movement may affect the heart. Although the surge of adrenaline has broadly similar effects, everyone reacts in their own unique way. One person's heart may become erratic whereas another person is more aware of the need to urinate. One person freezes, while another becomes agitated. The differing response is largely determined by the balance of *yin/yang* and the Five Elements.

> Like the climate sages are numerous and not alike ... This being so, physicians of high rank carefully consider the movements of *qi*, observe their patient's disposition and take these as the root of illness.
>
> (*I Hsien*; translated by Wang, 1990)

All emotions have profound effects on the body, which people can experience if the emotion is felt intensely enough. Practitioners working in Western society constantly see patients whose emotional life has been the cause of their illness. Ongoing difficulties in a person's life chronically unbalance the *qi*. People's health deteriorates as a result of failing to come to terms with stressful situations in their life such as divorce, redundancy, loneliness, disappointment or unresolved conflict with somebody close. In extreme cases, such as the death of a spouse, people's emotions can be so intense that they can lose the will to live. This is a complete negation of what is essential to the character *qing*; *sheng* the radical for life itself.

The seven internal causes of disease

In the *San-yin Fang*, Chen Yen gives seven internal causes of disease. These are anger (*nu*), joy (*xi le*), sadness (*bei*), grief (*you*), over-thinking (*si*), fear (*kong*) and shock (*jing*). Readers should note that contemporary Chinese books and most written by Western practitioners have changed the classification of internal causes from that proposed by Chen Yen. Where he listed *bei*, usually translated as sadness and associated with the Fire and Metal Elements, and *you*, customarily translated as grief and associated with the Metal Element, many writers have amalgamated these two emotions into sadness and given two meanings to the word *si*. Worry is the usual translation of one aspect of *si* and over-thinking or pensiveness of the other. In the changed classification both these meanings are included to make the number back up to seven.

Anger – *nu*

Anger is predominantly *yang* in its nature. It has many different forms and is an extremely common cause of illness. It is more precise to say as it does in *Su Wen* that when 'there is anger the *qi* rises up (*shang*)', as the relationship between an emotion and *qi* is more truly seen as a pattern than a causal relationship.

Anger is the emotion people feel when they want to bring about change in their external circumstances or in their personal limitations. When people are unable to generate the desired change, frustration and exasperation often follow. The Chinese word for frustration is *cuozhegan*, which literally means 'feelings of defeat'. People can feel frustration in many different situations. For example, being unable to create a better society, being in difficult circumstances in their working or personal lives, or finding their intimate and sexual relations limiting. Frustrations affect their *qi* adversely. This is especially so when people are unable to find a way to express or resolve the emotion and their *qi* fails to return to its normal movement. Instead of anger being a creative, productive, upward moving, *yang* force, it stagnates. (Stagnation is often the word used to describe the effect in the *qi* when the Liver becomes imbalanced.) Patients are often unaware of how strongly entrenched in their spirits these deep-seated feelings of frustration, exasperation, resentment and bitterness are.

Some people express anger by flying into a rage, although it often manifests as irritability, resentment and blame. This may be focused on other people, such as family members, work colleagues, car drivers, politicians, etc., but the underlying cause of the emotion lies in the individual's personal circumstances and history. Other people find it very difficult to get angry and need help in order to assert themselves. Both are imbalances that are detrimental to the Wood Element. Acupuncture can help to calm people's anger or enable them to become more adept at expressing anger and asserting themselves. This is especially true if people also realise that they need to change that aspect of their behaviour.

Joy – *xi le*

Whereas *xi* can be translated as elation, *le* is closer to the contentment aspect of joy. As a cause of disease most of the focus in the classics is placed on the deleterious effects of excess joy, excess *xi*. It is *xi* that is described in *Su Wen* as making the *qi* 'loose' (*huan*), which implies agitation and a loss of control. As it says in the *Guanzi*:

> Do not race your heart like a horse, or you will exhaust its energy. Do not fly your heart like a bird, or you will injure its wings.
>
> (Fruehauf, 1998, p. 17)

There is a well-known story in France that when some very old World War I veterans finally heard that they were to receive a special pension payment, several died within hours of hearing the news. A Chinese proverb states, 'When someone meets a joyful event, the *jing-shen* flags.' But life is not an endless series of joyful events.

> Sadness and joy follow each other and give birth to each other. The vital spirit moves in a disorderly way, without knowing a moment's respite.
>
> (*Huainanzi*, Chapter 1; quoted in Larre *et al.*, 1986, p. 96)

Although practitioners sometimes see patients who are manic and have excessive joy, they are more likely to see patients with an absence of joy (*bu le*) or 'disorderly' movements between the two states.

There is a truth inherent in the cliché, 'No man is an island', and in order to have a healthy Fire Element, people must have satisfying contact with other people. As a cause of disease lack of joy (*bu le*) is often the result of a person's life lacking fun, warmth and laughter. Although people can feel joy on their own, it is predominantly an emotion that is nourished by social interaction. Feelings of loneliness and isolation are epidemic in modern society and often lead to joylessness, and in turn people prone to a lack of joy often find it difficult to maintain intimate relationships.

Sadness – *bei*

The character has the Heart radical at the bottom and above it the character *fei* which is negation. What is implied is a kind of suppression of the Heart and therefore the 'radiance of the spirits' (*shenming*). *Su Wen* says that when there is sadness the *qi* 'disappears'. Sadness primarily affects the organs of the Metal and Fire Elements. The word grief (*you*) is used to describe the emotion associated with the Metal Element but does not describe the active expression of grief as people sometimes think. *Ai* is the Chinese word that conveys the howling and wailing that is normal behaviour during the mourning period in China, or the keening (wailing or lamenting bitterly) that people sometimes express when someone close to them has died. *Bei* is better described as sadness or melancholy.

Many patients carry terrible sadness within them and can be fairly described as 'broken-hearted'. Their spirits are crushed as they are assailed by feelings of resignation due to disappointments over past relationships, unfulfilled ambitions or their inability to live up to their youthful dreams and ideals. This is often due to a combination of frustration, primarily affecting the Wood Element, and *bei* suppressing the vitality of the Fire and Metal Elements. The similarity between *bei*, sadness, and *bu le*, lack of joy, is striking and it is often difficult for practitioners to diagnose whether sadness in a person is primarily centred in the Fire or Metal Elements. One may need to rely on other diagnostic criteria such as colour, sound and odour.

The antidote to sadness and feelings of resignation is to re-kindle a sense of lust for life, so that, whatever disappointments patients may have suffered in the past, they realise that life is precious. People need to maintain hope that they will again experience life as rich and fulfilling.

Grief – *you*

Grief is the word the *Nei Jing* and *Nan Jing* use to describe the emotion of the Metal Element. This feeling is often felt intensely and deeply whilst sadness (*bei*) is usually evident in the person's demeanour and especially in the eyes. Grief (*you*) is often repressed to such an extent that it is very difficult to discern, unless an intimate rapport has been has achieved and the practitioner is adept at eliciting it.

Grief, like anger, is an emotion people feel when their experience of life does not match how they would like it to be. People experience a sense of loss, regret or disappointment when outside circumstances, or their perception of themselves, do not match their expectations. In some situations it may be possible for people to develop sufficiently and no longer feel disappointed in themselves and their weaknesses. More often, however, people transcend painful feelings of grief, regret and disappointment when they re-evaluate their lives and begin to accept themselves and their circumstances.

Over-thinking – *si*

Si has been translated in different ways over the years. No English word does justice to the concepts described in the character (for more on the character, see Chapter 14, this volume). Some translators have used words such as 'pensiveness' or 'ponderousness' in an attempt to convey its sense of becoming worried, preoccupied or, in an extreme form, obsessed. Worry can become a major component of a person's stream of consciousness. Rarely is it beneficial to the person. As the commentary to one of the hexagrams in the *I Ching* puts it: 'A man's thoughts should restrict themselves to the immediate situation. All thinking that goes beyond this only serves to make the heart sore' (Hexagram 52 R; Wilhelm, 1951).

Si can also mean thinking too much in the sense of 'straining one's brain' through excessive studying or mental/intellectual activity. Because *si* is not a true emotion, it does not generate the same powerful movements of *qi* as, for example, anger and fear. Its effect is to 'knot' the *qi* and it is therefore neither strongly *yang* nor *yin* in nature. The effect of the *qi* 'knotting' is that it stops circulating. This makes it difficult for people to transform their thoughts into effective action: 'When there is *si* the *qi* is knotted (*jie*) ... the correct *qi* remains on the spot and does not circulate' (*Su Wen*, Chapter 39; Larre and Rochat de la Vallée, 1996).

Fear – *kong*

Fear primarily resonates with the Water Element, but the Heart and the other Organs of the Fire Element also often suffer when fear grips a person.

Fear as a cause of disease can range from low-grade anxiety to abject terror. Fear is predominantly a state of agitation about the future. People dread the prospect of suffering and it drives some people to compulsively dwell on disturbing situations that may or may not arise. This is usually an attempt to 'think through', and therefore be prepared, for all possible scenarios. The truth is that, 'Those who fear suffering are already suffering from what they fear' (Montaigne, Essays 3) and that 'freedom lies in being bold' (Robert Frost).

When people are afraid they usually attempt to reassure themselves by telling themselves that there is no point in feeling fearful. For example they tell themselves that statistics show that air travel is relatively safe or that if World War III is going to start there certainly isn't much they can do about it, etc. It is the strength of the person's *zhi*, their will, allied to the 'virtue' associated with the Water Element, wisdom, that largely determines whether fear becomes excessive or not. As a Japanese proverb puts it, 'Every little yielding to anxiety is a step away from the natural heart of man.'

Shock – *jing*

> When there is starting with *jing* the Heart no longer has a place to rely on. The *shen* no longer has a place to refer to, planned thought no longer has a place to settle. This is how the *qi* is in disorder (*luan*).
>
> (*Su Wen*, Chapter 39; Larre and Rochat de la Vallée, 1996)

Charles Dickens described the effects of the severe shock he experienced in a terrible train crash. 'For several weeks there was no such thing as 'I' in my knowledge. I was not I' (quoted in a BBC documentary on Dickens shown 25 February 2002). It seems that his *shen* truly 'no longer had a place to refer to'.

Shock is sometimes translated as fright and affects the Heart and Kidneys. Zhang Jiebin described it thus: 'With fear and dread (*jing*) the spirits are frightened, and they disperse ... Heart and Kidneys receive the attack' (Larre and Rochat de la Vallée, 1995, p. 127). Shock affects some people by making them agitated and by paralysing others. It can result from either emotional or physical trauma. It doesn't matter whether people have received deeply distressing news or have just emerged unscathed from a serious car crash; its effects are the same. In the short term people often feel disorientated, emotionally volatile, agitated or fatigued and experience unpleasant sensations in the heart. People who have experienced severe shocks in their childhood, in the form of violence, abuse, excessive melodrama, etc., commonly have an imbalance in their Fire and Water Elements. They may never have re-established a proper balance between their Heart and Kidneys. In the short term the Heart is often the most affected, but repeated shocks deplete the Kidneys significantly.

Movements of *qi* that resonate with the emotions

Su Wen Chapter 39 describes the movement of *qi* that occurs when a person feels a particular emotion. The practitioner attempts to discern these movements because pathological movement betrays imbalance of the Element. These movements can be observed in the changes to body language, voice tone, expression in the eyes, facial colour and in many other aspects of a patient (discussed further in Chapter 26, this volume). Excessive movement, for example the patient very easily becoming aggressive, is pathological. A lack of movement is also a sign of imbalance. For example, the patient may fail to respond significantly to warmth and joy. Erratic movement is also a sign of imbalance, for example the patient looks as if he or she is about to cry but denies feeling any distress and genuinely is unaware of any emotion being strongly felt at the time. The movements of *qi* outlined in *Su Wen* Chapter 39 are given in Table 5.1.

The five emotions and the role of 'sympathy'

Although there are seven internal or emotional *causes* of disease, the internal state of a person is usually *diagnosed* via five emotions. These are described in *Su Wen* Chapter 5, where each emotion is linked to one of the Five Elements. These emotions are joy, anger, fear, over-thinking and grief. These are sometimes referred to as the 'five minds' or 'five affects' and emphasis has always been placed on these five in Japan and other countries where the Five Elements are emphasised.

J. R. Worsley made one innovation in this system. Over-thinking or pensiveness is dissimilar to the others on the list, as it is not an emotion, more a state of mind. It 'knots' the *qi* and does not produce strong movements

Table 5.1 How emotions move the *qi*

Emotion	Elements primarily affected	Movement of *qi*
Anger (*nu*)	Wood	rises up (*shang*)
Joy (*xi*, *li*)	Fire	becomes loose (*huan*)
Sadness (*bei*)	Fire and Metal	disappears (*xiao*)
Fear (*kong*)	Water	descends (*xia*)
Over-thinking (*si*)	Earth	knots (*xie*)
Shock (*jing*)	Fire and Water	becomes disordered (*luan*)

Translations taken from Larre and Rochat de la Vallée, 1996. No movement of *qi* is given for grief (*you*) but it is very similar to sadness (*bei*) and is downward moving.

Table 5.2 The emotions that are commonly used in diagnosis

Emotion	Element	*Yin/Yang*
Anger	Wood	*yang*
Joy	Fire	*yang*
Sympathy	Earth	*yin/yang*
Grief	Metal	*yin*
Fear	Water	*yin*

of *qi*. It is interesting to note that Confucius, in the passage quoted in Chapter 4, refers to joy, anger, sorrow and fear but does not accord over-thinking a place. J. R. Worsley's perception, based on observation of many patients, was that when the Earth Element becomes dysfunctional, sympathy or the need to feel cared for or understood is the *emotion* that becomes imbalanced.

Everyone needs support at times in their lives. People who did not feel sufficiently supported in their childhood tend to crave and demand an exceptional and inappropriate amount of support and caring later on in life. Alternatively they may find it very difficult to accept care and support from others. When they receive sympathy or support, it produces feelings of disquiet, rather than the feelings of comfort intended (see Chapter 16, this volume, for more on this topic).

Practitioners of Five Element Constitutional Acupuncture therefore place particular emphasis on the emotions listed in Table 5.2 when making a diagnosis and are most interested in finding which of these are chronically imbalancing the patient's spirit.

Diagnosing the emotions

Internal and external causes of disease are diagnosed in a similar way. A practitioner of Chinese medicine diagnoses the presence of an external pathogenic factor by noticing the signs and symptoms of the patient.

Heat, cold, damp, wind and dryness can sometimes be directly felt or even seen, especially when they are lodged in the channels causing joint problems. Additionally, pulse and tongue diagnosis and questioning the patient should reveal whether the external causes of disease are still present in the patient. To this end an old Chinese saying states that the practitioner should 'Examine the pattern to seek the cause'. Ted Kaptchuk also describes this process when he says,

> Dampness is recognised by what is going on inside, not by knowledge of external exposure. The condition is not caused by dampness; the condition is dampness. The cause is the effect; the line is a circle.
>
> (Kaptchuk, 2000, p. 117)

As Westerners, however, we are conditioned to looking at the cause more lineally than this. A more 'Western' way of expressing the same concept is: 'The present contains nothing more than the past, and what is found in the effect was already in the cause' (Bergson, 1988).

Like external causes of disease, the emotions can be diagnosed by observing their presence or absence. The process is the same. If the practitioner discerns a particular emotion to an abnormal degree, then the diagnosis is made. A practitioner may diagnose that the patient's anger, for example, is extremely inappropriate. This does not inevitably mean that the angry state was caused purely by an internal cause. A 'miscellaneous' cause, such as alcohol or drugs, can also be a major factor. The anger is still a reflection of the state of a person's spirit, however. Some people respond to stimuli such as alcohol with intense change of emotion. Others may pay the price more physically. This is similar to the way that some people are more susceptible to invasion of external causes than others, depending on the strength of the 'upright *qi*' of certain organs.

Other causes of disease

The meaning of the words used when translating the internal causes should not be taken too narrowly. It has been pointed out above that there are many words that come under the umbrella of each of the seven emotions. There are some feeling states, however, that can destroy a person's health but do not fit easily into Chen Yen's seven-fold system. Often these states can be said to be a combination of the seven 'evils', but even this does not describe them adequately. Feelings of jealousy, shame and guilt, for example, can overwhelm some people. Practitioners must be particularly careful when making a diagnosis, as these feeling states may affect several different Elements. In spite of this, if the CF Element is treated this will usually have a more profound effect on the patient's emotional state than treatment on other Elements.

Not living in harmony with nature

As well as the traditional classifications of internal, external and miscellaneous causes, the Classics also comment on other factors that can be deleterious to a person's health. For example in the first chapter of *Su Wen* the Yellow Emperor asks why people's health was worse than it had been in 'antiquity'. Qi Bo tells him that people are 'enslaved by their emotions and worries'. Describing people in antiquity he goes on:

> Internally their emotions were calm and peaceful and they were without excessive desires. Externally they did not have the stress of today. They lived without greed or desire, close to nature. They maintained inner peace and concentration of spirit. This prevented the pathogens from invading.
>
> (Ni, 1995, p. 50)

There is no place in contemporary textbooks for considering whether people's illnesses have been caused by 'excessive desires', 'greed' or not living 'close to nature'. However, living in harmony with the energy of the seasons is a theme that recurs repeatedly in *Su Wen*. Chapter 2, for example, is largely devoted to the importance of living in harmony with the seasons. Ill health and a shortened life span are seen as the inevitable consequences of violating the laws of nature and not living in harmony with the time. *Su Wen* is unequivocal when it says:

> Going against the spring *qi* ... The Liver *qi* is injured internally. Going against the summer *qi* ... the Heart *qi* is empty internally.

And so on for all the seasons (Larre, 1996, p. 130).

What did the writers of the *Nei Jing* mean by 'going against' a season? Spring and summer are predominantly *yang* in nature. This meant that they were perceived as being a time when people should be at their most active and dynamic. Conversely the predominantly *yin* nature of autumn and winter were the appropriate times for resting and reflection. A later text put it like this.

> In spring and summer the *yang* energy is at its highest – human energy is also at its highest. In autumn and winter *yang* energy is at its lowest – human energy is also at its lowest.
>
> (*Da Cheng* 1601; quoted in Soulié de Morant, 1994, p. 48)

For Han dynasty practitioners the season of spring was virtually synonymous with the wind and the emotion of anger. They 'resonate' together (see Chapter 2, this volume, for a discussion of the concept of 'resonance' between seasons, climates and emotions). If people do not use the spring as a period of activity, change and transformation it can be injurious to their health, physically and psychologically. In the same way being buffeted by the wind or feeling intense anger can also have a deleterious effect.

'Going against' a season also means failing to adjust to the changes that are inherent in the transformations of *yin/yang* and the Five Elements. A central concept of Chinese thought in the Han dynasty was the inevitability of change: *yin* must always transform to *yang*, the Five Elements and seasons will always change into their successor in the *sheng* cycle, the cycle of creation. Nothing is permanent. It is people's inability to stay in harmony with these changes that leads to physical and psychological illness. As Kuo Hsiang wrote in the third century:

> Joy and sorrow are the results of gains and losses. A gentleman who profoundly penetrates all things and is in harmony with their transformations will be contented with whatever time may bring. He follows the course of nature in whatever situation he may be. He will be intuitively united with creation. He will be himself wherever he may be. Where does gain or loss, life or death, come in? Therefore if one lets what he has received from nature take its own course, there will be no place for joy or sorrow.
>
> (Chan, 1960, p. 245)

An unfulfilled life as a cause of disease

Chinese medicine also viewed people's health from other perspectives. Although it is not mentioned in the *San-yin Fang*, the Chinese considered it detrimental to people's health not to achieve their potential as human beings. One of the tenets of both Confucianism and Daoism was that each person has a *ming*, a contract with Heaven. Failure to fulfil one's side of the contract, to 'obtain oneself' (*zi de*) and to achieve one's potential, is bound to create frustration and disappointment.

On the subject of mental illness the Ming dynasty physician Yu Tuan, thought that: '*Dian Kuang* (mental illnesses) are mostly in people who have lofty aims that are not attained' (Dey, 1999, p. 6). Li Chan said, 'People who have unfulfilled plans, who get depressed because they have not accomplished their will, often get this disease (*dian-kuang*)' (Dey, 1999, p. 6).

The loss of self-esteem can be crippling. The great physician Sun Si-miao (+581−682) wrote in his final statement on healing that people have illness 'because they do not have love in their lives and are not cherished' (quoted in MacPherson and Kaptchuk, 1997). In our society work and love are the main focuses of most people's lives. Practitioners constantly see patients whose illnesses, psychological and/or physical, stem from their inability to derive satisfaction and contentment from these aspects of their lives.

Chinese thinkers and philosophers from antiquity to the present day have attempted to provide guidance to people on how best they can fulfil their lives, nourish their spirit and maintain health. In the *Ling Shu* it states, 'When the wise cultivate health ... they harmonise joy and anger and reside in quietude' (Dey, 1999, p. 95).

People's ability to cultivate their hearts is central to their ability to withstand the detrimental effects of the emotions on their health.

> The art of the heart consists of making the heart a centre that can receive all the incitements and yet remain in conformity with nature (*xing*).
>
> (Larre and Rochat de la Vallée, 1995, p. 47)

How people cultivate their own 'art of the heart' is an individual choice, largely determined by a person's nature and cultural background. It is up to every individual to take care of their spirit and therefore their health, if they wish to prevent disease: 'If a person's *jing shen* (spirit) is firmly established, no evil outside of the body will venture an assault' (*Xu ling tai yi shu quan ji*; quoted in Unschuld, 1992, p. 337).

The great philosopher Chuang Tzu wrote,

> In all things the Way (*Dao*) does not want to be obstructed, for if there is obstruction, there is choking; if the choking does not cease, there is disorder; and disorder harms the life of all creatures. All things that have consciousness depend on *qi*. But if they do not get their fill of *qi*, it is not the fault of Heaven. Heaven opens up the passages and supplies them day and night without stop. But man on the contrary blocks up the holes.
>
> (Watson, 1964, p. 138)

Discussion of aetiology with patients

It is presumptuous of a practitioner to give advice concerning someone's emotions and inner world, in the same way as they might offer dietary advice. It is another matter, however, to help patients to focus on the sources of their illness and explore with them what they might do in order to respond differently to emotional difficulties. Sometimes patients need encouragement to make changes that they have long known they should make and they know would be beneficial for them. This can then reduce the impact of the emotions on their future health. A practitioner's work is to help patients to be in charge of their bodies and spirits and to live a little closer to the *Dao*.

Summary

1 Practitioners of Five Element Constitutional Acupuncture place emphasis upon the emotions as causes of disease as these affect the person's spirit primarily.

2 The *San-yin Fang* gives seven internal or emotional causes of disease. They are anger, joy, sadness, over-thinking, grief, fear and shock.

3 Although these seven are considered to be important *causes* of disease, practitioners of Five Element Constitutional Acupuncture prioritise the five emotions associated with each Element *when making a diagnosis*. The exception is the Earth Element for which, in an innovation, sympathy is the main associated emotion.

4 *Su Wen* Chapter 39 describes the different movements of *qi* caused by each emotion.

5 Not living in harmony with nature and leading an unfulfilled life can be major causes of disease.

The inner development of the practitioner

6

Introduction

Throughout the history of Chinese medicine it has been understood that the individuality of the practitioner has an enormous effect on the efficacy of acupuncture treatment. With its emphasis on treating at the subtlest levels of the person's *qi*, it is natural that many practitioners of Five Element Constitutional Acupuncture place a great deal of importance on their internal state.

Wu was the ancient character for a healer or physician. This character depicts a female shaman below a quiver with an arrow and a spear (Weiger, 1965, lesson 82a).

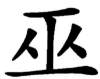

In the Shang dynasty, the era preceding the time of the *Nei Jing*, medicine was largely practised by shamans who lived in the community. It was accepted that certain people had the gift to be a shaman or a physician and that this talent was not available to everyone. The *Nei Jing*, however, ushered in an era where diagnosis was based on more systematic criteria such as *yin/yang* and the Five Elements. The gifts and skill of the person carrying out the diagnosis and treatment were still considered to be of crucial importance, however. The significance of this expertise is emphasised in the following quotation:

> If someone says that an illness that has persisted for a long time cannot be removed his statement is wrong. When someone who is an expert in utilising the needles removes such an illness, it is as if he has pulled out a thorn, as if he has cleansed what is soiled, as if he untied what is knotted, and as if he opened what is blocked. Even though an illness has persisted for a long time, it can likewise be brought to an end. Those who state that such illnesses cannot be cured have not yet acquired the respective skills.
>
> (*Ling Shu*, Chapter 1)

Sheng ren is the phrase used in the *Nei Jing* to describe the most accomplished physicians. Weiger translates it a 'sage' or 'wise man' who 'listened to and understood the advice given by the sage and thus becomes wise' (Weiger, 1965, p. 211). Richard Wilhelm says that a *sheng ren* 'through his power awakens and develops people's higher nature' (Wilhelm, 1951, p. 3).

Inevitably there are differences in how each individual practitioner's qualities are perceived (see Hsu, 1999, pp. 94–104). In the competitive world of Chinese medicine in China today, doctors who have a busy practice and a good reputation are said to have *jingyan*. Although usually translated as 'experience' the word means much more than that. An experienced but unpopular doctor does not have *jingyan*. 'Virtuosity' (*linghuo*), which can

DOI: 10.1016/B978-0-7020-3175-5.00006-1

be found in excellent physicians of any system, is part of what is conveyed by *jingyan*. Acquiring *jingyan* is a realistic goal for practitioners and a necessary one if they aspire to attain at least some of the attributes of a *sheng ren*.

> Whether a man goes on living in health, or whether a disease arises; whether it is in the human power to control it, and whether the patient can be cured; whether one is only at the beginning of the study of acupuncture (and moxibustion), or whether one has come to the fullness of it – all depends (on an understanding of the functions of) the twelve-tract network system of *yang* and *yin* channels. To the slap-dash practitioner or the tyro [a beginner, a novice] it all seems very easy; only the great physician knows how difficult it really is.
>
> (*Ling Shu*, Chapter 11; Lu and Needham, 1980, p. 28)

Why is inner development important?

Practitioners cultivate their virtuosity (*linghuo*) because it enhances their ability to make accurate diagnoses and give effective treatments.

Diagnosis

Signs versus symptoms

When carrying out a diagnosis, a practitioner needs to understand the patient's signs and symptoms. Diagnosis based on signs is far more difficult to practise than one based on symptoms. A diagnosis based on symptoms can be made from a transcript of a patient's case history, but it will not help the practitioner to understand subtler aspects of the patient. Diagnosis of the CF is made from observable signs and can only be made by using a combination of sensory acuity and intuition (*zhiguan*). This allows practitioners to perceive patients' emotional balance and temperament.

This was described by Chuang Tzu as follows:

> The hearing that is only in the ears is one thing. The hearing of the understanding is another. But the hearing of the spirit is not limited to any one faculty, to the ear, or to the mind. Hence it demands the emptiness of all the faculties. And when the faculties are empty, then the whole being listens. There is then a direct grasp of what is right there before you that can never be heard with the ear or understood with the mind.
>
> (translation from Merton, 1970, Chapter 4)

The emphasis on diagnosing the relative imbalance of patients' emotions requires practitioners to relate to the emotional life of the patient. Practitioners must be able to induce patients to reveal aspects of their inner selves in order to assess the balance of the key five emotions. To do this practitioners must make excellent rapport with their patients.

> If a man is brusque in his movements, others will not co-operate. If he is agitated in his words, they awaken no echo in others. If he asks for something without having first established relations, it will not be given to him.
>
> (Confucius; Analects)

The practitioner's internal state

Practitioners also need to be aware of their own emotions. Because of their own constitutional imbalances and emotional predispositions, practitioners may find it more difficult to experience some emotions than others. This is especially the case if they have emotions that are intense. Some practitioners, for example, are in denial of their own grief or sadness. They therefore do not feel comfortable exploring these areas in someone else. This can result in them having little idea of what really troubles the person. Some practitioners can find it hard to be very sympathetic or difficult to fully recognise the extent of fear in another person. If these limitations are overcome the practitioner's diagnostic abilities can reach their full potential.

Cultivating awareness

When using this style of acupuncture it is necessary to cultivate an attitude of highly focused awareness in order to make a diagnosis. The practice of Five Element Constitutional Acupuncture becomes sterile and inadequate unless practitioners are constantly vigilant. Practitioners need to listen to the nuances in the voice, observe the facial colour, attempt to discern an odour and perceive emotions arising in the patient. It is this vigilance and awareness that enables the practitioner to make diagnosis a stimulating ongoing process.

> If the patient has been separated from his relatives for long and has become worried as a result, then the emotions of worry, fear, joy and anger may undergo irregular changes which could cause an empty deficiency of the five viscera with the blood and *qi* departing from their usual guarding positions. A physician cannot be regarded as a good one unless he can detect such things in his diagnosis.
>
> (*Su Wen*, Chapter 76; Lu, 1972,)

Achieving and maintaining this level of awareness is dependent upon the internal condition of the practitioner.

Presence

Another important aspect of diagnosis is the quality of attention the practitioner gives to patients. When practitioners are completely present for their patients they can hear and accept what patients tell them without feeling a need to make their patients change. This special quality enables patients to feel accepted and acknowledged so that they can more easily accept themselves. Over time this allows patients to build trust in the practitioner so that they can open up and reveal parts of themselves they have previously kept hidden. By revealing these parts the practitioner understands and connects to deeper aspects of the patient's mind and spirit. (For more on making rapport, see Chapter 24, this volume.)

To develop presence the practitioner needs to cultivate a state of focused awareness, coupled with a quality of self-acceptance. Practitioners who strive to accept themselves are likely to also accept whatever arises from their patients. The quality of attention given to the patient by the practitioner helps to develop a deep level of rapport and trust which is of prime importance, not only for diagnosis but also for treatment.

Treatment

In the practice of medicine, rapport is often taken to mean that the practitioner and patient are getting along well and a therapeutic relationship has been established. Practitioners of Five Element Constitutional Acupuncture know that rapport needs to be significantly more than this. The contact between the practitioner and patient potentiates the treatment itself. This in turn evokes change in the patient's mind and spirit. The degree to which the *qi* of the practitioner harmonises with that of the patient influences the efficacy of each act of needling.

> If two are similar, they will coalesce. If notes correspond they will resonate.
>
> (Chun Qiu Fa Lu, approx. −200; quoted in Needham, 1956, p. 281)

Ideally at the moment of needling, the patient feels relaxed and secure with the practitioner. This enables her or him to be receptive to the change that is being initiated by needling the acupuncture point.

> In the mind of the physician there should be no desires, only a receptive and accepting attitude, then the mind can become *shen*. The mind of the physician and the mind of the patient should be level, in harmony following the movements of the needle.
>
> (*Da Cheng*; Zhen, 1996)

It is the inner development of practitioners that enables them to achieve the levels of awareness and depth of rapport needed in the treatment room.

Maximising rapport and increasing the efficacy of treatment

Practitioners accumulate *jingyan* through their own experience of life. It is not possible for a physician to lead an 'unexamined' life with no regard for morality or self-development and expect to attain significant amounts of *jingyan*. Sun Si-miao summed it up like this: 'The superior physician strives for a pure spirit and looks inward.'

Wu wei – non-action

Daoism has a concept of *wu wei* which has often been mistakenly translated as 'non-action'. What the Han dynasty Daoists meant by *wu wei*, however, was ensuring that all action was in accord with the nature of the particular time. One of the key emphases of the *I Ching* is to help a person gain an understanding of the particular time or situation present. *Wu wei* is action that is driven by the needs of the situation rather than by the person's needs or desires. For the Han dynasty Daoists living in harmony with nature was essential to living and acting in harmony with the needs of the time and situation. As it says in the *Huainanzi*: 'The sages in all their methods of action follow the nature of things' (Morgan, 1877).

The transition of the seasons, and the lessons learnt from them about humanity and the *dao* of Heaven and Earth are timeless.

Living in harmony with nature

The *Nei Jing* has many exhortations for people to live according to the principles that underpin the system of medicine.

In ancient times, people lived simply. They hunted, fished and were with nature all day. When the weather cooled, they became active to fend off the cold. When the weather heated up in summer, they retreated to cool places. Internally their emotions were calm and peaceful and they were without excessive desires. Externally they did not have the stress of today. They lived without greed or desire, close to nature. They maintained inner peace and concentration of spirit ... This prevented the pathogens from invading.

(Ni, 1995, Chapter 13)

Spending time outside being in direct contact with Heaven and Earth and observing the different energetic qualities of the seasons and the times of day, has been a source of inspiration for many practitioners. As well as helping them to maintain good health, it also helps them to create and sustain concentration and purpose. This is necessary in order to give high-quality acupuncture treatments as well as deepening their understanding of the Five Elements and *yin/yang*.

Stilling the mind and spirit

The *Nei Jing* makes it clear that one of the essential attributes of a *sheng ren* (sage) is the ability of practitioners to concentrate and still the mind and spirit. If practitioners are not able to put aside the preoccupations and suffering of their own life when they enter the treatment room then it is not possible for them to engage fully with the patient.

Su Wen makes the point that 'the *jingshen* of the *sheng ren* would not be dispersed' (Larre and Rochat de la Vallée, 1995, p. 34). This is not possible if practitioners do not actively seek to find a way to harmonise the turmoil of their emotional life and to still the ramblings of the mind.

> The reason that a physician fails to make a complete diagnosis is due to absence of mental concentration and irregular state of his will and sentiments which causes inconsistency between the internal and external and brings about the state of doubt.
>
> (*Su Wen*, Chapter 78; Lu, 1972, p. 634)

Qi development practises such as *qi gong*, and *tai ji*, as well as meditation, are all possible paths towards a more settled mind and spirit. Historically these have been used as self-development tools by practitioners from all areas of Chinese medicine. They are, however, especially beneficial to acupuncturists because they are working directly with a patient's *qi*.

Practising these arts enables acupuncturists to have greater awareness of their internal state while treating. Regular practice enables practitioners to have greater control over their *qi* and to relax and centre themselves before commencing treatment. *Qi* practices also enable the practitioner to develop greater sensitivity to their patient's *qi* and to focus their own *qi* on the patient while carrying out treatment.

Focusing attention

Because Five Element Constitutional Acupuncture has an overriding focus on diagnosis by signs, the development of sensory acuity and intuition is also part of the path towards a more focused mind and spirit. It is necessary to 'transcend the dulling of the senses', in order to develop the traditional diagnostic skills of seeing, hearing, smelling and touching to the level required for this style of acupuncture.

Just as artists or musicians hone their sensitivity in order to be able to express their nature more fully, the cultivation of these delicate and sublime parts of our humanity can lead to a more settled and refined spirit in the practitioner. Good pulse diagnosis requires that the mind is stilled. This is itself akin to meditation practices that require people to focus their attention on the subtle sensations that are felt in particular parts of the body, for example the Burmese Buddhist practice of *Vipassana* meditation. *Qigong* practitioners, who tend to be more concerned with their inner development than most acupuncturists, generally believe that it is the work they do in meditation and *qigong* exercises that is essential in order to replenish their own reserves of *yuan qi* (see Hsu, 1999, p. 74).

The Japanese acupuncturist Yanagiya was clear about what he considered the essential internal condition necessary for pulse diagnosis: 'Focus your attention to your fingertips. Do not speak, do not look, do not listen, do not smell and do not think. This is the key principle of pulse diagnosis' (Matsumoto and Birch, 1993).

Stillness while needling

A harmonious internal state is essential if the practitioner is going to receive the essential diagnostic information from the patient. Guo Yu, writing in the first century, was very clear that a practitioner needed to be both impeccable and experienced in order to practise acupuncture at the level required.

> Even the slightest hairline deviation when inserting an acupuncture needle is an inexcusable professional blunder. The skilful practice of acupuncture depends upon perfect coordination of the *shen* and hands. It can be learned, but not described in words.
>
> (Chuang, 1991, p. 27)

Practitioners must still their minds and be prepared to leave the concerns of their life outside the treatment room door.

> With nothing to be seen – your hands as gripping a tiger,
> No needs felt within – your attention on a noble fellow.
>
> (Bertschinger, 1991, p. 43)

The physician strives to practice acupuncture with 'no needs felt within', in keeping with the concept of *wu wei*. The closer practitioners come to the ideal state the more able they are to concentrate 'attention on a noble fellow'.

Intention

The Chinese word *yi* can be translated in several different ways depending on the context. In a Han dynasty text it refers to 'that which the physician desires and consciously conceives of, that which he wills, but also that which comes about through a kind of focusing of consciousness' (see Scheid and Bensky, 1998). This view of the importance of the internal state of the practitioner is well summed by the acupuncturist Guo Yu, who was famed for his needling skills.

> Now, when it comes to treating nobles, they look down on me from the heights of their distinguished places, and I am filled with anxiety that I might not please them. Though the acupuncture needles demand precise measure, with them I am often in error. I am burdened with a heart full of trepidation, compounded by a will reduced in strength. Thus intention *(yi)* is not fully there. Consider what influence this has on treating the disorder. This is the reason I cannot bring about a cure.
>
> (Zhou, 1983)

Most practitioners of Five Element Constitutional Acupuncture place a high value on the practitioner's intention and are in agreement with Sun Si-miao when he wrote, 'Medicine is intention *(yi)*. Those who are proficient at using intention are good doctors' (quoted in Scheid and Bensky, 1998).

There is a huge difference between being treated by a practitioner who is 'proficient at using intention' and one who is not. It is similar to the effect that a beautiful piano sonata has on the spirit when it is played by a sensitive and accomplished musician compared to the same piece of music used as a ringing tone on a mobile phone. In one instance the pianist has gathered his *yi* and imbued the music with his own spirit. In the other, the notes may be the same but the effect on a person's spirit is similar to being needled by a robot.

Su Wen hints at the kind of internal state and sensitivity necessary in the practitioner at the moment of needling: 'The physician must be like a crossbowman pressing his trigger at the exact time, not an instant too soon, not an instant too late – as if grasping a tiger – and the mind oblivious of all other things'.[1]

Interacting with the patient

In the treatment room the crucial factors are the rapport gained with the patient and the state of the practitioner's mind and spirit at the moment of needling. As well as being present with their patients, practitioners must also find ways to interact that satisfies patients' needs.

Five Element diagnosis may also be helpful. For example, some patients who are Fire CFs will need to feel warmth from the practitioner in order to feel truly relaxed and receptive at the moment of needling. A person who is a Wood CF may need to feel that the practitioner is assertive and in command of the situation. Any diffidence or indecision in the practitioner may set up a degree of anxiety and the required level of rapport is not achieved. Tenderness and gentleness are other qualities that enable patients to feel sufficiently safe and cared for so that they can be fully receptive to the treatment. In order to attain sufficient rapport it is necessary for practitioners to allow their spirit to radiate in such a way as touches the patient's spirit.

Understanding the patient's Five Element diagnosis may help the practitioner to understand what kind of relationship is best achieved with the patient. Physicians with excellent *jingyan*, whatever their system of medicine, have always been able to achieve the appropriate level of rapport. What is essential is that

---

[1]See, for example, translations in Merton, 1970, of Chuang Tzu's Chapter 19, 'The woodcarver', Chapter 13, 'Duke Hwan and the wheelwright', or Chapter 3, 'Cutting up an ox', for the kind of qualities needed in a craftsman in the execution of his work; see also Lu and Needham, 1980, p. 91.

practitioners are prepared to draw on all of their inner resources and are happy to try many different approaches in order to induce the optimum level of relaxation and trust in the patient.

Compassion

As well as stilling the mind and spirit and becoming 'proficient at using intention', another essential attribute is the cultivation of the Heart. Many of China's most respected practitioners came from the ranks of the Confucian 'gentlemen' (*ruyi*), One of the key qualities they traditionally cultivated was *ren*, which translates as 'a sensitive concern for others' (Elvin, M., in Carrithers, 1985, pp. 156–189) or 'humaneness' (Allan, 1997). The eminent Chinese practitioner Dr John Shen said that a practitioner must have a 'good heart' (lecture organised by the *Journal of Chinese Medicine* given in London in 1978). The physician's acceptance and care for the patient is an integral part of the healing process.

How can a practitioner cultivate *ren*? Awareness of its importance and creating a goal to develop it is obviously a start. In order to fully identify with the pain and suffering of another, however, practitioners benefit from having experienced and been aware of suffering themselves. As an Arabic proverb says, 'No man is a good physician who has never been sick'. To quote another saying: 'True kindness presupposes the faculty of imagining as one's own the suffering and joy of others' (André Gide).

For practitioners who are fortunate enough not to live in chronic physical pain it is a valuable experience to endure physical pain on occasions, as it gives some insight into what many patients suffer. This is also true at the level of the mind and spirit. It is largely through our personal experience of unhappiness and suffering that we develop our spirit and our compassion. Buddhism, China's third most important religion, teaches that the cause of suffering in people's lives is desire. Inability to satisfy their desires leads people to experience many painful internal states. People who deny their own suffering never experience their full humanity.

The combination of the constitutional imbalance and its effect on the other Elements makes it inevitable that certain emotions are more difficult to fully experience than others. The concept of the 'wounded healer' has become widely accepted in recent years. This idea assumes that it is through the experience of psychological wounds that physicians deepen their compassion and their understanding of the patient. As stated above, unless practitioners are prepared to explore uncomfortable areas of their own personality, they have little hope of recognising similar aspects in their patients' personalities.

Empathy

Similarly practitioners have little chance of fully developing their compassion for their patients' suffering if it does not resonate with their own experience of themselves. For example, many people find it relatively easy to empathise with the feelings of heartbreak and sense of loss that people experience when a loving relationship breaks up. It is often hard for practitioners, however, to have the same level of compassion if the patient has feelings such as jealousy, resentment, insecurity and self-loathing. These are regarded as less acceptable emotions and may incur disapproval from practitioners, especially if practitioners have repressed these feelings in themselves. Sun Si-miao wrote:

> Whenever a Great Physician treats disease, he has to be mentally calm and his disposition firm. He should not be swayed by his wishes and desires, but should first of all develop a marked attitude of compassion. He should commit himself firmly to the willingness to make every effort to save every living being.

Exasperation with patients for their personal weaknesses, their refusal to accept well-meant advice, excessive need for sympathy or whatever attributes or behaviour are most galling to the practitioner must never stand in the way of establishing a caring therapeutic relationship. As Bob Dylan rightly sang 'And remember when you are out there trying to heal the sick, that you must always first forgive them' (Bob Dylan, in 'Open the door, Homer', Basement Tapes, CBS records, 1975).

Forgiveness is only possible if practitioners maintain an attitude of humility towards the patient and the system of medicine they are attempting to practise. Whatever practitioners think they know about Chinese medicine and acupuncture, they delude themselves if they do not realise that they truly understand only a small amount about *yin/yang*, the Five Elements and *qi*.

> Alas medicine is so subtle that no one seems able to know about its complete secrets. The way of medicine is so wide that its scope is as immeasurable as the four seas.
>
> (*Su Wen*, Chapter 74; Lu, 1972, p. 635)

Cultivating virtuosity (*linghuo*)

In each treatment session there is a natural order of activity. The virtuosity of the practitioner affects the quality of the diagnosis and the efficacy of the treatment. Practitioners need to:

- Make excellent rapport with the patient. This is only possible if the practitioner is able to express sufficient compassion (*ren*). Excellent rapport allows patients to reveal the nature of their emotions and their suffering. Ideally this level of rapport is maintained throughout the entire encounter.
- Employ great sensory acuity and awareness to discern the colour, odour and voice tone.
- Use their own emotions to evoke emotions in the patient.
- Hone their intuition (*zhiguan*) in order to diagnose the patient's emotional imbalances.
- Still the mind and spirit and use sensory acuity to interpret the pulses.
- Consider the appropriate treatment
- Concentrate intention (*yi*) and *qi* to needle the patient.

In order to attain a measure of *jingyan* or virtuosity (*linghuo*) in this style of acupuncture these are the main qualities that need to be developed. Each person's path to this development is utterly individual. Traditionally acupuncture practitioners have often used various spiritual practices, including meditation, *qi gong* and *tai qi*. Others find communing with nature assists them, whilst others find they are helped by increasing their level of self-understanding.

The goal of the inner development is primarily to increase practitioners' ability to serve the needs of their patients. There is another goal, however. This is to make the experience of working with patients both a source of enjoyment in itself and a vehicle for the practitioner's own development as a human being. There is a huge difference between seeing patients when the practitioner's 'heart is not in it' and when the practitioner is stimulated and excited by the challenge of treating sick people. The latter is both considerably more therapeutic for the patient and a source of vitality and growth for the practitioner.

Some acupuncture practitioners report feeling 'drained' by their experience of seeing patients. It is open to question whether this is to do with 'giving away' their *qi*, or other factors common to all physicians, such as feeling burdened by feelings of responsibility and self-doubt. The exchange of *qi* at the moment of needling does not have to be one-way, but mutual. Many experienced practitioners know that they have contacted the patient's *qi* by the sensation of *qi* they feel in their own bodies. This can only be possible if *qi* is transmitted both to and from the practitioner. In order to be an acupuncture practitioner over a long period of time it is essential that practitioners do not allow the mutual exchange of *qi* and the difficulties of the situation to diminish their own *qi*.

The state the practitioner hopes to maintain for the vast majority of the time is one of feeling energised by the experience of treating patients. Without this it is difficult to maintain the level of awareness necessary for diagnosis, or the intention required for treatment. As the eminent American physician John Lettsom said, 'Medicine is not a lucrative profession. It is a divine one'. Or, as it says in the *Tao te Ching*,

> The sage does not hoard.
> Having worked for his fellow beings,
> The more he possesses.
> Having donated himself to his fellow beings,
> the more abundant he becomes.

(Chen, 1989)

Summary

1 Practitioners need to develop their virtuosity (*linghuo*) in order to accumulate *jingyan* or experience.

2 If practitioners wish to become excellent at Five Element Constitutional diagnosis, an important skill to develop is awareness.

3 The degree of harmonisation of the *qi* of the practitioner with the *qi* of the patient influences the efficacy of each act of needling. This is achieved by attaining a deep level of rapport and trust between practitioner and patient.

4 In order to develop as a practitioner it is necessary to still the mind and spirit, focus intention and develop a heartfelt attitude of compassion.

5 Honing sensory acuity and intuition concerning people's emotions is a path to greater sensitivity and refinement in the practitioner.

Section 2

The Elements and Organs

Introduction to the Five Elements

7

Introduction

The Five Elements lie at the heart of a Five Element Constitutional Acupuncturist's diagnosis. This chapter gives an overview of Chapters 8–23, which describe the Elements in detail. Each Element is described in three chapters:

- The first of the three chapters covers the Chinese character for the Element and the Element's 'resonances'. In many places we refer to the Chinese character and at the same time refer to a text where the character can be looked up. These references enable students to access some discussion of the various characters and thus broaden their understanding.
- The second of the three chapters explains the functions of the Organs associated with the Element.
- The third chapter of the three describes some aspects of the behaviour typical of the CFs of each Element.

Together, the three chapters about each Element provide the basis for diagnosing a patient's CF.

The first chapter – the Element and the resonances

The Elements

Each chapter begins with a discussion about the Element itself. Earth, Water, Fire, Metal and Wood all evoke powerful images. Understanding the Elements allows practitioners to gain deeper insight into patients who have that Element as their constitutional weakness. The Chinese character is analysed and its connection with the life of a person is discussed. There is further comment about how the Element appears in nature and the relationship of one Element to another via the *sheng* and *ke* cycles.

The resonances

In most translations of Five Element texts the areas connected by an Element are called either 'associations' or 'correspondences'. 'Association' suggests that the connection may be empirical or arbitrary. 'Correspondence', on the other hand, conveys something more about a relationship but does not suggest that the connection is energetic. Although 'resonance' departs from the usage of many writers, we prefer to use it because it suggests that there is an energetic link. For example, Wood, green, anger, wind and spring resonate together. Their *qi* has the same nature (see Chapter 2, this volume).

In the following chapters we describe two kinds of resonances:

- the 'key' or primary resonances
- the 'secondary' resonances.

Key or primary resonances

The key resonances used by a practitioner of Five Element Constitutional Acupuncture are colour, sound, emotion and odour. These are the primary resonances and provide the foundation of CF diagnosis. As *Ling Shu* Chapter 47 states: 'Examine the external resonances of the body to know the body's inner viscera' (Wu, 1993). These resonances can only be used in diagnosis if practitioners use their sensory acuity and intuition. Ideally the practitioner discerns all four of these resonances in order to make a diagnosis of a patient's CF. Table 7.1 sets out the key resonances.

Assessing the resonances

Each resonance expresses imbalance somewhat differently. Colour, for example, is present on the face. To assess the emotion, on the other hand, requires a context in which a topic is discussed and its 'appropriateness' assessed. The following are some comments about how the different resonances express balance and imbalance (see Chapter 26, this volume, for more on diagnosis using the key resonances).

Colour

When an Element is in balance, the face does not manifest the Elemental colour. When a colour is apparent, the associated Element is out of balance. The colour resonant with the Element appears on the face beside or under the eyes, in the laugh lines or around the mouth. Unlike the emotion or the sound in the voice, the colour is relatively constant.

The colour may change over time, for example, as the balance of an Element improves. It can also change very quickly after a shock, during an acute illness or while an emotion is intensely felt. In general, however, colour is the most constant of the four key resonances.

Sound

A person's voice normally manifests different and appropriate tones. Different voice tones occur because a person has a variety of emotions. When the emotion is felt the *qi* moves and this affects the voice tone. For example, a person shouts because anger makes the *qi* rise and this gives added force to the voice. The practitioner is listening for the sound that stands out as inappropriate or incongruent.

As the patient and practitioner talk, the content of the conversation and the rest of the patient's expression determine appropriateness. For example, if patients are speaking about events that gave them great pleasure the emotion they express would naturally be joy. It is therefore normal if the voice tone is laughing, the sound resonant with the Fire Element. If patients are talking about their grief about a loved one's death, then the fitting sound would be weeping, the sound resonant with the Metal Element. A sound that is not appropriate to the context, for example, laughing when the current context is painful, is a sign of an Elemental imbalance.

The voice tone is revealed during conversations between the patient and practitioner, so the practitioner must have skill and determination to ensure that several different contexts and emotions arise in those conversations.

Table 7.1 Key resonances

	Wood	Fire	Earth	Metal	Water
Colour	green	red	yellow	white	blue/black
Sound	shout	laugh	sing	weep	groan
Emotion	anger	joy	sympathy or worry	grief	fear
Odour	rancid	scorched	fragrant	rotten	putrid

Note that the translations from the Chinese vary slightly from one translator to another.

Odour

Ideally patients do not have a particular odour. When they do, the Element resonating with the odour is imbalanced. Odour is less constant than colour, but more constant than sound. Odours can change during a treatment by lessening or increasing. They are also more fragile than colour. A practitioner can look away from a colour and then return to it expecting it to still be there; on the other hand, practitioners easily habituate or become desensitised to an odour. Acutely ill or elderly patients tend to emit one or other of the odours strongly.

Emotion

An appropriately expressed emotion fits the context it is expressed in. During the practitioner–patient interaction the 'context' arises mainly from the content of the conversation. The practitioner must decide which of the five emotions is the least appropriately expressed. Like voice tone, appropriateness is measured by assessing whether the emotion is appropriate to the context in which it is used and the movement of the *qi* is smooth and of appropriate intensity. Emotions do not have a clear definition in modern psychology. The Rebers say 'Historically this term has proven utterly refractory to definitional efforts; probably no other term in psychology shares its combination of nondefinability and frequency of use' (see Reber and Reber, 1985, pp. 236–237). We would say that an emotion usually involves three things: 1, bodily sensations (to which people can become habituated and hardly feel); 2, some cognitive element, for example, interpretative perception based on memory; and 3, motivational properties in that the emotion tends to play a role in impelling activity.

The practitioner notices which emotion is the least fluent and least appropriate of the five. To use the previous example, if a patient is describing pain but has a laugh in the voice and appears to feel joyful, she or he is expressing an inappropriate emotion. By contrast, someone describing an upcoming and genuinely threatening situation would normally show some signs of fear, however mild.

Observing an emotion is somewhat different from observing a colour. From the practitioner's point of view, emotions are perceived as patterns that can be discerned from what the patient says, the tone of voice, the facial expression, the gestures and bodily stance. The emotion is not simple, like a colour, but is more complex and changes from one moment to the next. According to Ekman and Friesen (2003, p. 7), 'Our studies of the body, published in professional journals, have explored the differences in what the face and the body tell us. Emotions are shown particularly in the face, not in the body. The body instead shows how people are *coping* with emotions.'

Table 7.1 suggests that there are just five emotions. In the language of everyday life, this is not true. The concept, set out in the *Nei Jing*, of five key emotions posits that there are five emotional areas, each resonating with an Element. The resonance table labels the main emotion, but that emotion is really part of a continuum that has various extremes. For example, joy is a natural and normal emotion. But here its use spans both a complete absence of joy or misery on the one hand to euphoria on the other. Both are extreme and usually 'inappropriate' expressions.

Another issue about emotion is the language patients use to express what they feel. Practitioners cannot necessarily trust the patient's own perception of their emotions because emotional language was not primarily designed to *describe* feelings. For example, many patients who are obviously anxious and fearful in temperament do not perceive themselves to be that way at all. Verbal descriptions have their use, but even novelists when attempting to convey emotions rely less on the language of emotions and more on context, thoughts and the telltale, non-verbal signs of emotions.

The first chapter on each Element discusses the emotions associated with each CF, and Chapter 26 outlines how practitioners can gain a deeper understanding of their patient's *non*-verbal expression of their emotions. The practitioner's ability to feel what the patient is feeling and build intimate rapport is essential if the practitioner is to identify the patient's more hidden emotions. Gaining insight into these emotions enables the practitioner to understand how their patients *really* feel rather than listening to a *description* of their feelings.

The emotions associated with an Element are not simple or uniform. This is especially so when the patient moves from a more expected or appropriate emotion to the expression of emotions that are more pathological. It is the inappropriateness of an emotion that is the main factor in deciding if it is pathological. Practitioners need to ask themselves questions about their patient's emotions, such as:

• Is the emotion too intense or too prolonged for the situation?

- Is the person inclined always to have the same emotional response to many different situations?
- Which emotions create particularly disharmonious movements of *qi*, resulting in changes in the voice, facial expression or body language?

It is the subjective judgement of the practitioner in answer to these kinds of questions that makes the diagnosis.

The secondary resonances

As well as the primary resonances there are also other diagnostic categories that are described as 'secondary' resonances in the following chapters. These resonances assist the practitioner to gain a better understanding of the Element and they can also support the primary resonances when making a CF diagnosis. When the practitioner is assessing the balance of an Element the secondary resonances can indicate dysfunction, but *not* whether the Element is the CF. They are considerably less reliable than the key resonances and provide supporting, as opposed to primary, evidence for the CF.

For example, Wind is the climatic resonance for the Wood Element. Wind is invisible, it comes and goes and it makes the branches of the trees shake and sway. Understanding the nature of Wind helps practitioners to understand the nature of the *qi* of Wood.

Wind can also affect people who have an imbalance in their Wood Element. Such people are often disturbed by wind, even when they are protected from it. They may say that it bothers them or even that they *hate* it and they may become irritable if exposed to wind. The frequency of this occurrence, however, is not consistent. A majority of Wood CFs do not report this symptom. On the other hand those patients who *do* report this phenomenon definitely have a Wood imbalance and may be Wood CFs.

Another example is speech, which comes from the tongue, the sense organ associated with the Fire Element. 'Speech' means many things, from the act of speaking to the desire to communicate. Most Fire CFs will have no appreciable abnormality in their speech. However, people who speak awkwardly, stutter or mix words up probably have some problem with their Fire Element and may be Fire CFs.

If the secondary resonance of an Element is present in a patient in an imbalanced form, then it points strongly to that Element being out of balance. The secondary resonances are presented in Table 7.2.

The difference between key and secondary resonances

From the practitioner's point of view there is a major difference between key and secondary resonances. Colour, sound, odour and emotion are all diagnosed through the perceptions of the practitioner. The secondary resonances predominantly depend on the descriptions of the patient. It is the practitioner's sensory perceptions that must form the basis of the diagnosis.

Table 7.2 Secondary resonances

	Wood	Fire	Earth	Metal	Water
Season	spring	summer	late summer	autumn/fall	winter
Stage of development or power	birth	maturity	harvest	decrease	storage
Climate	wind	heat	humidity, damp	dryness	cold
Sense organ or orifice	eyes, sight and tears	speech and tongue	mouth and taste	nose and smell	ears and hearing
Tissues and body parts	sinews and tendons	blood and blood vessels	muscles and flesh	skin and nose	bones, bone marrow and hair on the head
Generates	nails, from sinews	hair, from blood	fat, from flesh	body hair, from skin	teeth, from bone
Taste	sour	bitter	sweet	pungent	salty

The second chapter – the functions of the Organs

The second chapters discuss the functions of the Organs for each Element. In Chinese medicine the Organ functions are predominantly drawn from the classical texts. Five Element Constitutional Acupuncture places particular emphasis on the descriptions given in *Su Wen* Chapter 8.

With the exception of Fire, each Element has two Organs. For example, the Wood Element includes the Liver and Gall Bladder and the Earth Element, the Stomach and Spleen. The Fire Element has two 'true' Organs – the Heart and Small Intestine – and two functions – the Heart-Protector (also called the Pericardium) and Triple Burner. Note that the convention of capitalising an organ has been followed when referring to the Chinese understanding. The Organs are listed in Table 7.3.

The chapters that follow discuss the functions of the Organs in this order:

- the functions of the *yin* Organ
- the functions of the *yang* Organ
- the time of day when the Organs are most active
- a comparison of how the paired Organs relate.

Five Element Constitutional Acupuncturists discuss the functions of each Organ in relation to how it affects the patient's body, mind and spirit. For example, one function of the Lungs is 'receiving *qi* from the Heavens'. Five Element Constitutional Acupuncturists interpret this not only as a way of describing breathing but also as literally taking in *qi* from the spiritual domain of the Heavens. The spiritual aspect of the *yin* Organ (in the case of Metal, the *po*) is also discussed.

The functions of the *yang* Organs appear to be less important than the *yin* Organs in many classical texts. Five Element Constitutional Acupuncturists, however, regard them as equal to the *yin* Organs and also consider them to have an impact on the body, mind and spirit. Thus, for example, the Small Intestine's function of separating the pure from the impure has an important effect on the mind and spirit as well as on the body. This point of view is useful in that often one of the *yang* Organs turns out to be crucial in treatment and the belief that the *yin* Organs are always more important could stop a practitioner from noticing this.

The third chapter – the behaviour typical of each Constitutional Factor

Behavioural patterns

The main substance of the third of the three chapters on each Element concerns the behavioural patterns that are typical of each CF. These are, effectively, additional modern 'resonances' based on practitioners' observations of patients. These associations do not directly derive from the classical texts. They are largely descriptions of how imbalanced emotions drive people's behaviour. In some cases they are extensions of what is set out in the descriptions of the Organs or Officials in *Su Wen* Chapter 8.

Although diagnosis based on colour, sound, odour and emotion is paramount, understanding the motivation behind certain behaviour can also be an important resource when making a diagnosis and when monitoring progress. This method is described more fully in the section 'Golden Keys' in Chapter 27. Understanding people's underlying drives and needs can also enable the practitioner to gain deeper rapport with a patient. In order to describe these behaviours it is important to give some background about these areas and discuss the following questions:

- What is meant by behaviour?
- How does an imbalance in an Element manifest in behaviours that are part of a person's personality?
- What behaviours will manifest as a result of an Elemental imbalance?

Table 7.3 The *yin* and *yang* Organs					
	Wood	**Fire**	**Earth**	**Metal**	**Water**
Yin Organ	Liver	Heart and Pericardium	Spleen	Lung	Kidney
Yang Organ	Gall Bladder	Small Intestine and Triple Burner	Stomach	Large Intestine	Bladder

What is meant by behaviour?

In everyday life people often use the word 'behaviour'. When trying to define this word, however, difficulties can arise. In this context, behaviour is what the practitioner can observe from the outside. For example, the practitioner may discern that a patient is timid, withdrawn and unwilling to give opinions. Another patient may be over-assertive, forthcoming and more than willing to give opinions. Behaviour in this sense is something that a patient's own description may corroborate. A patient may say, for example, 'Oh I don't like to be forward' or 'I always say what I think'. In this sense the practitioner may be noticing both single instances of behaviour as well as behavioural patterns that are discovered partly by the patient's own descriptions. Practitioners will watch in the treatment room for specific examples of behaviour, but will often also use their patients' accounts of other events in order to determine whether what they observed is a *typical* behaviour for the patient.

In order to allow this to happen it is essential that practitioners discuss a much wider range of topics with patients than the traditional 'ten questions' about their physical health. Patients need to be drawn out about areas such as their family, work and childhood in order to discover how they interact with others and behave in difficult situations (see Chapter 25, this volume, for more on these areas of diagnosis). In the treatment room the practitioner needs to be acutely aware, to observe accurately and ideally hear the patient's confirmation of a pattern.

The patient's perception of themselves may, however, completely contradict the practitioner's perception. This is especially common if the person is in denial of certain aspects of their behaviour or if their behaviour puts them in 'a bad light'. Many people, for example, would not describe themselves as lacking in joy, being excessively needy for sympathy or irritable, but the practitioner may well experience them as being so.

Examples of behaviours that a practitioner might observe are the person:

- being a clown and cracking a lot of jokes
- being very organised or very disorganised
- being excessively attentive to others' needs
- being distanced and cut off from emotional involvement
- taking part in dangerous pursuits, but with very little awareness of the danger.

A patient's behaviour is to some extent contrasted with what goes on in their internal world. Similar behaviours can have a very different underlying cause. For example, two people may tend to withdraw in order to protect themselves, but they do it for different reasons. One may withdraw because an imbalance in the Heart or Heart-Protector makes her or him feel vulnerable. The other may withdraw because of the fragility of the Lungs and feelings of excessive sensitivity.

How does an imbalance in an Element manifest in behaviour?

When considering the link between a person's behaviour and their CF it is important to consider why the constitutional weakness of an Element should have such an impact on a person's behaviour. It was stated earlier in the chapter that an imbalance in the Element manifests in small but detectable differences in a person's emotional state (as well as colour, sound and odour).

This emotional imbalance will cause people to react to situations in very different ways and will shape how they react to events during different developmental phases in their lives. For example, from birth to first schooling, children are extremely dependent on their carers. Early separation from the mother will have a different impact on a Fire CF as opposed to a Wood CF. Later when people start school they leave the almost complete dependence on their parental carers and enter the world of teachers and social groups. A Metal CF will respond to bullying differently from an Earth CF. A person's CF and the balance of the other Elements will largely determine their response because the CF influences emotional responses, core values and beliefs. The general pattern is shown in Box 7.1, while Box 7.2 shows how this might be manifested in a Fire CF. Patterns of the sort shown in Boxes 7.1 and 7.2 are attributable to each CF and are described in the third chapter.

The effect of the impaired or unstable emotions attributable to a person's CF is combined with the effect of their environment. Fire CFs with a loving family will probably turn out to be more stable and healthy than those who were unwanted and had unloving parents. In either case, the CF will shape the nature of the person's internal world and influence many core values and fundamental beliefs. The core values and beliefs in turn help to create people's experience of the world.

Box 7.1

How behaviour manifests from the constitutional imbalance

Constitutional weakness of an Element

↓

Impairment or instability of the associated emotions

↓

A pattern of repeated emotional states

↓

Core values and beliefs develop, partly in response to these imbalanced states

Box 7.2

How behaviour manifests from the constitutional imbalance of a Fire CF

The Fire Element gives the capacity for receiving love and warmth with appropriate degrees of openness and closeness.

↓

An imbalance of the Fire Element leads to a predisposition to feelings of hurt, abandonment and not being loved. There is a strong tendency for Fire CFs to doubt that they are loveable. They have issues around their lovability to a degree that other CFs do not.

↓

These states become habitual. They alter perception and the need for love, warmth, happiness and closeness becomes greater.

↓

Beliefs are formed, such as 'I must be happy to be liked' or 'I feel better if I don't spend too much time alone'.

What behaviours will manifest as a result of an Elemental imbalance?

Two people both watching a woman talking loudly in public might describe her differently. They may dispute what she said or did and disagree, for example, about the words she used or whether she pounded her fist on the table. A video recording, however, could soon sort what was factually right or wrong.

This becomes more difficult, however, when describing what is important to her or her deeper motivations. The woman may be described as 'showing off', 'trying to get attention', 'hoping to gain some recognition' or 'throwing her weight around'. If two people disagree with this kind of description, a video will not help and they cannot use the speaker's inner experience as a reference point. They

may be persuaded by someone else to revise their description, but there is almost always room for doubt. We have no direct vocabulary to describe these events.

The process of the weakest Element appearing in observable behaviours is supported by recent scientific research. In Chapter 1 of Eckman (2007) there is a summary of research proving the universality of facial expression in revealing emotion. Also discussed (Ekman, 2007, Chapter 4) is what are called 'affect programmes', the programme whereby an emotion gets expressed in behaviour. For example, when angry more blood goes to a person's hands and the person is predisposed to move towards the object of the anger. When fearful more blood goes to the legs and the person is predisposed to move away from the threat. The concept of 'affect programmes' is such that some part of the programme is pre-set and part is the result of learning. So part will be universal, like the facial expression, and part will be learned.

By understanding the different Elements and their behavioural 'resonances' practitioners can begin to gain a deeper and more accurate understanding of the reasons for different people's behaviours. Rather than just speculating on the person's motivation, the behaviour can be put into context and the practitioner can begin to understand the underlying patterns from which the person's behaviour may have resulted. This understanding is learned by the practitioner and reinforced over a period of time. Table 7.4 gives the main behavioural patterns of each CF. These are described in greater detail in the third chapters on the behaviours of each Element.

Table 7.4 describes how the patient's behaviour arises from the constitutional imbalance. The imbalance of the Element leads to a person having certain emotional responses. This in turn leads to issues of great concern arising. These 'main issues' are the areas practitioners might discover if they ask themselves, 'what does this person seem to be most concerned about day in and day out?' Each CF responds to these concerns with certain behavioural responses. Although there is no one behaviour that will define every CF, the patterns of behaviour described are the natural options people are likely to take given their inner state.

These behaviours tend to exist along a continuum from one extreme to another. For example, Earth CFs, in response to their 'issues', tend to vary from being excessively dependent to overly independent. Water CFs tend to be either inclined to recklessness

Table 7.4 The behavioural patterns of each CF

	Wood	Fire	Earth	Metal	Water
A balanced Element gives a person the capacity to:	Be assertive and yield appropriately in order to grow and develop	Give and receive love with appropriate degrees of emotional closeness	Give and receive appropriate emotional support and nurturing	Feel loss and move on. To take in the richness of life in order to feel satisfied	Assess risks and know the appropriate degree of 'threat'
The extremes and balance of emotion when this capacity is impaired are:	Meekness – assertiveness – rage/irascibility	Misery – joy – euphoria	Rejecting caring from others – centred – needing care from others	Melancholic – satisfied – no grief/ inert	Terrified – safe – fearless
This leads to main issues of concern about:	Boundaries Power Being correct Growth Development	Happiness Emotional volatility Closeness and intimacy Love and warmth Clarity and confusion	Feeling supported Getting nourished Being centred and stable Mental clarity Being understood	Recognition Approval Feeling complete Feeling adequate in the world Finding meaning	Needing to be safe Being reassured Trusting Drive Excitation in danger
The spectrum of behavioural responses to these issues may be:	Assertive/direct – passive/indirect Seekingt justice – apathetic Rigid – over-flexible Excessively organised – disorganised Frustrated and defiant – over-obedient and compliant	Compulsively cheerful – miserable Open and overly sociable – closed and isolated Clowning – earnest Vulnerable – over-protected Volatile – flat	Smothering/ mothering – not supporting Feeling needy – repressing needs Excessive independence – dependency Uncentred and dispersed – heavy and stuck Over-dependent on the security of the home – inability to put down roots	Fragile – unyielding Cut-off – seeking connection Resigned or inert – over-working and achieving Craving quality and purity – messy and polluted Deeply moved – nonchalant	Risk-taking – fearing the worst/over-cautious Distrusting – trusting Intimidating – reassuring Driven – no drive Agitation – paralysis

or extreme caution. People do not necessarily only behave at one end of the spectrum or the other, however. Some Earth CFs can be very dependent in some situations and independent in others. Some Water CFs are reckless in some ways and cautious in others. The practitioner observes which of these aspects are not balanced or appropriate in the person.

It is also important to remember that all people have all five Elements within them and may exhibit some characteristics of any of the Elements. Elements other than the CF Element will almost certainly be imbalanced to some degree.

Often a person's behaviour patterns will manifest as a direct result of their CF. Sometimes, however, people's behaviour may appear to be driven by the issues of one Element whereas it is motivated by other drives and needs. For example, a person may be cut-off and detached (a trait often associated with Metal CFs) but the behaviour is actually driven by an attempt to hide their fear (resonant with the Water Element). Noticing these behavioural responses is therefore useful but does not replace colour, sound, emotion and odour as the primary diagnostic indicators of the Constitutional Factor.

The chapters on the typical behaviour patterns of the different CFs look at the issues that arise when that particular Element is the constitutional imbalance. These issues are linked to fundamental uncertainties and questions deep within the person's character. The responses to these issues are as varied as there are people, but the chapter outlines some of the more common ways they manifest. These descriptions are not definitive. As more practitioners gain experience with this style of treatment it is to be hoped that even more patterns of behaviour will become apparent.

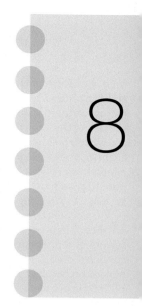

Wood – key resonances

Wood as a symbol

The character for Wood

The character for Wood is *mu*. This character represents a tree (see Weiger, 1965, lesson 119A). The vertical line is the backbone of the tree, the trunk and root. The line at the top represents the branches. The horizontal line is the earth, reminding us that much of the tree is below ground.

The Wood Element in life

The cycle of nature

The concept of Wood includes all forms of vegetation, from trees to flowers to grasses, but the tree is the archetypal representation. Consider an oak tree and its early manifestation, the acorn. In the autumn, leaves and acorns fall to the earth and some acorns become buried. During the winter the acorn, the seed, lies dormant in the ground. In response to the increasing *yang* of warmth and light in springtime, the acorn begins to sprout. It also requires moisture, sufficient soil and trace minerals in order to achieve its potential growth.

At this stage, the acorn has a plan within it. It is destined to be an oak or nothing at all. The young plant grows and encounters impediments such as rocks or nearby trees which frustrate it. It does not back off and consider giving up. It pushes upward but it is also prepared to change shape in order to maximise its growth. All the while it is forming itself, stage by stage, into an oak tree – the best, given the circumstances, that the acorn could have created.

Wood within a person

People also begin life with an internal map or plan as to their capabilities and direction. They strive to become

DOI: 10.1016/B978-0-7020-3175-5.00008-5

their own form of tree and they encounter obstacles and frustrations along the way. Depending upon the nature of their Wood, they may show flexibility in the face of these obstacles, thereby continuing to grow and develop. Alternatively they may have difficulty adapting and consequently become stuck. Like trees, people also require certain resources to fulfil their potential and they also require flexibility in order to adapt to changing circumstances.

For people the hindrances are often environments hostile to their growth. For example, a child with the talents of a mathematician may attend a school that supports drama and sports and has no committed maths teacher. Just as the oak requires resources, people require situations where their capabilities and directions are accepted, nourished and respected. Most of us know when we are not in the right environment, such as in the right school or doing the right work. Like the growing tree, our growth is frustrated and we need either to push harder or search out another context in which we are better able to thrive. The growing oak cannot pull up roots and transfer to a different field or meadow. Humans, however, frequently search out environments where the structures and resources available support their desire to grow and develop.

The manifestations of Wood

Although trees are the most obvious, any member of the plant world represents Wood. There are over 200 species of trees. Algae, lichens, moss, ferns, flowers and fungi all have a developmental cycle of growth in which maturity has a recognisable form at the end stage. Many plants (although not all) are green. They are usually rooted in the earth and respond to cyclical changes in the seasons. When acupuncture was developing, China was an agrarian society and doctors would have been well aware of the growth cycle of plants and what was required for them to flourish. Plant life provided many metaphors for early Chinese thinkers in their attempts to understand the human condition (Allan, 1997).

The Wood Element in relation to the other Elements

The Wood Element interacts with the other Elements through the *sheng* and *ke* cycles (see Chapter 2, this volume).

Wood is the mother of Fire

A fire needs fuel in order to burn well. In ancient times this fuel was usually the wood gathered from nearby forests. That Wood is the mother of Fire means that Fire symptoms, for example, heart pains, might be caused by one of the Organs of the Wood Element. When a symptom is manifesting from the Organ of one Element, it is always wise to look at the state of the *qi* of the previous Element. This is the 'mother' Element along the *sheng* cycle. An example of this is that Wood CFs can easily have heart problems arising from anger.

Water is the mother of Wood

Water is the 'mother' of Wood in the *sheng* cycle. It is easy to understand how Water can create Wood, as plants will not survive unless they are given enough moisture. Sometimes when patients manifest symptoms that appear to be connected to the Wood Element these are caused by imbalance in the Water Element, the mother. Treating the mother causes the symptoms to improve.

Wood controls Earth

Wood controls Earth across the *ke* cycle. If this relationship becomes dysfunctional it can easily create a wide range of symptoms. Physically there may be a tendency to digestive symptoms but it can as easily produce problems in patients' minds and spirits, especially in the relationship between their need for sympathy and their anger. For example, a patient may appear to be frustrated and angry but really be crying out for support and sympathy. Once the person feels supported the anger may lessen.

Metal controls Wood

The Metal Element controls the Wood Element. This is often described metaphorically with an example of a metal saw cutting down a tree. If a person's Metal Element becomes weak it can lose control of the Wood Element. The Wood Element in turn may become too strong and symptoms of fullness such as extreme anger and hostility may develop.

The key Wood resonances

The essential diagnostic resonances for Wood are a green colour, a shouting voice tone, a rancid odour and the emotion of anger. These are the key indications of a person's CF (Table 8.1).

The colour for Wood is green

The character for green

The character for green is *qing*. This character represents the hue of sprouting plants (see Weiger, 1965, lesson 79F).

The colour in nature

It is easy to understand why the colour resonating with the Wood Element is green as this is the colour seen in abundance in nature on the leaves of most plants and trees. Green especially resonates with spring, a time when green shoots emerge from the earth and green leaves appear on the barren branches of trees.

The facial colour

Green manifests on the face when the Wood organs are chronically out of balance. This colour is usually lateral to the eyes, under the eyes or around the mouth. There are many shades of green but the most frequent is a blue-green, a yellow-green or a bottle green.

As well as being the colour of Wood, a green colour is an indicator of *qi* stagnation, much of which occurs from the Liver's failure to ensure the smooth flow of *qi*. Green round the mouth is commonly seen when a person's Liver is temporarily struggling, for example, when a person is hung over. It is also common when a

woman has *qi* stagnation prior to menstruating. These are not indicators of the person's CF.

The sound for Wood is shouting

The character for shouting

The character for shouting is *hu* (see Weiger, 1965, lesson 72L).

A shouting voice

'Shout' is the sound resonating with the Wood Element. It is a sound naturally associated with anger, the emotion resonating with Wood. Anger makes the *qi* 'rise' and this upward movement of the *qi* gives the voice forcefulness.

A shout in the voice is an indication of assertion. The person who shouts wants to be heard and is often asking, explicitly or implicitly, for changes to be made. This voice tone frequently becomes louder at certain times, often at moments when the person is not really needing to be particularly assertive. Practitioners may feel that they are being talked at, rather then being talked to. There are also often moments when the practitioner and patient start talking at the same time and it is revealing to notice if the patient uses assertion and shouting in the voice to get their point in first.

As many people repress a great deal of anger, the voice often does not reflect their true degree of assertion. In this case the sound is therefore often clipped and abrupt. Two short experiments will give you an idea of this. For the first, say the words 'precisely inarticulate' with an abrupt emphasis on the 'cise' of 'precisely' and the 'tic' of 'inarticulate'. End the words abruptly. For the second, think of someone who makes you furious and imagine telling him or her exactly what you think. You should be hearing a similar emphasis or abruptness in your own voice.

Shouting in context

How does this sound connect with wholeness or imbalance? The shouting voice tone originates from varying degrees of frustration or anger. It expresses an assertion of the self. If the patient is expressing anger or assertion this sound is normal. Imbalance is indicated by the person's voice being clipped or forceful when it is not congruent with the emotion

Table 8.1 Key Wood resonances

Colour	Green
Sound	Shout
Emotion	Anger
Odour	Rancid

being expressed. It is also abnormal for a patient to be continually expressing anger for no good reason. A voice that is often shouting or clipped can be inappropriate based on the frequency with which the tone is present.

Lack of shouting

A different indication of imbalance is when there is a good reason for assertion in the voice and yet it is absent. This is called a 'lack of shout'. The *qi* fails to rise sufficiently. The sound seems to leave the person's mouth with insufficient power to travel across the room to the listener. It almost feels as though the practitioner needs to halve the distance from the patient in order to hear comfortably.

The odour for Wood is rancid

The character for rancid

The character for rancid is *sao*. This character is made up of two radicals (a radical is a recurring character used as a part of another character). The first, *jou*, represents flesh or pieces of dried meat gathered in a bundle. The second radical, *tsao*, represents birds singing in the trees. Together as *sao* these mean the odour of animals or urine (see Weiger, 1965, lesson 72A).

The odour resonating with Wood is rancid. In English, 'rancid' is applied to fat that is no longer fresh, for example, rancid butter. Rancid is also like the smell of new mown grass, but not so pleasant. Another description is 'slightly sour' like dried chives. The effect on the inside of the nose is somewhat prickling and makes people wrinkle their noses.

The emotion for Wood is anger

The character for anger

The character for anger is *nu* (see Weiger, 1965, lesson 67C). The character represents a female slave

under the hand of a master. The female would naturally feel angry, but in this case the anger would be held in. Rochat de la Vallée states that:

> One meaning of anger (*nu*) might be the effort made to raise something up from the earth's gravity. For example, the beginning of Chuang Tzu Chapter 1 has the description of a great fish in the ocean of the north, the northern abyss, which is the origin of life, the kidneys and so on. This great fish becomes a great bird. At the very moment of the passage from water to air the character for the effort of rising up, for the transformation from the swimming fish into a flying bird is *nu*. There is nothing pathological at this level. Here *nu* is not anger but the kind of violence proper to all beginnings.
>
> (Larre and Rochat de la Vallée, 1996, p. 64)

The importance of anger

Anger is often regarded as a 'negative' emotion owing to its sometimes painful and destructive consequences. It is a crucial emotion, however, found in all the higher primates. It is also the emotion required to initiate change. Anger makes the *qi* 'rise' (*shang*), a powerful expression of *yang*. Without these feelings there would be little or no growth, either personally or culturally.

For Wood CFs, however, anger lies at the heart of their suffering. Feelings of frustration, resentment, bitterness and rage are chronic and produce disharmonious movements of *qi*. Many Wood CFs find these feelings so painful that they do all they can to avoid experiencing them if possible. Keeping busy, withdrawing, being very physically active, using alcohol and drugs are some of the ways that people attempt to lessen the intensity of these feelings. 'God, I need a drink' seems to be the mantra of the person who resorts to alcohol to induce relaxation after the stresses of the day. Few people manage anger really effectively in their lives. As Aristotle wrote:

> It is easy to fly into a passion – anybody can do that – but to be angry with the right person to the right extent and at the right time and with the right object and in the right way – that is not easy, and it is not everybody who can do it.

The range of emotion for anger

Using a single term like 'anger' to represent the range of emotions resonant with Wood is convenient, but also misleading for two reasons. In the first place, anger is a key feeling, but it also covers a range of other connected feelings and some, at least to the outside observer, are subtly different from others. Secondly, Five Element Constitutional Acupuncturists assess emotions to determine balance or imbalance. Anger can be both appropriate and inappropriate depending on the context and the intensity of feeling. So it is necessary to consider the emotions of Wood in a wider context.

Frustration

Frustration is a key emotion for Wood (see Felt and Zmiewski, 1993, where, unlike almost all other English texts, they give 'discontent' as the emotion of Wood). Frustration (*cuozhegan*) describes a feeling of discontent arising from a person not achieving desires or expectations. Everybody feels frustrated at times and in each case this leads to a response and/or further emotion. There are three basic responses to frustration. One of these is a normal or appropriate response. The other two are pathological – the anger may escalate into rage or at the other extreme turn to apathy or depression. These three responses are discussed below.

A normal response to frustration

When a person initially experiences frustration, there are two normal responses that can take place. One is to produce a 'plan B', which is another way of getting what was wanted. To use a very simple example, a family have planned a picnic and at the vital moment it rains. They change plans and use a church hall where they can eat a packed lunch and play games with the children. They retain the picnic by having it indoors.

The second option is to reassess what was wanted. For example, with respect to the picnic, people may reassess what the picnic was intended to achieve. For instance, getting the children together with the grandparents, having a restful afternoon, observing how the prospective new nanny interacts with the children, etc. Flexibility is the key quality required.

In general flexibility involves people thinking of a 'plan B' or having the ability to do some re-planning based on the purpose behind it. People are still effectively striving to get what they want but the frustration is reduced and the mind and spirit are focused. These are signs of balanced Wood. As Bernard Shaw put it in *Man and Superman*,

> The reasonable man adapts himself to the world: the unreasonable man persists in trying to adapt the world to himself. Therefore all progress depends on the unreasonable man.

The pathology of anger – rage

One response to frustration is excess anger or rage. The Chinese, in keeping with Confucian views on the expression of intense emotions, tend to regard flying into 'a passion' as detrimental to the Wood Element. For example:

> Among the seven human emotions, only anger is of an intense nature. It dries up the blood and dissipates the *hun*. The person who understands the way of nourishing the Liver, therefore, never throws fits of anger.
>
> (Zhang Huang, quoted in Fruehauf, 1998, p. 4)

When the *qi* rises (*shang*) people struggle to contain its force. This may cause them to take a rigid, inflexible approach. People consumed with rage are no longer effectively striving to get what they want. The frustration has become excessive and the mind and spirit are no longer focused. Sun Tzu, author of *The Art of War*, was aware of this (Cleary, 1998, pp. 8 and 19). He recommended that one should cause the enemy's general to be angry, thus scattering his mind, making him unable to see clearly and therefore conceiving erratic plans. In the West we are just beginning to document the injury that can be caused by chronic anger. Goleman (2005, Chapter 11) deals especially with research on the adverse effects of various emotions, while a more prolific source is Martin (1997, pp. 195–196, 207–209 and 211–213). The following quotation is taken from Martin (1997):

> Hostility and anger consistently correlate with heart disease, poorer general health and increased mortality. This has been true in nearly every study in which they have been measured. A follow up study published in 1995 assessed the health of middle-aged women doctors who had graduated from the University of California School of Medicine at San Francisco in the 1960's. Women who had, in their initial assessment, been characterised as having low levels of hostility were in better health when middle-aged than their more hostile peers.

Resignation and apathy

The other pathway arising from frustration leads to resignation, apathy and depression. The original outcome, however important, is relinquished. The person exhibits little or no resourcefulness in overcoming the obstruction. The *qi* does not ascend and the person does not rise to the challenge of fulfilling their potential. When this becomes chronic, the *qi* in the Liver starts to stagnate. This can manifest as muscle tension and a range of other symptoms in the body. The mind and spirit are no longer focused on a clear outcome. The range of attitudes might be described as indifferent, apathetic, 'laid back' or blasé. 'I don't want any hassles' could be the person's motto. There are often tell-tale signs to help distinguish between a genuine benevolence (*ren*) and acceptance and the retreat from frustration into resignation. Genuine acceptance leaves the person's spirit and vitality undiminished, resignation leads to suppressed vitality and depression.

These two pathways are simply tendencies and both can manifest in the same person. People can feel resignation and rage at different times. Balanced Wood, however, usually manifests with the ability to express frustration, assert one's needs, consider alternative plans, go to higher ends, and not move too strongly towards rage or apathy. If either of the two paths becomes established as a long-term pattern, it is pathological. The two extremes were well summed up by Confucius.

> If you associate with those who are not centred in their actions, you will become too uninhibited or too inhibited. Those who are too uninhibited are too aggressive, while those who are too inhibited are too passive.
>
> (Cleary, 1998, Analects 13.21)

Both extremes provide evidence for the person's CF being Wood (Table 8.2).

The supporting Wood resonances

These resonances are considerably less important than the 'key' resonances given above. They can often be used to indicate that a person's Wood Element is imbalanced but they do not necessarily point to it being the person's CF (Table 8.3).

Table 8.2 Examples of the range of emotions associated with the Wood Element

Anger	Frustration, depression, resentment, irritation, bitterness, rage, wrath, ire, fury, outrage, crossness, indignation
Lack of anger	Unassertive, timid, meek, hesitant, depressed

Table 8.3 Supporting Wood resonances

Season	Spring
Power	Birth
Climate	Wind
Sense Organ/Orifice	Eye
Tissues and body parts	Ligaments and tendons
Generates	Nails
Taste	Sour

The season of Wood is spring

The character for spring

The character for spring is *chun* (see Weiger, 1965, lessons 79A, 47P and lesson 143A – sun). This character represents the germinating of plants by the effect of the sun.

Spring

After hibernation in the winter, the *yang* warmth of spring stimulates plants to grow and develop. The sap of the tree flows upward (just as anger makes the *qi* 'rise'; *Su Wen*, Chapter 39) and the green leaves emerge. Another year of growth begins. Many Wood CFs are very aware of the *qi* of spring. They resonate with and usually benefit from the increase of Wood *qi* in nature.

Claude Larre when speaking about the character for spring said:

> So spring is a time when life is sprouting . . . This is the way in Chinese characters to represent the condition of the universe when life is ready to come forth, to spring up and to sprout. There is tension in that movement as in a drawn bow.
>
> (Larre and Rochat de la Vallée, 1999, p. 12)

Elisabeth Rochat de la Vallée continues:

> The Liver is a manifestation of strength and the great and visible impulse of life, and in the natural world or in the universe this is the power of spring and of vegetation in the spring when flowers and herbs just spread out on the earth.
>
> (Larre and Rochat de la Vallée, 1999, p. 14)

The Wood Element creates the power that manifests in the *qi* of spring. It is the same *qi* that pushes the seedling upwards. It is the *qi* to give us a vision of our potential, to initiate growth and change and the determination to achieve that development.

For a practitioner to be outside in nature in the springtime and to feel the *qi* that is distinctive to that season is to directly experience the Wood Element. If the practitioner can understand how that expression of *qi* is manifested in a patient, then a diagnosis of the Element can be made.

The power of Wood is birth

The character for birth

The character for birth is *sheng* (see Weiger, 1965, lesson 79F). It corresponds with the season of spring in that plants are 'born' in the spring. The seedling pushes upwards from underground and begins its process of transformation from acorn to tree. The notion of birth resonates with spring, growth and development. For example, when we consider the qualities of a Wood CF, we may notice that they are likely either to be rather uncreative or, alternatively, rather innovative and creative. It requires upward rising *qi* to give birth to new projects, ideas and events. Some Wood CFs have this in abundance. It may be pathological but it certainly makes it relatively easy for them be creative and to initiate change. In others the upward rising *qi* has stagnated or has lost the force to initiate change and innovation.

The climate of Wood is wind

The character for wind

The character for wind is *feng* (see Weiger, 1965, lesson 21B). One part of this character represents a breath. Inside it is an insect. Insects have a hidden power to do damage, just like wind.

Wind

Wind by its nature is *yang* and dynamic. It 'induces an over-reaching in the rising and circulating movements which are those of the Liver' (Larre and Rochat de la Vallée, 1999, p. 101). So it is not surprising that Wood CFs often find strong wind uncomfortable. Many people become irritable when exposed to the wind and for some it provokes symptoms, such as a tightening of the neck muscles and headaches. Many Wood CFs feel affected by high winds even when they are inside and apparently protected. There is something about seeing the swaying of the tree tops and feeling the disturbance in the *qi* that often produces uneasiness and restlessness in people. On the other hand, some Wood CFs have a particular liking for the wind. They find it 'bracing' and experience feelings of exhilaration when it is windy.

Patient Example

A Wood CF patient who had been progressing well came in to report that three days previously he felt as if he had completely shut down. He said that he could no longer see any future and he had been sitting around, not knowing what to do. Wood resonates with eyes, vision, planning and having a future. The practitioner wondered why this ability to believe in and create a future had disappeared. Probing revealed that he had awakened the night before in this state. At the time there had been a tremendous storm blowing with high winds. The patient woke up frightened and afterwards had hardly slept. After the practitioner carried out treatment on his Liver, the patient said he felt back to normal.

The sense/orifice for Wood

The sense for Wood is the sight, the orifice is the eyes and the secretion is tears.

The character for eyes

The character for eyes is *mu* (see Weiger, 1965, lessons 158A and 26L). This character shows the human eyes with the socket, two eyelids and the pupil.

The eyes and sight

Eye problems are often traced to the Liver and Wood CFs will sometimes have diminished vision. The diminished vision may be mental, for example, the patient described above was unable to see where he was going in his life. The diminished vision may also be physical, for example, myopia, floaters, difficult night vision or vision that declines as the day progresses.

Five Element Constitutional Acupuncturists often observe a mental lack of vision in their Wood CF patients. The work of a general (the Liver is described as a general) is to plan and look ahead, to see the various options available and choose amongst them. This can manifest in a Wood CF's life in various ways. For example, some Wood CFs may fail to see opportunities, be unaware of the person in front of them or not have any vision about where they are going in life. At the other extreme some Wood CFs are very clear sighted and verge on almost being visionaries in some areas of their lives, but they may also lack vision or the ability to see ahead in other areas.

The judgement that someone cannot see in this way is usually the result of the practitioner making many observations. Culturally, we are loathe to make judgements about pathology in the context of a person's mental performance, but it is hard to practise this style of acupuncture well without a willingness to do so.

Tears

The secretion of Wood is tears. Crying can result from different emotions: for example, a person can have tears of grief, sadness or even of joy. However, tears can also be the overflow from held-in frustration. When a patient has frequent bouts of tears the practitioner might consider whether the reason is unexpressed anger.

Tissue and body parts for Wood – ligaments and tendons

The character for ligaments/tendons

The character for ligaments and tendons is *jin* (see Weiger, 1965, lessons 77B, 65A and 53A). Three radicals make up this character. Together they can be translated as elastic parts of the body that give a person strength.

The ligaments and tendons

Blood nourishes both the ligaments and tendons and when they are functioning well patients have a lack of clumsiness and adroit physical performance. It says in *Su Wen*,

> When the Blood nourishes the Liver, one can see. When Blood nourishes the feet, one can walk. When Blood nourishes the hands, they can grasp. When Blood nourishes the fingers, one can carry.
>
> (Ni, 1995, p. 43)

If the Wood Element is out of balance, the ligaments tend to be either too rigid or too flaccid and as a result become less functional. Movements are less precise and the joints may become sore and less stable. Many women suffer from problems with coordination and become clumsy if the Wood Element is imbalanced prior to menstruating.

The Liver 'stores the Blood'. When the Liver is functioning well, this means that when the body needs to move, the Liver can release Blood to move and nourish the ligaments, tendons and joints. Where the ligaments and tendons are tight and the Blood is slow in arriving, the movement of the body is less smooth. This lack of flow can often be observed from the way a person moves.

Dysfunction of the ligaments and tendons is not a good indicator of someone's CF, although it can indicate that the Wood Element is out of balance. It is noticeable, however, that the tendons on the feet of many Wood CFs are very prominent and rigid. Tightness in the musculature of the neck and upper back is also common.

Wood generates the nails

Nails are considered to generated from the sinews. Nails that are ridged, dry, soft, or brittle suggest that the Wood Element is imbalanced. The state of the nails is dependent upon the Liver's ability to store the Blood and the Blood's ability to nourish and moisten. Not all Wood CFs have nails that are of poor quality, but a person who does probably has a Liver imbalance even if she or he is not a Wood CF.

The taste for Wood is sour

The character for sour

The character for sour is *suan* (see Weiger, 1965, lessons 41G (*yu*) and 29E (*tsun*)). This represents a vase for keeping fermented liquids.

Sour

In Chinese herbal medicine the sour taste is astringent in action. Lemons, green apples, gooseberries and vinegar taste sour.

A strong liking or dislike of the sour taste is indicative of imbalance in the Wood Element, but will not necessarily indicate that a patient is a Wood CF.

Patient Example

A Wood CF patient who was Polish once said during the case history how much he loved borscht soup. This was not surprising. But later when asked if he liked vinegar, he beamed a smile and said, 'Of course, I put a full cup of vinegar in my bowl of borscht soup.'

Summary

1 Along the *sheng* cycle Wood is the mother of Fire and Water is the mother of Wood. Across the *ke* cycle Wood controls Earth and Metal controls Wood.

2 A diagnosis of a Wood CF is made primarily by observation of a green facial colour, a shouting or lack of shouting voice, a rancid odour and imbalance in the emotion of anger.

3 Wood CFs tend to easily have feelings of frustration.

4 Common emotional expressions arising from an imbalanced Wood Element are rage and excessive assertiveness, but so also are feelings of resignation and apathy.

5 Other resonances include the season of spring, the wind, the power of birth, the eyes, ligaments and tendons and the sour taste.

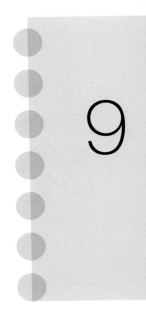

Wood – The Organs

Introduction

The two Organs resonating with Wood are the Liver, the *yin* Organ, and the Gall Bladder, the *yang* Organ. Although their functions are different, the two Organs exist close together and have some overlapping functions (Table 9.1).

The Liver – the planner

The character for the Liver

The character for the Liver is *gan*. This has the flesh radical on the left-hand side and a mortar and pestle on the right. The flesh radical means that the overall character refers to an organ or part of the body. The pestle indicates the power of a blunt instrument to grind and make changes to what lies in the bowl. The character is also interpreted as the stem of a plant and the manifest power of the plant to thrust upward (see Weiger, 1965, lessons 65A and 102A). We are reminded of the acorn's power to grow and develop into an oak.

Su Wen Chapter 8

Su Wen Chapter 8 says:

> The Liver holds the office of general of the armed forces. Assessment of circumstances and conception of plans stem from it.
>
> (Larre and Rochat de la Vallée, 1992b, p. 53)

As the commander of the armed forces, the general must be:

- aware of the ultimate goals, along with the outcomes relevant to any situation;
- strong and able to be forceful when necessary, like the emerging plant obstructed by a rock or at any time when new events are begun (birth);
- able to plan and devise strategies and to then create alternatives in the case of difficulties or an emergency.

A general has awareness of the ultimate goals

The awareness of ultimate goals is an important part of the planning process. All plans have intended outcomes, but ideally these outcomes themselves have

Table 9.1 The Wood Element Officials/Organs

Organ/ Official	Colloquial name	Description from *Su Wen* Ch 8
Liver	The Planner	The Liver holds the office of general of the armed forces. Assessment of circumstances and conception of plans stem from it
Gall Bladder	The Decision-Maker	The Gall Bladder is responsible for what is just and exact. Determination and decision stem from it

higher goals. For example, children like to play and enjoy themselves. Doing this develops motor and social skills. Developing these motor and social skills enables them to grow and develop into productive adults, and so on.

It is essential that people have these higher goals. A goal that cannot be negotiated becomes a burden and any frustration with respect to it is a dead end. In day-to-day life, people do not consider their higher goals very often. But the Liver holds in place a sense of these ultimate goals.

A general has strength and forcefulness when necessary

It is easy to make a connection between strength and the general. The archetype of a military commander is not a frail, spineless individual. This strength is the strength the seedling has when it is impeded by a stone or a competing tree. The seedling pushes through or, if that is impossible, it finds a way around the obstruction. In people this energy is focused and tied into the achievement of important goals.

A general is able to plan and establish strategies

People tend to think of planning as a mental and conscious process but it also exists as an unconscious process. For example, when menstrual blood is stored in the body and finally, on cue, begins to flow and be expelled, this is the end result of a highly organised plan. Planning which occurs in the mind is a more typical notion of planning. This may include, for example, thinking about what to do and how to do it and maybe also writing things down or even, like an architect, making drawings.

Planning is occurring all the time and on all levels of the body, mind and spirit. Indeed, we tend to notice the Liver's planning function more when it fails. For example, when the menstrual cycle becomes irregular, the mind becomes disorganised and unable to consider what needs to be done or the patient is waking at 2 a.m. and making plans that come to nothing during the day.

The Liver, therefore, allows us to meet the challenges of life with both vigour and flexibility.

The spirit of the Liver – the *hun*

All the *yin* Organs store a 'spirit'. The Liver houses the *hun*, which is usually translated as the 'Ethereal Soul'.

The character for the *hun*

The character for the *hun* has two parts (see Weiger, 1965, lessons 93A and 40C). One denotes clouds and the other shows a spirit or ghost. The character indicates the insubstantial nature of the *hun* and its ability to separate from the body. The spirit or ghost character is further broken down into a swirling movement and a head without a body (Maciocia, 2008, pp. 248–264, provides an excellent account of the spirit of both the Liver and the Lung).

The 'Ethereal Soul' is somewhat close to what people in the West call the soul. It is thought to enter the body shortly after birth and to survive death, leaving the body to return to wherever subtle *qi* or beings congregate.

The functions of the *hun*

The functions of the *hun* overlap with those of the Liver. As spirit, however, we are talking about a more refined level. Just as *qi* is more refined and subtler than *jing*, *shen* is more refined and subtler than *qi*. The mental functions affected by the *hun* are thinking, sleeping, consciousness and mental focus on the one hand and thinking and strategising with insight and wisdom on the other.

Thinking, sleeping and consciousness

The *hun* is said to be rooted within the Liver Blood. When the Liver Blood is not healthy, people can have a feeling of floating off when dropping off to sleep. They can also sleepwalk, have out-of-body experiences, experience 'astral travel' involuntarily and dream so that it is difficult to make a distinction between dreams and reality. The *hun* is easily upset by alcohol and drugs. When the Liver is relatively balanced, the *hun* remains rooted and people can distinguish reality from dreams. When the Liver is imbalanced, the symptoms arising can range from mild absent-mindedness to gross distortion of perceptions.

Patient Example

A Wood CF aged 32 mentioned in passing that he would wake up at night and find other people sitting in his bedroom. The first few times he was confused but he ended up getting to know them and having long conversations. He said he more or less knew that they were not 'real' people, but in their presence he responded as if they were visitors. For example, they had their own views, would express them and could argue their case. Over time, he had simply accepted that he could wake up and they would be there. His Liver Blood was deficient, allowing his *hun* to separate from his body.

Thinking, strategising with insight and wisdom

This function overlaps with what was said earlier about the Liver Official and planning. The 'general' not only functions on an everyday level by developing plans and working out how to achieve them, but also on a more spirit or psychic level. 'Insight' suggests that people's thinking is quick and the steps in their reasoning processes are enacted quickly. 'Wisdom' suggests that people's experience helps them to understand and have the ability to access and make sense of the patterns of events that occur in their lives. Like a football coach who has studied his players, the opposing teams and the wide variety of patterns that football presents, the *hun* can respond effectively to the key issues of life.

These issues are of varying degrees of importance and arise with varying degrees of frequency. They might be issues to do with whom a person should be friends, whether to choose a mate and which mate to choose, whether to follow a teacher, what subjects to study, whether to take a job, where to live and so on.

People with a well-rooted *hun* can make good decisions and plans, using their insight and wisdom. They can also accurately evaluate what the world might provide for them. Even more important, they match the choices they make to their long-term needs and capabilities. The challenge is for people to find paths that are appropriate to themselves and that allow them to fulfil their potential. If people fail to formulate such plans, frustration and disappointment are the likely consequences.

In a book edited by Thomas Cleary, subtitled 'A Course in Resourceful Thinking', there are many quotes from Chinese classics that are then commented upon by the editor. One of these says: 'Impulsive actions resulting in failure are faulty'. The commentary reminds us of the function of the *hun*.

> Successful endeavours are the result of strategic planning, adequate planning and appropriate timing. An arrow that is loosed before the bow is fully drawn will not likely reach the target; an arrow that is loosed before the aim is made certain will surely fly wide of the mark. When things go wrong, it is easy to blame other people or external conditions; but when failure is due to one's own impulsiveness, the responsibility belongs to oneself alone.
>
> (Cleary, 1996, p. 86)

We can assess the patient's *hun* with a simple question: 'To what degree is a person growing and developing towards his or her ultimate purpose or destiny?' This is often a difficult question to answer but it brings together many aspects or levels of the Liver. As the old joke goes 'Is life worth living?' 'It all depends on the Liver'.[1]

The Gall Bladder – the decision-maker

The character for the Gall Bladder

The character for the Gall Bladder is *dan* (see Weiger, 1965, lessons 1, 143B and 65A).

---

[1]A rare example of a pun that works in two languages. In French the answer is '*Question de foie*' (It depends on the liver) or '*Question de foi*' (It's a matter of faith).

Su Wen Chapter 8

The Official of the Gall Bladder has been described in various ways.

> The Gallbladder [sic] is responsible for what is just and exact. Determination and decision stem from it.
>
> (Larre and Rochat de la Vallée, 1999, p. 8)

or

> Official of wise judgement and decision making.
>
> (Felt and Zmiewski, 1993, p. 19)

The essential abilities of the Gall Bladder are discernment, judgement and decision making. As with the Liver, these functions are present in body, mind and spirit. These functions need to be understood on all levels of human functioning.

> There are choices in everything we do and it is through this Official that we are able to choose. . .Someone has to decide when to activate the blood clotting process, to release hormones, and to secrete bile. . .Every physical movement of our body is a collection of split-second decisions which keep us in balance and put our arms, legs and bodyweight in the right place.
>
> (Worsley, 1998, pp. 10–11)

The decision-maker works on behalf of the other Organs. In Su Wen Chapter 9 (Ni, 1995), it is said that the other Officials come to the Gall Bladder so that it can make decisions. The Chinese focus on how things interact, but this statement is remarkable. The other Officials cannot decide. Hence, the spontaneous choice when meeting someone on a narrow path to move to one side or the other, the decision to cross a busy street without a green light, deciding when to leave a party or when to write a letter of resignation are all in the domain of the Gall Bladder.

Patient Example

A patient once described throughout the case history a series of accidents for which he would give the exact location, time of day and date. After six such accounts, the practitioner wondered whether these were not 'accidents', but rather evidence for a lack of discernment and poor decision making. There is some dividing line between bad luck on one hand and bad judgement on the other. The patient was a teacher and his complaint, pain from a deep vein thrombosis, was brought on under conditions of both extreme anger and external wind. He taught history and would plan his lessons in great detail and then, at the last moment, teach from a different plan. He was a Wood CF.

Many of the functions of Gall Bladder points refer to regulation. When people are regulated they tend to take action that prevents them from going to extremes. The Gall Bladder regulates in a way similar to how the captain of a long ocean liner makes adjustments to his course well in advance. Gall Bladder points also have a similar effect and they often enable people to reach a more direct middle path leading them to a healthy balance. For example, the name of a Gall Bladder point, 'Sun and Moon', suggests by its name both extremes and the possibility of balance (see Chapter 43, this volume).

A common Gall Bladder pathology is extreme timidity, a definite lack of self-assertion and a lack of balance, regulation, and good decision making. As it says in Su Wen Chapter 8, 'determination' stems from the Gall Bladder and it is the absence of this forcefulness that is the same as the 'lack of anger' that is a crucial indication for some Wood CFs. In China the phrase ta ganzi da (meaning he has a big Gall Bladder) is used to describe someone who is courageous or successful.

The time of day for the Organs

Each of the Organs in Chinese medicine has a time when it is said to be at peak capacity. The time of day for the Gall Bladder is 11 p.m. to 1 a.m. and the time for the Liver is 1 a.m. to 3 a.m. It is very common for people whose Liver and/or Gall Bladder is under strain to wake in the early hours of the morning. They often report that they are quite wide awake and that their mind is very active at that time. This situation is often exacerbated by eating a heavy meal late in the evening or by drinking alcohol, as both of these activities strain the Liver. People who take recreational drugs often stay awake until the peak time for the Liver has passed. If people suffer from insomnia at this time of night they can often get back to sleep again much more quickly if they do something, like counting sheep or following their breathing. This stops their mind from planning and organising, an activity that often stimulates the Liver activity even further.

At the other end of the day, the Liver is at its weakest in the early afternoon. Some people feel especially tired at this time if their Liver is weak. Many feel a dip in spirits. This is often exacerbated by eating a big lunch, especially if the food is heavy or greasy. The difference in people's reaction to alcohol consumption at lunchtime compared to the evening is often very marked. Drinking alcohol when the Liver is at its weakest usually affects the person far more than if they drink later in the day.

How the Liver and Gall Bladder relate

The Liver plans and the Gall Bladder decides. It is said:

> The Liver analyses or assesses circumstances and decides the plan of action. The Gall Bladder being a *Yang* aspect of the Liver will have the firmness to make a clean decision and force through the situation so that the decision can be carried out, spreading the orders of the general far and wide.
>
> (Larre and Rochat de la Vallée, 1992b, pp. 71–72)

These functions are similar but different. The general has vision and can make appropriate plans, but plans without enactment are useless. Plans can include 'what ifs'. For example in a war, a general may look at many strategies. He may think about the opposing general's plans. He will consider the difference between sending his troops directly through a pass or making them wait on the sides of the hills. In the moment of battle, the general must decide the actual tactics to be used. His previously thought-through plans are the basis of what he does, but his judgements are made in the here and now.

Other decisions, like how many soldiers he should send, the effect of the weather and how much food to carry are also crucial. Hence there is a strong connection between these two Officials.

In practice, working with Wood CFs refines the Five Element practitioner's awareness of how plans and decisions interact. Because the Organs are paired and often treated together, it is rare for the practitioner to get a clear demonstration of the function of either Official on its own.

Summary

1 *Su Wen* Chapter 8 describes the Liver as 'The Liver holds the office of general of the armed forces. Assessment of circumstances and conception of plans stem from it'.

2 The *hun* is the spirit of the Liver and is responsible for aspects of:
   • thinking
   • sleeping
   • consciousness
   • planning with insight and wisdom

3 *Su Wen* Chapter 8 describes the Gall Bladder as 'responsible for what is just and exact. Determination and decision stem from it.'

4 The time of day associated with the Gall Bladder is 11 p.m. to 1 a.m. and the time for the Liver is 1 a.m. to 3 a.m.

Patterns of behaviour of Wood Constitutional Factors

CHAPTER CONTENTS

Introduction

This chapter endeavours to answer the question 'What is a Wood CF's behaviour like?' or 'How would I recognise a Wood CF?' It describes some of the most important behavioural characteristics that are typical of Wood CFs. Behaviour can be an indicator of a patient's diagnosis but in the end it can only be used to confirm the CF. It should always be used in conjunction with colour, sound, emotion and odour, which are the four primary methods of diagnosis. Once the CF is confirmed the patterns of behaviour may, however, support the practitioner's diagnosis.

The origin of the behaviours was described earlier in Chapter 7. The imbalance of the Element of the CF creates instability or impairment of the associated emotion. Thus specific emotional experiences are more likely to occur to one CF as opposed to another. The behavioural traits described in this chapter are often the responses to these negative experiences. In the case of Wood the person experiences feelings of frustration and she or he is responding to this.

Patterns of behaviour of a Wood CF

The balanced Element

The healthy Wood Element enables people to have a clear vision of their own unique path in life as well as the patience to allow it to unfold. This is a natural process which allows people to realise their potential. All growth has periods of activity followed by rest periods. People with a healthy Wood Element can judge when not to move forward as well as when the time is right for change to occur. They know that there is no need to push or force change or to try impatiently to speed things up.

In order to grow and develop, a person both consciously and unconsciously makes plans and decisions. The Wood Element allows people to consider their various options as well as to 'think through' the outcomes that are likely to occur from instigating plans. They will then fine-tune the plan so that it suits their own needs and the needs of other people who are involved. Some plans, especially short-term plans, can take only seconds to think through. More long-term plans may take longer.

In the event of a plan not coming to fruition, a person with a healthy Wood Element can reflect on what has gone wrong and if necessary initiate an alternative plan. How people assert themselves and make plans and decisions is 'patterned in' at an early age.

DOI: 10.1016/B978-0-7020-3175-5.00014-1

Formative events for a Wood CF

In the same way as the first shoots sprout from an acorn, babies start to change and develop as soon as they are born. They reach out and they explore. They recognise their mother and father and they cling to their favourite objects. Young children are renowned for stating what they want but inevitably it is not possible for them to have everything. Families deal with this by having rules and structures. These include who owns toys, where to sit, who gets second helpings, when to go to bed, how siblings are treated and almost everything of importance to a child. Some behaviours are rewarded and some are punished. There may be fights and negotiation over the rules, but no one ever doubts that we operate in contexts where rules exist.

When parents enforce these rules it ensures that children learn where their boundaries are. In consequence children discover both how to assert and move forward to get what they want and how and when to yield to a situation when this is not possible. Wood CFs frequently have difficulty dealing with the frustrations that occur when they are obstructed in getting what they want. This affects their growth and development as human beings. On the other hand in a world of few rules and boundaries they may find it hard to learn to be effective and to carry their plans through to fruition.

Although it is likely that people are born with their CF, many of their experiences, especially childhood emotional ones, tend to reinforce the imbalance. Wood CFs have less ability than others to make healthy plans and decisions. They may also be unable to recognise their inner goals. As a result many Wood CFs experience that their attempts to get what they want are thwarted.

People with other CFs often have fewer difficulties dealing with these issues. Their relatively healthy Livers and Gall Bladders allow them to make good plans and decisions. This enables them to adjust well to the frustrations of life. Their anger is less dysfunctional and they experience less of a struggle when they are obstructed.

The main issues for a Wood CF

For the Wood CF certain needs remain unmet. This situation creates issues that centre on these areas:

* boundaries
* power

* being correct
* personal growth
* development.

The extent to which someone is affected in these areas varies according to the person's physical, mental and spiritual health. Relatively healthy Wood CFs have less disturbance with these aspects of life, whilst those with greater problems end up with their personalities being more strongly influenced. Because of these issues they may consciously or unconsciously ask themselves various questions such as:

* Why can't I have what I want?
* Why do I not have the power?
* Why can I organise some things and not others?
* Why have I been blocked or stopped in this way?
* What do I really want?

Responses to the issues

So far we have described how a weakness in the Wood Element may lead to a lesser capacity to be assertive and yield appropriately. This hinders growth and development. The issues that subsequently arise lead to a spectrum of typical ways of responding to the world. These issues affect all Wood CFs, but are not exclusive to them. If other CFs have similar patterns of behaviour it may indicate that there is a different set of issues underlying them or that their Wood Element is imbalanced but is not the CF. Noticing these responses is therefore useful but does not replace colour, sound, emotion and odour as the principal way of diagnosing the Constitutional Factor.

The behavioural patterns of a Wood CF are along a spectrum and can go between various extremes:

1	assertive and direct	——————	passive and indirect
2	seeking justice	——————	apathetic
3	rigid	——————	over-flexible
4	excessively organised	——————	disorganised
5	frustrated and defiant	——————	over-obedient and compliant

Assertive and direct – passive and indirect

When the Wood Element is imbalanced a person's ability to grow and develop is affected. Wood CFs may either be continually asserting themselves and generating change or at the other extreme be passive and failing to create change. Sometimes a Wood CF may be overly assertive but fundamentally ineffective because of an inability to maintain a steady, focused purpose.

All people are driven to initiate change at some times but this drive is usually balanced by contentment with the status quo. This balance indicates a healthy Wood Element.

Forceful behaviour

Wood CFs are often aware that they can be very forceful people. How they use this force depends on the role they are in. If they are in a leadership role they tend to feel comfortable and often use their power in a positive and benevolent way. For example, a Wood CF who had trained in coaching skills would help people whenever she could. She said, 'People have come to me and I've stepped in and helped them. I can give them a vision then show them how to back it up. I know it's possible as my strength helps me to facilitate change and so I can impart that ability to others'.

It is often difficult for Wood CFs to be in a situation where they feel constrained. In this case one of the first things they do is check out, 'what are the rules, structures and boundaries?' and 'who holds the power?' This lets them know who tells them what to do, who can judge them and therefore who affects their welfare. This information is especially important when Wood CFs are in situations where they are not in control. Many find it easier to be the teacher than the student, the employer than the employee. The subtle boundaries defined by the practitioner in the treatment situation may also be challenged.

Sometimes being with strong Wood CFs can be a continual fight, especially if they are excessively forceful people. They may be so assertive and sure of themselves that they lose patience with others, finding it difficult to understand those who are not as assertive, organised or quick to react as they are. They do not 'suffer fools gladly'.

Generating change

Adventurousness is a positive aspect of this drive. The progress of the human race over the millennia has been driven by this expansive, innovative and assertive energy. In some Wood CFs it may take the form of having the vision and creativity to initiate change in all manner of stuck situations.

Many Wood CFs naturally assert themselves to generate change and find it hard to stop themselves continually pushing for something new to happen. Working practices, accepted methods of doing particular tasks, observing social niceties, the conventions that most people normally abide by, are all under 'threat' from the Wood CF's drive and assertion. This restless drive is, of course, largely unconscious. Once the person is thwarted, painful feelings may arise that thrust the issue into awareness.

The frustration of no change

People who have this tendency are, however, destined to struggle with feelings of frustration and exasperation. It is often not possible for a situation to be transformed in the ways they desire. A situation may be at a standstill because it is not yet the time for progress or it may be in conflict with the desires of other people. Some situations, for example, politically or in institutions, are not within the person's power to change. Everything changes at some stage, but not necessarily when or how a person wants. Unless a person can truly accept this, frustration or feelings of resignation follow. Dissatisfaction with the limitations of life in general, and the person's life in particular, can become chronic. In this situation the Wood CF may start blaming and complaining. Sometimes this behaviour becomes entrenched and may become a major component of the person's conversation. Contentment is elusive.

This chronic frustration may reveal itself in the issues patients choose to bring up with their practitioners. They may grumble about world events, their job, boss, partner, children or friends. They express their frustration with less inhibition if they feel that they occupy the moral high ground over an issue or conflict. This allows them to express their frustration with less inhibition than when they doubt whether their anger is justified or appropriate.

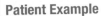
> ### Patient Example
>
> Some Wood CFs may be seen by other people as strong and powerful but feel insecure and weak in themselves. They have a lack of connection with their own inner strength. One Wood CF was surprised that she was perceived as angry and domineering by others. When told this she replied in a clear and loud voice, 'But you don't understand. I am not angry. I just want to get my point across clearly.'

In some cases the person suffers the constant pain of bitterness, resentment, depression and hopelessness. With no vision or plan of how to bring about changes in situations their *hun* becomes clouded and the *qi* of the Wood Element no longer flows harmoniously.

Indirectness, passivity, passive aggression

Everybody has had occasions when they were angry, but took care not to express it. Many Wood CFs continually do this. They may be cautious not to expose their anger, but feel frustrated and angry inside. They may not be aware that they are angry, only that they feel depressed, guilty, upset or tearful. Alternatively they may know that they feel angry but present as charming and pleasant, choosing to deal with a situation of conflict indirectly.

Indirectness

Some Wood CFs who are indirect are unable to ask for what they want and will hint or scheme instead. This does not reveal their true desires. This pattern usually starts in early life. For example, a child feels hungry and goes to the biscuit jar. The mother shouts 'no' and the child backs off. The child was being direct but this strategy has not worked. Because the desire is still there, the child decides to steal a biscuit instead. The child has learnt to become indirect in order to get what she or he wants.

Being indirect can take many forms. For instance, people may be extremely pleasant on the surface. If they become angry they may feel unable to express it. Consequently they may continue to be nice on the surface but make snide comments and talk behind the other person's back. Alternatively a person may decide to get their point across through other people. They might suggest that their friends or colleagues confront a person they are angry with but do not feel able to say anything to the person themselves. This can cause problems in a group situation with the Wood CF stirring others up to rebel but appearing to have nothing to do with the situation.

> ### Patient Example
>
> A Wood CF was going through a difficult time in her marriage but was unable to move forward. She had an especially hard time in the springtime and told her practitioner that she hated the springtime 'because the world is changing and I'm not'.

Depression

People who have not expressed their anger over a period of time usually become somewhat depressed. The anger has imploded and is stuck inside and consequently the person's life seems hopeless and without purpose. They may have no awareness of feeling angry. It may seem too hard to change and they repress any strong desires so that they can't feel frustrated by their lack of satisfaction. In this situation the anger has turned to passivity and they feel depressed, frustrated, uncreative and become resigned to never getting what they want.

Often Wood CFs who are trapped in this kind of depression feel better for physical activity. This is because the stagnant *qi* temporarily moves when they are active. Some Wood CFs find that if they exercise regularly they can stave off the depression for a period of time. If they stop being active, however, they relapse back into the depression because the underlying cause of the problem, which lies in the stagnation of the Liver and Gall Bladder, has not been dealt with.

> ### Patient Example
>
> A Wood CF described to his practitioner that in his teens he had so many rows that he 'decided' that his anger 'did not work'. He decided to allow himself to only be angry with himself and never with others. He managed to do this and ended up at a young age as a manager of a warehouse. Whatever his employees did, he would never get angry with them. However, he developed a problem with his neck and shoulders and was in constant pain. After having treatment he realised that his neck and shoulder pain eased when he expressed his anger and over the course of treatment learnt to assert himself in a more balanced way.

Sometimes Wood CFs swing between two extremes – they may push and assert themselves but if they think their efforts are being frustrated or a different idea is put forward they may decide to stubbornly resist it. In this case they may blame others for not letting the changes they wanted to occur happen. The middle way on this issue is best described by Lao Tse. While describing the 'sensible man', he says that 'He has his yes, he has his no' (translation from Bynner, 1962, Chapter 12).

Patient Example

Many Wood CFs say that they are passionate about trees and gardens and they feel that it is when they commune with that aspect of nature that they can grow and change. Often they find it difficult to meditate or relax but they gain their spiritual solace from the outside world. Some Wood CFs feel deeply moved by the greenness of nature in very simple situations. One Wood CF told her practitioner, 'When life was tough I used to say "let's head off for the trees". I'd seek out the biggest tree I could find and sit under it. The roots would ground me and the leaves would filter all my anger and frustration and it would dissipate those powerful feelings.'

Seeking justice – apathy

Dealing with injustice

Another trait of assertive Wood CFs is that they are often the first to act if they see an injustice taking place. Their sense of fairness is very strong and it is fuelled by a strong need to make change happen. Even if they find it difficult to assert themselves in relation to their own needs, it is often easy for them to fight for the rights of others and the chance to make the world a better place. Unconsciously or consciously their values might be those expressed by Henry Ward Beecher, the nineteenth-century preacher: 'A man that does not know how to be angry does not know how to be good. Now and then a man should be shaken to the core with indignation over things evil' (from *Proverbs from the Plymouth Pulpit*, 1887).

Historically, many important reforms have been brought about by Wood CFs who were fighting for justice for humanity. We can speculate that many of the people involved in reform movements such as the civil rights movement, for example, Martin Luther King, the early Trade Union Movement and also in the anti-apartheid movement in South Africa were Wood CFs. Change comes about by challenging authority and many Wood CFs feel compelled to make that challenge. This doesn't mean that all activists are Wood CFs. People of all CFs have seen the importance of making improvements in people's lives but Wood CFs are often at the forefront of these philanthropic organisations and movements and are willing to put their time and effort into the 'battle' for justice.

Fighting for justice is often acted out by lobbying politicians, by protesting at marches or by giving speeches at rallies and meetings. In the 1960s the protest song emerged with Bob Dylan and others singing songs such as *Masters of War, The Times They Are A-Changin'* and *Blowin' in the Wind*. Wood CFs have always found innovative and interesting ways to fight against injustice. Currently the internet has made protesting more global and there are many internet sites which reflect people's anger and righteous indignation in the movement towards justice.

Issues to fight for

In recent years different issues such as 'ban the bomb', women's rights, animal rights, gender issues or environmental issues have been important. Although the issues have changed, the Wood *qi* that has been channelled into them is the same.

Not all Wood CFs join groups in order to fight for justice. Many quietly get on with seeking justice for the sick, needy or the oppressed by direct contact. They may visit people in hospitals or prisons, and support those they see as downtrodden, oppressed or suffering from injustice in other ways. Others are busy with other enterprises but are nonetheless moved to jump in whenever they see something unfair. They may stand up to a boss, become active in their trade union, or stand up for a family member if there is a whiff of unjust treatment. Whatever the issue, whenever there is a large-scale fight for justice taking place, a Wood CF is likely to be involved.

Sometimes a Wood CF who is fighting for justice can be mistaken for an Earth CF who has the desire to give support to others. Both may have similar external behaviour but the motivation will be different for each.

Patient Example

A Wood CF came into treatment feeling very angry. She lived in a shared house and one of the men was not pulling his weight. 'We've now got someone else staying and this new person is doing all of the washing up and cleaning and my flatmate is sitting back letting her do it. When I see him leaving all of his rubbish in the house I get really angry because of the unfairness of it. It's not something that's really affecting me personally but when I see her doing his work I get upset. I know I'll have to challenge him. I can't let him get away with it.'

Apathy

At the opposite extreme, some Wood CFs find it almost impossible to stand up for themselves or others. Politically active people often despair and fail to understand why others seem so apathetic about causes that seem to them to be of self-evident importance and rightness. Whereas some Wood CFs have clear opinions and think they are right, others struggle to find any certainties in their life. Even when they think they know their views on an issue, they rapidly start to doubt them when confronted by an opposing opinion. The philosophy 'Better to live a day as a tiger than a lifetime as a sheep' expressed by Tippo Sahib, the warrior ruler of Mysore, is definitely not theirs. Their 'anything for a quiet life' mentality means that they become a pushover for anybody more determined, self-righteous or assertive.

This attitude inevitably leads to the mentality of the 'yes man' or 'yes woman', people who shirk conflict for fear of the painful feelings it produces in them. Their reluctance to stand up and be counted may be confused with fear or vulnerability, but in the case of Wood CFs it is predominantly because of their inability or reluctance to strongly assert themselves in the world.

Other Wood CFs can appear apathetic because their *hun* may be unable to envisage a viable strategy to initiate growth. Alternatively their *hun* may have a vision and a sense of purpose, but they lack the determination or ability to be flexible to bring about change for themselves or others. At the extreme they seem to look for a rut and make themselves at home in it. In the language of the *I Ching*, they find it easier to be receptive (*yin*) than creative (*yang*). Contentment can be less difficult for these Wood CFs but their lives may lack dynamism. Boredom, apathy and a life lacking in richness can be the result.

Rigid – over-flexible

Lao Tse wrote, 'Yield and you need not break' (Bynner, 1962, Chapter 22). A tree must bend when challenged by a wind stronger than itself. A tree that is dry and brittle will be rigid and can easily break in stormy, windy weather. In a similar way people need to remain flexible and supple when faced with life's storms and yet they also need to be firm. A tree that is at the mercy of every wind that blows will struggle to have enough resilience to grow to its potential. Similarly people who are too flexible will lack the structure and boundaries needed to grow and develop to fulfil themselves.

Patient Example

A Wood CF found it difficult when others were late. If people turned up late she would be rude and start to dislike them. She fell out with a friend who was meant to arrive at 9.00 a.m. and through no fault of her own arrived 4 hours late. The friend had even rung ahead to apologise. She was, however, working to become more flexible and said. 'In a situation when I'm hitting up against the wall I'll remind myself that there are many other ways of getting what I want. If I'm flexible I'll feel better in my body. I have to remind myself that flexibility is an option.'

Rigidity

Physical rigidity can most easily be diagnosed by examining the muscles, tendons and ligaments for tension. Wood CFs may develop stiff necks, tight shoulders, sore lower backs and/or hips and they may also have tight ligaments in their feet. They often find it difficult to relax physically. Sometimes tics or tremors may develop. The effect on the Organs is often more serious but this is less easy to perceive from a surface examination.

Rigidity of the mind and spirit

The effect of excess rigidity can more easily be recognised at the level of the mind and spirit. It affects a person's behaviour, attitudes and values. For example, the world of some Wood CFs is very black and white. They can be oblivious to many nuances of colouring in situations. Their internal rigidity means that they are unbending in their opinions about right or wrong or how other people should behave. They may be convinced that they are right. This can make some of their relationships difficult and they tend to 'take up a position' about something rather than look for common ground or compromise. Wood CFs can be so convinced about the rightness of their position that it may be a challenge for them to be tolerant of others. Often they are as hard on themselves as they are on others when they feel that they have not lived up to their own expectations of themselves.

They may also have a marked tendency to be excessively rigid in relation to matters of detail, especially in regard to time. Punctuality is often regarded as being of extreme importance. Wood CFs commonly become irritable if others are late for a meeting. The fear of not being on time themselves can also be a significant source of anxiety. They can also be often very precise in remembering dates and times of events. This tendency towards attention to detail can also show in other ways, such as coming to the initial consultation with a detailed list of all their medication and health history. As the Liver is responsible for planning and organising, precision and orderliness becomes a way of keeping the chaos of day-to-day life relatively under control.

If people are excessively rigid their spirits can become limited and impoverished. For example, if their life does not go according to plan, some Wood CFs find it difficult to reconsider and adapt their plans to the reality of the situation. This can also be a problem when Wood CFs grow old. There comes a time when it is appropriate and necessary to come to a gracious acceptance of the limitations of the mind and body. Many Wood CFs stubbornly continue behaving as though they are still young and consequently become depressed, frustrated and rage against their diminished capacity. It is not that they should become old before their time, rather that they have the flexibility to adjust their expectations where necessary. Rigid planning is particularly evident in the elderly but can often be seen in younger people whose need for planning has become excessive.

Rigidity affects many people's relationships. For example, marriages and long-term relationships can be diminished by the rigidity of one or more of the partners. Inflexibility on the part of parents towards their children can also have a detrimental effect and lead to conflict and estrangement. Asking patients about their relationships with work colleagues or family members often reveals the rigidity of a person's spirit.

Over-flexible

At the opposite end of the spectrum a person may be over-flexible. Physically this can take the form of flaccid musculature, loose tendons and ligaments and hyper-mobile joints.

At the level of the mind and spirit this resonates with the concept of 'lack of anger' or unassertive behaviour. In this case people can find themselves unable to stand their ground. When in a group, these Wood CFs may go along with what anybody else suggests rather than stick up for their preference. Very often they don't even have a preference. In a marriage they may prefer to concede to their spouse or children. They may not have the determination to stand up for themselves if they imagine that there will be a conflict and they may have sensitive antennae for any possible conflict that may arise.

Flexibility of this kind is often initially attractive as the Wood CF usually gives way to the demands of other people. There are drawbacks, however. The over-pliable nature of their behaviour means that they often fail to assert their personality. This means that they often seem bland and as a result relating to them can be curiously unsatisfying.

Passive aggression

In time the person may adopt passive aggressive behaviour in an attempt to avoid having to go along with other people's wishes. On the surface they appear to be flexible and compliant. Inside, however, they may be rigidly digging their heels in so that nothing changes. Passive aggression may cause them to become devious, agreeing to the person's face but secretly following a different course of action.

Over-organised – disorganised

Making long-term and short-term plans

If the Wood Element is healthy the Liver can make plans and the Gall Bladder can make decisions. A person can effectively organise and structure their life on a daily basis as well as being able to create a larger overview or 'life plan'. Daily plans may involve deciding what to eat, what to wear, when to sleep, when to exercise or how to set about many of life's daily tasks such as shopping, travelling or relaxing. Organising and structuring are activities that are carried out with relative ease by most people and generally go unnoticed.

A larger overview is more concerned about the direction of a person's life. It will involves issues such as what relationships to have, whether to have children or what career options to pursue.

On-going daily plans should fit in a person's overall life plan. For example, if a person decides that they want to change career they need to take small steps in order to set this in motion. This may involve finding out more about potential careers, deciding if they are really making the right choice, discovering how to re-train and if necessary going back to college and getting further qualifications. There may be many other steps to take, but the larger life plan of changing career cannot be fulfilled without the smaller plans being put into effect.

Of course, not all plans come to fruition. If the Wood Element is reasonably healthy and a plan does not work out, a person has the flexibility to move on to another option.

The need for structure

For some Wood CFs organisation can be more problematic. Their weakened Liver causes them to have less sense of an underlying pattern or structure in their lives and less ability to make plans. Their Gall Bladder is unable to make sound judgements, make appropriate decisions or give them the determination to initiate change. Wood CFs may compensate by spending time creating structures and over-planning in the hope that this will make up for their lack and cover all eventualities.

Alternatively they feel chaotic and unable to organise themselves. In this case if a plan doesn't work out they may feel they have no other options and become frustrated and confused. Many Wood CFs alternate between these two states.

Over-planning

If a Wood CF over-plans this may manifest in a number of different ways. For example, Wood CFs who tend to be over-assertive may try to control their environment by managing and structuring whatever and whoever is around them. This means that many Wood CFs become brilliant organisers as they devote time to producing rules, structures and boundaries for others to follow.

Many of this type of Wood CF can be found in administrative and managerial roles and they can become good leaders. A Wood CF who is a good organiser knows that a well-structured organisation

appears to run itself. It runs smoothly and efficiently in the same way that Liver *qi* should flow smoothly without causing any stagnation. When an organisation is badly run it will lurch from crisis to crisis. In this case there is usually a poor internal structure keeping it together. Being in a situation that lacks structure can be very unsettling for many Wood CFs who like to follow 'the rules' and have things carried out 'by the book'. They may become insecure, frustrated and angry in these situations and try to eliminate the chaos.

In a work situation it can be especially onerous if the boss is not running a tight organisation. The Wood CF may then jump in and try to organise the boss – usually creating friction and more frustration. Alternatively they may become resigned and depressed by the boss's lack of responsiveness. All people have their own different individual requirements for structure and some people need less than others. A lack of structure in others may be hard for some Wood CFs to tolerate. A Wood CF mother whose child is disorganised, a teacher whose pupils will not hand in their work on time or a disorganised work colleague can create much frustration and resentment.

Patient Example

A Wood CF described to her practitioner how she would go to bed (usually around 11 p.m.) and be unable to get to sleep at night. Instead she lay awake planning and scheming and generally thinking about everything she wanted to accomplish. She would finally go to sleep around 3 a.m. The practitioner pointed out to her that the horary time (see Chapter 9, this volume) for the Gall Bladder was between 11 p.m. and 1 a.m. and for the Liver was 1 a.m. to 3 a.m. It was at these times that the Liver and Gall Bladder were receiving a surge in *qi*, thus making her mind more active. On the suggestion of the practitioner the patient tried going to bed earlier at 10 p.m. If she woke up between 11 and 3 at night she was advised to think about anything other than plans for the future. Along with acupuncture treatment on her Wood Element this gradually resolved her problems.

Instead of organising everything so that it runs smoothly some Wood CFs tend to force their will on situations. They then appear to be insensitive to the needs of others within the structure. If this happens the rules and structures seem to become more important than the people concerned. This can cause others in the organisation to rebel against the draconian measures and against the Wood CF who is putting them in their place. Lacking the perception to see how they are behaving to others, they may feel that they are the 'victim' and that others are pushing them around. This can be especially upsetting for the Wood CF who knows that the structures have been made for the 'good' and effectiveness of those other people.

Disorganised

At the other end of the spectrum many Wood CFs lack a vision for their life and find organising their day-to-day lives difficult. Their lives lack direction and they may just fumble along as best they can. This can be worsened by smoking cannabis, which tends to particularly affect these aspects of the Liver and Gall Bladder. 'Going with the flow' sounds like an admirable Daoist way of living but in this case it just masks a person's inability to organise their life in a nourishing and meaningful way. Their Wood Element may fail to generate sufficient dynamism for them to move forward. Resignation, hopelessness and depression become familiar feelings to them. Many people like this are 'living lives of quiet desperation' and restoring their Wood Element to a better state of health is a crucial step to improved well-being.

Strategies to deal with disorganisation

Some Wood CFs deal with their internal disorganisation by joining a group that organises and provides rules for them. For example, they might join one of the armed forces or civil service or any organisation that provides people with a strong structure and discipline. Alternatively they might gain structure from joining a cult or religious organisation. This might provide strong rules and regulations and has the added bonus of also providing a life purpose. Some people choose life partners who are decisive and organised to compensate for their lack of ability to plan or make decisions.

It is important to remember that it is not the external behaviour which shapes the person's CF but the underlying reason for it. For example, people from all CFs may choose to join a religious community – but for different reasons. A Metal CF may want to connect to a higher source, an Earth CF to feel a part of the community, a Water CF to feel safe

and a Fire CF to connect with other people. They all have the same outward behaviour but their individual motives are different.

Sometimes taking on the outward form of a group may be enough to provide structure and support for the Wood CF. At other times the person's own lack of internal organisation makes it difficult for them to feel settled in their chosen environment. Although they appreciate the structure they may also feel frustrated by it and waver between loving and hating it.

Alternating between extremes

Many Wood CFs alternate between the two extremes of being organised or disorganised. They may, for example, be extremely well organised at work but at home they turn into 'slobs' who do nothing around the house. They rely on their partner to take charge of all plans and decisions involving household tasks, planning holidays and paying bills.

Other Wood CFs may be able to plan and organise to some extent but then not be able to follow their plans through to completion. For example, earlier in this chapter the small steps were described when a person wants to change career. Some Wood CFs might, for example, do all of the research about the chosen career but find it impossible to make the final push and go and retrain. In this case procrastination may become habitual. Others may enjoy planning and thinking about what they might do but never be able to put their ideas into action. This ability to initiate is a key function of the Wood Element.

Patient Example

An acupuncturist who was a Wood CF had been a fireman before learning acupuncture. While training he talked to his class about his CF in relation to being in the fire service. 'I loved the service life because things are very ordered and disciplined but at first I found the restrictions and the rules and regulations petty. For example, you would have to change into one rig for a drill and then into another rig for something else. As I rose higher through the ranks, however, it was me setting the rules. I then thought that maybe they were good rules after all! I also loved being in control. People would stand around waiting for me to make decisions. Everyone would be panicking and I'd come along and make a decision and it would sort it all out. I enjoyed that power.'

Frustrated and defiant – over-obedient and compliant

Some Wood CFs become chronically defiant when their efforts to assert themselves or create change are frustrated. At the other extreme they may become overly obedient and unable to create change.

Rebelling

There are times when it is appropriate for people to rebel. For instance, anyone who has been oppressed for a period of time might need to rebel. 'Rebel forces' in a country might overthrow a dictatorial regime to gain liberty from a tyrant. People who have been oppressed at work, in their personal life or in other relationships might stand up for themselves and gain freedom from their oppressor.

Children and teenagers often rebel. This is a necessary stage for the person to go through in order to assert their independence and grow into adulthood. Many Wood CFs, however, don't grow out of that rebellion and may tend to show defiance towards authority for many years. Earlier in this chapter we described Wood CFs fighting for justice and someone else's rights in an unfair situation. Wood CFs who are compulsively defiant, however, kick aside any constraint that lies in their path in the desire to assert themselves. They may appear to fight others for the sake of it and because they don't know of any other way to react.

Patient Example

A practitioner noticed that her patient seemed to be continually struggling with the situations that occurred in her life and banging up against things. She asked her what would happen if she had nothing to push against. This question stopped the patient in her tracks. She realised that if she had nothing to push up against she would find it 'really scary' and said 'I don't know who I am if I have nothing to push up against.' She explained that banging up against things, struggling, pushing and being surly was a way of trying her strength. It was like flexing her muscles and testing out who she was.

Wood CFs who are defiant are often in a quandary. On the one hand boundaries give them more of a sense of who they are and a better awareness of their internal structure, something they often lack. On the other hand they can often find it difficult to fit into other people's structures and kick and push against them whenever possible. This also gives them a better sense of their own boundaries. One Wood CF admitted that she always thought, 'I don't have to do anything I don't want to do' and so would compulsively do something a little different when out with her friends. 'I'll climb a fence or not pay the train fare, unless I'm asked. For me it's a way of having an adventure and fulfilling a desire to be free.'

The desire to challenge authority is often subtly tested in the practitioner–patient relationship. It is not an equal relationship and sometimes the patient is driven to defy the practitioner or engage in a struggle for power. For some people this dynamic is so powerful that they rarely seek help from authority figures of any kind, so practitioners rarely see such people as patients. In less extreme cases the patient is often compelled to test the boundaries of the situation, for example, over issues of lifestyle advice. In most cases the practitioner can only win the trust and respect of the patient if they can assert themselves and their role sufficiently and yet with enough skilful flexibility to avoid an outright triumph or humiliation on either side. It is somewhat similar to the way school bullies despise weakness in others and respect others that they perceive as strong.

In order to let go of rebelliousness, a Wood CF may need to learn to cultivate the 'virtue' of Wood, *ren*, benevolence or forgiveness. The habit of continually standing up to authority usually arises at an early age when an adult in authority puts too many constraints on the young Wood CF. Forgiveness is an important step towards letting go of the anger and rebelliousness that have fuelled this behaviour. This in turn may allow Wood CFs to become more flexible in their reactions and have more choices than rebelling.

Over-obedient

Some Wood CFs are at the other end of the spectrum and are over-compliant. They may be plagued by self-doubt and be uncertain of their own opinions. Because of this it can be difficult for them to make decisions and may leave them open to being influenced and dominated by others. Their passivity may make it hard for them to say 'no' for fear of upsetting another person. In order to avoid showing anger they may give in to other people's demands – thus avoiding confrontation. Chinese Medicine sometimes describes these people as having a 'deficient Gall Bladder'. In fact the expression 'to have a small Gall Bladder' in Chinese means a person who lacks courage, initiative or who is timid.

Often the main difficulty for such people is shouldering responsibility. This directly threatens their sense of self as it involves making decisions and implementing plans for which they are accountable. The idea of somebody criticising them for a mistaken strategy or poor judgement is abhorrent to them. They would often prefer to earn less in a less stimulating position than run that risk.

Wood CFs who are over-obedient may have such a strong sense of the importance of rules, structures and boundaries that they don't like to venture beyond any structures that are in place around them. They may be people who never broke the rules at school and are almost compulsively law-abiding as adults. To flout the conventions and customs of society or their own particular subculture is anathema. Because they find it difficult to assert themselves they can end up spending most of their time doing what other people want. Sometimes because of the weakness of their 'decision-maker' they may not even know what they want. Instead they always follow other people's will. For instance, they may stay in a job they don't enjoy, go into the family business rather than a career of their own choice or only take a job that involves little or no responsibility.

Patient Example

A Wood CF was having treatment for headaches. She had one child but her mother-in-law wanted her to have more and would continually 'hassle' her about it. The patient did not know how to stand up to her. She was happy with one child but would pretend to agree that she and her husband would be having more children just to pacify her mother-in-law. The patient worked in a library and loved her job as it gave her peace and quiet. She found any form of confrontation extremely painful and found it hard to watch the news as she found it too violent. She was surprised when her practitioner suggested she switch off the TV as that idea had not occurred to her!

Summary

1 A diagnosis of a Wood CF is made primarily by observation of a green facial colour, a shouting or lack of shouting voice, a rancid odour and imbalance in the emotion of anger.

2 Wood CFs tend to have issues and difficulties with:
   • boundaries
   • power
   • being correct
   • personal growth
   • development.

3 Because of these issues a Wood CF's behaviour and responses to situations tends to be inappropriate concerning:

   • being assertive and direct   —————   passive and indirect
   • seeking justice   —————   apathetic
   • rigidity   —————   over-flexibility
   • being excessively organised   —————   disorganised
   • feeling frustrated   —————   over-obedient and compliant

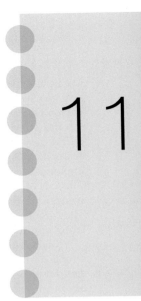

Fire – key resonances

Fire as a symbol

The character for Fire

The Chinese character for Fire, *huo*, represents ascending flames (see Weiger, 1965, lesson 126A). This is a simple representation of a fire, such as might be used for cooking. When this character was chosen to represent the Element, fire would have been used for cooking and undoubtedly for warming too. People would gather around fires as a source of heat and social contact would result. The hearth is symbolic of the heart of the home in all cultures.

The Fire Element in life

Fire in the world

The sun is clearly the Fire Element of nature. As the central focus of our solar system, it is the ultimate Fire. It burns and provides heat and light for almost all animals and vegetation. People are totally dependent on the sun for warmth and even minor variations in temperature can have catastrophic effects. Too much sun (and too little rain) can cause crops to fail, resulting in famine. Polar caps can melt, causing land to flood. Established species that are accustomed to a particular range of temperature are suddenly vulnerable and poorly adapted.

Fire within the person

The Fire Element manifests on a physical level through people's sensitivity to heat and cold. One of the most crucial variables in people's ability to function is being at the right temperature. Everyone has an acceptable range and as they go beyond that range their performance deteriorates. Personal range of temperature is often widest when people are young. This is because they have a balanced source of Fire within and a balanced source of Water to control the Fire. As people get older, their Water decreases and their Fire becomes less steady. They may discover that their ideal range of temperature has narrowed.

Emotionally the Fire Element manifests in being joyful. There are many factors contributing to people's happiness, but the joy associated with Fire is significant. To be with others, sharing and communicating, generates and maintains the Fire within us. The pleasure in having satisfying human contact both nourishes the Fire Element and is made possible by the Fire being balanced.

An upward or downward cycle occurs according to the health of the Fire Element. Balanced Fire enables people to reach out and be nourished by human contact. The human contact, in turn, helps to keep the Fire nourished and in balance. Diminished Fire can discourage people from reaching out for more human contact and the lack of Fire nourishment further depletes the Element.

Strengthening the Fire Element with acupuncture treatment can make profound changes to a person and enhance their ability to connect with others. From this contact they become more able to nourish their own Fire. Chronic loneliness is not life enhancing. People need to allow the emotional rays of the sun to touch them. Those with depleted Fire Elements begin to crave for the rays of the sun to penetrate and warm and even melt them at their core. Such are the issues associated with Fire.

The Fire Element in relation to the other Elements

The Fire Element interacts with the other Elements through the *sheng* and *ke* cycles (see Chapter 2, this volume).

Fire is the mother of Earth

On the *sheng* cycle, Fire creates Earth. This relationship is not as obvious as Wood creating Fire, but when Fire burns, ashes are left and they become Earth. This means that when treating patients who have obvious Earth Element symptoms, such as digestive complaints, they may have originated in the mother Element, Fire. A practitioner may treat the mother to assist the child.

Wood is the mother of Fire

On the *sheng* cycle, Wood is the mother of Fire and creates Fire. For those who have built a camp fire by gathering wood, it is easy to understand how Wood creates Fire.

That Wood is the mother of Fire means that a symptom, for example, heart pain, which apparently arises from the Fire Element, may be the effect of the Wood Element upon the Fire Element. Thus, when a symptom is manifesting from the Organ of one Element, it is always wise to look at the state of the previous Element (for more on this, see Chapter 2, this volume). This is the 'mother' Element on the *sheng* cycle.

Water controls Fire

A fire hose illustrates how water can be used to control fire. In general, there are many body–mind functions that involve heat and which can be spoiled by too much fire. The control of inflammation, the drying out of joints and the rising up of excessive joy and excitation are all examples. In these cases, Water will contain, control and regulate the excesses of Fire.

Fire controls Metal

Fire controls Metal. It softens it and helps to shape it. When fashioning beautiful objects in gold, the gold must be heated in order to mould it to the desired shape. Should the Fire Element become deficient, then the balance of the Metal Element is harder to maintain. In this case the Lung itself is more likely to weaken, fail to distribute protective *qi* and fail to receive *qi* from the Heavens.

The key Fire resonances
(Table 11.1)

The colour for Fire is red

The character for red

The character for red is *chi* (Weiger, 1965, lessons 60N and 126B). As well as being a simple colour word, this character is also used as the technical term for the facial red that accompanies too much heat in

Table 11.1 Key Fire resonances

Colour	Red
Sound	Laughing
Emotion	Joy
Odour	Scorched

the Heart. 'Heart-fire' is a pathological pattern where the Heart has accumulated excess heat.

Colour in nature

Had a divine artist painted the world, she or he used red sparingly. Sometimes the sky manifests beautiful tones of pink and red. Within species of flowers, red and its various variations appear frequently. The most common association with the colour red is probably blood. Later in the chapter it will be described how Blood is clearly connected with the Fire Element.

On an emotional level, red is associated with passion and especially with the Heart. No one draws a valentine with a green or blue heart on it. The Heart and the colour red are associated with love and relationships in many cultures. Significantly, the Chinese traditionally married not in white, but in red, the colour of love. In the West, it is a common custom on Valentine's day to give red roses or cards with red hearts to our loved ones.

Facial colour

Fire can manifest either as too much red on the face or too little. This facial colour manifests under and beside the eyes, in the laugh lines or around the mouth. When red appears on the face in other areas this may indicate excess heat and may have nothing to do with an imbalance of the Fire Element. Because of this, where there is a red colour, the practitioner's observation needs to stick strictly to the relevant facial areas. Practitioners rarely see red under the eyes, beside the eyes in the laugh lines or around the mouth, however. It is more common for patients to manifest 'lack of red'.

What is lack of red? Practitioners expect there to be a normal amount of pink or red in the face. At certain times, for example when someone faints, people may say that the blood has drained out of someone's face and the person has become ashen or grey. The practitioner is noticing an absence of the normal pink of a complexion, a rather dull bloodless colour. With respect to a longer-term and serious Fire imbalance, the dull lack of red can become greyer. This is generally the colour practitioners are looking for when examining the face. They look to the side of the eye and there is a patch where the usual pink seems to have been drained. On some patients lack of red is detected by a general dullness and lack of vitality in the colour of the face overall.

The sound for Fire is laughing

The character for laughing

The Chinese character for laughing is *xiao*. On the top of this character is the radical for bamboo. Underneath this is the character for a man who is bending forward, possibly as someone having a belly laugh (see Weiger, 1965, lessons 77B and 61B).

Laughter in life

Laughter is the sound that naturally emanates from the Heart. The Chinese have many expressions about happiness and laughter. For example, one proverb states that, 'A person should laugh three times a day to live longer'. Another says, 'A good laugh makes you ten years younger, while worry turns the hair grey'. This suggests that laughter eases the Heart, increases relaxation and restores balance.

This principle is used in Chinese *qi gong* exercises. For example, 'the inner smile' is a simple exercise to smile and then let the feeling of the smile drop downwards in the body to relax the Organs. Laughing is an extension of this feeling. A good belly laugh can massage and relax our organs and raise our spirits. One well-known *qi gong* teacher purposely laughs loudly in his teaching sessions in order to increase the relaxation of the group.

The context of laughter

The time for laughter to be present is when pleasure or joy is being expressed. This may be during personal interaction where warmth is being exchanged or people are talking about remembered pleasurable experiences. Inappropriate contexts would be when there is loss, fear or feelings of anger or sympathy.

The voice tone of laughing

When a person has a laughing voice there is not necessarily actual laughter present, as in the notion of a belly laugh. The sound of laughing is almost a 'pre-laugh' without an actual laugh emerging (although it might). Fire is a very *yang* Element, so it is natural that in the same way that laughter seems to rise upwards and outwards, so does this sound. It is close enough to a laugh that listeners might easily feel that, were they to apply a gentle tickle, the sound would develop into a laugh. It doesn't have to, however, because laughter is there in the sound of the voice.

The quickest way to appreciate this voice tone is to listen to people who are talking about enjoyable events or exchanging funny stories. While doing this they will usually have a laughing sound in their voices. If this sound is missing from their voices, the event or story sounds less funny. Another way to detect a laughing voice tone is to talk out loud as if enthusiastically telling someone you like about a really enjoyable time you had. You will feel your voice rise up and feel your face on the edge of a smile.

Five Element practitioners listen and notice if the voice tone and its content matches. For example, laughter should be present in the voice when a person is talking about things that are funny. If a person is often laughing out of context this is inappropriate. For example, a person may laugh whilst talking about painful experiences, or laughter may be completely absent when the subject is one of enjoyment or pleasure. In this case the sound in the voice may be indicating that the person is a Fire CF. There is a tendency for people to laugh in order to hide their nervousness. Practitioners need to be aware of this and not succumb to thinking all nervous laughter is evidence of the person being a Fire CF.

Lack of laughter

Some Fire CFs, especially those who tend towards lack of joy, have voices that have no sparkle or gaiety in them. The tone is monotonous and is easily mistaken for the groan of a Water CF. It has a tendency to sound rather croaky and flat.

The odour for Fire is scorched

The character for scorched

The character for scorched is *zhuo*. The left-hand side is the character for fire and the right-hand side that of a 'kind of spoon' (Weiger, 1965, lessons 54H and 126A). Except for the inclusion of the character for fire, the character does not seem especially significant.

The odour of scorched is probably the easiest to describe of all the Five Element odours as it actually resembles what in ordinary life a person would describe as scorched. Some scorched smells to consider are:

- burnt toast
- clothes coming out of the tumble dryer
- a shirt that has just been scorched while ironing
- vegetables in a steamer which have just burnt dry

The scorched smell varies according to what is burning. In the same way, scorched will also vary from person to person according to their underlying *qi* (for more on diagnosing the odour, see Chapter 25, this volume). An elderly person's scorched, or any other odour, smells quite different from that of a young child.

This odour can often be detected on a person who is feverish. The heat of the fever places a strain on the Pericardium and Triple Burner especially and this temporary imbalance produces a scorched odour. This scorched odour from a fever will not necessarily indicate that a person is a Fire CF.

The emotion for Fire is joy

The characters for joy

The emotion corresponding to Fire is joy. There are two main characters for this emotion. One is *xi* and the other is *le*.

Xi (Weiger, 1965, lesson 165B) translates as elation and *le* (lessons 88C, 119K and 119) as joy (see also Larre and Rochat de la Vallée, 1996, p. 106). Another term is also used – *bu le* (see Weiger, 1965, lesson 133A for *bu*), which means an absence of joy. Elisabeth Rochat de Vallée notes the atypical nature of this phrase. The pathology of an emotion usually lies in its excess, not its absence (Larre and Rochat de la Vallée, 1996, pp. 106–108 and 118–120). She puts the two together in the following way. When the *xi* is out of balance people tend to become over-elated. When the *le* becomes imbalanced people tend to go into lack of joy (*bu le*).

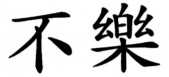

The description of these characters is helpful and enables the practitioner to gain a deeper understanding of joy. *Xi* describes the right hand striking the skin of an ancient drum. At the bottom of the character is a mouth depicting singing. The whole character describes singing and making music – the ability for people to enjoy themselves and have a good time. Based on the drum, the nature of the occasion is informal. *Le* is also related to music and shows a great drum with bells on either side. These are drums used in rites and ceremonies that are more formal occasions. They have a deeper sound than the drum of *xi* and make contact with the spirit. This character depicts a harmony and unity inside a person (Larre and Rochat de la Vallée, 1996, pp. 107–108).

Appropriate joy

Practitioners of Five Element Constitutional Acupuncture observe a person's capacity to regularly and normally experience joy. Joyful incidents may occur at a social gathering interacting with friends, recounting a pleasurable event, enjoying food, watching a favourite striker score a goal or being in close contact with a lover or soul-mate. They vary enormously in their nature and intensity and are judged mainly by how they are experienced. They 'feel good', bring a smile to a person's face and quicken the heart.

Five Element Constitutional Acupuncturists assess their patients' capacity to feel joy and whether they can appropriately and smoothly move in and out of joy.

What are the pathological movements of joy?

Ling Shu Chapter 8 gives us a clue:

> The Heart is in control of the blood vessels and the spirit resides in the blood vessels. A hollowness of the energy in the Heart will cause the emotion of sadness; a solidness of the energy in the Heart will cause incessant laughter.

> (Lu, 1972, p. 101)

The more robust the functioning of a patient's Fire *qi*, the more it will support and facilitate a person's ability to express joy appropriately.

Imbalanced Fire *qi* can have two consequences. One is that the Heart is too weak to allow the Fire *qi* to move through it and express all the stages of joy. These stages are entering into joy, going to the peak of the feeling and then descending out of joy back to a base level. A person who is unable to move through all of these stages has *bu le*, an absence of joy. For example, joy is in the air; other people in the group laugh, but one individual appears unable to join in, looks sad, and may have the additional distress at feeling left out. The Heart is responsible for the 'radiance of the spirits'. Sometimes people try to join in and laugh with others but they are only going through the motions. Their joy has no conviction or radiance. It does not communicate genuine joy or warmth.

Another consequence of pathological Fire *qi* is an excessive or erratic movement in expressing joy. This might be described as fullness, but it can be better described as instability. The Fire *qi* does not flow in a steady manner and flashes up into elation in the form of slightly uncontrollable laughing or excitation. It can also be accompanied by internal agitation. This joy may flare up and become excessive but equally it can flare up and as rapidly fade away. The essential observation is that the joy and therefore the Fire *qi* does not flow smoothly. On the outside there is an appearance of joy but from the inside a person does not have the experience of feeling good.

Patient Example

A Fire CF patient described how when she was particularly low she could be with people that she really liked but be unable to join in. 'Everyone may be having a good time but I can't seem to feel happy although I desperately want to. It's worse if there are strangers around. I am just missing some spark and I feel desperately unhappy.'

Which emotions injure the Fire Element?

(Table 11.2)

The Fire Element is easily harmed by several of the emotions. Excess joy, *xi le*, harms the *qi* by making it 'loose' (*Su Wen* Chapter 39). This creates instability in the *shen* and tends to make many Fire CFs particularly volatile emotionally. Lack of joy, *bu le*, is also deleterious to the Fire Element. It is very difficult for a person to maintain their *joie de vivre* without joy, warmth and stimulation from others. Everyone needs contact and intimacy with others to lead complete lives and realise their potential. When a person becomes isolated and lacks companionship over an extended period of time, their Fire Element is cut off from a crucial source of nourishment. This is similar to when a plant has to endure too much shade. It usually survives, but it doesn't thrive.

Sadness, *bei*, is probably the emotion that most affects a patient's Fire Element. *Bei* makes the *qi* 'disappear'. Sadness is an inadequate translation of the wide range of painful feelings that people feel in their Hearts. In childhood the pain of feeling unloved by parents, siblings or classmates can be devastating to a person's Fire Element.

In adulthood the Fire Element can be devastated by the heartbreak associated with the decline and ending of intimate relationships and in this case it can be a major source of physical and psychological illness. The current trend of 'serial monogamy' can create a cycle of falling in and out of love that severely strains the Fire Element. 'Falling in love' is often accompanied by excess joy and excitation, as well as feelings of vulnerability. This is usually followed by intense pain as the relationship fails to live up to the unreal expectations placed upon it. Literature, pop songs, opera and much conversation is now dominated by this theme. It can also play a prominent part in the discussion between patients and practitioners. Exploring the emotional life of the patient is essential if the practitioner wishes to diagnose the health of any of the patient's Elements.

The Fire Element is also easily imbalanced by shock (*jing*). Trauma, abuse and emotional upsets make it difficult for the Heart to remain settled. Shock predominantly attacks the Organs of the Fire Element, but also depletes the Kidneys. This is a common cause of a breakdown in relationship between the Water and Fire Elements.

The supporting Fire resonances

These resonances are considerably less important than the 'key' resonances given in Table 11.1. They can often be used to indicate that a person's Fire Element is imbalanced but they do not necessarily point to it being the person's CF (Table 11.3).

The season of Fire is summer

The character for summer

The character is *xia* (Weiger, 1965, lesson 160D). *Xia* indicates a countryman walking with his hands down and his work done. He is allowing his plants to grow by themselves.

Summer

Summer is the most *yang* and expansive time of year. Plants are at their most developed and animal life is generally at its most active. In temperate climates,

Table 11.2 Examples of the range of emotions associated with the Fire Element

Joyousness	Excitement. elation, euphoria, exhilaration, excessive enthusiasm, mania
Sadness	Misery, unhappiness, despair, gloom, sorrow, flatness, melancholy, downheartedness

Table 11.3 Supporting Fire resonances

Season	Summer
Power	Maturity
Climate	Heat
Sense Organ/Orifice	Tongue
Tissues and body parts	Blood vessels
Generates	Hair
Taste	Bitter

summer typically brings people out of their dwellings. They wear fewer clothes and are ready to sunbathe, sit in cafes, chat with friends or go to the seaside. People talk more and have many opportunities for pleasure and joy. This time of year clearly connects with the Fire Element.

Because summer is normally warmer, questioning people about their preference for the seasons does not yield consistent and therefore useful information. It is hard to separate preference for a certain temperature from the preference for the energy of the season. Many Fire CFs, however, experience a craving for the warmth and light of summer more than other CFs.

In addition, it is said in Chinese medicine that the Heart hates heat. In practice, many Fire CFs have a dual experience of summer. Many of them crave the sun and love the heat. But as the heat increases, the blood vessels dilate to cool the body. This puts an extra burden on the Heart and depending on a person's health it can cause difficulties. All people, including Fire CFs, can have issues with heat and therefore the summer.

The power of Fire is maturity

The character for maturity

Cheng is the character for maturity, the power for Fire (Weiger, 1965, lessons 50H (*cheng*) and 75 (*shu*)).

Maturity

Maturity is at the peak of the cycle from birth to storage. While the countryman leaves his arms by his sides and allows the plants to grow, everything else in nature is also developing and reaching maturity. Fruits absorb the rays of the sun and become ripe. Compared to the cycle of a day, summer is equivalent to the moment that the sun reaches its zenith. As long as the moisture, the right soil, the minerals and especially the warmth are present a plant will evolve. No special effort is necessary – they do it all by themselves.

The climate of Fire is heat

The character for heat

Re is the character for summer heat. The top of the character depicts the sun, while the lower part is a grammatical term meaning a document, phrase or speech (Weiger, 1965, lesson 79K).

Summer heat

Summertime is when the heat of the sun is strongest. Plants require this final application of heat in order to complete their growth. In a similar way to the countryman with his hands by his sides, there is nothing to do but let the warmth of the sun do its work. This can be compared to sunbathers on resort beaches who do nothing but soak up the sun's rays and feel better for it.

Although the connection between the summer and heat is obvious, what Fire CFs make of heat is less obvious. Some love it and others hate it. Many Fire CFs crave summer and adore the heat. Others manifest the notion that 'the Heart hates heat' and avoid sitting in the sun, sun-soaked holidays and even central heating.

There are two notions of heat or warmth that Five Element practitioners consider. One is that which typically comes from the sun and can be measured by a thermometer. The other refers to the internal warmth that comes from human contact and communication. Practitioners of Five Element Constitutional Acupuncture will pay more attention to the latter form of warmth (see the discussion of the Fire Organs in Chapter 12, this volume).

The first notion of heat (actual temperature) affects people of all CFs. Fire is controlled by Water and our moisture diminishes slowly as we age. Thus older people, who at one time might have enjoyed lying in the sun, begin to prefer the shade.

The second notion of heat or warmth is more related to Fire CFs. This is described earlier in this chapter and is to do with Fire CFs' ability to receive love and warmth from others. Often Fire CFs have more difficulty with this than people of other CFs. Unfortunately there is no easy measuring tool (like the thermometer) for this kind of warmth and practitioners have to rely on their own developed sensitivity to feel this aspect of the person. The practitioner needs to be warm to the patient and perceive the effect it has on the person's Fire Element. Did it create intense change in the patient by meeting a deep need in them? Was the patient reluctant to let that moment go as it was so delightful? Did it meet a void in the patient's *shen*, making it impossible to fully enjoy warmth from another? It is by these means rather than by asking questions about a patient's response to temperature that the practitioner can determine the CF (for more on warming the body, see Chapter 12, this volume).

The sense organ/orifice for Fire

The sense organ for Fire is speech and the orifice is the tongue. Literally, in English, speech is not a sense organ and the tongue is not an orifice. Their resonance with Fire, however, is clear.

The character for tongue

She is the character for tongue. It has an open mouth for the lower part and the upper part is an extended tongue (Weiger, 1965, lesson 102C).

Tongue and speech

A practitioner can appreciate two connections between the tongue and speech. The first connection is the ability to speak using the tongue. This connection is obvious. Speech means both the ability to express oneself in words and the physical ability to create words, which specifically involves the tongue.

The second connection is between the speech-tongue and the Heart. The Heart, which is the key Organ of the Fire Element, has a strong role in generating joy by reaching out to others to communicate and share love and warmth (compare with the description above of the character for joy, *xi*, with an open mouth in the centre). We can communicate through touch and looking, but speech is the most common way that people reveal their innermost world and thus merge with another at a deeper level. In this context, speech is a crucial tool for the Heart.

If the Fire Element is deficient, and as a result is less stable, then practitioners often observe irregularities of speech. For example, speech easily falters or the person becomes tongue-tied, babbles away, stutters, mixes up words (as in malapropisms) or frequently forgets words and names.

Our Western approach is to ask 'what exactly is wrong here?' The Chinese approach is to say that speech and the tongue resonate with the Fire Element (and the Heart specifically) and if there are other indications of a Fire imbalance, then this Element should be treated. By so doing, the speech problem will be regulated.

A practitioner may ask if all speech impediments are found in patients with Fire CFs. The answer is no, but they may indicate that a person has an imbalance in the Heart. Speech problems are only supportive evidence for a person being a Fire CF when colour, sound, emotion and odour, the key resonances, are present.

The tissues and body parts for Fire are blood and blood vessels

The resonating tissues and body parts for Fire are blood and blood vessels. There are various references for this resonance. In some cases, just the blood is mentioned and in others the blood and blood vessels, for example, *Su Wen* Chapters 10 and 44.

The character for blood vessels

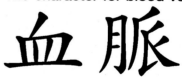

The overall character for blood vessels is made up of the character for Blood, *xue* (Weiger, 1965, lesson 157D; note that the modern *pin yin* spelling for blood is *xue* rather than *hsueh*) and the two characters for vessel, *mai* (Weiger, 1965, lessons 65A and 125E). The character for Blood is a picture of a vase full of a sacred red fluid. The character is similar to the Western symbol of the Holy Grail. The character for vessels is similar to that for water (see Chapter 20, this volume), but also has the flesh radical attached, indicating that it is a part of the body.

Blood and blood vessels

The Heart is said to govern the blood and the blood vessels, thus providing the link between the Organ, tissues and body parts. It is helpful to think of the Heart, blood and blood vessels as one system. The Heart pumps the blood through the blood vessels and this allows the flow of Heart *qi* to manifest as balanced joy. The Heart's function of governing the blood also emphasises the Heart's role in creating the blood and pumping blood to all the tissues in the body in order to nourish and moisten them. The *shen* is 'housed' in the Blood (*Ling Shu* Chapter 32; Wu, 1993), easily becoming disturbed when the Blood is not healthy. Blood and blood vessels are an intimate part of the Fire Element.

Other Elements have important influences on both the blood and the blood vessels, so any specific pathology does not necessarily point to a person being a Fire CF. There is, however, an important conceptual link between the Heart, the blood and blood vessels as described above and problems with the blood and blood vessels may provide supportive evidence for a person being a Fire CF.

Fire generates hair

Hair, blood and Fire Hair is also described as the surplus of the blood (Wiseman, 1993, p. 76). The connection between hair and Fire is via the blood. Blood's function is to nourish and moisten. Thus the quality of a person's hair will reflect the quality of their blood. In turn, the blood reflects the Fire Element. Sometimes this connection will be short term and obvious. For example, a woman's hair can become drier and of poorer quality as her menstrual blood gathers ready for the period to flow. Then, further into the cycle when her blood has been renewed, the quality of her hair improves. The connection is less obvious when a man's Fire and Blood are deficient and where the dryness of the hair is constant and therefore assumed to be normal.

The taste for Fire is bitter

The character for bitter

Ku is the character for bitter (Weiger, 1965, lessons 78B and 24F). The top part of the overall character means 'plants' and the lower part indicates 'that

which has passed through ten mouths, i.e. a tradition dating back ten generations'. The reference here is probably to old or processed plants that often have a bitter flavour.

Bitter

In Chinese herbal medicine, the bitter taste has two functions. It can drain or dry dampness or it can disperse or clear excess heat. Examples of ordinary foods with a bitter taste are coffee, burnt toast, pumpkin seeds, rhubarb and watercress. The clearest example is Angostura bitters. These are available in most bars and can be added to whisky. (Gentian, which is the main herbal ingredient of bitters, also appears in the Chinese herbal *materia medica* as *long dan cao*, a herb used to clear damp and heat generated by the Liver.) Beer is also bitter but the drink beloved of some Fire CFs is Campari, red in colour and very bitter in taste.

Some Fire CFs enjoy a bitter taste but others don't. It is therefore not a reliable indicator of a person being a Fire CF but may be used as supportive evidence.

Summary

1 Along the *sheng* cycle, Fire is the mother of Earth and Earth is the mother of Metal. Across the *ke* cycle, Fire controls Metal and Water controls Fire.

2 A diagnosis of a Fire CF is made primarily by observation of a red or lack of red facial colour, a laughing or lack of laughing voice tone, a scorched odour and an imbalance in the emotion of joy.

3 Fire CFs tend to easily swing between being very joyful and being rather sad.

4 The Fire Element is easily imbalanced by excessive joy (*xi*), shock (*jing*) and sadness (*bei*).

5 Other resonances include the season of summer, heat, the power of maturity, the tongue, blood and blood vessels, hair and a bitter taste.

Fire – The Organs

12

Introduction

Fire is different from the other Elements. It has two *yin* Organs and two *yang* Organs. Two of these are not ordinary Organs and are often referred to as functions. The two Organs are the Heart and Small Intestine and the two Organ/functions are the Heart-Protector and the Triple Burner.

The Heart-Protector is also known as the Pericardium, which is the sac around the heart and is a physical part of the body, if not an organ. The Triple Burner gets its name from the division of the torso into three 'burning spaces'. The Upper Burner is from the solar plexus up, the Middle Burner is from the solar plexus down to the navel, and the Lower Burner is from the navel down (see Figure 12.1).

The four Organs are divided into pairs, each with one *yin* Organ and one *yang* Organ (Table 12.1). The pairing on one 'side' of the Fire Element is the Heart and Small Intestine and on the other is the Heart-Protector and the Triple Burner. In general Fire CFs tends to be treated on one of the *yin/yang* pairs, either the Heart and Small Intestine or the Heart-Protector and Triple Burner. This is not a rigid rule and there are patients where other combinations are more clinically effective.

The discussion that follows will first centre on the two *yin* Organ/functions and then on the two *yang* Organ/functions (Table 12.2)

The Heart – the Supreme Controller

The character for the Heart

The Chinese character for most Organs contains the 'flesh' radical, indicating that it is a part of the physical body. The character for the Heart, *xin*, is different (Weiger, 1965, lesson 107A). It has no flesh radical but instead shows a space. This demonstrates that the Heart is not merely a muscle which pumps the blood, but more a space that our *shen* or mind-spirit shines through. The heart is more to do with 'being' than with 'doing'.

Su Wen Chapter 8

Su Wen Chapter 8 says: 'The Heart holds the office of lord and sovereign. The radiance of the spirits stems from it' (Larre and Rochat de la Vallée,

DOI: 10.1016/B978-0-7020-3175-5.00012-7

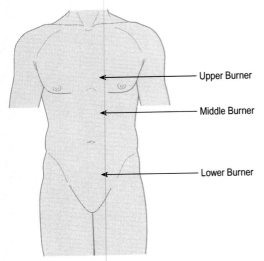

Figure 12.1 • The Three Burners

Table 12.1 The Fire Organs

	Organs	Organ/functions
Yin	Heart	Heart-Protector
Yang	Small Intestine	Triple Burner

Table 12.2 The Fire Element Officials/Organs

Organ/ Official	Colloquial name	Description from *Su Wen* Ch 8
Heart	Supreme Controller	The Heart holds the office of lord and sovereign. The radiance of the spirits stems from it
Pericardium	Heart-Protector	The Envelope of the Heart (Pericardium) represents the civil servants; from them can come joy and pleasure
Small Intestine	Separator of pure from impure	The Small Intestine is responsible for receiving and making things thrive. Transformed substances stem from it
Triple Burner	The Official of Harmony and Balance	The Triple Burner is responsible for opening up the passages and irrigation. The regulation of fluids stem from it

1992, p. 33). Thus the Heart has a special relationship to all the other Organs. The welfare of all other Organs is dependent on the sovereign. *Su Wen* Chapter 8 continues:

> If then the sovereign radiates (virtue), those under him will be at peace. From this the nurturing of life will give longevity, from generation to generation and the empire will radiate great light.

> But if the sovereign does not radiate (virtue), the twelve charges will be in danger, which will cause the closing and the blocking of the ways, finally stopping communication and the body will be seriously injured. From this the nurturing of life will sink into disaster. Everything that lives under Heaven will be threatened in its ancestral line with the greatest of dangers.

> (Larre and Rochat de la Vallée, 1992, p. 34)

The Heart is important because it governs every other Organ. The Organs are like the officials of a court. If the emperor is settled and well, the officials can do their jobs. If the emperor is weak or disturbed, the officials are unable to function well.

Historically, the emperor of China was regarded as being halfway between human and divine. It was through the emperor and specifically through his *ling* (see Appendix A) that the people had a connection to the heavens and the spirits. The emperor had total authority over his people yet his role was to do nothing other than reflect the will of the heavens. A healthy heart with no obstructions does nothing other than allow our spirit to rest peacefully within it.

The spirit of the Heart – the *shen*

All the *yin* Organs store a 'spirit'. The Heart houses the *shen*.

The character for the *shen*

The character for the *shen* is composed of two characters. On the left is *shih*, which suggests an 'influx coming from heaven' (Weiger, 1965, lesson 3D).

On the right is *shen*, which gives the notion of 'two hands extending a rope; the idea of extension, or expansion' (Weiger, 1965, lesson 50C). Both characters together help us to understand something about the power of the *shen*. It emanates from heaven and is capable of unfolding with infinite expansive power from within us.

The functions of the *shen*

Shen

The *shen* enables people to radiate outwards. *Shen* gives a person a sparkle in the eyes, an inner vitality, *joie de vivre*, and an alertness of the mind. This brightness and radiance is called *shen ming* in Chinese texts. *Shen ming* is the glow and radiance of Fire. Practitioners often notice after a treatment on the Fire Organs that patients' *shen ming* has been enhanced. Their eyes sparkle more, their mind is more settled and their pulse improves. The change reminds us of the description of the Heart. It is like an empty space, just being, needing to do nothing and influencing simply by being there.

> When the luminous radiance of the Spirit's *shen ming* is stored within the Formless, and when the essences/ spirits *jing shen* return to the Supreme Authenticity, then the eye is radiant and no longer oriented towards vision, the ear is fine and no longer just for hearing, the heart spreads out, is propagated far and wide, and is no longer for preoccupation and worry.
>
> (*Huainanzi*, Chapter 8; Larre and Rochat de la Vallée, 1995, p 88)

Relationship with the other spirits

Each *yin* Organ has a 'spirit' associated with it. Thus as well as being the spirit of the Heart, the *shen* is also the spirit of the whole Element. The other spirits are the following:

- Wood   *hun* or spiritual soul
- Earth   *yi* or intellect
- Metal   *po* or corporeal soul
- Water   *zhi* or will

One of the functions of the *shen* is to be the overseer or leader of the other spirits. This means that for each of these to thrive, they will to some degree depend upon the state of health of the *shen*. If the *shen* itself is healthy the other spirits may then perform their roles perfectly.

Other functions

The *shen*, which the Heart stores, has other more specific functions. Like many of the Organ functions in Chinese medicine, these are not exclusive to the Heart. They are primarily a function of the *shen*, but the spirits of the other Organs also influence them.

The *shen* affects our ability to sleep, especially to go off to sleep. The *shen* goes outward during the day and engages with the world. At night, when it is time to rest, the *shen* returns to the Heart. The *shen* rests in the Blood of the Heart. When the Heart Blood is not healthy, then the *shen* is not 'rooted' and becomes agitated. This is somewhat like a dog that circles its blanket time and time again and cannot settle. Going off to sleep depends upon a settled *shen*. If the *shen* is unsettled, then the unconscious can be sufficiently disturbed for dreams to break through into consciousness and wake the person up.

The *shen* affects our short-term memory. When the *shen* is disturbed or deficient it often manifests in ways such as not knowing why we came into a room, not remembering the name of someone to whom we were just introduced, or forgetting where we put our pen or car keys. Scatty, vague, absent-minded are the usual terms to describe these mental states. This often deteriorates with age or if the person is upset or preoccupied.

The *shen* also governs our ability to think clearly and have clear consciousness. Thinking clearly means that there is a purpose to one's thinking and that a person can concentrate without wandering off. When the *shen* is weak or agitated the mind easily strays. Clear consciousness is similar to the function of thinking clearly. Anyone who has meditated knows the tendency for the mind to wander, to disappear into foggy gaps and then re-emerge. Consciousness is also affected or lost when a person has a fit or is in a coma. The *shen* has no 'residence'. At the same time the person often becomes extremely 'lack of red', indicating that the Fire Element is out of balance.

Imbalance of the Heart

A Five Element Constitutional Acupuncturist's diagnosis is largely made by observing 'signs' such as colour, sound, emotion and odour. These signs can reveal the person's CF but not which Organ is primarily in distress. This is especially important in the case of the Fire Element as there are four Organs as opposed to two. Pulse diagnosis is crucial but the nature of the symptoms can also be revealing.

The hallmark of Heart dysfunction is lack of internal control, especially when the *shen* is affected. Difficulty getting off to sleep and dream-disturbed sleep are also common. Seeing someone in an acute state of shock can give some insight into disturbance of the Heart's *shen* in an extreme form. Excessively volatile emotions, uncontrollable tearfulness and internal desperation are common. Lack of stability of the emotions is the key diagnostic indicator. The person usually finds it difficult to stabilise the intense movements of *qi* induced by mild shocks and upsets. This is especially so when brought on by difficulties in relationship to other people but can arise in other situations. Tearfulness is often very transient, arising and departing in a flash. Feelings of rejection are often extremely intense. The person can also be panicky, and may experience intense feelings in the chest.

The Pericardium – the Heart-Protector

The character for the Pericardium

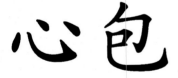

The character for the Pericardium is *xin bao*. The character on the left-hand side is for the Heart, *xin*, and has been described above. The character on the right, *bao*, indicates a wrapping up and containment (Weiger, 1965, lesson 54B). Thus we have the basis for the name, the Heart-Protector.

Su Wen Chapter 8

The description of the Pericardium in *Su Wen* Chapter 8 is as follows:

> The Envelope of the Heart (Pericardium) represents the civil servants; from them can come joy and pleasure.
>
> (Anonymous, 1979b, p 24)

(The Han dynasty Chinese obviously had a more positive image of civil servants than we do nowadays!)

The concept of 'representing civil servants' suggests that the Pericardium is a servant of the Heart, and that the Pericardium has a function to look after and protect the Heart. This statement reinforces the name, the Heart-Protector. The question arising is how the Heart-Protector evokes joy or pleasure. (Note that in *Su Wen* the function which later came to be known as *xin bao*, the Pericardium, was still referred to as *tan zhong*, a centre of *qi* in the chest.)

The function of the Heart-Protector

Protecting the Heart

The Heart-Protector can be described as the guardian of the Supreme Controller. The Supreme Controller is like an emperor who does nothing but act as the spiritual link, half-human and half-god, between the Earth and the Heavens. This delicate role requires protection. The emperor's subjects cannot just drop in to see him to make complaints. The Heart-Protector protects the Heart and decides who should get in, who should be kept out.[1] When the Heart is properly protected, joy and pleasure can arise.

How does the Heart-Protector work?

The Heart-Protector's job requires flexibility. Close friends, advisors and confidants need to be admitted. Strangers and hostile petitioners need to be excluded. The Heart-Protector works like a pair of doors, opening to allow appropriate people in and closing to keep inappropriate people out. For example, in one day, a mother might pay a bill presented by the deliveryman, talk to her child's teacher at school, have lunch with an old school friend, deal with a hostile neighbour over pet problems, talk to the children about school and whisper sweet nothings to her husband after the children have gone to bed. She requires a subtle difference of openness or closedness in each case. She would definitely talk about some subjects with her old friend that she would not talk about with the deliveryman. A healthy

---

[1]Many contemporary Chinese medical books suggest that the functions of the Heart and Pericardium are identical. By contrast, the experience of Five Element practitioners is that treating a Fire CF on Pericardium or Heart can achieve different results. Indeed, when the practitioner is sure that the patient is a Fire CF, it is essential to determine which of these Organs is more important. This experience indicates that there must be a difference in function between the two (see Chapter 45, this volume).

Heart-Protector manages the variations in openness and thus produces what we might call 'appropriate behaviour'.[2] When the Heart-Protector is weak, a person will often demonstrate a lack of awareness of context.

A simple metaphor for the Heart-Protector's function is that the doors maintained by it can get stuck open or stuck closed. When stuck open people may have the propensity to get easily hurt and to behave in inappropriate ways. For example, falling in love and wanting to get married in one evening – nicely romantic but a little too quick. The Heart is left exposed, when it should be protected. The excessive emotions as discussed in the previous chapter are often a consequence.

On the other hand, when the Heart-Protector is stuck closed, a person may be unable to let others in and make deep-level, heartfelt contact. The result is difficulty in making friends, building relationships and being available to receive love and warmth from others. Sometimes this appears as a seemingly odd commitment to superficial contact only. This can also produce what was described in the previous chapter as a 'lack of joy'.

The Pericardium's relationship to *ming men*

In Five Element acupuncture, the source of physical warmth is regarded as derived from the Fire Element. A contrary view is held by those more influenced by *yin/yang* practice. They say that the source of warmth is the Kidney's gate of vitality or *ming men*.

The Heart-Protector also acts as a servant to the Heart and an intermediary between the Heart and the *ming men* of the Kidneys. It is interesting to note that the *ming men* is also sometimes called the 'Ministerial Fire'. From this viewpoint, both the Heart-Protector and the *ming men* work closely together. The Heart-Protector works to connect the *qi* from the *ming men* and the Heart and to transform and harmonise both a person's inherited and acquired *qi* and essence. Harmony between the Heart and Kidneys is very important in order for a person to be at ease mentally and spiritually (Larre *et al.*, 1986, pp. 170–17; this text provides a discussion

of the relationship amongst the Heart, Pericardium, the *ming men* and the Kidneys). For more discussion about the *ming men*, see the section of the Triple Burner later in this chapter.

Imbalance of the Heart-Protector

The role of the Heart-Protector is so similar to that of the Heart that it is often difficult to tell them apart. In theory as long as the Heart-Protector is healthy, the Heart cannot suffer. In practice some people are born with constitutional imbalances in the Heart and treatment needs to be focused on the Heart.

The most obvious manifestation of the Pericardium as the primary Organ to treat is patients' inability to protect their Heart from feelings of rejection. A tendency to be 'over-sensitive' and to easily feel hurt is a common indication. The person may live their life with their 'heart on their sleeve', often experiencing feelings of rejection. Despite the pain, the need to feel loved is so strong that they are compelled to attempt to achieve intimacy whenever remotely possible.

Others may have found the feelings so excruciating in the past that they now ensure that they will not have to feel those feelings again. They are not prepared to take the risk of embarking on an intimate relationship, preferring an impoverished life to a painful one. In these cases pets often provide a welcome source of safe intimacy.

The Small Intestine – the separator of pure from impure

The character for the Small Intestine

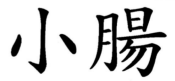

The character for the Small Intestine is the *xiao chang*. The first part of this character, *xiao*, means small. The second part, *chang*, contains two parts. First is the 'flesh' radical, which indicates that it is part of the body. Next to this is the character for *yang*. This indicates that it is an Organ, where much movement and activity is occurring (Weiger, 1965: *xiao*, lesson 18H; *chang* is made up of *jou* (flesh), lesson 65A and *yang*, lesson 101B).

---

[2]Some authors list a virtue for each Element. Kaptchuk (2000, p. 439) lists 'propriety' as the virtue of Fire. We would see that 'fitness' or 'rightness' comes from the combined efforts of the Heart and Heart-Protector as described above.

Su Wen Chapter 8

Su Wen Chapter 8 says:

> The Small Intestine is responsible for receiving and making things thrive. Transformed substances stem from it.
>
> (Larre and Rochat de la Vallée, 1992, p. 107)

This quote suggests the ideas of receiving material from another Organ and transforming it and through the process of separation, sorting what to keep from what to discard. This could easily be a brief description of the small intestine's function from the viewpoint of Western medicine.

The functions of the Small Intestine

Physically

The Stomach passes rotted and ripened food and fluid on to the Small Intestine, which separates pure from impure. All food and fluids that we take into our body need to be transformed and sorted out during the process of digestion. The relatively pure fluid is passed on to the Bladder for re-absorption while the impure goes to the Large Intestine for elimination (note that these are the functions of the Organs, and not the actual route of the fluid). Nutrients are absorbed into the blood and food waste is passed to the Large Intestine. As we can see from the character for the Small Intestine, the function of this Organ requires active *yang* energy and therefore heat.

Mentally and spiritually

Food is not just physical. Our minds and spirits are also constantly being nourished. Indeed, in our current world, with respect to our mind being nourished, we have more to sort out than at any other time in history. The world is changing rapidly. We have an extraordinary range of choices with respect to lifestyles, reading material, listening options, holiday locations, job opportunities, clothing, leisure activities, sporting activities, entertainment and food.

With respect to our spiritual nourishment, compared to 100 years ago, we also have an extraordinary number of influences. Almost any Westerner is subject to many more choices as to what to take in and what to exclude, what to absorb and what to let go of than ever before. Two major activities of modern life, shopping and watching TV, endlessly strain our Small Intestine.

One Small Intestine channel point is called Heavenly Ancestor (SI 11). A story about the Heavenly Ancestor is that when the world was created and *yin* and *yang* were separated, the Heavenly Ancestor was given the job of holding *yin* and *yang* apart so that they would not merge back into oneness (see Chapter 40, this volume, for more on Small Intestine points). The Small Intestine, in separating the pure from the impure, has an important job of discrimination. When we listen to the language, jokes and preoccupations of some people, we can detect an inability to separate pure from impure, clean from turbid and what we need to retain and what we should separate from.

The inability to separate the pure from the impure can mean that people easily become confused or indecisive. When the Gall Bladder is imbalanced the person often finds it difficult to decide between two or more choices. When the Small Intestine is indicated it is more that the person struggles to even see what they are supposed to be choosing between. The tendency to be ambivalent is also marked, as it is hard for people to commit to a course of action as the pros and cons swirl about in their mind.

The Small Intestine and our relationships

It might appear that the Heart and the Heart-Protector are always imbalanced when relationship problems are the main issue. The Small Intestine, however, can also be an important factor in relationship difficulties. At times in relationships we develop closeness and almost merge. At other times we separate and turn our attention to others. This movement back and forth can be a strain for the separator of the pure from the impure.

The associated internal states vary. The person may become mentally fuzzy, unable to make decisions or have difficulty evaluating what to do next. The person may be convinced that others do not understand them (and they may be correct), but not realise that it is due to their confusing comments.

Patient Example

A quote from a male Fire CF who was treated mainly on the Small Intestine. 'When it comes to women I can get bowled over by certain types who are really inappropriate for me. I know I am being stupid, but I just get carried away.'

Going towards extreme purity can also be the result of a Small Intestine imbalance. A person can be strongly drawn towards purity of food, water, mind, spiritual practice, air, or exercise.

The Triple Burner – the Official of balance and harmony

The character for the Triple Burner

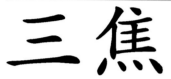

The character for the Triple Burner is *san jiao*. It has two parts to it. The first part, *san*, comprises three lines and denotes the number three. The second part, *jiao*, shows a bird with a short tail, usually thought to be a chicken, roasting over flames. This character probably denotes the heat and nourishment that the Triple Burner brings to the three '*jiaos*' or three burning spaces (Weiger, 1965, lesson 3A for three, and lesson 126A for the roasted bird). Missing is the character for flesh which indicates a physical Organ.

The three *jiao*

The Triple Burner is a function without an Organ. There is no body part to point to and say 'this is the Triple Burner Organ'. There are, however, the three burning spaces. The idea of a 'burning space' comes from the notion of a transforming process, like cooking meat to make it edible, or stir-frying herbs to change their properties. The burning spaces are areas of transformation and each has a particular location and function. The three burning spaces cover the process of a body taking in food, drink and air, transforming them, separating them and absorbing part and excreting the remainder.

The upper *jiao* (burning space) lies at the level of the chest and contains the Heart, Lungs and Pericardium. The middle *jiao*, which is at the level of the solar plexus, contains the Stomach, Spleen, Liver and Gall Bladder. The lower *jiao* lies in the lower abdomen and contains the Small Intestine, Large Intestine, Bladder and Kidneys (see Chapter 24, this volume, for the method of diagnosing imbalance of

the heating function of the Triple Burner). Sometimes the Liver is placed in the lower, rather than the middle, *jiao*.

With respect to the fluids, the upper *jiao* is compared to a mist. The middle *jiao* is compared to a maceration chamber or muddy pool and the lower *jiao* is described as a drainage ditch (see Table 12.3).

Su Wen Chapter 8

Su Wen Chapter 8 says:

> The Triple Burner is responsible for opening up the passages and irrigation. The regulation of fluids stem from it.
>
> (Larre and Rochat de la Vallée, 1992b, p. 129)

The key phrase here is the 'opening up of the passages and irrigation'. Rivers in China have a special significance. The welfare of millions depends on flood control and the use of river water for irrigation. One Chinese writer believes that the fundamental idea behind acupuncture arose in the minds of those who regulated the water of the Yellow River. He relates the famous story of Great Yu who was appointed by Emperor Shun to control the flooding of the Yellow River. After thirteen years, Great Yu had been so effective that Emperor Shun abdicated the throne in Great Yu's favour and Great Yu became the first emperor of the Xia dynasty (*c.* −2000 to −1500) (Xinghua and Baron, 2001).

Table 12.3 The three *jiao*

Burner	Resembles	Significant Organs	Organ functions
Upper	Mist	Lung	Distributing protective *qi*
Middle	Maceration chamber	Stomach, Spleen	Transformation, rotting and ripening, transportation
Lower	Drainage ditch	Kidneys, Small Intestine, Bladder and Large Intestine	Separating pure from the impure. Receiving, storing and excreting urine. Absorbs water from solid wastes and excretes

The functions of the Triple Burner

Moving fluids through the three *jiao*

The Triple Burner regulates the flow of fluids throughout the three burners. It is the supreme hydraulic engineer. Imbalance in the Triple Burner often only manifests indirectly. If the Triple Burner Official is not functioning well, then it may be the performance of the Lungs in spreading protective *qi* or the Stomach in rotting and ripening that goes awry. This indicates the importance of CF diagnosis. The practitioner will give priority to treating the CF and not to treating the Organ whose function appears impeded.

Spreading *yuan qi*

Yuan qi is a form of *qi* which develops from *jing*. An acupuncturist contacts it through the use of the *yuan* 'source' points (see Chapter 36, this volume). The Triple Burner spreads the *yuan qi* from the Kidneys through the three burning spaces and into the channels and specifically to the *yuan* source points that exist on the wrists and ankles. The spreading of this *qi* is similar to the regulation of fluids described above. So in general terms, it can be said that the smooth flow of *qi* through the whole body and specifically the three burning spaces is in part a function of the Triple Burner Official (see Birch, 2003).

Because *qi* is also warmth, the assessment of the three burners (described in Chapter 24, this volume) involves feeling the temperature of the skin on the surface of each burner. Evaluation involves judging whether the temperature is normal, hot or cool. For example, if the Middle Burner is cool, this suggests that either the Stomach, Spleen, Liver or Gall Bladder Officials are imbalanced. Alternatively it may mean that the Triple Burner is not properly regulating the water passages, thus smoothing *qi* and also temperature. The title, 'the Official of Balance and Harmony', accurately describes the crucial regulatory functions of the Official (Felt and Zmiewski, 1993, p. 19).

Warming the body

In Five Element theory the Organs of the Fire Element are largely responsible for providing the *yang qi* required to create and maintain life. Without warmth, there is no life. According to Chinese medicine theory the function responsible for creating the warmth in the body is the Gate of Life or *ming men*. Chapter 36 of the *Nan Jing* states:

> The two kidneys are not both kidneys. The one on the left is the kidney. The one on the right is the Gate of Life (*ming men*).
>
> (Unschuld, 1986)

For many years the *ming men* was regarded as purely a function of the Kidneys, but in the Ming dynasty theoreticians started to think about the *ming men* differently. The *Nan Jing* had laid down that, 'The *ming men* is where the spirit-essence (*jing-shen*) resides' (Unschuld, 1986, Chapter 36).

The *jing* resides in the Kidneys (Water Element) but the *shen* is housed in the Heart (Fire Element). Zhang Jiebin affirmed that the *ming men* was situated between the two Kidneys and that, 'The *ming men* is the organ of Water and Fire' (Anonymous, 1979a). Zhao Xian He called the *ming men* the 'Minister Fire' (*xiang huo*), a term also applied to the twin functions of the Pericardium and the Triple Burner (see Maciocia, 2005, p. 160).

Nan Jing Chapter 66 identified the area between the two Kidneys as the site of the Triple Burner. Although it has no physical form (*xing*), its energetic focus has always been regarded as being in the area between the two Kidneys. Although the *Nei Jing* focused on its functions regarding fluid distribution in the body (for example *Su Wen* Chapter 8), its role in providing warmth throughout the body is crucial (see Mole, 1994). Li Shi-Zhen wrote that 'the Triple Burner is the function of the *ming men*' (Matsumoto and Birch, 1993b, p. 125) and Zhang Jiebin stated:

> The Triple Burner, although it is the *fu* of all drainage and irrigation of the middle, is also that which gathers together and protects all the *yang*.
>
> (Larre and Rochat de la Vallée, 1998, p. 44)

The Japanese writer Sawada wrote:

> In what way can we describe the Triple Burner? The reaction of the burner is as heat. Heat is the fire; fire is the body temperature. Therefore, this also is the regulator of the body temperature.
>
> (Matsumoto and Birch, 1993b)

Five Element Constitutional Acupuncture is consistent with other Five Element styles that emphasise the role of the Fire Element, in particular the Triple Burner and Pericardium, as more important than the Kidneys in the creation of body heat.

The time of day for the Organs

Each Organ has a time of day connected to it. The times for the four Fire Organs are:

Heart	11 a.m. to 1 p.m.
Small Intestine	1 p.m. to 3 p.m.
Heart-Protector	7 p.m. to 9 p.m.
Triple Burner	9 p.m. to 11 p.m.

The *qi* of the Organ is at its peak during these intervals.

Many nurses and doctors confirm that cases of heart failure take place at night during the low time for the Heart – between 11 p.m. and 1 a.m. Heart attacks, where there is too much energy, occur more frequently at midday (Beinfield and Korngold, 1991, p. 91).

People whose Heart-Protectors are deficient often feel an increase in vitality in the evenings. The evenings are also the time when people spend time socialising and make contact with each other.

How the Heart, Heart-Protector, Small Intestine and Triple Burner relate

The Heart and Heart-Protector have a well-defined relationship. The Heart is the Supreme Controller which is half-human, half-divine. This Official resides in its palace housing the spirit and keeping people in contact with the divine. Because of the sensitivity of the Heart, the Heart-Protector exists to defend and protect it by both opening up and closing down its contact with the outside world. The Heart rules, the Heart-Protector protects.

The Small Intestine shares some of the role of the Heart-Protector. By separating impure from the pure, the Heart is protected and a morally impeccable Supreme Controller is maintained.

The job of the Triple Burner is to maintain the flow throughout the three burners and as such to create harmony. When the Heart and/or the Heart-Protector are weak, people often have a tendency to have emotional ups and downs. When the Triple Burner is healthy, it moderates these fluctuations. In contrast, when the Triple Burner is deficient, the fluctuations may be exaggerated.

Summary

1 *Su Wen* Chapter 8 describes the Heart as 'The office of lord and sovereign. The radiance of the spirits stems from it.'

2 The Heart houses the *shen*, which is responsible for governing the spirits of the other Organs.

3 *Su Wen* Chapter 8 describes the Pericardium as 'The Envelope of the Heart (Pericardium) represents the civil servants; from them can come joy and pleasure.'

4 The Pericardium's main responsibility is to protect the Heart. It is sometimes known as the Heart-Protector.

5 The Small Intestine is responsible for 'receiving and making things thrive. Transformed substances stem from it'. It is known as the 'Separator of the Pure from the Impure'.

6 'The Triple Burner is responsible for 'opening up the passages and irrigation. The regulation of fluids stem from it.' It is known as the Official of Balance and Harmony.

Patterns of behaviour of Fire Constitutional Factors

13

Introduction

This chapter describes some of the most important behavioural characteristics that are typical of a Fire CF. Some aspects of a person's behaviour can be observed in the treatment room. Others can only be discerned from patients' descriptions of themselves and their life. As stated in the previous chapters, behaviour can be an indicator of a patient's diagnosis but it can only be used to *confirm* the CF. It should always be used in conjunction with colour, sound, emotion and odour, which are the four primary methods of CF diagnosis. Once the CF is confirmed the patterns of behaviour may, however, support the practitioner's diagnosis.

The origin of the behaviours was described in Chapter 7. The imbalance of the Element of the CF creates instability or impairment of the associated emotion. Thus specific emotional experiences are more likely to occur to one CF as opposed to another. The behavioural traits described in this chapter are often the responses to these negative experiences. In the case of Fire the person experiences more frequent feelings of being unloved and she or he is responding to this.

Patterns of behaviour of a Fire CF

The balanced Element

People with a healthy Fire Element are able to give and receive love with appropriate degrees of emotional closeness. This enables them to cope with a wide range of differing relationships and to appreciate how and when to open up or close down to other people.

The variability and range of closeness in people's relationships is enormous. Some relationships are usually extremely close, for example a spouse or 'life partner', in which case there is usually physical, emotional and spiritual closeness. Others are friendships which can be either with people of the same or a different sex, but which involve no physical intimacy. Some relationships are ones we don't consciously choose, although they may be close. For instance, people become close to relatives because they are 'family' or to colleagues because they see them on a daily basis. Other relationships will be more distant and formal, such as with a doctor, shopkeeper or builder.

A healthy Fire Element enables people to know how and when it is appropriate to open up or shut down to people. It also helps them to decide how much to open up to others. This ability partly arises from experience, but if people have a well balanced Fire Element they cope with this aspect of life.

Formative events for a Fire CF

Because it is likely that people are born with their CF, many of their experiences, especially emotional ones, are coloured by it. If they are born with their Fire out of balance, then their ability to give and receive warmth becomes impaired. This can lead to many Fire CFs experiencing being rejected, abandoned or unloved at an early age. In comparison, people who have more balanced Fire Elements are less likely to have this experience.

Many Fire CFs feel this rejection strongly and a vicious circle develops. Children who easily feel hurt or rejected can over-compensate and protect themselves by keeping their heart closed off from other people. They may then find it difficult to take in warmth and respond to intimacy. As a result they start to feel that others do not like them or that they are unloveable. The more this occurs, the more their Fire Element becomes out of balance. This results in them becoming more and more desperate for love and attention to compensate for their feelings of not being loved.

When the Heart or Heart-Protector is imbalanced the Fire CF may not know when to open up or shut down to others. When these Organs are stuck open, the smallest offence, for example, being let down, ignored momentarily or mistakenly left out, causes hurt and pain. When these Organs are kept closed, intimacy is not achievable and the Fire CF will be unable to get close to others. Sometimes the Fire CF may swing between these two extremes and alternate between being too open and too closed. Fire CFs often feel very changeable, swinging from happiness to misery and back again.

Patient Example

A Fire CF told her practitioner that she was the third child and her mother had only wanted two children. She had always known that she was unwanted and had often felt rejected by her brother and sister as well as by her mother. When young she would often cry because her brother made fun of her. But she felt that her mother would always stick up for her brother and tell her off. She responded by learning to hide her feelings of unhappiness and pretend to feel happy all of the time. She succeeded so well that people often made remarks about what a happy child she was. After having acupuncture treatment she began to feel better about herself. 'I think I was ashamed for much of my life because I thought I was not a very loveable person.'

The main issues for a Fire CF

For the Fire CF certain needs are not fully met. This situation creates issues that centre on these areas:

- love and warmth
- emotional volatility
- closeness and intimacy
- happiness
- clarity and confusion

The extent to which someone is affected in these areas varies according to the person's physical, mental and spiritual health. Relatively healthy Fire CFs will have less disturbance with these aspects of life, whilst those with greater problems end up with their personalities being strongly influenced by this imbalance. Because of these issues they may consciously or unconsciously ask themselves various questions such as:

- Am I loveable?
- Why do I go up and down so much?
- How can I truly relate to others?
- How can I find true happiness?
- Why can't I sort things out?

Responses to the issues

So far we have described how a weakness in the Fire Element leads to a lesser capacity to give and receive love and to cope with a wide range of different relationships. The issues that subsequently arise lead to a spectrum of ways that people typically respond to the world. These responses are common, but not exclusive to Fire CFs. If other CFs have seemingly similar patterns of behaviour it may indicate that there is a different set of motivations underlying the behaviour or that the person's Fire Element is imbalanced but is not the CF. Noticing these responses is therefore useful but does not replace colour, sound, emotion and odour as the principal way of diagnosing the Constitutional Factor.

The behavioural patterns are along a spectrum and can go between these extremes:

1. compulsively cheerful ——————— miserable
2. open and overly sociable ————— closed and isolated
3. clowning ——————— earnest
4. vulnerable ——————— over-protected
5. volatile ——————— flat

Compulsively cheerful – miserable

Fire CFs often swing between the two extremes of being joyful and sad. Many of them, however, only show the happier side of their personality to the world. Their sadness is often kept more private. Other people might describe them as having a sunny disposition, a cheerful nature or being a friendly person or a 'nice guy'.

Patient Example

A 56-year-old nurse who was a Fire CF worked in a care home for the elderly for over 30 years. Her nature was so bright that her boss nicknamed her 'Susie sunshine'. She told her practitioner, 'One of the patients says whenever I walk into the room it's like a breath of fresh air and the sun's shining. I have a laugh with people if I can and I try to get them to look on the bright side.' Underneath her bright exterior, life had not always seemed as good for her. She was very tired when she first came for acupuncture treatment and often felt fed up and miserable but she rarely showed this side of herself.

When some Fire CFs are feeling joyful, they can have such enthusiasm that they fill everyone they meet with warmth and excitement. Their ability to 'sparkle' can be infectious and on a good day they can 'light the fire' of those around them. For example, a teacher who feels 'fired up' may bring a usually uninteresting subject to life and infect the students with this enthusiasm and passion. Other Fire CFs, like the patient described above, may have the ability to cheer others up when they are feeling a bit down. People naturally gravitate towards the cheerful Fire CF's warmth and friendliness.

Compulsive cheerfulness

The habit of cheering others up can become compulsive, however, and the Fire CF may feel compelled to try to cheer others up. Fun can become the be-all and end-all. They often find it difficult to believe that anyone would rather be in any state other than a jolly one. The person they are 'cheering up' may prefer to stay with their feelings and in this case the Fire CF's attitude of 'looking on the bright side' can be annoying rather than pleasing. If pushed away the Fire CF may end up feeling rejected.

Being happy is an important issue for many Fire CFs. Deep down they think that if they can make other people happy it will result in them being happy and contented too. If they are in a bad atmosphere, for example, if they think a person doesn't like them, they may find it difficult to function well and may be unable to think clearly or to work.

Although they have this ability to be happy, many Fire CFs know that their joy does not run deep. When a Fire CF is asked 'when did you last feel *truly* joyful?' they will often find it hard to think of any time at all. They may have been 'happy', 'playful', 'enthusiastic' or 'optimistic', but real joy, joy that comes from an open and peaceful Heart, eludes them.

Patient Example

A Fire CF told her practitioner that she had difficulty finding joy in her life, 'but that doesn't mean I'm walking around feeling miserable all the time'. She also said that she liked to feel jolly and happy but underneath this she felt lonely. The loneliness was not because she was on her own, in fact the more people who were around the more isolated she would sometimes feel. 'Sometimes I put the barriers up and I don't want to let anyone in.'

At the extreme, Fire CFs can become too stimulated and over joyful. In this case they may seem to be on a 'high' for a period of time. When they are feeling 'up' they may be always on the go and constantly talking and laughing. In small amounts this can be stimulating but in larger doses it can become too much for others to be around. People who are 'up' in this way tend to be insensitive to other people's difficulties or needs. One Fire CF described that she would go up 'like being on a cloud' and would float along feeling high, always knowing she might fall off. She did not mind this, however, because it was so good to be on top of the cloud, even if it was only for a while.

The *Huainanzi*, Chapter 1, describes how joy and sadness follow each other:

> The great drum and bells are set up, the orchestra of flutists [sic] and lutinists [sic] are in position, the cushions and ivory-poled canopies are arranged and seductive courtesans take their places. Out come the wine flasks as goblets are passed round over the course of feasting which joins day to night. Soaring birds are downed with bow and arrow; hunting dogs flush hare and fox. This

is called pleasure. Certainly excitement and violent agitation stir up our hearts and work their seductions upon us. But no sooner have the wagons been unhitched and the horses turned out to rest, the flasks emptied and the music ended, when suddenly the heart contracts as if in mourning. We feel the bereavement of great loss.

How is that possible? Because instead of bringing joy from inside to outside, we have tried to bring rejoicing from outside to inside. The music rings out and we are full of joy, but when the tune ends we are distressed.

Sadness and joy follow each other and give birth to each other. The vital spirit moves in a disorderly way, without knowing a moment's respite.

(quoted in Larre et al., 1986, p. 96)

Miserable

The desire to show a happy face can be deeply ingrained in a Fire CF's psyche. When they are sad they are likely to hide their feelings and pretend that they are feeling happy by showing a bright smile to the world. Deep inside they may be hiding a lack of self-confidence and suspect that they won't be liked or loved if they show their real feelings. In this case it is only when Fire CFs feels very 'safe' that they can show their sadness. This may not always make it easy for their partners.

Patient Example

A Fire CF commented to her practitioner that her husband sometimes got upset because when she was with him she was 'as miserable as sin'. Later when she went out to see somebody she suddenly became the life and soul of the party. 'We can have a good time together, but he doesn't understand that he is one of the few people I feel safe to show my sad side to as well.'

Because they have a self-image of being a 'happy person', many Fire CFs cut themselves off from their sadness. It sits inside them. In time their misery builds up. It then only takes a small incident or an upsetting remark for all the unhappiness that has previously been hidden to come to the surface. It may come out in one giant wave and Fire CFs may need to cry in order to let out their sad feelings. The person who appears to have induced the sadness with a trivial remark may be left feeling bewildered and may not understand why the person has had such a strong

reaction. When Fire CFs experience and release their sadness this may allow them to reconnect to their inner happiness.

Like their enthusiasm, a Fire CF's sadness can be catching too. They can drag others down with their gloom and misery.

Self-obsession

Fire CFs can become so low that they become rather self-obsessed. Their Heart, the Supreme Controller, can be so disturbed that they can only think, feel and talk about themselves. The most inconsequential remarks can be blown up to become a serious slight. When not talking about themselves they may cry in desolation and despair. If this happens Fire CFs can find it impossible to laugh or even begin to be able to raise a smile on their faces. It is as if the facial muscles just won't move upwards. If they ever felt happy it is a vague and distant memory.

When a Fire CF is feeling so low, others who have previously enjoyed their warmth may try hard to support them, but may find the Fire CF pushing them away. Although Fire CFs want reassurance that they are loveable, this is often the time when they can least take it in. Once they've rejected all those around them and no one makes contact anymore they have proved to themselves that no one loves them.

Open and overly sociable – closed and isolated

Most Fire CFs put a high value on personal connections and relationships. At the same time connections and relationships can seem threatening. If the Heart-Protector does not open and close appropriately, the Fire CF can be wide open to others. This may cause them to crave intimacy and relationships to such a degree that they miss out on some important 'stages' of making contact.

The stages of relating

In order to have intimate sexual relationships people go through many of these 'stages' and will often proceed carefully. First they might feel attracted to a person. Next they might make contact and get to know the person better. If things go well they may go on to have a relationship and later the relationship may become more committed. It is usually when they share more intimacy that they also may go on to develop a sexual relationship.

The Fire CF may miss out on some of the middle stages of relating and jump right into an intimate relationship. This is sometimes referred to as 'unearned intimacy'. In the desire for closeness they may not have stopped to consider all of the implications of having a close connection with the person in question. The result may be relationships that start with great passion, but later fail.

Overly open

Some Fire CFs, however, may want to be open with everybody and think that everyone they meet is their best or intimate friend. At best this can be charming, but it can seem inappropriate to those at the receiving end. For example, earlier in the chapter it was mentioned that it is normal to have more formal relationships with some people than others. Most people will have a formal relationship with their bank manager. A Fire CF may feel hurt and rejected when turned down for a loan even though the bank manager's decision is not personal but is based on objective criteria.

A practitioner, who was not a Fire CF, talked about her experiences when treating Fire CFs. She said she found that they often opened up too much and revealed everything about themselves too soon. 'I find that they can sometimes tell me too much. Everything about them comes out before I even know them. I end up feeling like I have to put them back together again because they've been too open and have lost all sense of their boundaries.'

Because of a compulsion to be liked, some Fire CFs try to please everyone and are even friendly to the people that they don't particularly like. As one Fire CF said, 'Even if I don't like someone I still value their opinion of me so I do my best to be nice to them and make them like me.'

Patient Example

A student talked about her partner who was a Fire CF. She said she found him confusing and amusing at times. He ran his own business and would often be doing things such as having a conversation about the finance of the company with the cleaner, 'People think he can't keep secrets but he's just sorting out his own thoughts. He's probably having an open conversation with himself!'

Because of their openness many Fire CFs can become skilled at quickly making contact with other people. For example, some can talk to strangers and make deep connections. Others just enjoy chatting to whoever they meet. The person holding the attention of everyone in the launderette, hairdressers or local store may well be a Fire CF. When they get home they may be sad and miserable, but while they were out they had an enjoyable time brightening up others' lives.

Isolated and withdrawn

Some Fire CFs find it difficult to relate to those around them at all. Outwardly they may seem friendly but inwardly they are withdrawn and closed off. Not relating closely means that they don't have to strain themselves whilst in other people's company. They might wish they had an intimate relationship but the benefits of not having one are greater. If someone hurts them, they may find it difficult to deal with the pain so this will be a further reason to push people away.

Patient Example

An elderly Fire CF patient was prone to atrial fibrillation. This most often happened after she felt that she had 'strained' herself entertaining. She felt obliged to be the perfect hostess and create a happy atmosphere, but it exhausted her and was sometimes at a high price.

Some Fire CFs like to be alone and find security and relaxation in their own company as they lack confidence around other people. As a result they may rarely socialise and have difficulties going out to social events such as dinners or parties. Because of their outward gaiety it is easy to assume that Fire CFs love to party. This is true for a few Fire CFs, especially when they know the people they are meeting. Meeting new people, however, makes many Fire CFs unsure of themselves. These Fire CFs find being outgoing and chatty a real strain and like to have a few drinks to give their Fire a temporary boost. Many Fire CFs prefer to have a few people around them that they know and trust. Trusted friends are less likely to hurt them. New acquaintances are an unknown quantity.

> **Patient Example**
>
> Some Fire CFs think they don't need others around, at least until they are no longer with them. One Fire CF patient admitted that she loved being on her own, as long as people rang to check that she was OK. She would never ring them because she assumed that they would not want to hear from her.

Some Fire CFs swing between making good connections with others then breaking off contact. One Fire CF told her practitioner that she thought she had set herself up for a fall. She had recently moved to a place where she didn't know anyone and although she felt it was not appropriate for anyone to look after her, she felt very hurt when the new neighbours didn't come round and make contact. This was in spite of the fact that she never attempted to contact them. Consequently she was very lonely for a while.

Some Fire CFs withdraw into themselves and find it difficult to relate to people, especially ones they don't know and trust. Others find that they feel better if they perform to an audience. This may be performing on a stage or taking centre stage in some other area of their life.

Clowning – earnest

Natural performers

The Heart governs 'the radiance of the *shen*'. Many Fire CFs are natural performers. It is not surprising that many of British comedy's most famous names – Benny Hill, Eric Morecambe, Frankie Howerd, Tony Hancock, Billy Connolly, Lenny Henry, Tommy Cooper, Kenneth Williams and Les Dawson, to name a few – were or are all probably Fire CFs. Making people laugh can make a Fire CF feel more loveable and give them a better sense of their worth. Some of these comedians, Tony Hancock, for example, made people laugh by showing the funny side of being depressed. Billy Connolly has also gained many laughs by joking about his appallingly abusive childhood. Others such as Tommy Cooper, Les Dawson and Eric Morecambe have made people laugh by playing the fool.

Many of these comedians are now dead and died of heart conditions. People have said that Tommy Cooper and Eric Morecambe died 'in the way they would have most wanted to'. Both had heart attacks: Tommy Cooper on stage and Eric Morecambe in the wings of a theatre. Some died in sadness. Benny Hill was said to have died of a 'broken heart'. He died soon after being told that his TV contract would not be renewed. He was out of fashion and could no longer do the thing he loved the most.

Most Fire CFs are not famous, but many still love to entertain in their own environment. These people may perform by playing the fool in their place of work, by lecturing in a classroom, by making their friends laugh or by entertaining their children. It doesn't matter as long as they have an audience. Many Fire CFs played the class clown when they were young or enjoyed making others laugh at their crazy antics. As one Fire CF said, 'I was like an electric circuit. I was only switched on when there were other people around.'

> **Patient Example**
>
> A Fire CF related to his practitioner that he had had a difficult time when he was 9 years old. He had moved to a new school and couldn't make friends. No one liked him, partly because he was intelligent and did well in his exams. When he started to get bullied he found an innovative way of dealing with the situation by playing the class fool. 'Suddenly I was popular, but I didn't do well in my school work any more. It wasn't until I was in my teens that I realised that in order to be popular I had missed out on a large part of my education and I had a lot of catching up to do.'

It is hard for some practitioners to understand that 'having a ball' may be a good indicator of their patient's constitutional imbalance. Having missed a diagnosis of Fire many students have commented that, 'I thought that their Fire was really good', not realising that if the patient is being extremely entertaining and making them laugh more than usual, this may be the clowning end of a Fire spectrum.

Being earnest and serious

At the other end of the spectrum some Fire CFs are extremely solemn and take themselves very seriously. When other people are in the presence of Fire CFs who are earnest they notice that there is very little laughter around. If others make a joke Fire CFs may not even perceive that anything has been said in jest or if they did they pretend they didn't notice. A heavy atmosphere can be created that is hard to lift.

Vulnerable – over-protected

When a patient's Fire Element is out of balance their ability to have 'heart contact' with another person can become strained. This may be particularly reflected in their relationships. This is especially true when the predominant Organ in distress is the Heart or Heart-Protector and may be less marked in people whose Small Intestine or Triple Burner is the primary Organ.

Exposed and unprotected

When a person 'falls in love' the mutual attraction and good feelings can create a feeling of well-being and happiness and a person can feel 'high'. Fire CFs can be especially affected, but the usual opening and closing of the Heart and Heart-Protector can come under even more strain than usual. Sometimes Fire CFs can 'love' with such complete passion and abandon that they wish only to please their partner in everything they do and say. At first this may be fine, but later when the initial 'honeymoon period' has finished it creates problems.

The more Fire CFs try to please the more they can become dependent on their partner. Their sense of their own self diminishes. They then become increasingly vulnerable and may feel out of control. The likeable and cheerful person that the partner was first attracted to may have disappeared leaving a vulnerable 'people pleaser' who seems to have no identity at all.

Often in this situation the Fire CF is able to back off and regain a sense of themselves as separate from their partner. If both partners want the relationship to succeed, the Fire CF must then come back into the relationship with a renewed sense of independence.

Overly open

In certain situations, however, a downward spiral in the relationship may begin. The partner finds she or he is 'walking on egg shells' around the Fire CF, who demands never to be criticised or even momentarily ignored. Any negativity from the partner will cause the Fire CF to feel battered and 'kicked' emotionally. In effect this stops the partner from being true to him or herself and the relationship comes under threat. The Fire CF starts to walk around with what amounts to a 'kick me' label hanging around her or his neck and the resulting strain on both partners may cause the relationship to break down.

Fire CFs who are in reasonably good health in their spirit and are less vulnerable may be able to open up and close down appropriately. When the Heart and Heart-Protector are wide open a vicious circle of feeling kicked and being too open to protect themselves can make the Fire CF feel even more vulnerable.

Feeling easily hurt

The vulnerability described above doesn't only happen in close relationships. It can also occur with anyone who is important to them, such as a friend, a boss or relations. It can especially happen when the Fire CF feels a strong need to please or be liked. For instance, Fire CFs may be so sensitive to other people that they take offence when others are only mildly teasing. One Fire CF described how as a child she would often get upset by her friends' light-hearted antics. She burst into tears when they played tricks on her like making her an 'apple pie' bed. She thought that this was their way of showing that they no longer liked her. She subsequently had a history of breaking up and then making up in friendships. Many years later, after she'd had acupuncture treatment and felt less vulnerable, she realised that it was she who had had the problems, not them.

Earlier in the chapter it was said that Fire CFs can be vulnerable in some group situations. They may desire to be liked so much that if, for instance, they don't immediately feel welcomed by a new group, they may retreat into a shell. Fire CFs may want to be involved but be shy of pushing themselves forward. As a result they may feel as if they have been invisible to the group and go home feeling devastated because they have been left out. Making new friends takes time and the desire of the Fire CF for immediate intimacy may make them impatient.

Over-protected

Fire CFs who have felt hurt or abandoned too often may react by keeping their hearts tightly closed off to other people. If this is the case they may find it difficult to have any form of close relationship. On the surface they may appear to be easy to relate to but as soon as a relationship appears to be going deeper the gates of the Heart-Protector immediately close down. The Fire CF may then end the relationship because it is too threatening or may withdraw and stop showing affection. An intimate relationship feels too risky for them. On the surface the Fire CF may seem invulnerable and to have no emotions. The 'iron bars' on the chest are keeping people out ensuring that the Fire CF is not hurt. But no love can reach them either.

Patient Example

A Fire CF told her practitioner that she had had a happy childhood. Her mother, however, always said that 'she had never got to the bottom of me, as I always remained slightly aloof.' The patient said that she could still be aloof and that her relationships had been difficult. 'If I had a new relationship now I'd cope better but I've been told that I'm very closed and cold. I'm think I'm very scared of people getting too close to me. It takes a long time for me to trust them.'

Some Fire CFs prevent relationships from arising by hiding their attraction to others. At a party or social event if someone who looks interesting catches their eye they may immediately look away or feign a lack of interest. All eye contact is then cut off and the interested person thinks they have no appeal and goes away. It can seem too dangerous for the Fire CF to show that any attraction could be mutual. Fire CFs who don't love themselves can't imagine that another would find them likeable (or loveable) in return. The Fire CF might even think that anyone interested in them can't be very special. A special person would look for someone else.

Volatile, passionate – flat

Fluctuating emotions

Many Fire CFs lack stability in their emotions and find that they are constantly going up and down. The change from feeling very high to very low may happen in a matter of only a few moments. They may become rather like Jekyll and Hyde and forget how they were before. When they feel down they feel as if they've always been miserable. When they feel up they forget that they were ever unhappy. For some Fire CFs the sudden switch from being joyful to being sad may happen for no obvious reason. For others, the changes in their emotions often relate directly to their relationships with other people. For example, they might wake up feeling miserable. They might then be boosted by someone who is nice to them or who gives them a compliment. Later in the day their mood may vary according to the warmth of the contact they have with others.

For some Fire CFs their emotions going up and down feel so overwhelming that they may struggle to find stability. Others, however, may prefer to have the excitement generated by the ups and downs.

Feeling flat

Some Fire CFs experience feeling flat and low for lengthy periods. This is more a state of monotony and dullness than the state of being actively sad and miserable as discussed earlier in this chapter. They may find it difficult to raise themselves up out of this gloom and life becomes uninteresting and grey. When the Fire CF feels this way, the practitioner may correspondingly feel flat and uninspired when she or he is with them.

Patient Example

A Fire CF described how her emotions could fluctuate in the space of 10 minutes. 'I can go from feeling fine to not feeling fine and in that time I can change quite fundamentally.' She described herself as being a 'mass of contradictions' in relation to people. She sometimes liked people to be around but sometimes not. 'I want to choose. I might suddenly want my own space. It can come on suddenly. I can have a house full of people and suddenly I want them to go. I must be hell to live with!'

In order to counteract this feeling of flatness it is not surprising that some Fire CFs continually look for sensation. To do this they may continually search for activities that keep them stimulated and excited. Whatever they do, they may do with great passion but this may later fizzle out as their Fire can't hold the intensity.

To stimulate their excitement they may watch exciting films, read romantic novels or just live through other people's lives on TV soaps or other programmes. Alternatively they may enjoy the feeling of falling passionately 'in love', but be looking around for a new love interest when the initial excitement disappears. As a result relationships never develop beyond the initial stages.

Patient Example

A Fire CF described going on holiday with her father for 10 days. 'At the end of the 10 days I felt sluggish, heavy, had toe ache and a sore back. It was no fun. It wasn't negative, just not positively good. It made me realise how many props I had in everyday life like radio, TV, phoning people and seeing people. When I'm positive I feel more energy, brighter, happier and it's easier to relate to people and I'm more relaxed. When I'm feeling low I hide behind other people in social situations and need my props more.'

Sometimes Fire CFs succumb to finding excitement and stimulation through drugs, drink or stimulants. The buzz that these give can become addictive. Although any CF has the potential to become dependent on stimulants, the reason for each will differ. For the Fire CF it is often the craving for excitement in order to cover up the underlying state of feeling that life is flat and monotonous.

Creating stability

As they become healthier Fire CFs can usually find ways to help them to retain their stability and stop their emotional lives from seeming like a roller coaster. Some may find that meditation or deep relaxation helps them to find a more comfortable and peaceful place to settle inside. It has been said that 'meditation is the exercise for the heart' (Hill, 2000, p. 164) and that to settle and calm the Heart is better than physical exercise for keeping the Fire CF healthy.

Creating good relationships with friends, family or partners can help Fire CFs to retain their stability. When entering a committed relationship the Fire CF may 'test' their partner's love by continuously questioning whether they are really loved or by pushing the partner away for periods of time. A Fire CF who admitted sabotaging her relationships commented, 'A person has to keep saying they love me, but if they say it too many times I won't believe it'.

Over time, if the partner proves that they are willing to stay in the relationship, the Fire CF may feel more secure and stable. The Fire CF may, however, never trust that they are *truly* loveable until they learn to love themselves.

Summary

1 A diagnosis of a Fire CF is made primarily by observation of a lack of red or red facial colour, a lack of laughing or laughing voice tone, a scorched odour and imbalance in the emotion joy.

2 Fire CFs tend to have issues and difficulties with:
   - love and warmth
   - emotional volatility
   - closeness and intimacy
   - happiness
   - clarity and confusion

3 Because of these issues Fire CFs' behaviour and responses can become inappropriate and swing between these extremes:

   - compulsively cheerful ＿＿＿＿＿ miserable
   - open and overly sociable ＿＿＿＿＿ closed and isolated
   - clowning ＿＿＿＿＿ earnest
   - vulnerable ＿＿＿＿＿ over-protected
   - volatile ＿＿＿＿＿ flat

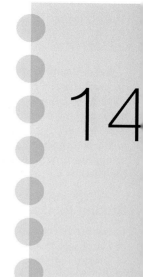

Earth – key resonances

Earth as a symbol

The character for Earth

The Chinese character for Earth is *tu*. This character is composed of two horizontal lines and one vertical line. The top horizontal line represents the surface soil and the second line the subsoil. The vertical line represents all things that are produced by the Earth (Weiger, 1965, lesson 81A). The character therefore represents the two key qualities of Earth – nourishment and stability.

The Earth Element in nature

The Earth as a provider

Seeds lie in the soil, seemingly inert, throughout the winter. In the spring they start to burst forth and grow and by the summer the plants are in full bloom. In late summer farmers harvest their crops. This is the time when Europeans hold the Harvest Festival and people traditionally give thanks for the products of the earth.

Caring for the earth

If the seeds are of high quality, the weather favourable and the soil well prepared and nourished, then the earth bears many fruits and people feast on them. In order that the fruits of the earth are nourishing and of high quality, the soil needs to be fertile. At one time farmers worked with nature and respected the needs of the earth. For instance, they would regularly allow the land to rest by alternating the crops and by leaving some fields to lie fallow. Farmers would also nourish the soil using natural compost derived from animal and vegetable waste products that were fed back into the earth. This would create a continuing ecological cycle and allow the soil to feed us with wholesome and nutritious crops.

DOI: 10.1016/B978-0-7020-3175-5.00014-9

Recently, however, many farmers under pressures of productivity have strained the capacity of the earth by poisoning the soil with chemical fertilisers, not returning compost to nourish it and not allowing it to rest by lying fallow. The earth becomes less fertile and the harvested crops are of a less nourishing standard, sometimes toxic with pesticides. Although the earth is a provider, it also needs to be cared for.

Storing food and energy

Foods are harvested in one season, often to be used in a later season. Our ancestors developed many ways of preserving grains and fruits so that the produce of the harvest could be spread over time. Several points on the Stomach and Spleen channels refer to this process. Stomach 14, Storehouse, and St 4, Earth Granary, are examples. Storehouses and granaries indicate that the function of Earth includes the storage of nourishment.

The Earth Element in life

An imbalanced Earth Element can also create famine. This can be a physical one with the Earth Organs unable to transform our food into nourishing *qi*. The phrase 'you are what you eat' is only a partial truth. 'You are what you make of what you eat' is more accurate. When the Earth Element struggles to transform food into flesh and *qi*, people may feel tired and suffer from a wide range of physical symptoms.

The famine can also be on a mental or spirit level. Can we concentrate or remember what we have heard or read? Can we bring the projects of our life into harvest, give and receive support from others and raise our children? We may have difficulty 'reaping a harvest' in our lives and never feel that what we have put into our lives has borne fruit. Chronic feelings of dissatisfaction often afflict Earth CFs. Being unable to reap on the level of mind and spirit can be as important as any physical symptoms.

Humans stand 'between Heaven and Earth'

Humans stand 'between Heaven and Earth'. Our head should be in the heavens so that we can take in the 'heavenly' *qi* and our feet on the earth so that we can be grounded and stable.

An earthquake or tremor is one of the few times when the earth is not stable beneath us. It induces strong feelings of shock and insecurity. After an experience of an earthquake it can take a long time to recover equilibrium and feel balanced again. When people have an imbalance in their Earth Element they can easily feel unstable in a way that is similar to the instability aroused when there is an earthquake.

People may also feel insecure and unsafe inside for many other reasons. The Earth Element may be too dry, in which case it may be crumbling and cracking or feeling as if it is collapsing. At the other extreme the Earth may have become waterlogged, making us 'damp' and as if we are muddy inside. Damp can make us feel heavy in our bodies and we may have difficulty thinking clearly or wanting to move.

The Earth as our mother

The Earth Element is often compared to a mother. The character *tu di* is often used in this respect (see Weiger, 1965, lessons 81A (*tu*) and 107B (*di*)). This character often represents the Earth when it is coupled with Heaven. It signifies the soil on which plants grow, but also the ability of the earth to be like a mother (Larre and Rochat de la Vallée, 2004, p. 20).

The mother and nurturing

Like the earth itself, our mothers or main carers provide us with support and security when we are young. Over time, and especially in the context of a family, we learn how to care for others and to care for ourselves.

In the womb we are connected to our mother via the umbilical cord which is attached at the physical centre of the body. When the cord is cut we are put to the breast and our mother nourishes us with her milk. After we have been weaned our mother helps to connect us to the world and we gradually learn to have our own identity. In the best situation our mother feeds, supports and loves us unconditionally. She also gives us tactile comfort by holding and caressing us. By taking in nourishment from our mother we gain stability. We slowly make the transition from dependence to independence.

If a person is born as an Earth CF the relationship with the mother may be affected. The Earth CF may be less able to receive nourishment and care from the mother. This can make a balanced relationship between the mother and the child more difficult.

The Earth Element in relation to the other Elements

The Earth Element interacts with the other Elements through the *sheng* and *ke* cycles (see Chapter 2, this volume).

Earth is the mother of Metal

Along the *sheng* cycle Earth hardens to create Metal. The metal lying within the earth is often compared to trace minerals that give the soil extra quality and richness. When patients have signs and symptoms associated with the Metal Element this may be caused by imbalance in the Earth Element, the mother. For example, chest problems and/or asthma can be caused by an Earth imbalance. If the Earth is the original cause, treating it will benefit the person more permanently whilst treating the Metal will have only a temporary effect.

Fire is the mother of Earth

When a fire burns ashes are left and these become part of the Earth. Patients with obvious Earth symptoms such as digestive complaints or a sense of insecurity may have developed these because the Fire, the mother, was out of balance. The practitioner may treat the mother to assist the child and give it more stability.

Wood controls Earth

The most common situation occurring between Wood and Earth is one of Wood over-controlling the Earth. When Wood invades Earth in this way it can cause many symptoms including a churning feeling in the stomach, indigestion and/or nausea. By calming the Wood and strengthening the Earth, the Wood settles and the balance returns to normal.

Earth controls Water

If a river has burst its banks or is flowing too rapidly, the situation can be rectified by damming the river up with earth. In patients the Earth may not control the body fluids and the water, causing symptoms of 'dampness' and oedema. This can cause signs and symptoms physically, mentally and spiritually and patients may complain of feeling heavy, tired, listless, muzzy-headed and demotivated.

The Earth in the centre

As well as being situated between the Fire and Metal Elements in the *sheng* cycle, the Earth Element is sometimes placed in a central position between all the other Elements. *Su Wen* Chapter 4 states that, 'The central region is the Earth' (Larre and Rochat de la Vallée, 2004, p. 16).

In its central position the Earth is the pivot for all of the other Elements which encircle and spin around it. It is a place of stability within the body, mind and spirit. From this stable anchor, change and growth can take place. Our food can be transformed and processed by the Stomach and Spleen and turned into *qi* that nourishes the body, mind and spirit.

The key Earth resonances
(Table 14.1)

The colour for Earth is yellow

Su Wen Chapter 10 states that, 'Yellow corresponds to the Spleen' (Anonymous, 1979a, p. 27). The Chinese word for yellow is *huang*.

The colour in nature

In China the colour 'yellow' is associated more with the colour of soil or ploughed earth than, for example, the colour of a lemon. The Yellow River is called the Huang He and to many Chinese people *huang* is

Table 14.1 Key Earth resonances

Colour	Yellow
Sound	Singing
Emotion	Sympathy
Odour	Fragrant

Singing

The singing voice tone occurs naturally when we sing a lullaby with a child in our arms, or when we try to soothe an anxious or distressed animal or person. It might also occur when we are holding a baby, speaking to someone who is ill, or supporting a work colleague who is going through a difficult time. When this voice tone consistently occurs out of context it indicates an Earth imbalance.

always associated with the colour of this river. The Yellow River is famous for silting up and the efforts both to unblock and rechannel the flow are thought to provide a conceptual background for understanding the flow of *qi* in the body and the need to guide and unblock it (Xinghua and Baron, 2001, pp. 12–15). Other examples of yellow in nature are the colour of millet and a field of grain ripe for harvesting.

The voice tone of singing

The singing voice has an increased variation in pitch. The voice goes up and down in pitch more frequently and to a greater extreme than normal. One way to detect a singing voice tone is to imagine a situation where you might use it. For example, a child has been hurt through no fault of her own. She is now resting comfortably, but in some pain and has been confined to bed. She is going to miss her best friend's birthday party and is very disappointed. In your mind, say to her, 'I am so sorry. You're a poor old thing.' Your voice will naturally become more singing than usual.

The facial colour

When a person's Earth Element is imbalanced it will manifest as a yellow or earthy colour on the face. Yellow indicating that the Earth is out of balance will be seen beside or under the eyes. It may vary in colour from a bright yellow to the muddier, earthy yellow.[1]

The sound for Earth is singing

The norm of singing

Some languages and dialects naturally have a singing tone. This is especially true of the accents of country people more than town-dwellers. Welsh people, for example, have very sing-song voices. Many Welsh people also sing a lot and they probably have more choirs per head of population than in any other country. When assessing the voice of someone from Wales, it is useful to have a norm based on other Welsh people. Within Welsh speakers, there will be those who sing more and have a singing tone out of context. The norms against which the practitioner measures the speaker will have to take the norms of the language and culture into consideration.

The character for singing

The character for singing is *chang*. This character is made up of two radicals. The first, *kou*, represents a mouth and the second, *chang*, represents splendour or glory (Weiger, 1965, lesson 72A (*kou*) and lesson 73A (*chang*)). Together this can be translated as 'splendour emanating from the mouth'.

The odour for Earth is fragrant

The character for fragrant

---

[1]Yellow on the face can also indicate the presence of excess body fluids causing Dampness in the body. Yellow indicating Damp will be seen more around the mouth and on the cheeks. Because an imbalanced Earth often leads to Damp, the practitioner will frequently find yellow in both places.

The Chinese character for fragrant is *xiang* (Weiger, 1965, lessons 73 or 121I). This character can be translated as an agreeable savour or odour of fermented grain or the odour of fermented millet.

This is probably the most ineptly named odour. 'Fragrant' is usually applied to flowers and is thought to be pleasing, but this odour is usually a less than pleasing smell. It is cloying, sickly-sweet and with a tendency to linger in the nostrils and the room.

The emotion for Earth is over-thinking, worry and/or sympathy

The character for worry or over-thinking

si

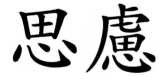

si lu

Si is one of the emotions associated with the Earth Element. This is sometimes translated as over-thinking or obsessive thought, and can also be called preoccupation, rumination or cogitation. Weiger (1965, lesson 40A) says of this character, 'When one is thinking, the vital fluid of the Heart ascends to the brain'. *Si* is sometimes combined with *lu* as in *si lu*, where *lu* means to meditate (Weiger, 1965, lesson 40A for *si lu*).

The character for *si* consists of a brain with the Heart radical below it. It demonstrates the nature of thinking – which the Chinese believed required the brain to be in communication with the Heart. If the Heart/brain connection is lost, the images of the mind do not constitute focused thinking. There is a difference between directed, purposeful thought and random images floating through the mind. When the connection between the brain and the Heart is lost, thoughts can become obsessive and repetitive. *Su Wen* Chapter 39 states, 'When there is obsessive thought, the *qi* is knotted' (Larre and Rochat de la Vallée, 1996, p. 159).

It is not that worry produces intense movements of *qi* as do the emotions of fear, anger, joy and grief. In this sense si does not truly describe an emotion.

Sympathy

Another emotion commonly associated with the Earth Element is sympathy. Although this is not mentioned in Chinese texts, J. R. Worsley observed that this emotion becomes affected when people have an imbalanced Earth Element. This is an innovation in Chinese medicine in Five Element Constitutional Acupuncture. It is a significant contribution to an understanding of the Five Elements.

There are two directions for sympathy, giving it and receiving it. Both the ability to give sympathy and the ability to receive it are related to Earth. When Earth is in relative balance, both of these, the giving and the receiving, are smooth and function appropriately.

What is the core emotion for Earth?

As with the other Elements there are emotions or feelings that are natural, appropriate and resonate with the Element. It is not so easy to label Earth's core emotion. 'Worry', 'over-thinking' and 'concern' describe an aspect of Earth's dysfunction, but they do not touch the heart of the Earth emotion. J. R. Worsley introduced the term sympathy, which is as good a word as we have in English.

It helps to consider the context of sympathy. It comes out of mankind's social nature. Although there are odd exceptions, humans cannot or do not live alone. Individuals belong to various communities, for example, families, tribes, groups of friends, neighbourhoods, gangs, fans of a sports team, the team itself, work colleagues, professional associations, committee members, citizens of a country, and so on.

People within a group have either common aims and/or an emotional bond. These bonds increase the person's awareness of others' welfare and can stimulate mutual support. Support can range from physical help to verbal and non-verbal acknowledgement of another's predicament. Slightly different 'feelings' are associated with giving and receiving 'sympathy'. But both are resonant with a person's Earth Element.

These feelings are more easily understood by going back to our first dependence, the relationship to our mother or initial carer. Babies who are never held or touched can die. Our early receiving of 'sympathy' is being held and fed. In the mother there is a natural urge to hold, feed and care for. As we get older, the nature of sympathy or support changes, reflecting our varying degrees of dependence and independence. One challenge is to maintain a balance between being independent and allowing ourselves to be cared for when appropriate. Another challenge is to maintain a balance between caring for ourselves and being sensitive to the needs of others.

Sympathy at different ages

It is useful to consider how the nature of appropriate sympathy or support changes with age. When a 4-year-old falls and scrapes a knee, the sympathy expressed by the mother will probably involve both attention to the injury and some physical comfort. For example, the mother may find out if it's serious and ask if it needs a bandage or plaster. She may also kiss it better, sit her child on her lap and/or give her or him a hug.

When an adult complains about a hard day at work with an even worse prospect tomorrow, another adult does not behave like the mother. Instead, they give some acknowledgement, for example, 'Yes, this sounds like a difficult time for you.' If the feeling is authentic and heartfelt the voice tone and facial expression will be congruent. Sometimes a hug and a cuddle may well be appreciated. The naturalness of what the mother does seems obvious. What the acknowledgement does for the adult is similar and also different. For adults, the net result is that the burden is somewhat eased and they often feel better knowing that someone appreciates their situation.

A writer, on the subject of emotions, describes a feeling he had at 15 when he was welcomed into a rock band. He had various descriptions, but, in short, it was a 'feeling of acceptance, of belonging, of being valued by a group of people whom I was proud to call my friends'. He later discovered that the Japanese had a word for this which he says is 'comfort in another person's complete acceptance'. He also refers to the original Chinese character, a breast on which the baby suckled. This suggests a feeling that is based early on in the act of suckling and that evolves and exists in a different form, as we grow older (see Evans, 2002, pp. 1–3).

As the child grows up two abilities arise. One is knowing how to give support, that is, expressing it at the right level. People do not usually put a 35-year-old on their laps and say 'There, there, it will be all right.' The other is for people to create a balance between getting support and giving it to others. Only taking or only giving does not indicate a balanced Earth.

The varieties and extremes of 'sympathy'

What happens when the natural flow of giving and receiving sympathy is not supported by a balanced Earth? The four most obvious patterns are:

1 excessively wanting sympathy and support
2 rejecting any help, support or sympathy from others
3 excessively feeling and giving sympathy
4 being untouched by others' distress.

These indicate an imbalanced Earth

Excessively craving sympathy and support

This pattern is not being able to truly receive sympathy in such a way as to satisfy the person. The way in which patients tell the practitioner about their symptoms is an excellent time to observe this aspect of a person. Sometimes, when the Earth *qi* is weak, food can appear in the stools undigested or not transformed. Similarly, a person can take in sympathy, but does not appreciate or benefit from it. It is similar to being given a box of chocolates and eating one after another and then, looking down at the empty box, wondering where they all went.

It is this lack of deep satisfaction that characterises this pattern. The person is often perceived as 'needy' owing to their compulsion to seek support and care from others. Their response to what they feel as others' lack of consideration and sympathy can be anger, withdrawal, agitation or depression.

Patient Example

A patient says: 'When I am not well, I just want someone to pay attention and listen to me. I go on and on and whinge and complain and I can't stop. I know I have lost friends, but I am very demanding and behave a bit like a spoiled brat. The rest of time I am fine with others.'

Rejecting sympathy

There are times and situations when it is normal to accept support or sympathy from others. Some Earth CFs find it difficult to accept sympathy. They might, for example, complain about their situation, but when they are given sympathy they decline it by denying that they complained or readjusting the information so their situation does not sound so bad. Other people do this because receiving care and sympathy was outside their experience as a child. They might feel the neediness but unconsciously feel that it is a sign of weakness. Thus, when given sympathy or support, they feel the need for it but in response they feel a stronger need to deny the neediness and behave as if they are independent. This is probably more common with men, but also occurs in women.

This pattern is often easy to miss. It is usually necessary for the practitioner to give sympathy and see if it evokes discomfort in the patient. Many people can take or leave sympathy, but when this pattern is marked, sympathy will provoke an awkwardness in the patient.

Excessively expressing sympathy

A common pattern demonstrated by Earth CFs is to be overly sympathetic. An example is people who are always looking after others, especially when their own needs are not being met. As C. S. Lewis wittily wrote about a character 'She is the sort of woman who lives for others – you can always tell the others by their hunted expression.' (*The Screwtape Letters*).

People with this tendency often find others' distress almost unbearable. The idea that their children or other family members are unhappy is often a source of great concern, frustration or sadness. Sad movies, the idea of cruelty to animals or the harsh fact of world poverty and famine are examples of situations that evoke intense feelings in such people.

This is not to suggest that caring for others is pathological. There are many situations in life when offering sympathy or assistance to others truly 'meets the needs of the situation'. It is pathological when people need to care a lot for others and especially if they do not care appropriately for themselves.

The stereotype of the Jewish mother illustrates a combination. She is excessively caring so as to be smothering ('eat an extra portion, you need it') and at the same time she puts out a very strong 'poor me, no one really cares' message.

Being untouched by others' distress

This pattern is most common in people who reject sympathy themselves. When other people are in need of some support or care, for example when ill, it evokes little feeling of sympathy in the person. It can even induce slight feelings of contempt or disdain. In extreme cases they are completely unmoved by suffering, especially if it is a consequence of the sufferer's own behaviour.

This hardening is characteristic. Whereas people who crave sympathy or who care a great deal for others can usually be described as tending to be 'soft', the hardness of those who reject sympathy and feel little for others is often striking.

Summary

Worry, over-thinking and over-concern are definitely part of the pathology associated with the Earth Element. We find, however, that sympathy and its variations also describe the normal and pathological emotional expressions that resonate with the Earth Element. In practice there is a range of words associated with the emotions of this Element (Table 14.2).

The supporting Earth resonances

These resonances are considerably less important than the 'key' resonances given above. They can often be used to indicate that a person's Earth Element is imbalanced but they do not necessarily point to it being the person's CF (Table 14.3).

Patient Example

An Earth CF was on a postgraduate training course. She disappeared every lunchtime and came back a few minutes late for the afternoon session. When asked about this she said that she was seeing patients who she was unable to accommodate in the evenings. It turned out that she worked 70+ hours a week, frequently didn't charge, and rarely had time for lunch or a proper evening meal. When asked what would happen if she didn't do her caring with such fervour she said she thought 'the whole world would collapse'.

Table 14.2 Examples of the range of emotions associated with the Earth Element

Worry	Obsession, over-thinking, fixation, fretfulness, angst, over-concern, insecurity
Sympathy	Over-concern, over-supportive, needy, over-condolence, commiseration
Lack of sympathy	Unsympathetic, uncaring

Table 14.3 Supporting Earth resonances	
Season	Late summer
Power	Harvest
Climate	Dampness/humidity
Sense Organ/Orifice	Mouth
Tissues and body parts	Muscles and flesh
Generates	Fat
Taste	Sweet

The season for Earth is late summer

The character for late summer

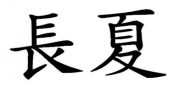

The character for late summer is *chang xia* (Weiger, 1965, lessons 113A and 160D). This character represents abundant long hair tied back by hand. This is an image of luxurious growth, suggesting that this time of year is when the harvest can be taken.

Late summer

As stated above, Earth is sometimes located in the centre of the other Elements but usually it takes its place in the *sheng* cycle between Fire and Metal. The latter arrangement is used by Five Element acupuncturists. It comes after the peak of high summer and before the leaves drop in autumn. This season is very marked in Northern China but in some countries it barely exists. The actual times will vary from country to country, but the growth of most plants has peaked and the harvesting of grains and fruits is taking place. (For example in Southern England, where the authors live, it usually starts in mid August and finishes in early October.)

What is most striking about this season is the sense of time standing still. The peak of *yang* is over and the days are getting shorter but the leaves are still on the trees and the weather can still be extremely warm. The melancholia of autumn is yet to begin. It is a time when *yin* and *yang* are finely balanced.

The power for Earth is harvest

The character for harvest

The character for harvest is *shou*. This character is made up of two radicals. The first represents tangled or creeping plants, and the second the right hand. By extension this might be translated as a hand picking the crops when they are fully grown (Weiger, 1965, lessons 45B and 43B).

Harvest

This is the time of year when crops come to fruition. At one time the harvest also meant carefully storing the crops so that there was a plentiful supply throughout the winter. If there had been adverse weather conditions there might have been no harvest. Nowadays we would import more food from other countries but at one time this would have led to a famine and not enough food for the winter months. At this time of year people traditionally gave thanks for an abundant harvest.

Practitioners might consider if their patients are reaping a harvest. For example are they gaining the benefits from eating good quality food. They may also ask whether they have psychologically benefited from what they have experienced. Does their study go into their mind and bear fruit? Can they transform what they take in into thoughts or ideas or whatever will be useful? Are they satisfied with what they have received or are they still hungry for more?

The climate of Earth is dampness or humidity

The character for dampness

The Chinese character for dampness is *shi* (Weiger, 1965, lessons 125A and 92E).

Humidity and dampness both refer to the atmosphere where there is a higher degree of moisture than normal. When people have 'Damp' then their body has a higher than appropriate degree of fluids. They may have oedema, a bloated abdomen or a muzzy feeling in the head. Like a humid atmosphere outside, they have too much moisture on the inside.

There is a relationship between good quality Earth and the occurrence of Damp. Earth transforms and, as it transforms, food and drink are moved and fluids distributed. When the Earth is weak, the transformation process is weak and fluids can accumulate.

One diagnostic consequence is that people with deficient Earth Elements usually dislike damp or humid weather. Too much Damp on the inside makes them more likely to complain about the excess damp on the outside. Such people are susceptible to joint pain, aching muscles, headaches or lethargy that is worsened by damp or humidity.

It is useful to ask patients how they respond to damp or humid weather. If they 'hate' it, then this suggests that their Earth is imbalanced.

In Chinese medicine, certain foods are classified as 'damp-forming'. Dairy products, all greasy foods and alcohol increase the damp in the body. Thus it becomes important to check a patient's food intake. The Earth cannot be expected to deal with an abnormal balance of foods that cause us to retain fluids. In the same way, in a location where the rain is excessive and the run-off from the soil poor, the earth becomes too sodden to grow many crops.

Patient Example

A practitioner had been struggling to help an Earth CF, who also had Damp. Progress had been slow, but in the process of a consultation the patient mentioned keeping the windows open during the winter. When asked why, she said that the walls of her flat were so wet that it was better to be cold and get them somewhat drier than it was to be warm. Her practitioner responded by encouraging her to buy a de-humidifier. Ultimately she changed her living situation.

The sense organ/orifice for Earth

The character for the mouth

The character for the mouth is *kou* (Weiger, 1965, lesson 72A).

The mouth and taste

The sense organ of Earth is that of taste and the orifice is the mouth. That the mouth and taste resonate with Earth is not surprising. The sustenance of the Earth enters our mouth and its taste is crucial. Taste guides what we eat. Unfortunately, people today are guided by many factors other than taste. The ability to taste foods for their freshness, nutritional value and relevance for oneself is often limited. *Ling Shu* Chapter 17 says:

> The energy of the Spleen is in connection with the mouth, when the Spleen is healthy, the mouth is able to absorb nourishment normally.
>
> (Anonymous, 1979a, Chapter 17)

If the Earth Element is healthy, people have a good sense of taste. If it is weak, people may lose their taste, have a sticky taste in the mouth or have difficulties with digestion.

The colour of the lips should be bright, red and moist. It is a poor sign when the lips are dry, dull and of a pale colour. Saliva should not be excessive or deficient. None of these confirms a CF diagnosis, but they do suggest some weakness of the Earth Element.

The tissues and body parts for Earth are muscles and flesh

The character for muscles and flesh

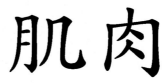

The character for muscles and flesh is *ji rou* (Weiger, 1965, lessons 65A (*jou*), 20A (*ji*) and 65A (*ju*)).

The muscles and flesh

The quality and function of the muscles and flesh depend on the *qi* of the Earth Element. Poor muscle tissue will indicate a weakness of the Earth Element. Lumps and swelling under the skin indicate poor transformation and thus a weakness of Earth.

The practitioner can feel the flesh for its smooth consistency in order to gauge the efficiency of the Stomach and Spleen's transformation process. This will give some insight into the balance of the patient's Earth Element, though it may not be the CF.

Earth generates fat

Fat is said to be generated by flesh. Excess fat, which sometimes occurs in lumps under the skin, is interpreted in Chinese medicine as Damp or as Phlegm, which is a thicker form of Damp. So any excess fat on the body suggests some weakness of the Earth. There are other weaknesses that might lead to fat, but imbalance in the Earth Element is one major one.

The taste for Earth is sweet

The character for sweet

The character for sweet is *kan* (Weiger, 1965, lesson 73B). This character literally means 'the sweetness of something held in the mouth'.

In *Su Wen* it states that, 'The Earth produces sweet flavours' (Veith, 1972, p. 119). Most people associate the sweet taste with the strong sugary taste of sweets, candies, cakes, chocolate and other foods commonly eaten in the West. The sweet flavour described by Chinese medicine is pre-white sugar and is a more subtle flavour. The sweet taste is found in many different foods – rice, carrots, corn, chicken, cabbage, pumpkin and peanuts – to name a few. In the herbal *'materia medicas'* of Chinese herbal medicine, the sweet taste is said to have a strengthening effect on the body.

Sweet is also the predominant taste of breast milk. It is the sole nourishment for babies in the first few months of their life and enables them to grow strong and healthy. If people eat a balanced amount of this subtle taste it will, like breast milk, be strengthening to their *qi*.

Many people do not stop at eating a small amount of this flavour, however, and start to crave it in large quantities. Eating too much sweet food will weaken the Earth Element and the Stomach and Spleen. Weakness of the Stomach and Spleen in turn creates a stronger craving for the sweet taste. A vicious cycle is produced. Often, the more depleted the Earth becomes the more we crave sweetness and the Stomach and Spleen correspondingly become even more deficient.

Summary

1. Along the *sheng* cycle Earth is the mother of Metal and Fire is the mother of Earth. Across the *ke* cycle Earth controls Water and Wood controls Earth.

2. A diagnosis of an Earth CF is made primarily by observation of a yellow facial colour, a singing voice, a fragrant odour and imbalance in the emotion of sympathy.

3. Worry and a lack of caring support are detrimental to the Earth Element.

4. When the Earth Element is imbalanced, the following tendencies arise:
   - excessively wanting sympathy and support
   - rejecting any help, support or sympathy from others
   - excessively feeling and giving sympathy
   - being untouched by others' distress

5. Other resonances include the season of late summer, humidity, the mouth, muscles and flesh, fat, the power of harvest and the sweet taste

Earth – The Organs

15

Introduction

The two Organs or Officials resonating with Earth are the Spleen, the *yin* Organ, and the Stomach, the *yang* Organ. Although their functions are different, there are also similarities.

The Spleen – the controller of transforming and transporting

(Table 15.1)

The Chinese understanding of the functions of the Spleen differs a great deal from the Western view. The Spleen functions according to Chinese medicine are greater and more fundamental to the healthy functioning of the body, mind and spirit. They tend to include some of the functions of the pancreas, which will be obvious as we proceed. Thus we continue to capitalise the first letter of 'spleen' to remind readers of the difference.

The character for the Spleen

The Chinese character for the Spleen is *pi* (Weiger, 1965, lessons 152C and 46E).

The character has the flesh radical on the left, indicating that is it an Organ, and a character on the right that means 'ordinary' or 'vulgar'. The character was originally a picture of a water vessel. This could be contrasted with a sacrificial vessel used only on special occasions. The ordinariness or vulgarity comes from the vessel's everyday use, which is like the work of the Spleen. The Spleen functions to control the digestive system and as such is as ordinary or common as a cook who is on duty 24 hours a day. Its work is basic. It does not have the glamour of the Liver, which is a general, or the Lung, which is a chancellor. We can compare this job to that of a mother who is always available to care for and support her family. A mother's job is an important one, often unacknowledged until she is ill or away.

Su Wen Chapter 8

Su Wen Chapter 8 says:

> The Stomach and Spleen are responsible for the storehouses and granaries. The five tastes stem from them.
>
> (Larre and Rochat de la Vallée, 1992b, p. 97)

DOI: 10.1016/B978-0-7020-3175-1.00015-8

Table 15.1 The Earth Element Officials/Organs

Organ/ Official	Colloquial name	Description from *Su Wen* Ch 8
Spleen	The Controller of Transforming and Transporting	The Stomach and Spleen are responsible for the storehouses and granaries. The five tastes stem from them
Stomach	The Controller of Rotting and Ripening	

This passage indicates how closely the Stomach and Spleen work together. All the other Officials in *Su Wen* Chapter 8 are listed separately.

The Spleen as transformer and transporter

The Spleen is primarily involved with transformation and transportation.

> Its functions [the Spleen's] are to master transportation and transformation, *yun hua*, to transmit and diffuse the *jing wei* (food essences) which supply nutrition, to raise the clear and lower the unclear. It is the source of transformations that produce the Blood.
>
> (Larre and Rochat de la Vallée, 2004, p. 152)

Thus the Spleen is described as the Official of transformation and transportation (see Felt and Zmiewski, 1993, p. 19; Maciocia, 2005, pp. 144–145). Transformation is mainly thought of as the conversion of food and fluids into *qi*. Hence the notion that the Earth Element is the main source of basic *qi*. Although the process goes through various stages, the Spleen is the Official overseeing this function. The mechanical breakdown of food in the mouth with the addition of saliva, the more extensive breakdown of food and fluids in the stomach, the movement of digesting material through the small intestine and into the large intestine and finally the movement of material to be excreted through the large intestine and out of the anus are all broadly under the control of the Spleen.

Although Five Element Constitutional Acupuncture does not use the understanding of the Substances (the 'Vital Substances', which are *qi* Blood, body fluids, *jing* and *shen*) and speaks only of *qi*, the Spleen is responsible for the transformation of food and fluids into Blood as well as *qi* (Maciocia, 2005, pp. 60–64).

The notion of transportation reflects the movement that accompanies the transformation process. It refers specifically to the movement of food essences, the various stages in the breakdown of food, and the capacity of the body to move fluids and prevent various imbalances of the fluids of the body, for example, oedema, fluid on the lungs, and joints that are 'damp' and prone to stiffness.

A breakdown in the transport system can also reflect mentally and spiritually. Thoughts also have to be processed and distributed throughout the body, mind and spirit. When the Spleen is weak, the moving and transforming power of the mind and spirit can deteriorate. Thinking may be poor and not convert into action. Concentration and memory are affected. People may also have obsessive thoughts or they may start worrying or become preoccupied. They can become obsessive or feel muzzy in the head.

Patient Example

An Earth CF patient said that sometimes she couldn't think clearly or think through something. When describing how this felt she said, 'My head feels like an impenetrable thicket. It's too much effort to think things through. My thoughts go round and round and I don't get anywhere. It's best to wait until I feel clearer.'

J. R. Worsley compares the Spleen to a transport manager controlling a fleet of lorries. When people are healthy the Spleen's job is easy. It receives the 'rotted and ripened' substances from the Stomach and then transforms and transports them. The lorries carry *qi* and other substances such as Blood and body fluids to every part of the body and mind–spirit (Worsley, 1998, p. 13.7). This allows all parts of the system to be nourished.

If people are unwell it can be compared to a breakdown in some of the lorries. The transport system doesn't work properly and the food and fluids don't reach their destination. Everything comes to a standstill. Physically this may result in the fluids not moving. Damp and Phlegm are formed and clog up the system, especially in the lower half of the body where people often accumulate fat. They may also feel tired and lethargic and not want to move around as a result of the breakdown in the transport system.

The direction of the Spleen

The main direction of the Spleen *qi* is upwards and it raises the clear *yang qi* to the head. If the Spleen is not creating good quality *qi*, then a person will probably feel tired. The direction of a tired person is clearly downward, wanting to sit down, lie down, slump and flop. This can be accompanied by a feeling of physical heaviness and emotionally by low-grade depression. Diarrhoea is an example of failure of the Spleen to move in an upward direction. When the Spleen is weak and fluids are not fully transformed, then the head can become unclear, reflecting the failure of the Spleen to raise clear *qi* to the head.

As well as taking the *qi* upwards, the Spleen also has a 'holding' function. For example, it helps to hold the Blood in the blood vessels. If the Spleen is weak, people may develop symptoms of bleeding, for example, uterine bleeding, nose bleeds, bruising or petechiae (red spots of blood in the skin). Characteristically, bleeding due to Spleen weakness is usually dribbling rather than gushing, and pale and watery rather than bright red and thick. The Spleen *qi* also holds the Organs in their correct positions. Prolapses can occur, for example, if the Spleen fails to hold the Organs in place.

The spirit of the Spleen – the *yi*

Yi is the spirit of the Spleen and can be translated as thought or intention.

The character for the *yi*

Li at the top of the character means 'to establish'. This is placed over the character *yue* meaning to speak – pictured as a mouth with a tongue in the middle. These, in turn, are on top of the character for the Heart (Weiger, 1965, lesson 73E). Overall, this character means 'the process of establishing meaning in the world with words that come from the Heart'. In the West we may assume that thinking should be separated from the Heart because the Heart introduces emotion and therefore irrationality into the thinking.

In Chinese medicine, however, the involvement of the Heart means that the thinking is grounded and the person is being true to themselves. The Spleen is responsible for 'applied thinking, studying, memorising, focusing, concentrating and generating ideas' (Maciocia, 2008, pp. 272–273).

The ability to think clearly and study

In practice, the nature of the *yi* means that the Spleen is responsible (along with the Heart) for our ability to think and study with clarity. The excessive use of the mind, for example, when cramming for exams or spending many hours a day thinking and writing can weaken the Spleen.

One of the major problems when the Spleen is imbalanced is the tendency for the person to become preoccupied, or at worst obsessed. *Si* or 'knotting' of the *qi* occurs and diminishes a person's ability to think one thought and then move on to another. This inability to think clearly can diminish a person's creativity, spontaneity and happiness.

Intention

Yi also describes 'intention'. This is a person's ability to focus the mind on a desired object. It is what has been described as the 'consciousness of potentials' (Kaptchuk, 2000, p. 10). If the Spleen and therefore the *yi* is weak, the ability to concentrate on work, or even another person's conversation, can be affected. In relation to the spirit, however, it diminishes people's ability to remain steadfast to their purpose. Agitation, insecurity or lethargy of the spirit can make it difficult for many people to stick to the paths they have chosen for themselves. This in turn easily leads to depression, anxiety and despair. Voltaire remarked: 'Madness is to think of too many things too fast, or of one thing exclusively.' He appears to be describing a pathology of the *yi*.

The ability of the *yi* to form ideas is used in the practice of *qi gong*. In some *qi gong* exercises a person's intention is to move *qi* through their body. For example, *qi* may be projected from the shoulder blades out through the arms projecting beyond the fingers or dropping down through the legs and feet to below the ground. The ability to project *qi* often starts with a person having an image of *qi*, light or water flowing through the chosen path. The *yi* enables the *qi* to move. One quote about the *yi* says, 'when the *yi* is strong the *qi* is strong; when the *yi* is weak the *qi* is weak' (Yang, 1997, pp. 30–31). The applications in terms of motivating oneself and directing *qi* are obvious and all involve the *yi*. (For more on *qi gong* exercises, see Hicks, 2009, p. 109 and Hicks A. and Hicks J., 1999, p. 139.)

Patient Example

A patient, an Earth CF, came for treatment because of depression, drug addiction and some digestive problems. Initial treatments included the Internal Dragons (see Chapter 31, this volume) and basic treatment on the Spleen and Stomach. After three months the patient was well and returning to his work as a musician and songwriter. He had achieved what he asked for, but said that he wanted to continue treatment. When asked how he would then evaluate treatment, he said that he would like to regain his ability to think. He explained that as a songwriter and poet, he took his life experience, expressed it in words and then expressed these through his songs. He said he was regaining this ability, but more than anything else he wanted to be able to think. Six months later he gave his practitioner his latest CD.

The Stomach – the controller of rotting and ripening

The character for the Stomach

The character for the Stomach is *wei* (Weiger, 1965, lesson 122C). This character is a simple picture of a stomach with food inside it. The Chinese describe the Stomach as the great granary or storehouse for our food. As the source of our nourishment, the Stomach is one of the most important of all of the *yang* organs.

Rotting and ripening

The action of the Stomach is to rot and ripen. The mouth breaks up food and drink, adds saliva and warms the total mixture before swallowing. The Stomach carries on this process of breaking food

down so that the food essences, or the part of the food to be retained, can be separated out and used to create *qi*. There are various descriptions used to account for this process. Sometimes the activity of the Stomach is compared to a maceration chamber.

J. R. Worsley compared the Stomach's rotting and ripening function to a concrete mixer (Worsley, 1998, p. 13.1). In order to make good concrete, people need the right ingredients and a good mixer. If they have the correct amount of cement, sand and water and mix it well, it will make strong concrete that is capable of building a sturdy building which will last for hundreds of years. If, however, it is the wrong consistency or poorly mixed, the concrete will be of poor quality.

Another analogy is cooking. In order to bake bread people need the correct ingredients and to mix yeast and sugar with the correct quantities of flour and water. They also have to knead the loaf well. If this isn't done correctly then the bread will not rise. Finally, the bread must be cooked at the correct temperature otherwise it may be inedible. It could be too sticky or lumpy or too hard. This combination of the right ingredients plus correct kneading and cooking is similar to what the Stomach requires.

The correct food is important but we also need a strong and healthy Stomach Official in order to digest physical, mental and spiritual nourishment. It is notable that in everyday language we frequently use phrases from the digestive system – for example, 'I find that hard to stomach!' or 'I can't digest it', when referring both to food and ideas. A person can suffer nausea wholly from the mind or emotions. Students do better when served the right-sized portions of information and being given breaks in which to mull over and absorb it. Study of the Chinese understanding of Earth suggests these are more than clever metaphors.

Patient Example

A student who was an Earth CF said that before exams she'd just 'worry, worry, worry' and she'd feel it in her solar plexus. 'Everything is unsettled and jittery in there and I eat to try and calm myself down. But I can't eat because I am too jittery in there. I think that if I ate I would throw up.'

This relation between the mind and Stomach goes both ways. If we go back to a pathological expression of Earth emotion, worry, then severe worry can easily disrupt the transformation process. (For an account of how the Chinese saw good eating habits, see Hicks, 2009, p. 9.)

The Stomach as the origin of fluids

It is the Stomach that filters and processes fluids when they first enter the body. The Stomach also requires a wet environment in which to flourish, which is why the phrase 'the Stomach likes wetness and dislikes dryness' is sometimes used. When an imbalance of fluids occurs in the body the Stomach may be involved.

The direction of the Stomach

The Stomach's direction is downward. It receives food from above and passes on the food it has rotted and ripened to the Small Intestine. Any failure to send food downwards results in a movement in the opposite direction and a movement upwards. Alternatively there might be stagnation especially in the Middle or Upper Burner. Symptoms may be belching, hiccups, nausea or vomiting. These symptoms are all manifestations of the 'wrong direction' and are sometimes called 'rebellious' *qi*.

The time of day for the Organs

Each Organ in the body has a 2-hour period of the day associated with it. During this time the Organ has extra *qi* flowing through it. The 2-hour period for the Stomach is 7–9 a.m. and for the Spleen 9–11 a.m. It is interesting to note that the period of 7–9 in the morning is when most people eat their breakfast. This is the time when our digestion should be at its best. If the Stomach is reasonably healthy, eating a good hearty breakfast will set a person up for the rest of the day. Many people, however, have no appetite at this time.

From 9 to 11 a.m., which is the period associated with the Spleen, we digest the food we ate earlier in

the day. From here it will be transported to all the other Organs in the body in order to nourish us.

Many people whose Earth Officials are weak struggle to maintain vitality between 7 and 11 p.m., the low time of day for these Officials. Eating at this time, as opposed to earlier, is an abuse of the Stomach. It is like a worker who has gone off his shift being called back to do more work.

How the Stomach and Spleen relate

The functions of the Stomach and Spleen are closely related and may even overlap. Both Organs have important functions in the digestive process and they enable people to digest food as well as their thoughts. The Spleen's role is to transform and transport food and thoughts and the Stomach's to rot and ripen them.

The Stomach and Spleen also have some opposing functions. For example the Stomach is a *yang* Organ. Its *qi* has a downward direction, it likes wetness and prefers cooler temperatures. The Spleen on the other hand is a *yin* Organ. Its *qi* has an upward direction, it likes dryness and prefers warmth.

Summary

1 *Su Wen* Chapter 8 describes the Stomach and Spleen as 'responsible for the storehouses and granaries. The five tastes stem from them.'

2 The Spleen is sometimes known as the 'controller of transforming and transporting'. The Stomach is sometimes referred to as the 'controller of rotting and ripening'.

3 The *yi* is the spirit of the Spleen and can be translated as thought or intention.

4 The *yi* gives us the ability to think clearly and concentrate. It also gives us the ability to focus our attention and intention.

5 The time associated with the Stomach is 7–9 a.m. and that with the Spleen is 9–11 a.m.

Patterns of behaviour of Earth Constitutional Factors

16

Introduction

This chapter describes some of the most important behavioural characteristics that are typical of this CF. Some aspects of a person's behaviour can be observed in the treatment room. Others can only be discerned from the patient's description of themselves and their life. As stated in the previous chapters, behaviour can be an indicator of a patient's diagnosis but it can only be used to *confirm* the CF. It should always be used in conjunction with colour, sound, emotion and odour, which are the four primary methods of diagnosis (these are described in greater depth in Chapters 2 and 25, this volume). Once the CF is confirmed the patterns of behaviour may, however, support the practitioner's diagnosis.

The origin of the behaviours was described in Chapter 7. The imbalance of the Element of the CF creates instability or impairment of the associated emotion. Thus specific negative emotional experiences are more likely to occur to one CF as opposed to another. The behavioural traits described in this chapter are often the responses to these negative experiences. In the case of Earth the person experiences feelings of being unsupported and nurtured and she or he is responding to this.

Patterns of behaviour of an Earth CF

The balanced Element

Patients with a healthy Earth Element can easily give and receive emotional support and nurturing. The health of a person's Earth Element is largely dependent on the quality of the relationship with the mother. As was stated earlier in Chapter 14, it is no coincidence that the earth is often referred to as 'Mother Earth'. This is because the fruits of the earth nourish and support us, much as a person's mother does.

In a healthy relationship a mother or main carer provides a child with support when it is young. The mother feeds, holds and comforts the child if it is distressed. If children fall and hurt themselves they usually run to their mothers for comfort. The mother will rub the wound better or do what is necessary to console the child. Once comforted the child feels safe enough to be independent again. She or he knows that when the going gets tough the mother will be at hand for more support. This external security in the early years enables children to create their own internal security and become independent later on in adult life. Research with monkeys shows that the young become independent more quickly and completely when they have received stable and supportive parenting in infancy (Harlow and Harlow, 1962).

Having been provided with this early support, people are usually capable of nourishing themselves.

They learn to ask for help when they need it and take in nurturing and care offered by others. They are also able to give support and nourishment to others and to distinguish between when it is appropriate to look after their own needs and when to care for the needs of other people.

Formative events for an Earth CF

Although it is likely that people are born with their CF, many of their experiences, especially emotional ones, are also coloured by it. The need to feel supported or cared for when distressed is a very basic human need, that in itself is not pathological. When the person's need for support goes out of balance, however, it becomes pathological.

Many Earth CFs feel that they never really bonded or received sufficient nurturing from their mother. This means that their Earth Element never received adequate nourishment to achieve good balance. Sometimes the mother or main carer was not available to give support when the need arose. Even if she was available, the manner in which it was given may have meant that the person was unable to take it in and felt deprived.

Others were dominated by their mothers and were overly dependent upon them for caring and intimacy. This can create significant problems when the time comes for the child to build a life independent from the family. It can also cause difficulties when the person's mother dies.

Patient Example

A patient who is an Earth CF was the third child in a family of ten. She described to her practitioner that she didn't get very much attention from her mother. 'By the time I was eighteen months old another child had come along and after that they just kept coming. I never felt I got my needs met and was always left wanting more.' As a result of this situation the patient struggled later on when it came to bringing up her own daughter. 'I think I overcompensated and overfed her. I was so worried that she wasn't getting enough from me. At some level I also didn't let her in. She's eighteen now and I'm still trying to get close to her.'

Many Earth CF children may have lost touch with their own needs. For some people it means that they only think of the needs of others. They have lost the ability to receive support when appropriate and act independently when it is called for. When having

acupuncture they may feel uncomfortable about doing something for themselves and being supported. Others only think of themselves and don't consider others' needs. They feel so insecure inside that they may be oblivious if others are also having difficulties.

Sometimes the practitioner temporarily takes on the role of the mother or carer for the patient. This can be a difficult situation for physicians and carers. If patients become dependent they may be getting the support they need but an unhealthy dependency could develop that will be hard for the patient to transcend. The goal is to enhance the patient's Earth Element sufficiently for the patient to be able to let go and care for her or himself.

The main issues for an Earth CF

For the Earth CF certain needs remain unmet. This situation creates certain issues which centre on these areas:

- feeling supported
- getting nourishment
- feeling centred and stable
- having mental clarity
- being understood

The extent to which someone is affected in these areas varies according to the person's physical, mental and spiritual health. Relatively healthy Earth CFs will have less disturbance with these aspects of life, whilst those with greater problems end up with their personalities being strongly influenced by this imbalance.

Because of these issues they may consciously or unconsciously ask themselves various questions such as:

- Who will give me the support I need?
- How can I get nourished?
- How can I become centred and stable?
- How can I get what I want from the world?
- How can I feel I belong?
- Who will really understand me?

Responses to the issues

So far we have described how a weakness in the Earth Element leads to a lesser capacity to give and receive emotional support appropriately. The issues that subsequently arise lead to a spectrum of typical ways of responding to the world. These are common, but not exclusive to Earth CFs. If other CFs have patterns of behaviour that seem similar it may indicate that there is a different set of motivations underlying them or that the Earth Element is also imbalanced but is not the CF. Noticing these responses is therefore useful but does not replace colour, sound, emotion and odour as the principal way of diagnosing the Constitutional Factor.

The behavioural patterns are along a spectrum and can go between these extremes:

1	smothering/ mothering	not supporting
2	feeling needy	repressing needs
3	excessive dependency	over-independence
4	uncentred and dispersed	stuck and heavy
5	over-dependent on the security of the home	inability to put down roots

These are discussed below.

Smothering/mothering – not supporting

Earth CFs who would like to receive more support and nurturing often start caring for and mothering others. For some Earth CFs this can be almost compulsive and they find it hard to resist any waif or stray who comes to them for help or whom they perceive to be in need of their assistance.

Patient Example

A patient came for treatment describing herself as feeling 'worn out and depleted'. She had a busy counselling practice and said she had difficulty saying 'no' to people. 'If I'm asked for anything I'll automatically say "yes" and try and fit it in. My reason for existing is giving to others and for them to need me'. She also described that she could be so over-empathetic with her clients that she could completely lose herself in them and take on all of their problems. 'Sometimes I'll almost merge with people and lose a sense of who I am.'

Some Earth CFs may channel the tendency to 'mother' into their families and children. One Earth CF, for example, described knowing she 'had a purpose in her life' once she had become pregnant and this left her 'deeply satisfied'. Unfortunately this also had a negative side and she felt desolate and depressed when her child-rearing days were over. She also found it difficult to let go of the children as they grew up and became independent.

Sometimes the person on the receiving end of this kind of mothering can find it excessive. What is perceived as supportive behaviour can turn into interference. An Earth CF who compulsively looks after others may forget to check whether the person they are caring for actually wants support from them. In this case the need to care can be so great that mothering becomes 'smothering'.

Patient Example

A patient who was 35 continually complained about her mother's meddling. Her mother would phone her every day to see if she was 'all right' and to find out every detail about what she had been doing that day. When the patient tried to assert her independence and said she'd rather not have so many calls, her mother became ill until the behaviour pattern had re-established itself.

Mothering and work

The compulsive need to care for others may lead Earth CFs to take jobs in caring professions such as nursing, counselling, social work or complementary medicine. Other caring jobs can be pastoral work, teaching or voluntary work, but the need to mother can be channelled into *any* work. The office worker that everyone turns to for support and sympathy, the hairdresser who listens to her clients' troubles or the childminder who cares for everyone else's children can all be using their mothering skills. People often find it easy to talk to them and tell them their troubles as they are adept at creating an atmosphere of acceptance and caring.

This extremely caring attitude can create difficulties for the person. Because the behaviour is compulsive and driven by the imbalance in their Earth Element, many people sublimate their own needs in order to be helping others. For example, they may continue to rush around supporting everyone when they are ill and needing to rest.

When Earth CFs find they are unable to make things better, they can start worrying excessively and can obsessively go over and over any of the smallest problems in fine detail. Watching suffering on the television news night after night can often be overwhelming for people who are excessively sympathetic.

Not supporting

Alternatively Earth CFs may go to the other extreme and find they are unable to give support to others. This might be because they had little experience of sympathy or support when they were young and they in turn feel awkward, depleted or resentful when called upon to give it to others. They are largely untouched by other people's distress. This may manifest as a harsh belief system that values self-reliance above all else. They may think that people who ask for support are 'whingers' or are 'wallowing in self-pity' and that people should 'get on with their life' or 'pull themselves together'. They have forgotten that people ask for help because they are struggling and need a small amount of sympathy and acknowledgement.

That is not to say that there aren't times to encourage someone to stop indulging in their distress. The challenge lies in knowing when to give support and when to withhold it. An imbalanced Earth Element means that people may be unable to make the appropriate judgement as they are driven by their own needs and neuroses. *Wu-wei* means acting spontaneously in accord with the needs of the situation. If one's own needs are too pressing then this becomes impossible.

Unlike the more common overly soft and sympathetic Earth CF, Earth CFs who are unsympathetic tend to be hard and ungiving. Metaphorically their Earth Element is like barren and rocky soil rather than a rich productive loam. Their experience of life is not one of having needs which they struggle to satisfy, but of finding themselves distant from other people.

In a close relationship, if an Earth CF's partner needs support the Earth CF may appear unsympathetic. This can be because Earth CFs feel that their needs and stability are threatened. They are worried that they will no longer get support if the partner is distressed. Over time this can cause their relationships to become empty and desolate.

Being unsupportive is really the other side of the coin from being overly sympathetic. Some Earth CFs

go between these two ends of the spectrum of sympathy in different situations.

Giving in order to receive

Some Earth CFs cut off support when they feel tired or if they have given out 'too much'. They may feel exasperated that they have received nothing in return. For many Earth CFs asking for something in return is anathema to them. It would spoil the enjoyment of giving if they had to say they wanted something back – so they carry on giving. In this process they are demonstrating, often unconsciously, the way they would like others to give them what they need. When others don't get the 'hint' the Earth CF might give out still more. They hope that someone will finally see what they need and do the same for them in return. However, if no one gets the hint the Earth CF can start to become very resentful or feel unsupported.

Some Earth CFs may appear to be very angry – to such an extent that they may be mistaken for a Wood CF. Sympathy and understanding is the key to softening their anger.

Patient Example

An Earth CF who was usually very supportive to others described at times having 'compassion fatigue'. In this case she could be listening to someone who was complaining and instead of feeling sympathetic she would tighten up inside and start to wonder what they could do to help themselves. 'If people tell me their problems I start to feel resentful and think "you think you've got problems – what about me". I don't say anything though.'

Many Earth CFs who mother and care for others may appear to be almost saintly in their capacity to give out so much. It's clear that most Earth CFs *do* want to get something back from those they give out to – the problem is how to get what they want.

Feeling needy – repressing needs

Any nurturing relationship involves both giving and taking. In the pattern described above the Earth CF does a lot of giving without much taking. This creates a very real risk of becoming burnt out.

Seeking attention

Rather than not asking for what they need, some Earth CFs will go to the other extreme. Often Earth CFs feel that they didn't get nurtured at an early age and were left to 'scream' when they needed the help of their mother or main carer. Subsequently as adults they may continue to 'scream' whenever they feel the need for support. In this case they may try to get their needs met by making excessive demands on other people's time and attention. This may take the form of endlessly talking about their problems or using attention-seeking behaviour. Sometimes they can seem so 'needy' that others find it impossible to satisfy them. An extreme version of this is Munchausen syndrome – a psychiatric disease when people make themselves ill and gain admittance to hospitals in order to win other people's attention.

More commonly attention seeking may take the form of 'whinging' and 'whining'. Some Earth CFs are aware that they talk about their problems excessively. For example, an Earth CF told her practitioner, 'I know it would be better if I could get to the point quicker. It's just that I need to make sure that somebody else understands where I'm coming from.' Often Earth CFs are completely unaware of how demanding they are and if this pattern is extreme they may wonder why their desire to see their friends is not always reciprocated.

There are occasions when some Earth CFs have been accused of taking up more time than is necessary in the treatment room. A simple question like 'How are you?' may lead to a 20 minute discussion about a person's problems. A practitioner may find it difficult to finish a treatment as the patient seems to incessantly talk about their illnesses in great detail. Practitioners speak of the 'door handle syndrome'. The treatment is finished and the practitioner is about to leave. At the moment when the practitioner's hand is on the door knob, the patient brings up another problem they are having, pulling the practitioner back.

Some Earth CFs are driven to extract every last drop of sympathy from a situation. For others, it is not so much the emotion of sympathy they are craving. In fact they sometimes don't know how to respond if the practitioner is sympathetic. In this case the need to communicate every last detail is driven by the need to feel 'understood' and that their needs are being considered and taken into account. The drive is to engage the practitioner's mind rather than his or her feelings. Sometimes it is not just the time taken to discuss the problems that is striking. What reveals that the patient is an Earth CF is the enjoyment evident when they find an ear for their problems.

Patient Example

A patient noticed that as soon as he woke up he felt sorry for himself. He described how as a child he was told not to whine or he'd be sent to his room. This led him not to whinge directly. 'I don't say "Oh poor me please help me," it's more "Oh I'm so tired and I've got this to do or that to do."'

Disguising their needs

Some Earth CFs may feel that no one gives them the appreciation, support or caring that they deserve. They might find it difficult to ask for what they want and disguise their needs. In this case they may have a hidden agenda and try to get support without actually asking for it.

Patient Example

An Earth CF patient was continually complaining that he didn't receive enough support from other people. The practitioner suggested that he ask for what he wanted but it was clear that this was difficult for him. Later on in the treatment he admitted that he expected people to know what he needed without having to tell them. He told the practitioner, 'I get upset when people don't second guess my needs.' Over time and with many more treatments centred around his Earth Element he became more able to ask for the support directly.

Not expressing and asking for their needs to be met can become a vicious cycle. The more Earth CFs give out, the more they may feel unappreciated. The more they feel unappreciated the more they feel unable to ask for what they want.

Suppressing needs

Some Earth CFs suppress their needs and reject any sympathy offered to them. If they have not had their needs met when young they may feel undeserving of other people's support or may worry that they are in danger of becoming too dependent on others. The intimacy that another person attempts to create when being supportive engenders feelings of agitation and insecurity. These feelings are uncomfortable so the person pushes the support away in order to avoid these difficult feelings.

One patient told his practitioner that he hated it if people said things like 'take care' or asked him how he was. When offered any support of this kind he would immediately tense up and try and push it away by behaving brusquely. He said that 'caring' behaviour was much too 'syrupy' and made him feel too dependent on others.

Patient Example

An Earth CF patient who had multiple sclerosis was severely disabled and had difficulty dressing himself. After treatment he wouldn't allow the practitioner to give him any help and he would struggle to dress and tie his shoe laces. Although this behaviour was admirable and helped him to maintain his independence, it was also difficult for those around him. They could see that he needed assistance at times and were gruffly pushed away when they offered to help.

The two types of behaviour described above can run concurrently. Having felt extremely needy, some Earth CFs may flip into the other extreme and try to show that they have no needs at all. Ultimately the Earth CF may reach a balance between these two states. This is a more stable centre point from which they can relate to the world.

Excessive dependency – over-independence

People who feel nurtured when young are often more able to develop a sense of 'belonging', both to family and to the community around them. Later on in life this enables them to build their own homes and families and to integrate into communities of colleagues, neighbours and friends. Without this sense of belonging people always feel somewhat uncomfortable in their relationships with others. They will tend to push others away or to be driven to feel a part of a community. They may also fluctuate between these two modes of behaviour.

The need for a sense of community is important in most people's lives, but it is often especially so for those who are Earth CFs as it may provide them with

a sense of family. This is especially true if they didn't feel nurtured by their own family when they were young. In this way the community can become a very positive contact for the Earth CF.

If Earth CFs don't feel a part of any community they may move from group to group searching for contact with others but be unable to find it. In consequence they continually feel alienated and separate from other people. One Earth CF described that she felt either 'linked' to others in a group or disconnected from them and she would always be at one extreme or the other. She said, 'When I'm disconnected from myself I'm also disconnected from others. I can also merge with people I've been intimate with. Then it's terrifying. It's like I haven't got an identity.'

Melting and merging

Merging can be an important issue for many Earth CFs. Some Earth CFs have an urge to merge with others but the downside of this is that they may find it hard to be independent and they can lose their identity. Some Earth CFs have described a sense of 'melting' into another person. This can be so extreme that they actually feel as if they become the other person and are no longer two separate people.

Patient Example

An Earth CF described being in relationships where the intimacy was very intense. 'At first it's just unbelievable, but then it starts to get not so good. He's having PMT pains or I'm having his headache! Then his mood becomes my mood and I can't be in my own mood. If he's in a particular state I can't help him to get out of it because I'm so affected by it.'

Ultimately an Earth CF may find merging with another a pleasurable experience as long as she or he is able to separate from the person again when appropriate. Otherwise the person finds it hard to remain an individual. One Earth CF patient said that if she was around people for too long she would lose a sense of who she was. She found that the best way to deal with this was to go off on her own for a while so that she could 'feel where I begin and end'. She described that she could then 'drop down from my head to my insides and regain the important sense of being myself again'.

Feeling disconnected

Other Earth CFs may find it difficult to achieve intimacy with someone else. Feelings of separateness and alienation often begin in early childhood and continue to be an issue throughout a person's life. If children do not feel understood or cared for they often harden themselves and cut off from others. They may unconsciously say to themselves, 'Why allow myself to need support when no one responds when I reach out?' They may think it is far better to be independent than let themselves be disappointed and rejected again.

An Earth CF who feels disconnected may be mistaken for a Metal CF who is distanced or cut off but the underlying cause is different. An Earth CF's experience arises from feeling unsupported or a lack of nurturing whilst Metal CFs distance themselves when they feel fragile and need to defend themselves.

Uncentred and dispersed – stuck and heavy

Good nurturing gives people strong foundations. Without this a person may feel that they lack a centre inside. This may manifest in a number of different ways. For example, some people physically feel that they have an empty space in their centre, usually in the region of the stomach. Others just feel generally dissatisfied and feel a need to give themselves some kind of reward in order to cheer themselves up. They will try and deal with this in a number of different ways.

'Comfort' eating to fill the centre

Many Earth CFs have a difficult relationship with their appetite and food. When a person feels insecure one reaction is to 'comfort' eat. A person may feel they have a void inside which never gets filled. In this case the void makes them feel hungry but the underlying cause may be insecurity or lack of a centre. It can never be adequately filled by physical food.

One patient described how, when her relationship was breaking up, she would raid the fridge in the middle of the night – but it only filled the gap for a while. Another described how 'sinking hunger leads to sinking energy'. If she didn't have food to eat her 'middle would disappear entirely' and her mind felt clouded.

Other people easily lose their appetite if they are anxious, angry or unhappy. They have to be reasonably content in order to want to eat. In extreme cases this can create major problems such as anorexia or bulimia.

Becoming dissipated

Another way Earth CFs may lose their centre is by paying so much attention to others that they lose touch with themselves. This can happen when they worry about other people. Sometimes it is easy for them to give to others because they have little sense of their own needs. If they satisfied themselves instead they would gain a better sense of their individuality. This pattern can often be seen in mothers who have lost their sense of self after years of putting their own needs in the background in what they perceive to be the interests of their family.

At other times Earth CFs may need to make some conscious effort to find themselves again. This may entail discovering ways to become 'grounded'. Each person finds the best way for themselves. Some need to get away from other people and spend time by themselves. Others may wish to lie down on the earth and take in the 'earth energy'. Some may 'earth' themselves by doing *qi gong* exercises. Others may wish to walk in a natural environment and commune with nature.

When the Earth is unstable some Earth CFs have the desire to pamper themselves in an attempt to fill the void that arises. Trips to the hairdresser, long hot baths, a cigarette, a drink when the person gets home from work are all examples of ways they might try to give themselves a little 'present'. For some people shopping is a necessary evil, for others it is 'retail therapy'.

Patient Example

A patient who was an Earth CF made a lot of progress from treatment and no longer had many of her original symptoms. She had more energy, better digestion and she also felt much better in herself. One important symptom remained – she felt that she didn't have a centre. She found this hard to describe so she used the metaphor that her body felt like a 'hollow tree trunk' and that she had a space from the solar plexus down to her lower abdomen. She said that she had had it all of her life and it worsened when she was tired and especially when she ignored her own needs and looked after other people. Over a one-year period of treatment and with her practitioner's encouragement she gradually learned to nurture herself better. During this time the feeling lessened to a great degree.

When people become dissipated their internal feelings of stability are often precarious. They are inclined to be rather emotional and easily upset. Without strong feelings of internal stability it is easy for them to have a dramatic view of life, where molehills become mountains and problems seem like crises. In this case the tendency to feel dissatisfied is strong. They may become restless in regard to their work, relationships, home or interests as they slip into the unconscious belief that the 'grass is greener' elsewhere.

Feeling stuck and heavy

At the other end of the spectrum, instead of feeling uncentred and dissipated, many Earth CFs can feel stuck and heavy inside. The feeling of stuckness can manifest on many different levels. Physically the Spleen's lack of transportation and transformation may make them feel that they don't want to move. They may feel weighed down, flat and clogged up. One patient told her practitioner that her most frequently used saying was 'why stand if you can sit and why sit if you can lie down'.

Other patients may experience feeling clogged up mentally. Their thoughts may be stuck inside their heads because the Stomach is not assimilating and the Spleen not transforming and transporting on a mental level. This may make it difficult for them to think clearly. Different patients have described this in various ways. One patient said, 'I have thoughts in my head which can't get through. It's like there's something in there stopping me thinking properly.' Another patient described it as feeling like spaghetti 'where all of the spaghetti gets knotted up and I can't separate the strands'. Other descriptions have been a 'feeling as if there is a tight band around my head' or feeling 'as if my head is stuffed with cotton wool'.

The state of feeling stuck and the state of being dissipated and uncentred are two ends of a spectrum which may alternate. Many Earth CFs have to be careful about what they eat as it affects them mentally and emotionally as well as physically and this may exacerbate the swing between these two extremes. In these cases if they don't eat properly they may feel disorientated whilst if they have too much they go to the opposite extreme and feel full, heavy, tired and unable to function.

This internal feeling of stuckness also means that they can also lead to a rather stolid and phlegmatic temperament. If this is the case Earth CFs experience very little of the highs and lows of life. They are neither very enthusiastic nor very upset about anything. Life is bearable but diminished.

Over-dependent on the security of the home – inability to put down roots

Lack of stability and uncertainty

Our sense of belonging extends further than to those around us. We can also get a sense of belonging to the earth itself. Lack of nurturing on the inside may send people searching for a home on the outside. Children ideally grow up in a stable, loving and nourishing family and environment.

When these qualities are missing it can create difficulties. For example, some people grow up in families that move around a great deal. This is particularly common when one of the parents is in the Armed Forces or moves around because of their occupation. A consequence of this is that the child may then grow up with no strong feeling of being rooted or having a real sense of home. Often they also had little continuity of friendships. Constantly changing schools meant that they had to often make new friends and adjust to changing circumstances. While this is not a problem for some people, it is a serious problem for others.

Problems can also arise if children grew up with a sense of uncertainty. For example, they may wonder if the parents are going to stay together or the life expectancy of one of the family may be very uncertain. In this case it is then very difficult for a child to feel secure. This lack of stability often contributes towards a person's Earth Element becoming imbalanced.

Constant moving

Many Earth CFs move from place to place searching for a connection to the earth. The problem is internal and they never find the 'right' place. Often later in life they might settle. If this is the case it may have profound significance for them and enable them to feel more grounded and gain more of a sense of belonging.

Some Earth CFs report having moved a large numbers of times. For example, one patient told her practitioner, 'I travelled a lot in my youth and I always felt like a fish out of water – like a refugee or a foreigner. Wherever I lived I felt I had more community somewhere else and wanted to move on again.' This patient is now working on settling in one place: 'I'm trying to stay put at the moment and am hoping that it will help me to gain more stability.'

Remaining in one place

At the other extreme some Earth CFs get so attached to one place that they become very insecure if they have to move. One patient described travelling 100 miles a day so that she could continue being with her old workmates after she had moved when her husband changed jobs. After two years she became tired and ill and she begrudgingly realised that she had to stop and find a job closer to her home.

Others can be reluctant travellers as being away from their home for any period of time gives them deep feelings of unease. Foreign parts are all very well if you like that kind of thing but really they would rather be snuggled up in front of the fire at home. People of this disposition might also generate physical symptoms when they travel. Sleep, bowels and the menstrual cycle especially can become disturbed.

Feeling at home is important for everybody but it can be especially important for an Earth CF. Being able to build a home and make a nest can give an Earth CF a sense of being centred and can help to build more stability inside them. The Chinese visualised people standing on the earth with their heads in the Heavens. The feet being on the ground is a sign of being 'down to earth', practical and grounded. Many *tai ji* and *qi gong* exercises encourage people to 'develop a root' and these can be especially beneficial to an Earth CF. By connecting with the ground they can gain nourishment from the earth and in turn feel more centred and balanced.

Gaining equilibrium

Some Earth CFs may find it difficult to develop a sense of equilibrium and be unable to reach a stable and centred place. They may think they have found stability for a while only to find that they are swinging over to another extreme again. One patient described feeling either 'brilliant' or 'overwhelmed' and that it was hard to stay in a centred state.

Over time it may be possible for some Earth CFs to develop more internal stability. One Earth CF recently described how she can now feel that she has a balance from where she can 'act in a positive way'. This is a sense of equilibrium that many Earth CFs try to find. Acupuncture treatment may be an important key to helping them to achieve this.

Summary

1 A diagnosis of an Earth CF is made primarily by observation of a yellow facial colour, a singing voice, a fragrant odour and imbalance in the emotion of sympathy.

2 Earth CFs tend to have issues and difficulties with:
   • feeling supported
   • getting nourishment
   • feeling centred and stable
   • having mental clarity
   • being understood

3 Because of these issues Earth CFs' behaviour and responses to situations tend to fluctuate between:

   • smothering/ mothering _____ not supporting
   • feeling needy _____ repressing needs

   • excessive dependency _____ over-independence
   • being uncentred and dispersed _____ stuck and heavy
   • over-dependent on the security of the home _____ inability to put down roots

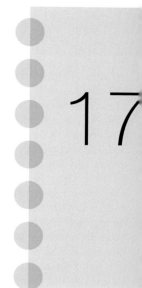

Metal – key resonances

17

Metal as a symbol

The character for Metal

The character for Metal is *jin*. *Jin* includes the character for Earth (see Chapter 14). The Earth character has only two horizontal lines – a base line and one other. The Metal character has an extra horizontal line. The third line indicates that metal is deep within the earth, under many layers. This depth has been described 'as if in a mine shaft'. The top of the character is a sloping roof indicating in addition that something is covered over. The two shorter lines at the bottom represent nuggets of gold buried deep within the earth (Weiger, 1965, lesson 14T).

The meaning of the character

Many Elemental systems have been created, but only the Chinese included a Metal Element. This Element was named in antiquity before the invention of steel mills, aluminium production or the discovery of many of the metals we use today. So what does this character reveal about the nature of the Metal Element? The character suggests something small in quantity, but of great value, buried deep within the earth.

The Metal Element in life

Metals have always been valuable. For centuries, gold has been regarded as the most precious metal. Its scarcity is one reason for its value. Buried within each of us there is something scarce, hard to find and at the same time very valuable.

We can also think of Metal as the minerals or trace elements in the earth or in our food. Four per cent of our bodies are made from trace minerals. These are used to regulate and balance our body chemistry. For example, a person may require 400 or more grams of carbohydrate a day, but less than a millionth of that amount of chromium. Yet chromium is also essential. The valuable Metal is deeply buried within.

The Chinese also sometimes described the sky as an inverted metal bowl and the stars as holes in that bowl (Hicks, 1999, p. 11). Our Lungs draw in *qi* from the Heavens and thus a link is made between air, Metal and the breath of life.

The Metal Element in nature

'Metal in nature' demonstrates something interesting about this Element. The other Elements – Water, Wood, Earth and Fire – have very obvious manifestations

DOI: 10.1016/B978-0-7020-3175-5.00017-6

in nature. Tidal waves, forest fires, giant redwood trees and soil all manifest something elemental. But what is Metal's manifestation in nature? After all, the ancient Chinese had not developed metals to the extent that modern people have.

In nature, Metal revitalises the earth. In autumn, leaves and fruits fall off the trees and fall to the ground. They rot and enter the earth, providing minerals and nutrients that nourish and enrich the earth's capacity to grow new plants. Today, we are increasingly aware of the dangers of industrialised farming where we attempt to accelerate the natural process. We take the maximum from a field by using it every year and fertilising it artificially. 'Natural' farming would allow fields to lie fallow and for part of the plants to rot and almost invisibly return vital nutrients to the earth. The agrarian Chinese understood this kind of farming and appreciated the necessity to return essential minerals and nutrients to the earth. Metal provides the quality for the earth.

Metal also describes the role of impervious rock within the earth. Without rock all the water would soak through to the centre of the earth. For life to be possible on earth it is essential that water is returned to the surface in order to nourish animals and plants. It is in this way that Metal creates Water along the *sheng* cycle.

The Metal Element in relation to other Elements

The Metal Element interacts with the other Elements through the *sheng* and *ke* cycles (see Chapter 2, this volume).

Metal is the mother of Water

Along the *sheng* cycle Metal creates Water by containing it. Water has no shape unless contained by the impermeable rocks in the earth. If patients have obvious Water Element symptoms, such as urinary symptoms, these may have originated in the mother Element, Metal. A practitioner may treat the mother to assist the child.

Earth is the mother of Metal

Along the *sheng* cycle Earth hardens to create Metal. So there is a close relationship between Earth and Metal. Metal provides the minerals and nutrients that give Earth its quality and at the same time Earth creates Metal. When patients have signs and symptoms associated with the Metal Element these may be caused by imbalance in the Earth Element, the mother. For example, loose bowels or chest problems can be caused by an Earth imbalance. If the mother is the original cause, treating it will permanently help with the signs and symptoms whilst treating the Metal will have only a temporary effect.

Metal controls Wood

The Wood Element is controlled by Metal. A common symbol of this is of a metal saw cutting down a tree. If a person's Metal Element becomes weak it can lose control of the Wood Element. The Wood Element in turn may become too strong and symptoms of fullness such as extreme anger and hostility may develop. An apparent imbalance in the Wood Element may therefore actually stem from the Metal Element.

Fire controls Metal

Fire controls Metal. It softens it and helps to shape it. When fashioning beautiful objects in gold, the gold must be heated in order to mould it to the desired shape. Should the Fire Element become deficient, then the balance of the Metal Element is harder to maintain. In this case the Lung itself is more likely to weaken, fail to distribute protective *qi* and fail to receive *qi* from the Heavens.

The key Metal resonances

(Table 17.1)

The colour for Metal is white

The character for white

The character for white is *bai* (Weiger, 1965, lesson 88A). This character describes the sun which has just appeared in the sky. This represents the dawn in China where the Eastern sky has become white.

Table 17.1 Key Metal resonances	
Colour	White
Sound	Weeping
Emotion	Grief
Odour	Rotten

Colour in life

The colour for Metal is white. In the West people often wear black clothes or a black armband when someone dies. In contrast, in the East white is worn as an outward manifestation of the grieving process. The 'celebration of the white' is a three-day funeral party. Wreaths are placed outside the entrance of the home and over the three-day period, which is the established time for the passing of the dead, the guests eat, drink, play mah-jong and talk (Zhang and Rose, 2000, p. 73).

Facial colour

A white colour manifests on the face when the Metal Element is chronically out of balance. This colour usually appears under and beside the eyes. Unlike a simple paleness or lack of a healthy pink, white often appears 'shiny' with the colour appearing almost off the face. It is not just the paleness of 'lack of red', but a distinct colour in its own right.

The sound for Metal is weeping

The character for weeping

The character for weeping is *qi* (Weiger, 1965, lessons 125A and 1F). This character is made up of two parts. The first represents water (*shui*). The second part describes a man standing on the ground (*li*). Together these two radicals represent a person weeping or sobbing.

Weeping in life

This voice tone is based on an emotionally expressive but non-verbal sound, that of weeping or crying.

These expressions are normally associated with loss or grieving so the 'sound' resonates with the emotion of Metal, which is grief. Metal CFs often have difficulty expressing their grief and it then remains locked inside their chest. If practitioners hear their patients expressing a weeping sound when the conversation is totally unrelated to loss, this may be labelled inappropriate weeping and could indicate that the patient is a Metal CF.

When sadness is induced or arises, the intensity of the weep can be indicative of the extent that the Element is out of balance.

The voice tone of weeping

It is easier to demonstrate a sound, through a recording or mimicking, than a verbal description. The weeping sound has, however, some distinctive characteristics. There is a hint that the person speaking with a weep might easily begin to cry or weep in the ordinary sense. Sometimes there is a slight faltering in the words, almost a choking back, as the person struggles to stop the underlying emotion breaking through. There is also a weakness or lack of density in the voice and it may trail off at the end of a sentence.

Were the voice box like a flute, it would be a flute that was partially blocked and could not play at full volume.

To experience the sound of weeping, sit with the head dropped and the chest squeezed in order to prevent the free flow of *qi* through the chest. Think of anything sad and let yourself feel the sadness or the loss of what 'might have been'. Then say to yourself 'This is awful and I can't do anything about it.' Then say it again out loud. Speak slowly and let the voice crackle, break and drift off.

The odour for Metal is rotten

The character for rotten

The character for rotten is *lan* (Weiger, 1965, lessons 126A and 120J).

The odour resonating with Metal is rotten. Like some of the other odour translations, 'rotten' is not consistently used in English to describe a specific smell. There is, however, a characteristic odour of animal or vegetable matter that is rotting. Probably rotting meat is the best verbal description, but the odour of a rubbish bin or garbage truck where many different substances are decomposing is also close.

The best way to learn odours is by smelling Metal CFs, but there are some descriptions of rotten which might be useful:

- like rotten meat
- fills the inside of a person's nose with tiny prickles
- clenches the inside of a person's nose

The emotion for Metal is grief

The character for grief

The two main characters that are used to express grief are *you* and *bei*.

The Chinese term for grief is *you* (Weiger, 1965, lesson 160). At the top of this character is a head. Below this is a heart and at the bottom a pair of dragging legs that accompany the troubles in the head and heart (Larre and Rochat de la Vallée, 1996, pp. 145–149). '*You*' is sometimes translated as oppression or worry and can be associated with more than one Element.

Sadness, *bei*, is also associated with Metal. The character has two parts to it (Weiger, 1965, lessons 170A and 107A). The first, *fei*, means the notion of something in opposition or not communicating. Instead the two sides are back to back. The second radical, *xin*, represents the heart. Together they represent the negation of the Heart and a brutal sadness, desolation or loss.

Grief in everyday life

Many people's everyday notion of grief is that it is the emotion felt when, without warning, a loved one dies. There is often shock and then an outburst of grief. This extreme emotion is sometimes seen on TV, when there has been a plane crash, 'terrorist' attack or a passenger ferry sinks. The bereaved wail and cry and their faces show the typical 'collapsing downwards' of grief. *Ai*, not *you*, is the Chinese word that conveys the howling and wailing that is normal behaviour during the mourning period in China or the keening that people sometimes express when someone close to them has died.

Such extreme grief is not typical. Everyday life brings many instances of loss from very small to large and for each of these there is an appropriate emotional response associated with the ability to let go. The range of people's losses varies from physical objects (some highly valued, others less so), to loved ones or friends, to dreams about what they might have done or who they might have become. Over the course of people's lives, possessions wear out, relationships change, people's prestige or self-worth can lessen and, indeed, people are all getting a little older with all the potential loss of abilities, possibilities, health and future. Of course, as time moves on, many aspects of life may get better, but in the end all that people have acquired in a lifetime will be lost, if not during the passage through, certainly by the end.

It is natural for people to own or possess or in some sense hang on to 'things'. Concepts of ownership and private property are well entrenched in most cultures and most people. 'Mine' seems to be one of the first words that children learn. The acquiring of material possessions is one of the most powerful driving forces in many people's lives. However much spiritual teachers recommend that people continuously let go and simply pass through life, humans tend to hold, possess and hang on to things. A farmer may have a caretaker role with respect to his farm, but he nevertheless believes it is *his* farm, if only for this lifetime (Kornfield, 2002; see pp. 15–16 for one of many anecdotes about passing through).

Grief and letting go

Attachment to other people or things is inevitable. As people get older it is probable that many of those they have loved during their lives will die. If people love someone it meets a deep need and that inevitably creates a degree of dependence. Intense or prolonged emotions often arise when people lose something or someone they depend upon. For many children intense feelings of abandonment, of grief or loss will be the most powerful cause of disease that they will face. A sense of loss is the most intense emotion that some people have to endure. Whether a person's spirit remains alive or becomes deadened and diminished by this has a huge effect on the person's Metal Element.

Loss can, of course, evoke other feelings such as anger or anxiety. But grief is the emotion most appropriate to the process of letting go of, or mourning what has been lost in preparation for moving on. After all, people think it odd for someone, after a heavy loss, just to shrug it off, apparently feeling no intense emotions and carry on in the changed circumstances as though nothing had happened.

The range of expressions of grief

Grief is experienced in many different ways. In some people, feelings of disappointment and yearning are intense. In others, regret is powerfully felt. When these feelings are intense or prolonged, it is often too painful for a person, especially a child, to fully experience.

Su Wen says that when grief is present the *qi* 'disappears' (*xiao*). This *yin* expression of an emotion implies a withdrawal of the *qi* leaving a void behind. This entirely fits with the feelings of emptiness which are common in Metal CFs. Many would not perceive themselves as 'empty' at all but there is a deadened, inert aspect to them. As Havelock Ellis wrote, 'Pain and death are a part of life. To reject them is to reject life itself' (*On Life and Sex: Essays of Love and Virtue*, Volume 2).

A life with something missing, and a part of the spirit that is not fully alive, is the price that people pay if they repress this aspect of their being.

Grief in health and sickness

The Metal Element, the Lungs and Large Intestine, gives people the capacity to confront loss, let what they once possessed go, feel the pain and then move on. When the Metal Element is reasonably balanced, this process happens smoothly. The 'disappearing' movements of the *qi* run through the face, chest and abdomen and dissipate. Tears may flow and sobbing may occur. The movements of *qi* are fluent. When the Metal Element is out of balance, grief is less fluent and people can get stuck, not having truly

let go. This stagnation, or inability to come to terms with change, has the oppressive effect on the spirit depicted by the dragging legs in the character *you*. A person's physical health may be affected.

The chest in particular holds tight in order to stop the feeling. One of the most common descriptions of stuck grief is that of 'choking up' where the chest and throat tighten up, impeding the flow of *qi*.

Dealing with feelings of grief

For many people the need to numb the pain of grief and sadness is an emotional necessity. To deny that anything is amiss can become compulsive. If something has gone wrong apologies are seldom offered as that would involve admitting to themselves and others that they failed to behave appropriately to the needs of the situation.

The tendency to be somewhat inert and lacking in passion is a key characteristic of many Metal CFs. They can be inclined to be somewhat withdrawn and morose. Others maintain a perfectly bright exterior in an attempt to convince themselves and others that everything is fine. (A character in literature that comes to mind is Dr Pangloss in Voltaire's *Candide*. Despite experiencing much suffering he was stubbornly determined to maintain that 'All is for the best in the best of all possible worlds.') This bright exterior, however, has a quality of brittleness that hints at its function of masking or holding in the underlying grief. It should not be confused with the joy of a Fire CF which although often brighter and more joyous than that of a Metal CF, can also be more precarious and more easily move to the other extreme of joylessness (Table 17.2).

Patient Example

A Metal CF had suffered from endometriosis since 21. When asked whether anything had happened around that time she said she was sure that there was nothing she was aware of. When asked what had been the most difficult time in her life so far, she replied that her boyfriend had committed suicide when she was 21. She laughed nervously as she talked about it and said that she had not grieved at all. She had moved away but when she returned to her home town five years later had had 'a bit of a nervous breakdown' as she started having 'panic attacks' and having nightmares about his death.

Table 17.2 Example of the range of emotions associated with the Metal Element

Grief	Loss, emptiness, resignation, longing, regret, remorse, mourning, feeling bereft

The supporting Metal resonances

These resonances are considerably less important than the 'key' resonances given above. They can often be used to indicate that a person's Metal Element is imbalanced but they do not necessarily point to it being the person's CF (Table 17.3).

The season for Metal is autumn

The character for autumn

The character for autumn is *qiu*. The first part of this character, *ho*, represents an ear of corn that is so heavy it is bending over. The second part is the character for fire, *huo* (see Weiger, 1965, lessons 121C (*qui*), 121A (*ho*) and 126A (*huo*)). Autumn is the season when the leaves of the trees and plants become golden like fire and everything needs to drop and be cut down. It can also be translated as the season when the grain is burned.

Autumn

The yearly cycle of growth was close to the hearts of the agrarian Chinese. Any plant goes through

Table 17.3 Supporting Metal resonances

Season	Autumn/Fall
Power	Decrease
Climate	Dryness
Sense Organ/Orifice	Nose
Tissues and body parts	Skin
Generates	Body hair
Taste	Pungent

different phases and manifests a different quality of qi according to the season. Autumn is the time that the *yang qi* of the summer becomes more *yin*.

The leaves of the tree wither and drop to the earth – it is a time of death and a falling downward. The acorns of the oak tree, the seeds that will carry on the species, fall to the ground with leaves attached. Thus what has fallen contains both the seeds for the next generation and the material which will rot, enter the soil and provide nourishment and quality for the new plants.

This *yin* phase in the growth cycle is the opposite of Wood with its emphasis on birth and upward movement. Many people feel a sense of melancholia, an indefinable slight sense of sadness, at this time of year. 'The melancholy days are come, the saddest of the year' (William Cullen Bryant).

The power for Metal is decrease

The character for decrease

The character for decrease is *jian* (see Weiger, 1965, lessons 125A and 71P).

Decrease

After the thrusting up of spring, the growth of summer and the harvest of late summer, autumn is a time of decrease. It is the time of letting go, when the *qi* is drawing in. At this time of year the nights draw in and the temperature becomes cooler. Stillness often accompanies the dropping leaves and seeds. Grief resonates with this phase, as there is death, a letting go and a preparation for new life.

The climate for Metal is dryness

The character for dryness

The character for dryness is *zao* (see Weiger, 1965, lessons 126A (*huo*) and 72L (*tsao*)). This character combines the character for fire, *huo*, with the character for a tree with three singing birds in it, *tsao*. It can be assumed that when it is hot the birds singing in the tree will get very thirsty and dry.

Dryness

Dryness is considered to be an external 'evil', which can invade and cause illness. It is more likely to occur in autumn in Northern China, although it rarely occurs in Britain. A comparison with Earth is useful. For the Earth Element, the opposite or too much fluid is often the problem. External humidity attacks and causes the already Damp person to feel worse, often with stiff and aching joints or a muzzy head. In a similar way, external dryness causes dryness patterns that are treated via the Lung, hence the connection with Metal. The main symptoms of dryness are a dry nose, throat and skin, a dry cough and possibly thirst. For those who are already dry, living in a desert region or one with very low humidity can cause this pattern to occur.

People living in extremely dry climates are especially prone to respiratory illness. For those, however, who suffer from asthma or recurring bronchitis, brought on by a damp environment, a holiday in a dry climate can be therapeutic.

The sense organ/orifice for Metal is the nose

The character for the nose

The character for the nose is *bi* (Weiger, 1965, lesson 40C).

The nose

The Metal Element is associated with the nose and the sense it governs is the ability to smell. The connection between the Lung and the nose is an obvious one and free communication should take place between them. Breathing through the nose both warms and filters the air before it enters the Lungs. This protects against pathogens entering the fragile Lungs. If the nose is blocked and a person can only breathe through the mouth the air is not filtered or warmed and pathogens are more likely to enter the Lungs. If a person continually breathes through the mouth rather than the nose the lung *qi* will become weakened and the person will begin to feel depleted and low in energy.

The tissue and body part for Metal is the skin

The character for the skin

The character for the skin is *pi* (Weiger, 1965, lesson 43H).

The skin

The body part resonating with Metal is the skin. Naturopaths have often said that the suppression of a skin disease, for example by steroids, may drive the disease into the lungs. The connection between asthma and eczema is well known. Chinese medicine does not make this particular connection, but a weakness of the Lungs leads to weak 'protective' (*wei*) *qi*. One function of this *qi*, which flows between the skin and the muscles, is to ward off external 'evils' or pathogenic factors such as Wind, Cold and Damp. At the same time, however, it nourishes the skin and thus the quality of the skin depends on having good quality Lung *qi*.

When a patient has poor quality skin, for example, dry skin, clogged or inelastic skin, this may indicate a weakness of the Lungs or Large Intestine. This is not a reliable factor in diagnosing Metal CFs, however, as there are too many other factors that can affect skin.

Metal generates body hair

The body hair, like the skin, is connected to the Metal Element via the protective energy. The state of the body hair may, like the skin, indicate a weakness of the *qi* of the Metal Element.

The taste for Metal is pungent

The character for pungent

The character for pungent is *xin* (see Weiger, 1965, lesson 250H).

The pungent taste

Garlic, cinnamon and ginger are examples of the pungent or acrid flavour. Anything pungent is said to move or scatter *qi*. For example, when a person has a cold or flu, the energetic pattern may, depending of course on the symptoms, be called an 'Invasion of the Lung by Wind-Cold or Wind-Heat'. In both cases, a pathogenic factor is stuck at the level of the skin and muscles. In this situation the *qi* needs to be moved to expel the Wind and scatter the Cold or expel the Heat.

Foods with pungent flavours move the *qi*. They also frequently produce sweating, which is one of the ways the pathogenic factors are released. If, however, the Lung *qi* is weak but not invaded, it could be a mistake for the person to eat too much pungent-flavoured food. Expelling or scattering is appropriate only when pathogenic factors have invaded.

Some Metal CFs enjoy pungent food. A craving for this taste may sometimes indicate that people have problems with their Lungs. This is not, however, a reliable indicator of the CF.

Summary

1 Along the *sheng* cycle Metal is the mother of Water and Earth is the mother of Metal. Across the *ke* cycle Metal controls Wood and Fire controls Metal.

2 A diagnosis of a Metal CF is made primarily by observation of a white facial colour, a weeping voice tone, a rotten odour and an imbalance in the emotion grief.

3 Metal CFs rarely express grief forcibly as might be assumed from the use of the word in English.

4 A sense of loss or a feeling of melancholy and longing or alternatively being 'cut off' from feelings of sadness are common emotional expressions arising from an imbalanced Metal Element.

5 Other resonances include the season of autumn, dryness, the power of decrease, the nose, the skin, body hair and a pungent taste.

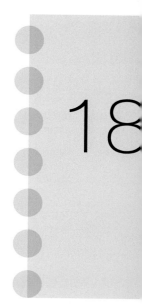

Metal – The Organs

Introduction

The Metal Element embraces two Organs. The *yang* Organ is the Large Intestine and the *yin* organ is the Lung. In ancient texts, the Chinese, probably because the writers were more function oriented, usually spoke of the Lung as a single organ. From the *Nei Jing* onwards, however, they often say that the Lung is divided into two parts (Larre and Rochat de la Valleé, 1989, p. 56). People in the West speak of the lungs, in the plural. The trachea divides into the left and right bronchi, which divide into bronchioles that in turn are designated as the left and right lungs. For this reason we tend to say that we have two lungs. In this book we will sometimes refer to the Lung and sometimes to the Lungs (Table 18.1).

The Lung – receiver of *qi* from the heavens

The character for the Lung

The character for the Lung is *fei* (see Weiger, 1965, lessons 79G and 65A).

This character has two parts. On the left is the flesh radical. This indicates that the Lung is not just a function, but also a part of the body. The right part of the character represents plants branching up from the soil. These are not plants that grow upwards but are ones that creep along the earth multiplying indefinitely (Larre and Rochat de la Vallée, 2001, p 1).

The multiplying branches of the plant are probably a physical analogy with the trachea that branches into the bronchi that in turn branch into smaller bronchioles. The trachea is a tube that, by branching, ends up in many extremely thin-walled sacs or alveoli. In books on Western medicine this structure, rather than being plants proliferating along the ground, is sometimes described as an upside down tree (Thibodeau and Patton, 1992, p. 372).

DOI: 10.1016/B978-0-7020-3175-5.10018-6

Table 18.1 The Metal Element Officials/Organs

Organ/ Official	Colloquial name	Description from *Su Wen* Ch 8
Lung	Receiver of *qi* from the Heavens	The Lung holds the office of minister and chancellor. The regulation of the life-giving network stems from it
Large Intestine	The Drainer of the Dregs	The Large Intestine is responsible for transit. The residue from transformation stems from it

Su Wen Chapter 8

Minister and chancellor

In *Su Wen* Chapter 8, the function of the Lung is described as follows:

> The Lung holds the office of minister and chancellor. The regulation of the life-giving network stems from it.
>
> (Larre and Rochat de la Vallée, 1992b, p. 45)

The location of an organ is relevant to its function. The Lung is in the upper part of the body close to the Heart. Functionally, the Lung begins in the nose and ends in alveoli. Being in the upper part of the body, the Lung connects more with Heaven than Earth.

The notions of a minister and chancellor suggest a hierarchy. If the Heart is the sovereign, then the Lung is the minister to the sovereign. The minister (Lung) converses with the sovereign (Heart), takes instructions and carries these out. There is an image here of the closeness between the beating of the Heart and the rhythm of the respiration. Although the sovereign is higher in the hierarchy, the two are interdependent. What is a sovereign with no officials to carry out any work? What is an official like a minister and chancellor who has no instructions to perform? The interdependence is obvious when we consider that the Heart controls Blood and the Lung controls *qi*, two of the key 'substances' that constitute a person.

The receiver of *qi* from the heavens

In other contexts, the Lung is said to be 'The Receiver of *qi* from the Heavens' (Larre and Rochat de la Vallée, 1992b, p. 54). Within this brief phrase there are at least two important ideas. The first is that the Lung is important in the act of breathing and is given credit for bringing in air for the creation of *qi*. The control of breathing is shared, however,

with the Kidney, which is said to 'grasp the *qi*' and hold it down when we breathe in.

The physical level of the Lung

If the Lung is weak, and thus the physical taking in of breath is weak, people will end up with weak *qi*. Shallow breathing leads to weaker *qi*. If the Lungs are weak, people can breathe more consciously and this will partially compensate. Without stronger Lung *qi*, however, people's energy will remain low. Strong Lung *qi* enables people to naturally breathe deeply and make use of the additional air they take in.

The Lung and inspiration

The second idea relates to what people take in on a spiritual level. The Lung receives from the Heavens and what it takes in is broadly covered by the word 'inspiration'. People frequently consider the world in terms of how it may satisfy them in a material way. They look at goods in a store and feel a desire to own them. In contrast, however, people may look at a scene in nature, observe a painting, listen to music or be given a compliment by someone they trust and feel lifted in their spirit. In this case there is nothing to own and nothing to possess or use up. The essence within them has been touched. They are nourished in their spirit and those elusive nuggets of gold in the Chinese character have been brought within their sight. They thought they saw the mountain, heard the music or received some heartfelt appreciation, but really they felt their own nuggets of gold.

The healthier the Lung *qi*, the easier it is to be inspired and feel vital about life. People's contact with their sense of quality, or their nuggets of gold, is a condition of feeling vital and alive. When the Lung *qi* is weak, access to the nuggets of gold is much more difficult. It is blocked by clouds of oppression and sadness. How appropriate that the second acupuncture point on the Lung channel is called 'Cloud Gate' – a gate in the clouds through which we can see the Heavens.

J. R. Worsley connected the functioning of the Lungs with contacting our Father in Heaven. He says:

> The Metal Element represents the Father within us, the connections with the Heavens, which gives our lives a sense of quality and higher purpose. The Receiver of Pure Qi Energy from the Heavens is the Official [Organ], which establishes and maintains this connection. Examples draw us to religious experience for illustrations, where an almost literal spiritual void has been filled suddenly and completely.
>
> (Worsley, 1998, p. 14.7)

It is this lack of feeling of connection to Heaven, this lack of inspiration, which is one of the characteristics of Metal CFs. They may try very hard to compensate for this feeling by searching for meaning in their lives or by forming relationships with people they respect and admire. The drive to fill that void becomes one of the most powerful influences on their lives.

The Lung and 'Defensive' *qi*

The Lung also has the function of spreading or dispersing what is called 'Defensive' or 'Protective' (*wei*) *qi* all over the body. This Defensive *qi*, a subcategory of our overall *qi*, lies just under the skin and protects us from climatic conditions such as Wind, Cold and Damp. If these conditions penetrate through the Defensive *qi*, they can result in infections and achy joints. A person with weak Defensive *qi* (through weak Lung *qi*) will frequently catch colds and flu and be more likely to have allergic responses.

The Lung as the 'fragile' Organ

The Lung takes in air directly from the outside. If airborne pollutants or harsh climatic conditions are taken in, these go directly to the Organ. Hence, the fragility of this Organ. When the weather is cold in China, Chinese people are frequently seen wearing facemasks to protect themselves from the entry of the cold into the lungs. The Lung's fragility can also be sometimes seen in the person's spirit as they struggle to come to terms with the grief and sadness that lies deep in their personality.

The spirit of the Lung – the *po*

The character for the *po*

The Lung houses the '*po*' or physical (corporeal) soul. The character for the *po* has two parts (see Weiger, 1965, lessons 88A and 40). On the left is the character for 'white', the colour resonating with Metal. On the right is the radical for *gui* or spirit or ghost.

So the *po* is a white ghost (see discussion of the *po* in Maciocia, 2008, pp. 264–272). This 'corporeal soul' is linked to the body and might be described as the organisational principle of the body.

The functions of the *po*

The *po* and physical activity

With reference to movement, the corporeal soul 'Gives the capacity of movement, agility, balance and co-ordination of movements' (Maciocia, 2008, p. 265). Any physical activity that is designed to improve the alertness of the senses, develop awareness of the body and promote the ability to move in a co-ordinated way, helps to develop the *po*. Martial arts training is one example of this so it is not surprising that many martial and meditation traditions include breathing exercises.

Two other functions of the *po* are of particular importance.

The *po* and psychic protection

This function is similar to the 'Defensive' (*wei*) *qi* referred to above. On a physical level the Lung gives us the ability to ward off infections like coughs and colds. Because they are vulnerable to these 'attacks' by infections they are called the 'fragile' Organ. On a mental and spiritual level we are also fragile and the *po* gives people protection from attack on these levels.

People who have strong Lung *qi* often have a natural ability to protect themselves. People with weak Lungs, however, are often more sensitive to criticism or emotional assault. This is often hidden by the fact that many Metal CFs appear to cope well and be very competent in many areas of their lives. Their somewhat deadened spirit is often capable of lessening the intensity of the feelings to the extent that they can avoid revealing much to others and possibly to themselves.

The *po* and animation

The *po* also gives people the capacity to have clear sensations. A strong *po* means that people's physical senses are keen and this in turn allows them to be physically and spiritually alert and animated. The Chinese say that someone has '*po li*' when they have high spirits that lead them to become vigorously involved in an activity.

The Large Intestine – the drainer of the dregs

The character for the Large Intestine

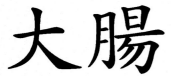

The character for the Large intestine is *da chang* (see Weiger, 1965, lessons 60 (*da*), 130A (*jou*) and 101B (*chang*)).

Su Wen Chapter 8

As always in Chinese medicine, the *yang* paired Organ has a much simpler description than the *yin* Organ. In *Su Wen* Chapter 8, it says:

> The Large Intestine is responsible for transit. The residue from transformation stems from it.
>
> (Larre and Rochat de la Vallée, 1992b, p. 103)

In Chinese medicine texts, this function is broken into three separate functions: the Large Intestine:

- receives transformed food and drink from the Small Intestine;
- absorbs the remaining pure food and nourishment;
- excretes the dirty wastes

Another shorthand description used in Five Element Constitutional Acupuncture is that the Large Intestine is the 'drainer of the dregs'.

The drainer of the dregs

The 'drainer of the dregs' works by eliminating physical matter and fluids from the body as faeces. In the same way as the Lung works on the mind and spirit as well as the body, so the Large Intestine also works on all three levels. It also drains the dregs from the mind and spirit.

This Organ can be compared to dustmen or garbage collectors who regularly empty people's bins. They receive very little recognition for the important work that they do. If the dustmen go on strike, however, people begin to appreciate what they do. After a few days overflowing bags of rubbish fill the streets. This builds up and in time the rubbish starts to rot and the smell starts to pervade the area. If this waste isn't cleared it rapidly becomes a health hazard, creating yet more illness and disease.

We can compare the situation arising when the dustmen strike to what happens if the Large Intestine becomes imbalanced and no longer 'lets go' of rubbish inside us. Instead of being evacuated the waste matter starts to physically build up inside the body and cause internal pollution. This may result in many symptoms especially in areas such as the bowels, skin and hair. It is also reflected at the level of the mind and spirit. People start to become congested and 'mentally constipated' and unable to let go and move on in their lives. They may also become increasingly negative in their thoughts and feelings.

As J. R. Worsley says:

> We are surrounded in our modern society by all kinds of sordid and unpleasant material... Many people with sick Large Intestines may literally become foul mouthed, the bad language, dirty jokes and nasty comments about friends and colleagues all point to the garbage piling up inside.
>
> (Worsley, 1998, p. 14.3)

Deciding what to discard and let go of is therefore the role of the Large Intestine. Some people find it difficult to fully access their grief. For others the struggle is to come to terms with the loss, accept that the situation is now changed and be prepared to move on and form new attachments. When a patient appears to be struggling to 'let go' in this way this may indicate that the Large Intestine is in need of treatment.

The time of day for the Organs

Each Organ in the body has a 2-hour period of the day connected to it. During this time the Organ is at its peak and it has extra *qi* flowing through it. The 2-hour period for the Lung is 3–5 a.m. and for the Large Intestine is 5–7 a.m.

Impaired breathing that consistently occurs around 3 a.m. may point to a weakness of the Lung, but does not necessarily point to Metal as the CF. It is interesting that 3 a.m. has traditionally been the time in many monasteries and convents throughout the world for the monks and nuns to rise. At this time they may meditate, pray or focus on their breathing. This time is favoured as the time when people can most easily receive inspiration from the Heavens and concentrate awareness on the rhythms of breathing and of the body.

On a more mundane level, it is striking that, in countries where people rise with the sun, between 5 and 7 a.m. is the time when people generally open their bowels.

How the Lung and Large Intestine relate

The Lung takes in both air and inspiration from the heavens and the Large Intestine lets go of the dregs. There are many ways to describe the relationship between taking in and letting go.

- Both Organs, although predominantly either taking in or letting go, do some of both. The Lung exhales as well as inhales. It lets go of toxins in the process of exhaling. The Large Intestine absorbs fluids and thus takes in.
- The Lung contacts Heaven. The Large Intestine, as the final stage in the digestive process, contacts the Earth.

The practitioner can often observe the relationship between the Lung and Large Intestine by the ways in which the people relate to change in their lives. The tendency to withdrawal is common in Metal CFs. For some this is predominantly due to their difficulties in receiving. This may manifest, for example, in regard to intimacy, taking on board new ideas, accepting praise or receiving gifts. Some, however, struggle to take on something new because they cannot find a way to let go of what is no longer relevant to them. They cling to what they feel they might lose. This may be a belief or a relationship, and it is as though there is no room for something new to be created.

On the other hand some people are reluctant to let go of their attachment to something until a replacement has been found. For example, when a much-loved pet dies, some people immediately obtain a new pet in order to help them come to terms with their loss. They choose to receive in order to help them let go. Others feel that getting a replacement is almost disloyal to the memory of their beloved pet and may continue to feel the loss for an extended time. It is inappropriate for them to receive until they have managed to let go.

Sometimes it is difficult to understand these kinds of processes, but if the practitioner can gain insight into how the process of taking in and letting go operates much can be revealed about the nature of a patient's Metal Element.

Summary

1 *Su Wen* Chapter 8 describes the Lung as holding 'the office of minister and chancellor. The regulation of the life-giving network stems from it'. It is sometimes known as the 'Receiver of *qi* from the Heavens'.

2 The *po* is the spirit of the Lungs. It gives the capacity of movement, agility, balance and co-ordination of movements.

3 *Su Wen* Chapter 8 describes the Large Intestine as 'responsible for transit. The residue from transformation stems from it.' It is sometimes known as the 'drainer of the dregs'.

4 The time of day associated with the Lung is 3–5 a.m. and that for the Large Intestine is 5–7 a.m.

Patterns of behaviour of Metal Constitutional Factors

19

CHAPTER CONTENTS

Introduction

This chapter describes some of the most important behaviour patterns that are typical of a Metal CF. Some aspects of a person's behaviour can be observed in the treatment room. Others can only be discerned from the patient's description of themselves and their life. As stated in the previous chapters, behaviour can be an indicator of a patient's diagnosis but it can only be used to *confirm* the CF. It should always be used in conjunction with colour, sound, emotion and odour, which are the four primary methods of diagnosis. Once the CF is confirmed the patterns of behaviour may, however, support the practitioner's diagnosis and be used for feedback.

The origin of the behaviours was described in Chapter 7. The imbalance of the Element of the CF creates instability or impairment of the associated emotion. Thus specific negative emotional experiences are more likely to occur to one CF as opposed to another. The behavioural traits described in this chapter are often the responses to these negative experiences. In the case of Metal, people often experience feelings of loss and being worthless and are responding to this.

Patterns of behaviour of a Metal CF

The balanced Element

People with a healthy Metal Element can both feel loss and move on. They take in the richness of life in order to feel satisfied and accept that when something is over they must let go. The Lungs allow people to take in *qi* from the heavens. The Large Intestine allows them to let go of all that they have accumulated and that is no longer of use. When a person is able to take in and let go, their life has quality and meaning. If they don't take in, they feel empty inside. If they don't let go they become congested with waste.

People form attachments as they move through their lives. They become especially attached to the things that are important and nourishing to them. The attachment may be to people, such as parents, friends and partners, but can also be to a beloved pet or possession, to a religious belief, or to certain beliefs or ideas. The Metal Element allows people to connect with these aspects of life and to experience their significance and value. This connection allows people to fully participate in life.

At different stages of life people change their attachments. They must be able to let go and move on. For instance, when children leave home both the parents and children may experience sadness and a sense of loss. Experiencing the sadness allows them to loosen the bonds of their attachment. They can grow and mature from the experience and move on to become connected to whatever becomes significant in the next stage of their life.

Formative events for a Metal CF

Metal CFs may feel that something is lacking in their lives but find it difficult to put their finger on what it is. This is because they may not have really lost anything at all. Their longing is for something that is there but of which they are unaware.

Although it is likely that people are born with their CF, many of their experiences, especially emotional ones, are also coloured by it. Many Metal CFs feel that they weren't given positive acknowledgement as children, however much they actually received. As a result they reach adulthood never really knowing that they are worthwhile human beings. They may grieve that this quality is missing, although they may only be aware of a vague sense of melancholy and lack of self-worth.

Traditionally it is the father's role to instil in children a sense of their own value. It can be early events in relation to the father or a 'father figure' that are connected to the Metal CF's feelings of worthlessness. Metal CFs may have been given cuddles, love and security as children but they especially need to be told how well they did and how important they are. Because Metal is their constitutional imbalance, they may always feel they lack true value, but sensitive parenting can partially compensate for this.

Often, from the viewpoint of a child, the father is the ultimate authority and arbiter of right and wrong. The relationship to the father is vitally important to Metal CFs. A few lose their fathers early in their lives and may be unable to come to terms with the loss. Some may have a distant connection and be aware of a lack of closeness. Many yearn to feel more connected with their father during childhood. They may still yearn for that intimacy when they are adults.

Sometimes there has been a strong bond but they are in awe of their father. They may have difficulty letting go of this as they fail to see him as an ordinary flawed human being. Later in life nobody can ever live up to the idealised vision they have of their father. This can create difficulties in their marriages and working lives.

Patient Example

A Metal CF described her relationship with her father as a contradiction. He was a great influence on her as well as a huge problem. He complimented her in front of other people but never gave her personal attention when they were on their own. Later on she realised that she always tended to turn other people into father figures and put them on pedestals. 'It takes a long time for me to see people as human beings – I give people far too much respect and I tend not to see their failings. I put them beyond criticism, though I can be very hard on myself.'

Partly as a result of these issues, many Metal CFs feel a little distanced and disconnected from other people. They may struggle to take in acknowledgement but at the same time crave it. People with other CFs may find this easier. Their healthy Lung and Large Intestine allow them to take in recognition and to feel connected to others, as well as allowing them to grieve and move on when it is appropriate. Metal CFs often have more difficulties. They may be continually searching for something that will give them a sense of their own value to make up for what they feel they were not given when they were young.

The main issues for a Metal CF

For the Metal CF certain needs remain unmet. This situation creates issues that centre on these areas:

- recognition
- approval
- feeling complete
- feeling adequate in the world
- finding inspiration

The extent to which someone is affected in these areas varies according to the person's physical, mental and spiritual health. Relatively healthy Metal CFs have less disturbance with these aspects of life, whilst those with a greater energetic imbalance end up with their personalities being strongly influenced by this imbalance.

Because of these issues they may consciously or unconsciously ask themselves various questions such as:

- What will give my life meaning?
- Am I really OK?

- What do I need to be complete?
- How can I connect to the world?
- How can I find inspiration and meaning?

Responses to the issues

So far we have described how a weakness in the Metal Element leads to a lesser capacity to accept loss and move on or to take in the richness of life and feel satisfied. The issues that subsequently arise lead to a spectrum of typical ways of responding to the world. These are common, but not exclusive to Metal CFs. If other CFs have patterns of behaviour that seem similar it may indicate that there is a different set of issues underlying them or that their Metal Element is also imbalanced but is not the CF. Noticing these responses is therefore useful but does not replace colour, sound, emotion and odour as the principal way of diagnosing the Constitutional Factor.

The behavioural patterns are along a spectrum and can go between these extremes:

1	fragile	_____ unyielding
2	cut-off	_____ seeking connection
3	resigned or inert	_____ over-working and achieving
4	craving quality and purity	_____ feeling messy and polluted
5	deeply moved	_____ nonchalant

These are discussed below.

Fragile – unyielding

Thin-skinned and delicate

Chinese medicine refers to the Lungs as the 'fragile' or 'tender' Organ. The skin is also associated with the Lung. When the Lung is weak the Metal CF can feel very 'thin-skinned' and delicate.

This emotional fragility is also connected with the *po*, which is the mental-spiritual aspect of the Lungs. In the previous chapter it was discussed that the *po* protects us from unwanted mental or psychic influences. Physically we are protected by the Lung's defensive (*wei*) *qi* and psychically by the *po*.

When the Lungs are weak a person becomes more vulnerable to outside influences.

Many Metal CFs describe being easily wounded. Some show this vulnerability whilst others appear to feel confident. Underneath, however, they may feel inadequate and lacking in self-esteem. If they admit how they feel many Metal CFs say that few people understand the depth of their fragility and weakness.

Over-protected and unyielding

Because most Metal CFs hate to show how delicate they are they will over-protect themselves. This enables them to appear to be 'normal' to the outside world even when they are feeling fragile inside. Whilst Fire CFs often leave themselves vulnerable, Metal CFs usually go to great lengths to defend themselves *before* the attack comes. It is almost as if they carry a shield over their lungs or have put up a 'Keep Out: Private' sign on their chest.

Patient Example

A Metal CF talked to his practitioner about his lack of self-confidence. He told her that he often felt like a failure. He hated to show how bad he felt and would come over to others as very arrogant sometimes. 'It's important not to show my vulnerability to others as it runs very deep. I can easily feel wounded by things others say and do. Then I don't let them in. It makes me feel very alone at times.'

To other people Metal CFs can seem critical, harsh, cold or brittle. They may push people away by putting up a hard front and sometimes even cut off communications completely. This is in an effort to try to show that they don't care and they may even believe their own story. It reduces the intensity of feelings of disappointment and lack of self-esteem. Denial is a marked characteristic of many Metal CFs. They may keep defending themselves even when it is unnecessary and no attack is being made.

One form of defence can be 'nit picking'. For example, a Metal CF may feel hurt and criticised by some idle or imprecise comment that has been said about them. A person with a different CF might recognise the comment as incorrect but let it go or gently rebut it. Fragile Metal CFs, however, may feel injured and misjudged. On the surface they might not show their feelings but may immediately ask specific questions about the truth of this 'judgement', picking out any aspects of language or content that are incorrect. If all goes well the critic backs down and takes back the comment. The Metal CF may even be able to turn the criticism back on to the person who is finding fault and 'prove' that it is not the Metal CF who is in the wrong but the one who has made the comment.

Similarly many Metal CFs may feel personally threatened when someone attacks their opinions and/or beliefs. In this case they may not be able to 'let go' or give any ground about what they believe in. Stubbornness becomes an emotional necessity. By digging their heels in they prove to themselves that they are OK. If they give way they feel fragile and weak.

Criticising to protect

A more aggressive form of protection can be putting other people down. For example, in a situation where a Metal CF doesn't feel comfortable in a group, they are likely to become defensive. The tendency for Metal CFs to feel cut off from others makes this a common situation. They may say to themselves or others, 'I didn't like those people anyway'. In this way they feel better about themselves and avoid looking at their responsibility for the situation. They may have missed the fact that to be accepted by the group they need to be pleasant. They may also defend themselves by fantasising. For instance, if not included in the group, they may convince themselves that it is because people are jealous or feel threatened by them. It is easier to fantasise that they are powerful than to admit that deep inside they are bruised and feel inadequate.

These behaviours may leave them feeling like an outsider and always slightly distanced from others.

Patient Example

A Metal CF talked to her practitioner about how she criticised other people if she felt hurt or badly treated. In general she preferred to get on with others but if she felt slighted it would eat away at her and then she would become critical. She admitted that this was because she felt diminished by the other person's behaviour. Being critical made her feel stronger.

Cut-off – seeking connection

Feeling alienated

Metal CFs distance themselves because they feel fragile and their chests are weak. A weakened chest affects a person's breathing, causing less qi to travel through the bloodstream. Consequently the other Organs don't get revitalised, so the person may feel depleted in energy.

Weak breathing also affects people at the level of the spirit. Breathing connects us to the qi of Heaven, so if people don't breathe properly they often feel cut off and alienated from the world around them. They are unable to make connections or receive what others try to give them. Consequently they begin to feel lonely and isolated. It is as if they have built a wall around themselves. Others can't get in and they can't get out.

When Metal CFs distance themselves, they can appear to be 'cut-off'. Even when they are apparently fully engaged in activities or conversation, other people can feel that they are holding a part of themselves back. One result of this is that others often don't quite know where they stand with Metal CFs. They might ask themselves: "What is going on in there?' or 'Who is this person?' There are many degrees of distancing and many different observations that lead to this description.

How Metal CFs might cut off

Sometimes the cut-off quality will manifest as an inability for Metal CFs to express themselves in an open way. As a result some Metal CFs find work that requires a professional attitude or a clear role to play. Owing to their difficulties with being really present they may then stay in that role outside work so that they don't have to be open and personal. Others spend more time than usual on their own, even though the rest of the family, social group or community are together. Another way that they might be cut off or distanced is by holding back or becoming more intellectual when others are expressing personal feelings. They can then avoid direct expression of feeling. This is a common tendency and is often the way that a Metal CF fails to meet the 'needs of the situation'. There are times when people are distressed and require warmth, compassion and humanity. The inert nature of some Metal CFs makes this difficult.

Metal CFs rarely reveal their deepest concerns nor wear their hearts on their sleeve. Sometimes they may talk a lot, but rarely about themselves. They often keep their personal feelings very private. Often they are unable to immediately take in and deal with the feelings generated by an experience and they need to go away and process them by themselves. It is not that they have no feelings, in fact their feelings are often deep and intense. Keeping distanced from them, however, prevents them from becoming overwhelmed and most Metal CFs would hate to show that they are unable to cope.

Patient Example

A Metal CF described how throughout her life she had felt different from other people. When she was younger and healthier she felt there was something special about her and it was a pleasant feeling. Later in life she became depressed and a feeling of dullness set in. She commented that whether she felt well or not she always felt separate. 'Some people say I seem slightly aloof. Other people might feel a separation from others but it's more palpable with me. I love to be in relationship to other people but a part of me is always a little distant as well.'

It is interesting to note that in almost every spiritual tradition where people meditate in isolation they also focus on breathing. Breathing can stop people from feeling isolated and alienated and allows them to connect to something greater than themselves. This can stop them from getting depressed. Strengthening the Lungs and learning to breathe can help Metal CFs to connect to themselves and the world and enable them to become less cut off and alienated.

Seeking connection to the heavens

Because many Metal CFs feel distanced and cut off they have a strong desire to feel more connected. In order to do this they may search for inspiration more intensely than others. In the Chinese tradition the heavens represent the feeling of quality given by one's father and the earth represents the feeling of being nurtured given by one's mother. Humans beings stand between Heaven and Earth and need to be in contact with both. People can nourish themselves with food from the earth but still be lacking something because they have lost contact with heaven. They literally lack inspiration. Some compensate for feeling cut off and inert by seeking a connection with an image of a father or something inspirational outside themselves. This may be expressed through a need to adopt a religion or spiritual path or by finding teachers, mentors or other 'father figures' to guide them.

Traditionally, Christians have always prayed to the 'Father in Heaven'. All the major monotheistic religions believe in a male God who resides in the heavens. Although this emphasis on the male archetype is changing, the quality brought by his role is still often seen as one that gives acknowledgement and recognition as well as authority and guidance. By receiving *qi* from the heavens the Lungs can be thought of as the main contact with the higher guiding part of ourselves. The earth satisfies people's more basic needs, but the heavens are the location of their mental and spiritual nourishment and inspiration.

When people make contact with Heaven through meditating, chanting or praying they may feel more connected and experience greater satisfaction and fulfilment. Spending time in nature, especially being on mountains, can also nourish a person's spirit in a similar way. Once the communication cord to Heaven is in place it can spill over into the rest of a person's life. If the Lungs are weak, however, it may be difficult to make this connection. People may easily become disappointed, pessimistic and critical. They struggle to find anything that gives them a feeling of genuine fulfilment.

The experience of losing religious faith exemplifies how some Metal CFs feel. People who have had a strong religious conviction from early in life can encounter bleak and desolate feelings of emptiness, loss and lack of meaning if they lose their faith. They may experience deep feelings of grief but it is unusual for them to show this overtly or publicly. Such people usually keep their feelings well hidden and go about their life as normal. Their feelings of being cut off from their source of inspiration and their sadness, however, may stay with them for the rest of their lives.

Father figures

Rather than turning to a spiritual father some Metal CFs may strive to become as powerful as a father figure and gain respect from those around them. This is often a powerful drive for a Metal CF. Just as a Fire CF craves warmth, Metal CFs need the feeling that others respect them. They may outwardly shrug it off if people pay them a compliment or adopt a respectful attitude, but it is this recognition that they crave.

Alternatively they may find father figures to turn to. They may hold these people in high esteem and turn to them for support and advice. They may have a conflict between becoming independent from a father figure and at the same time wanting more dependence and connection. Independence temporarily makes them feel more whole. They don't have to rely on another person – but they are isolated. Dependence temporarily gives them a feeling of being connected – but they can't always rely on that person to be there.

When Metal CFs connect to their own spirit, they feel more connected to life and more comfortable in the world. Connecting makes them feel whole. Treatment on the Metal Element helps Metal CFs to establish and deepen this connection.

Patient Example

A Metal CF commented that although there were a lot of things that other people seemed to find fun, she couldn't really be bothered with any of them because the spiritual path was so important. Rather than being connected to other people it seemed more essential for her to be connected to a 'higher truth' that was not to do with God or a religion. 'It's not that I don't like other people, it's more that people are not a primary thing for me. Finding my spiritual path and following it – that's the only thing that seems worthwhile.'

Resigned or inert – over-working and achieving

Resignation

Many Metal CFs may feel that they are in a situation that is similar to that of Sisyphus, a character in Greek mythology. He was given the task of pushing a round stone up a mountain on which there was no level place for the stone to rest. When he came to the top and rested momentarily, the stone would roll back down. He would then retrace his steps down the mountain and push the stone up again. Like Sisyphus, Metal CFs want completion and connection but whatever appears to answer the quest never seems to work and the stone rolls down the hill again. If this happens too often the Metal CF may give up. What seemed like it might reveal the 'gold nuggets' that appear in the character for Metal has not worked. The consequence is often a state of resignation and cynicism.

Resignation is a natural response to continued failure. People feel sad and in despair and this results in a feeling of emptiness inside. Grief makes the qi 'disappear', leaving a void in its place. The glass is half empty rather than half full. Sometimes resignation can seem similar to the attitude of detachment prescribed by spiritual teachers, but it is not the same. People who are resigned will passively endure whatever comes their way because they have given up. They are surviving life rather than meeting it full on. They may complain of tiredness, which feels very physical to them. They are suffering from a resignation of the spirit and a lack of zest for life. Their eyes often lack vitality and sparkle whereas a true state of spiritual detachment is accompanied by an inner radiance that beams out through bright, shining eyes.

Cynicism

A common consequence of resignation is cynicism and a tendency to criticise. The effect of the belief that they are flawed can be taken by some Metal CFs to mean that all their efforts are worthless. They may feel that everything they do is futile and doomed to failure and they may project this on to others by becoming disdainful and critical. They may also be as critical of themselves as other people and set impossible standards that no one can reach.

The resignation and cynicism can easily become associated with arrogance, a quality sometimes attributed to Metal CFs. It is well known that arrogance always masks feelings of inadequacy. One way of coping with the Sisyphean failure is to claim success or a special understanding of life. This may compensate and make Metal CFs feel that they have internal quality. In the process of attributing this to themselves they may insinuate that others are not this way and are inferior.

Continual achieving

At the other extreme to being inert or resigned many Metal CFs strive to achieve. They may work harder than everyone else, to compensate for feeling that they have no real worth and value. Metal CFs might still be working when everyone else has gone home and in order to give themselves an additional sense of worth may also work at weekends. This can be contrasted with some Earth CFs who also work excessively hard but for a different reason. This is because they are unable to say 'no' to people who want their sympathy and support.

Becoming successful or the 'best'

Metal CFs might also decide to try and gain a sense of worth and self-respect by becoming successful and gaining recognition. They think that if they are successful it will make them feel more complete. Recognition is a basic need for many people. Compared to other people, Metal CFs might already be getting more recognition but be having difficulty taking it in. They then try to obtain even more as a way to lessen the feeling of not having enough.

Metal CFs may also try to feel complete by becoming the 'best' at whatever they do. They are often more competitive than others and may become experts with specialist knowledge in certain aspects of their work. As it may be impossible to be good at everything, Metal CFs often try to be outstanding at one specific area. They may completely throw themselves into whatever they are trying to achieve. This search for excellence has many positive aspects but it easily becomes compulsive. The task in hand may be being a research scientist, a housewife and mother or a window cleaner. The theme running through all of these is the motivation to do well. Unfortunately Metal CFs may set themselves such impossibly high standards that they never quite do it well enough and always feel as if they are falling below their expectations.

Because they are constantly criticising themselves many Metal CFs always feel dissatisfied. They find it hard to acknowledge what they have achieved. Satisfaction and contentment are normal and nourishing states for most people. They may result from having helped a child to read, supported and listened to a friend in need, from having written ten letters or from having put up a garden fence. After putting effort into something there is a normal time when people stop and allow themselves to say, 'Yes, I've done that well.' Metal CFs may find it difficult to reflect on what they have done and subsequently to take in praise or feel satisfaction. They often cut this time short and reject acknowledgement, from the inside or outside, and thus they stay hungry.

Craving quality and purity – messy and polluted

Searching for quality

Some Metal CFs might choose to assert their quality and worth by living a luxurious lifestyle and owning 'classy' possessions. They might buy expensive designer clothes, own a deluxe model car, send their children to the most expensive schools or live in the most upmarket part of town. They think that the 'right' accessories can also indicate that a person has quality and value. Metal CFs may become obsessed with wearing valuable jewellery, having high quality shoes or even an 'accessory' such as a handsome man or beautiful woman on their arm. They may want to be seen in the right places, doing the right things. A high status job may also be important. All of these things can give the impression of quality and at times at least it may make a Metal CF feel that they are important and better than other people. At other times it can still leave them feeling empty and dissatisfied as of course there are always going to be richer, more successful people to emulate.

The question the Metal CFs might ask themselves is: 'Does this activity just generate attention and look good or does it give me internal satisfaction?' The more they have on the outside does not mean more on the inside, so the quandary remains the same. Taking in the achievement is the issue, not generating massive amounts of it.

Finding meaning

Another deeper way to gain internal richness is for Metal CFs to ask themselves questions about the meaning of what they are doing. They may ask, 'Why should I do this?' 'What purpose does it serve?' These questions are not exclusive to Metal CFs, but whatever activity is happening, whether they are playing cards, working at the office, baby-sitting or sitting on the beach on holiday, they may be unconsciously evaluating if it is meaningful. They may then try to find a greater sense of purpose in what they do. This may be through things such as seeking knowledge, truth, beauty, the right organisation to join or the right exercises or developmental practice to follow. Fulfilment will probably still elude them, so they continue to search.

Some Metal CFs may be acutely aware of the lessening quality of life generally. They may also look around them with regret as they see falling standards and increasing superficiality in the world. They easily become nostalgic. Where the major influence on people was once their culture, family and work, they now see TV, fast food and being famous as prime influences. It used to be better before. The special quality that was there is now gone.

As a result of their search for quality, some Metal CFs may frequently appear to chop and change and may go through a number of different professions, spiritual practices or friends. This can give the impression to others that their life is very erratic. Externally things might be changing but on the inside it is the same search for connection.

No quality

Many Metal CFs flip back and forth between feeling that they have no quality and feeling that they are better quality than other people. Some may have an inner sense of poverty and deprivation because they think they are worthless and unimportant. This feeling may lead to them feeling depressed and self-critical. How they look, feel and take care of themselves may reflect this. Rather than buying the best quality they may think and act as if they are poor. They may buy cheap clothes or ones that come from second-hand shops and may even prefer to wear clothes that are worn. Anything immaculate doesn't feel quite right.

Feeling polluted

Some Metal CFs feel polluted. This is especially true if the Large Intestine is sluggish. In this case waste materials in the body are stored instead of eliminated. In order to try to clear out the pollution they may fast or take enemas or may eat health foods in order to 'de-toxify'. They may feel unclean inside and, despite washing, always feel or look a little dirty. Their skin may not be clear and their hair may be lifeless.

Mentally they may be just as congested and they might hold on to rigid beliefs or old grudges and find it hard to let in new thoughts or ideas. They may compare themselves to others and find themselves wanting. They may feel that they may never be as good, powerful or clever as other people.

The tendency to feel inferior to others is a reflection of a Metal CF's lack of feelings of self-worth. Self-criticism is often insistent and harsh. These feelings are not usually shown to others so the practitioner may need to win an especially deep level of trust if Metal CFs are to open up. It is easy for this kind of Metal CF to dwell on their shortcomings in particular situations and they often find it hard to forgive themselves for their perceived inadequacies. This is the opposite end of the spectrum from those Metal CFs who hate to admit to any failings and therefore find it easier to blame others.

Deeply moved – nonchalant

Special moments

It is normal for everyone to have special moments. At these times extra *qi* runs through the chest as people take in and acknowledge the wonder of what they are experiencing. For some Metal CFs these feelings can be so overwhelming that they find it easier to avoid them and play them down. At the other extreme some Metal CFs attempt to capture the specialness in every moment to make up for the lack of richness they normally feel inside.

Some Metal CFs can easily feel tearful and overwhelmed by ordinary events in life. They may feel a person's pain and suffering. The grief and melancholy inside them is often so strong that when they feel the tears well up it is painful and they instinctively push them down again. Many rarely actually let go and fully express their tears. Crying in this way would be too overwhelming so they are more likely to choke up or weep a small amount at a time.

They may choke up if they or others are rewarded for something they have done well. This may be pleasurable but at the same time overwhelming.

> **Patient Example**
>
> A Metal CF said that she was often feeling that she'd lost something and that she'd had something but it had now gone. For example, she said that she often wished she could go back to when her children were little. Because she had these feelings it increased the specialness of other moments in her life. She would think, 'Oh, this is really nice so I'd better treasure it right now.' She said she thought she felt the moment more acutely than other people and would often feel pleasure tinged with poignancy.

Some Metal CFs can feel totally overwhelmed by the beauty and special qualities of life. Some may express this artistically and see a beautiful sculpture in an ordinary piece of wood or feel moved to paint a picture of a golden sunset. Others may feel stirred to write poignant poetry about a special moment. Their experience may be extremely emotional and affect them deeply. Some Metal CFs savour these profound experiences. They may keep them to themselves but feel them deeply. Others may want people to partake in the experience. If the special times are expressed creatively, Metal CFs may want to be recognised by the outside world for their unique gift. Some may gain this recognition but, of course, others don't.

Some people may see Metal CFs as too serious about themselves and rather 'precious'. What Metal CFs find extraordinary might seem mundane to other people. If others do not recognise the special quality of the Metal CF she or he may feel disappointed. They may be dismissive of others for their lack of depth, rather than recognising that everyone has different tastes and experiences.

> **Patient Example**
>
> A Metal CF 'confessed' to her practitioner that she adored watching the Academy Awards on TV and would stay up all night watching them. She loved to see the look of joy on people's faces as they experienced their special moments of fame on receiving their rewards.

Nonchalant

Some Metal CFs underplay their experiences. If something special comes up it can be easier to deny it than to acknowledge it. By ignoring their feelings they can avoid becoming overwhelmed.

> **Patient Example**
>
> The grown-up son of a Metal CF used to become exasperated and at the same time amused by his father. They would regularly meet for lunch and catch up on what had been happening in their lives. The Metal CF would always understate what had happened to him and would almost forget to mention that he had been promoted at work or had changed his job. The son (who was a Fire CF) would, on the other hand, be bursting with the news of a job change or other life event and couldn't wait to tell his Dad, and anyone else who would care to listen.

Metal CFs can behave nonchalantly by speaking about important events and experiences as if they are commonplace occurrences. Everything is 'no big deal'. They may have had an accident, have lost their job, their best friend died, or on the positive side won an important competition. These might all be spoken about with the same matter-of-factness as going for a walk, eating a meal or taking a shower. The nonchalance is a protective measure. It stops them from becoming overwhelmed by the awe and wonder of special feelings and also stops them from being overpowered by feelings of grief and sadness. *Any* feelings that go through the lung area can be difficult for the Metal CF to experience fully.

Sometimes a Metal CF may act nonchalantly to avoid showing how worthless they really feel. If they stood up and talked about themselves they wouldn't expect people to be interested and if people did take notice it might be too overwhelming anyway. Those who did not feel acknowledged when they were young may still not expect their feelings to be acknowledged now. Because of this they may continue to ignore how they feel, especially if they think they may need support from others when expressing their needs. It is easier to show that they are independent and can look after themselves and they may look ahead to the next activity or project rather than looking back at any grief or loss. This ensures that life can remain on an even keel with no one suspecting what is really going on inside.

Summary

1 A diagnosis of a Metal CF is made primarily by observation of a white facial colour, a weeping voice, a rotten odour and imbalance in the emotion of grief.

2 Metal CFs tend to have issues and difficulties with:
- recognition
- approval
- feeling complete
- feeling adequate in the world
- finding inspiration

3 Because of these issues Metal CFs' behaviour and responses to situations tend to fluctuate between being:

- fragile   _____ unyielding
- cut-off   _____ seeking connection
- resigned or inert   _____ over-working and achieving
- craving quality and purity   _____ feeling messy and polluted
- deeply moved   _____ nonchalant

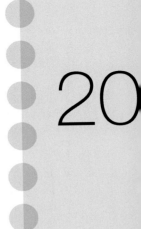

Water – key resonances

Water as a symbol

The character for Water – *shui*

The character shows a central current of water with side streams or whirls beside it. It suggests the flow of water in a river where the main current is bordered by small whirlpools. The whirlpools arise from the difference in flow between the central stream and the edges where the current may be slower or even running in the opposite direction (see Weiger, 1965, lesson 125). Acupuncture points are often thought to arise in a similar situation, where the flow of *qi* is bent or redirected and as a result a vortex develops.

The Water Element in nature

Water is the most *yin* of all the Elements. It is everywhere, but has no shape, taking only the form given by containers, river banks and the beds of the oceans. Although it is the softest of substances, it can wear away the hardest rock and move around any obstacle to penetrate beyond. It appears both as a solid and as a gas. Water filters through the earth, enters roots of trees and flows upwards. In response to warmth it turns into a gas and appears in the sky as clouds, ultimately to fall as rain moistening wherever it falls and reappearing in streams, rivers, lakes and oceans.

Floods and drought

Water has the capacity to cause havoc. People who have experienced flooding or powerful waves understand how water can penetrate and sweep away all that lies in its path. After the initial surge, flood water will often become stagnant. Disease and pollution follow, resulting in illness.

At the other extreme a drought can be just as devastating. Climatic changes can leave a degree of dryness that inhibits crops, resulting in famine. Adults and children shrivel up and die of thirst and starvation.

Water within a person

Water makes up 55–60% of an adult's body weight (Thibodeau and Patton, 1992, pp. 474–476). Most of this water is enclosed in or surrounds individual cells and the remainder is plasma, that is part of our blood. These fluids have many functions, but most involve movement and flexibility.

A newborn baby, who has emerged from living within water, is roughly 80% water. This percentage declines rapidly in the first year of life and gradually as we age our water content diminishes.

The skin and hair of children and young adults is naturally moist and the joints and bones are resilient and pliant. Injuries heal rapidly. Young people's minds are also flexible and have the capacity to take in enormous amounts of information. Languages can be learned very rapidly. They can flow and change in whichever way life takes them.

As people age their bodies become dryer, their hair more brittle, their skin withered and their movements less smooth. Their minds lose flexibility. They have difficulty with new information and accepting changes in the world around them. Ageing is partly a drying up process, a sign that the Water Element is weakening and that we are losing our water reserves. In spite of Water's flexibility, when it is constrained and not moving, toxins develop and function is diminished. The newborn with the maximum amount of clean water has the maximum flexibility and softness; the octogenarian will be fluid deficient, harder and less flexible.

The Water Element in relation to the other Elements

The Water Element interacts with the other Elements through the *sheng* and *ke* cycles (see Chapter 2, this volume).

Metal is the mother of Water

On the *sheng* cycle Metal creates Water by containing it. Water has no shape unless contained by the impermeable rocks in the earth. This means that when treating patients who have obvious Water Element symptoms, such as urinary symptoms, these may have originated in the mother Element, Metal. A practitioner may treat the mother to assist the child.

Water is the mother of Wood

The close relationship between Water and Wood is often stressed in Chinese medicine. Hence

practitioners will sometimes have difficulty in deciding whether to focus treatment on the Wood or the Water. Five Element practitioners mainly use colour, sound, odour and emotion to decide. The mother–child law, based on the *sheng* cycle, stresses that symptoms arising from the Wood Element often indicate a weakness of the mother and that treatment of Water is required.

Water controls Fire

On the *ke* cycle Water controls Fire. A fire hose illustrates how water can be used to control fire. In general, there are many body–mind functions which involve heat and which can be spoiled by too much fire. The control of inflammation, the drying out of joints and the dampening down of excess emotions are all examples. In these cases, Water will contain, control and regulate the excesses of Fire.

Water is controlled by Earth

In nature it is clear how water is controlled by earth. River banks and dams are obvious ways in which Earth contains or directs the flow of water. Earth controlling Water means that a balanced Earth helps Water to also be balanced. For example, if the Spleen is failing to move fluids these may accumulate and in so doing create a disturbance within the Water Element.

The key Water resonances

(Table 20.1)

The colour for Water is blue/black

Colour in nature

Ask ordinary people, 'What is the colour of water?' and they would probably say 'blue'. In a drinking glass

Table 20.1 Key Water resonances	
Colour	Blue/black
Sound	Groan
Emotion	Fear
Odour	Putrid

water is transparent and colourless. At the lake or seaside, water can appear different colours because of its ability to reflect light from the sky. Divers describe the colour deep under water as black, more from the lack of light than any inherent colour of water itself.

The character for blue, blue-black or black

The character for blue or blue-black is *kan* (see Weiger, 1965, lessons 92A and 73B).

Alternatively the character is black, *hei* (see Weiger 1965, lesson 40D).

This character refers to the colour of soot. The character shows it deposited around a window through which smoke escaped in Chinese huts.

Su Wen Chapter 10 states that: 'Black (or blue-black) corresponds to the Kidneys (or Water)' (Anonymous, 1979a, p. 27).

Facial colour

When the Water Element is out of balance a black, dark blue or occasionally a lighter sky or powder blue will manifest on the face. This colour can appear at the side of the eyes, under the eyes or around the mouth. The lighter blue is more confined to under or beside the eyes.

Blue/black can appear for reasons other than Water being the CF. Kidney disease is one. Many of the patients in a kidney dialysis ward have a blackish facial colour, but not all will be Water CFs. Their illness, manifesting in poor kidney function, may well have originated in another Element. In a similar way, anyone who fails to sleep well, or who becomes very tired through excess activity, may appear dark under the eyes. The lack of sleep or overwork is depleting reserves that are normally said to be stored in the Kidneys. So it is important when observing a dark colour to enquire about a patient's sleep patterns and lifestyle and whether there is any history of kidney disease.

The sound for Water is groaning

The character for groaning

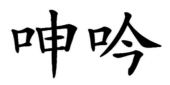

The character for groaning is *shen yin* (see Weiger, 1965, lessons 72A (*kou*), 50C (*shen*) and 14K (*chin*)).

The context

The voice tone resonating with Water is groaning. The context in which it would normally occur is when a threat has appeared and the person speaking is anxious or afraid. There are, of course, other appropriate tones when fear is present. For example, with a shock or a situation of intense fear the person may be screaming or crying out. In most situations of fear or anxiety, however, it would be said to be normal for a person's voice to modify and begin to flatten into a groan. There is little movement or modulation in the quality of the sound.

People often have a groaning voice when they are afraid, but Water CFs groan at other times when the context is not threatening or dangerous. For example, if someone groans when discussing the pleasure of a recent party or the recent loss of a relative, this might be said to be expressing inappropriate groaning. A pattern of groaning in these contexts would indicate evidence of a Water CF.

The sound of groaning

The sound of groaning is one of flatness as if the more normal ups and downs of the voice have been squeezed or flattened out. In some people this is more marked at the end of sentences. It can sound a bit like an old reel-to-reel tape that has become stretched so that the speech or music plays slightly slowly. It sounds as though it is dragging and lacks animation.

Groaning can also be visualised. To visualise a groaning voice, imagine a line on a graph which moves up and down according to the changes of pitch in a person's voice. Then imagine that a boundary line comes down from above and up from below cutting out the higher and lower reaches of the voice. This makes the voice flatter.

To experience the effects of fear that lead to a groaning voice, imagine being in a room with a group of people. The group leader tells you that a deadly snake has escaped and is somewhere on the floor. The snake will respond to any abrupt movement or loud noise. You need to ask the leader for the next best move in order to make your escape. You flatten your voice in order not to create more disturbance. You are groaning.

Groaning indicates an imbalanced Water Element but it can easily be confused with the flat voice that is known as 'lack of laugh' which indicates a Fire CF. Careful attention to the context in which it is used will help to differentiate.

The odour for Water is putrid

The character for putrid

The character for putrid is *fu* (see Weiger, 1965, lessons 59I (*yen*), 45C (*fu*) and 65A (*ju*)). The first parts of this character represent a shed (*yen*) and building (*fu*). The second part means pieces of dry meat in a bundle (*ju*). The character gives the sense of the putrid odour arising from keeping dried meat in a building.

Putrid

The smell of processed or rotting meat is one of the descriptions for putrid in English. But putrid also describes the smell of water in a stagnant pond or the smell of stale urine. Bleach and ammonia smell putrid. It can be a sharp, aggressive odour. Some practitioners say it makes the inside of their noses clench or seize up.

The emotion for Water is fear

The character for fear

The character for fear is *kong* (see Weiger, 1965, lesson 11F). The character shows a hand carrying a tool poised above the heart. There is stillness here as well as the potential for agitation. Below this is the Heart. The effect of fear when it feels as though something is repeatedly beating or knocking on one's heart is conveyed. This is fear that could cause us to feel palpitations on the inside and be frozen and unable to move forward on the outside.

If a person becomes fearful or anxious it is natural for this to be accompanied by symptoms of *qi* 'descending' (*Su Wen*, Chapter 39; see Larre and Rochat de la Vallée, 1995). If instead the person attempts to suppress this movement of *qi*, then the *qi* may move upwards, causing symptoms in the upper part of the body, for example palpitations, indigestion or asthma.

The character for fright

The character for fright is *jing*.

The Water Element is also especially affected by fright. *Jing* means shock or fright (Weiger, 1965, lessons W54G and W137A). *Jing* affects both the Kidneys and the Heart. It is made up of two characters, *chi* at the top and *ma* at the bottom (see Weiger, 1965, lessons 137A (*ma*) and 54G (*chi*)).

Chi means to restrain oneself or be self-possessed. It shows a ram's horns, because a ram excels at standing motionless. On the upper right-hand side there is a hand holding a rod. This signifies authority. Both these images symbolise stillness. In contrast, *ma* represents the head, mane, legs and tail of a horse. The horse is a powerful symbol to the Chinese. It is very *yang*, moves fast and is also regarded as sensitive, nervy and jumpy. The whole character suggests a state similar to, but also subtly different from, fear (*kong*). The person is trying to be self-possessed, but is shaking and trembling on the inside.

With respect to the causes of disease the significance of the two terms is that fear is the emotion most often associated with Water and fright or shock is the emotion which might occur only once, but even so can cause lasting imbalance. For example, it is believed some forms of epilepsy are caused by the mother being shocked while the foetus is in the womb. For others, their life is characterised by shocks and traumas which 'scatter' their *qi* (*Su Wen*, Chapter 3; Larre and Rochat de la Vallée, 1995).

Fear as an appropriate emotion

When some people first encounter the emotions resonating with the Elements, they think that some emotions seem 'negative', while others seem 'positive'. For example, fear is usually regarded as a negative experience, whereas joy seems positive. Fear, however, is one of our most primary and necessary emotions because it allows us to survive. *Ju* is often used by the Chinese along with *kong* to describe fear.

懼

This character shows the Heart radical on the left. On the right we can see two eyes and below them a small bird (see Weiger, 1965, lesson 158G). Small birds symbolise vigilance, which is the positive benefit arising from our fearful feelings.

The ability to survive is one of the strongest instincts we have. Without fear we would not be alive and human life as we know it would not have been able to continue. Fear alerts animals to protect themselves from predators and other dangers. Fear of illness is what leads to the discovery of new medicines and ways of staying healthy. Fear of being destitute leads people to find ways of earning a living. Fear of death is a human's most basic fear as it threatens one of the key functions of the Water Element, the drive to survive. Caution and prevention are the positive aspect of this emotion.

There is also a very fine line between excitement and fear. Physiologists can detect no difference between the two adrenalised states. One is pleasurable, one is not, however. Without fear there would be no excitement or sense of adventure and humanity would be the poorer for it.

The mental aspect of fear

The natural process of fear runs through these stages:

1 awareness of a threat

2 feeling of fear

3 mind considers solution(s)

4 action

5 safety (or if not return to 3)

If someone is about to be run down by a car and jumps to avoid it, the process is short. If a person notices a tile about to fall from the roof, possibly onto where the children play, then they think about what to do and the overall process is extended. The feeling of fear is simply the initiator and it is helpful to think of the whole process.

Fear tends to involve the mind in two ways. People perceive something, for example, the roof tile, as a threat. So the mind is important in even noticing the roof tile and forming the judgement that it may be dangerous. What some people find threatening, others hardly notice. The mind is also involved in devising solutions. For example, 'can I reach the tile from an upstairs window and temporarily make it safe?' or 'can I ring up my handyman and get him over before the children return from school?' Chinese medicine states that the Kidneys create cleverness and wisdom (see Chapter 21, this volume). One interpretation is that a healthy Water Element leads to a balanced approach to the presence of danger that in turn requires the mind to work quickly and effectively.

Abnormal patterns of fear

There are two main ways that fear manifests and these can appear to varying degrees. The first way is for people to be intensely fearful, the second is for people to anticipate 'danger' so that they avoid experiencing fear. Some Water CFs tend to excessive fearfulness, others to an absence of fear.

Fear

When people feel intensely fearful profound changes take place in the body's physiology. Adrenaline production increases, muscle tone tightens, heart rate and perspiration increase. The mind may be overwhelmed and the person struggles to function well. The extremes of this pattern are phobias and hysteria. We are using the word 'hysteria' in the dictionary sense of morbidly or uncontrollably emotional. A person with agoraphobia cannot leave the house and no amount of reasoning will make a difference. They cannot *hear* potential solutions even when they are generated by others. Someone behaving hysterically with fear does not appear to access their mind in order to consider solutions.

Or if they do, the messages it gives are overwhelmed by the intensity of the feelings. Everybody knows that a small spider cannot harm anybody, but for someone who is terrified of spiders this knowledge makes little or no difference. The Water Element is out of balance and the intensity of the emotion overwhelms the mind.

Much of the time, people hide their fear from others. Being joyful, sad or even angry does not seem as shaming as letting others see the fear within them. Diagnosing Water CFs, therefore, can often be particularly difficult. Fear, however, produces increased physiological activity and this often shows in the patient as agitation. Some tend to be physically restless and find it hard to keep their bodies still. Others have found ways to quieten the agitation in their bodies to such an extent that the fear is only really visible in their eyes. They somewhat resemble a rabbit caught in the headlights as the intensity of their fear paralyses them.

Fear makes the *qi* descend. When fear is intense this often makes people need to go to the toilet in a hurry. In chronic cases it often leads to strong physical sensations in the torso as the movements of *qi* create agitation. Some feel this in the heart and chest primarily. Others feel it in the 'pit' of their stomach and others feel it more in the lower abdomen.

Patient Example

One Water CF, who inclined to this pattern, described the following: 'I'm scared most of the time to some degree or another. At times I may feel a contraction in my lower belly. I think it's to do with not knowing why I'm scared. If I know why I'm scared I'll have other symptoms. I'll feel a rush of adrenaline – my heartbeat increases, my mouth goes dry and I need to pee.'

The patient's response to reassurance can sometimes be revealing. Some patients will attempt to allay their anxiety by looking for reassurance. Health issues are obviously a common theme where this manifests. In order to assess the person's degree of fear it is often necessary to evoke a degree of anxiety and then gauge the patient's response to the reassurance offered. Whereas most people would be relieved by reassurance, or at least take it in, it is usually impossible to reassure a Water CF. This

is because their fear is deeply irrational and cannot really be touched by words or information. It is as if a block has occurred between their mind and feelings. Water CFs naturally often find it difficult to trust others. There is a wariness about them that is rarely relinquished.

Some Water CFs find that fear agitates their body, mind and spirit, so they attempt to reduce these feelings. To do this they may avoid situations that generate excitement, as the extra adrenaline produces feelings of discomfort. Fun fairs, scary movies and dangerous activities are also generally avoided. Acupuncture, regrettably, is also often avoided for the obvious reason concerning needles. Often it is only desperation or extreme health anxiety that drives them to come for treatment. Practitioners, therefore, see these kinds of Water CFs less often than some other CFs.

Lack of fear

Some people have learnt to repress their feelings of fear. They become hyper-aware and attempt to anticipate threats and deal with them before they appear. Why do people do this? Some have felt frightened in early childhood and hated the experience. Over time they evolve coping strategies that involve suppressing the intensity of the emotion, often to the extent that they have become unaware of the feeling. Whatever the origin of the pattern, we label these people 'lack of fear' as they rarely appear to be frightened and do not admit to situations causing them to be frightened. They may invest a lot of energy in anticipating what could go wrong and thinking through their responses before any threat appears. Such people are often very competent in their work. For example, the essence of entrepreneurship is to assess risks and increase the money-making aspect while avoiding failure. People with a lack of fear pattern often excel in such an activity. They draw on a skill that has been refined since childhood.

People with this pattern also frequently take what the rest of the world thinks of as unnecessary risks. They drive too fast, ride motor bikes, bungee jump, parachute or hang glide. Excitement is one thing, recklessness another. They usually do not describe what they do as frightening. It is fun, exciting, gives them a sense of feeling alive, but whatever it is it is not scary. A female Water CF of this type drove her powerful car at what most of us would consider excessively high speeds. When questioned, she said that it was exciting, but not dangerous. When

Table 20.2 Examples of the range of emotions associated with the Water Element

Fear	Fright, terror, anxiety, dread, panic, trepidation, apprehension, horror, foreboding, cowardice, wariness
Fearlessness	Bravado, unafraid, adventurous, courageous, daring, risk taking, recklessness

Table 20.3 Supporting Water resonances

Season	Winter
Power	Storage
Climate	Cold
Sense Organ/Orifice	Ear
Tissues and body parts	Bones
Generates	Teeth
Taste	Salty

challenged that the excess speed did increase the risk of a serious accident, she said that the increased speed made her more alert and therefore safer. She also said that the only time she felt scared was in a scary movie, when of course she could easily walk out (Table 20.2).

> **Patient Example**
>
> A friend describes an example of a calculated risk-taker: 'She has the most scars of anyone I have ever met. She likes to go and walk along under the cliffs and get stuck in the tide and risk her neck. She really enjoys being on the edge. She denies that what she does is dangerous and says only that it is exciting.'

Lack of fear is a pattern that is often hard to diagnose as it is the absence of the emotion rather than its obvious expression. Questioning the patient about their leisure activities may give an indication, but it needs to be supported by colour, sound, odour and the practitioner's direct experience of their emotion. Often these patients tend to be almost motionless in their bodies, but their eyes are alert for every possible danger. There is also a tendency for practitioners to feel anxious in their presence although they may struggle to understand why.

The supporting Water resonances

These resonances are less important than the 'key' resonances given above. They can often be used to indicate that a person's Water Element is imbalanced but they do not necessarily point to it being the person's CF (Table 20.3).

The season of Water is winter

The character for winter

The Chinese character for winter is *dong* (Weiger, 1965, lessons 17A and 17F). The character represents a skein of thread that is fixed by a tie or a brooch to keep it closed. This gives us a sense of loose threads that are tied up or something that is tied up and finished. Winter is the time of year when everything in nature slows down. It is the end of the cycle of the seasons when the sun diminishes, hence the character representing the tied up threads symbolises completion. The lower part of the character represents water crystallising into ice. So we have the ideas of the last season in the cycle and the stillness of ice.

Winter

Life slows down in the winter. It is a time when nature rests. Water freezes over, the fields lie fallow, animals hibernate and the seeds of plants lie dormant ready to sprout forth in the next season. *Su Wen* Chapter 2 states:

> In winter all is hidden, this is the season of retirement into the depth, because it is cold outside. It is necessary at this moment not to disturb or disperse the *yang* energy, thus complying with the energy of the Winter.
>
> (Anonymous, 1979, p. 3)

Su Wen urges us to follow the cycle of the seasons in order to stay healthy. In the wintertime the days are short and darkness falls early. This means that in the winter we should go to bed early, slow our activity to a minimum and preserve and protect our reserves of *qi*. This conserves our *qi* and helps us to remain healthy when the time for movement arrives in the spring.

The power of Water is storage

The character for storage

The character for storage is *cang* (Weiger, 1965, lessons 78B (*tsao*) and 82E (*tsang*)). This character is not illuminating, being made of two other characters, the upper one denoting herbaceous plants and the lower one the notion of compliance, which is said to be the virtue of ministers.

Storage

What was said about the season of winter reveals the nature of storage. In winter our *qi* will naturally flow deeper inside us. If we rest and take life slowly we will preserve it. By being too active we will waste it. Animals demonstrate storage by hibernating and by storing food for the winter. Humans also store food for winter. People store crops, fruits and vegetables through cooling, bottling and preserving in order to have reserves for winter.

Maintaining an appropriate balance between activity and rest is crucial to the health of the Water Element. This Element stores much of people's reserves of energy. That is why over-work and lack of sleep easily depletes this Element and the Kidneys especially. Tiredness due to severe deficiency in the Water Element often has a particular characteristic. When people feel tired they often have a desire to stop completely. They have nothing in reserve; nothing to fall back upon. This is especially common in pregnant women, the elderly and when people are convalescing.

In nature the seeds are the archetype of storage. The potential of the plant is stored within the seed.

During winter the seed lies dormant, waiting for the warmth of spring before sprouting. This is resonant with the concept of *jing*, the human seed, which is stored in the Kidneys. Human life begins when the *jing* of two people unite. The person is created from the stored up potential inherent in a microscopic seed.

The climate of Water is cold

The character for cold

The character for cold is *han* (Weiger, 1965, lessons 78G and 47U). This character depicts a man who is trying to protect himself from the cold by remaining in his hut and burying himself in straw.

In cold conditions the mortality rate can increase drastically. In France the winter of 1963 was one of the coldest since the beginning of the century. In that year the mortality of people over 60 years increased by 15.7% compared to the previous winter. Another study of 1,600,000 cases of circulatory disorders in Germany and another in the Netherlands showed a similar trend. The colder the weather, the greater number of fatalities from angina pectoris, coronary thrombosis, cerebral haemorrhage and myocardial infarction. The warmer the winter the lower the mortality rate (Gauquelin, 1980).

Cold is *yin* and heat is *yang*

Cold induces a slowing down, where the movement of *qi* is diminished and even contracted. The cold of winter makes our *qi* run slowly and pull inwards. Unless we protect ourselves well this can become extreme and can result in pain from the contraction, greater susceptibility to colds and infections and a diminished flow of Kidney *qi*. Cold closes the pores of the skin, reduces sweating and increases urination. In the twenty-first century, we have much better protection against the cold than at any time in history. The man in the Chinese character who buried himself in straw reminds us how devastating cold can be, especially in the northern parts of China. In any society, those who are frail, especially the aged, dread the cold. Cold is a ruthless pathogenic factor and those who do not protect themselves damage the *qi* of the Kidneys and open themselves up to a wide range of illnesses.

People whose Water Element is deficient in *yang qi* often feel the cold intensely but it is far from a reliable diagnostic indicator of a Water CF. Diagnostically it is significant, but more for the need to use moxa to reinforce the treatment. It is useful to question how patients respond to cold, both in themselves and with respect to their symptoms. For example, when someone says 'I *hate* the cold and all my problems are worse when it's cold', this suggests that it may be important for the practitioner to warm the patient. This may be carried out using moxibustion.

The sense organ/orifice for Water is the ear

The character for the ear

The character for the ear is *er* (Weiger, 1965, lesson 146).

Hearing and the ear

The sense of the Water Element is hearing and the orifice is the ear. The connection between Water and the ears and hearing is not immediately obvious. It has been suggested that the shape of the ears is like the shape of the Kidneys. This may be true, but there is also a more significant connection through the emotion of fear.

Whenever a person is afraid, they will ordinarily look for some action that will avoid any violation and remove the threat. Seeking reassurance from others can be part of this process but when they ask for this, many people who are chronically afraid (and are probably Water CFs) have a hard time hearing and taking it in. Their difficulty is not to do with the physical hearing mechanism, but with the mind. It is as if when the mind is immersed in fear it cannot get free enough to take in useful information. The person who is afraid will show this through slightly turning away, closing the eyes or making other similar gestures.

Water CFs often report that they had ear infections as children more often than people with other CFs. It is of limited use, however, to ask if the patient has had childhood ear infections because they could still be another CF.

The tissues and body parts for Water are the bones

The character for bones

The character for bones is *gu* (Weiger, 1965, lesson 118).

The bones

Bones are the 'tissues and body parts' for Water. The strength and function of the bones depends on the *qi* of the Water Element. Water CFs may not appear to have problems with their bones unless their Water Element is extremely deficient. Were we to routinely measure people's bone density, however, then the connection between bones and being a Water CF might be more obvious.

Problems with bones early in life, for example, irregular or abnormal bone growth before 10 years old, do suggest a problem with the Water Element, however. To some degree these conditions do support a diagnosis of a Water CF – because they are conditions that arise early in life. Problems with bones that occur later in life, for example osteoporosis, can be linked to a weakness of the Kidneys, but do not necessarily support the patient being a Water CF. The decline of Kidney *qi* after menopause, for example, is a normal event and is often accompanied by a weakening of the bone structure.

Water generates the teeth

Teeth are generated from the bones. Effectively, what we have said about bones is also true of teeth. Tooth disease does not support a CF diagnosis, although very early deterioration of the teeth might be supportive evidence. The decline of teeth associated with ageing supports the general Chinese view that the strength of the Kidneys tends to decline in later life.

The taste for Water is salty

The character for salty

The character for salty is *xian* (Weiger, 1965, lesson 41).

The taste connected to the Water Element is salty. It is easy to associate salt with Water as the largest bodies of water, the oceans, are salty. Western medicine also takes the view that excess salt, which inclines the body to retain water, is not good for a person with hypertension. This should be taken into consideration when giving dietary advice.

Water CFs sometimes have a passion for the salty taste. This can manifest in eating an excessive amount of seaweed, but more frequently it manifests as a strong desire for crisps, salted nuts, yeast extract, bacon or simply lots of salt distributed over whatever is on the person's plate.

There are probably proportionally more Water CFs amongst those with a craving for the salty taste, but this inclination, because of its infrequency, is not useful in determining a CF. A passion for the salty taste will indicate that the Kidneys are out of balance and should be taken into consideration in the overall diagnosis.

Summary

1 Along the *sheng* cycle Water is the mother of Wood and Metal is the mother of Water. Across the *ke* cycle Water controls Fire and Earth controls Water.

2 A diagnosis of a Water CF is made primarily by observation of a blue-black or light blue colour on the face, a groaning voice, a putrid odour and an imbalance in the emotion of fear.

3 Water CFs tend to often feel fearful or anticipate danger in such a way as to reduce feeling fear.

4 Some Water CFs exhibit a lack of fear.

5 Other resonances include the season of winter, cold, the power of storage, bones, teeth, the ear and the salty taste.

Water – The Organs

21

Introduction

The Bladder and Kidney are paired Organs associated with the Water Element. Like the Organs in other Elements their functions overlap and yet are different. The similarity between their functions is illustrated in their 'nicknames' – 'Controller of Water' for the Kidneys and 'Controller of the Storage of Water' for the Bladder. (J. R. Worsley (1998, pp. 15.1–15.12) calls the Kidneys, 'The Official who Controls the Waterways', whereas Felt and Zmiewski (1993, p. 19) call the Kidneys the 'Controller of Water'.) (Table 21.1)

The Kidneys – the Controller of Water

The character for the Kidneys

The character for the Kidneys is *shen* (Weiger, 1965, lesson 82E). The lower part of the character indicates that this is an organ of the body. The upper part indicates both a minister who is prostrate before his master and someone taking a firm hand.

The significance is that the Kidneys are the servant of life and that they both have control and the strength to keep life on a firm footing. The firmness can also denote the firmness and hardness of the innermost structures of the body, such as the bones, teeth and marrow, which are controlled by the Kidneys. In addition, the Kidneys are the lowest *yin* organs in the body and lie at the back of the body. These lowly organs lie waiting to be of service to all of the other Organs and provide the *qi* for people to go about their daily activities.

Su Wen Chapter 8

> The Kidneys are responsible for the creation of power. Skill and ability stem from them.
>
> (Larre and Rochat de la Vallée, 1992b, p. 119)

This quotation stresses the power the Kidneys create. When people are young and well, they have strength. Their muscles are strong, their hair is shiny and they can work and play hard. As life progresses, the strength of the Kidneys declines and overall vigour and stamina diminish.

We now consider what is the connection between the 'creation of power' and the Kidneys.

Table 21.1 The Water Element Officials/Organs

Organ/ Official	Colloquial name	Description from *Su Wen* Ch 8
Kidney	Controller of Water	The Kidneys are responsible for the creation of power. Skill and ability stem from them
Bladder	Controller of Water Storage	The Bladder is responsible for regions and cities. It stores the body fluids. The transformations of *qi* then give out their power

The Kidneys store the *jing*

An essential part of the association of strength and the Kidneys is through the Kidneys' function of storing the *jing*.[1]

The character for *jing*

The left-hand side of the character is four grains or seeds bursting forth with life. The right-hand side is the colour *qing*, which is the colour of sprouting plants. The character presents an image of transformation and life bursting forth. It signifies that the essence that is stored in the Kidneys is the foundation of our *qi* and is the seed of life itself (Weiger, 1965, lesson 122A). Sperm is also the seed of life itself and for this reason sperm and *jing* have the same Chinese character.

The role of *jing*

Jing has various characteristics that say much about the nature of the Kidneys.

- *Jing* is people's constitutional bequest from their parents and ancestors: it is one of the 'three treasures' (see Chapter 1, this volume). In so far as

it is possible to refer to someone's *inherited* constitution in Chinese medicine this is the *jing*. Because the Kidney stores it, the welfare of a person's constitution partly comes about through the welfare of their Kidneys.

- Acupuncture is extremely effective at enabling a person's body, mind and spirit to operate to its greatest potential. Some people, however, are born stronger than others. There are limits to how much improvement can be made to significant *jing* deficiency. Sometimes a person needs to adapt to their situation rather than alter it through treatment. As the old saying goes, 'What can't be cured must be endured.' A person's aim should be to preserve and nurture *jing*. Lifestyle advice needs to take *jing* into consideration with respect to diet, exercise, work and rest (*tai ji*, *qi gong* and breathing exercises are said to nourish *jing*; see Hicks, 2009, Chapter 4, p. 88).

- *Jing* operates a bit like a credit card. People can borrow on it, but in the end they need to make repayments. Excess expenditure does not go away when they return to normal expenditure; instead it accumulates and interest is charged. People deplete their *jing* by working too hard, ejaculating too frequently (for men) or having too many childbirths (for women), taking drugs, eating a poor diet and not getting enough rest or appropriate exercise. Luckily it takes time for people to deplete their *jing* and a healthy lifestyle will prevent this from happening. *Jing*, however, is hard to replace. When the credit card total has mounted up, the interest charges then become an additional burden. Worse still, if people have depleted their reserves, they become less able to cope when a crisis arises. There will be no reserves to draw on and they perform without 'cleverness', thus increasing their likelihood of becoming ill.

- *Qi* moves quickly, but *jing* moves slowly and governs the longer-term cycles of growth, reproduction and sexual development (fertility, conception and pregnancy). Women have seven-year cycles and men eight-year cycles. After seven cycles for women (49) or eight for men (64), the *jing* is expected to be declining.

The balanced functioning of the Kidney is therefore essential for people to have abundant energy and power. Skill, ability and cleverness can also be gained through the Kidney's effect on the brain and mind.

---

[1] J. R. Worsley did not use the language of Substances or specifically '*jing*'. On the other hand, in his book on the Officials (Worsley, 1998, p. 15.7) he refers to the Kidney being the storehouse of ancestral energy which is passed to each person by their parents (see also Maciocia, 2005, pp. 51–52).

Patient Example

A patient to whom the practitioner had explained the concept of *jing* said: 'I knew I always did more and worked harder than other people. At the time I thought I was very strong but in retrospect I think I was needy for a lot of things. I think others who didn't work as hard were more comfortable with themselves. In the end I wore myself out. I over-worked, didn't get enough rest, ate irregularly and had a poor-quality diet. I became ill and I knew I had to change.'

The *ming men*

The idea of *ming men* or 'gate of vitality' is also an essential part of how the Kidney is understood in Chinese medicine. The gate of vitality provides the heat or fire for the rest of the Organs. This view is somewhat at odds with the notion that the warmth of the body comes from the Fire Element, but both views can be held (see section 'Warming the body' in Chapter 12, this volume.)

When treating a patient who is cold, practitioners may decide to use moxa (see Chapter 35, this volume). They will also consider which points should be treated with moxa. The Fire Element is not the only way that a practitioner can access the body's own ability to warm itself. For example, the acupuncture point *Du* 4 is an important point to increase the warmth of the body and is located between and somewhat below the physical kidneys. The Kidneys are important for the warmth of the body and for the warmth of the other Organs.

The spirit of the Kidneys – the *zhi*

The *zhi* is the spirit of the Kidneys. It has been translated as will, willpower, ambition, drive or motivation.

The character for *zhi*

The character for *zhi* shows something that is able to stand firm and upright – the ability for a person

to stand their ground and not be deflected from their goals. *Zhi* gives us the push or drive that enables people to be motivated to achieve things in life (Weiger, 1965, lesson 79B).

The functions of the *zhi*

The drive to survive

At the most fundamental level the *zhi* gives people the 'drive to survive'. This drive, although usually not evident except in extreme situations, is regarded as the most powerful drive in people. The drive to reproduce, and thereby ensure the survival of the species and the family, is certainly an immensely powerful force in all living creatures. The resonance with *jing*, humans' life-giving seed, is obvious.

How do we understand *zhi* and willpower as part of Water? In the first place, willpower requires goals and the determination to push towards them. The Kidneys give people the strength to push consistently towards what they want.

The *yin* and *yang* of the Kidneys and the *zhi*

The Kidneys are thought of as having a *yang* and *yin* aspect. The *yang* is the outward-moving, warming *qi* and the *yin* is the inward-moving cooling *qi*. The will of those with balanced Kidneys is reasonably normal. Those with deficient Kidney *yang qi* tend to be listless, weak and lacking in movement, physically and mentally. At an extreme, they are cold, shivery and lie curled up in bed. Those with deficient Kidney *yin qi* tend to be restless, active and overly determined. At an extreme, they are hyperactive, hot and moving relentlessly towards their outcomes. These imbalances can both be seen as distorted patterns of will.

Fear and the *zhi*

Another way of understanding the relationship between the will and the Kidneys is to consider the resonating emotion, fear. The previous chapter described how fear can manifest when it is imbalanced. One pattern will lead to no action and feeling too much fear to act and the other pattern to hyperaction and anticipating threats and dealing with them beforehand. Both can be seen as patterns of imbalanced will as much as imbalanced emotion.

Patient Example

A Water CF with an imbalanced *zhi* said, 'When I was younger I was determined to learn to sail even though I was scared of the water. It was like a driven determination. I drove myself because I was so determined and then I could break through my fear.'

A balanced *zhi*

The paragraph above gives examples of how the will can be out of balance. It is also important to describe what a balanced will is like. Ted Kaptchuk (2000, p. 62) describes a balanced will as 'the will that can't be willed'. The will works independently from a person's conscious volition. It gives people a sense of moving towards their destiny without carrying out too much conscious processing. This unobtrusive will, which operates under the surface, is the result of healthy Kidney *qi*. Significantly, it goes unnoticed because it is expressed appropriately.

The virtue associated with Water is wisdom. If people have moved through life, enacting their destiny and doing so in part because of balanced Kidney *qi*, then wisdom accumulates (Kaptchuk, 2000, pp. 62–63). There is no better breeding ground for understanding the world and gaining wisdom than gradually, through time, to have achieved a series of interconnecting goals. Ideally when people grow older, although their *jing* declines, their wisdom increases.

The Bladder – the Controller of the Storage of Water

The character for the Bladder

膀胱

The character for the Bladder is the *pang guang* (Weiger, 1965, lessons 117A (*jou*), 24J (*pang*) and 29I (*kuang*)).

The first radical depicts a space with three dimensions – probably representing the Bladder Organ, that is, a space that stores water. The second represents light or lustre or a man carrying a torch. Together these describe the power of the Bladder – it is a storage space with *yang* power.

Su Wen Chapter 8

The Bladder is responsible for regions and cities. It stores the body fluids. The transformations of *qi* then give out their power.

(Larre and Rochat de la Vallée, 1992b, p. 133)

The Bladder has its own *qi* and one of the key functions of *qi* is to transform and move. The analysis of the section in *Su Wen* Chapter 8 that relates to the Bladder gives us some clues as to its function. The Bladder is responsible for keeping dry areas separate from wet areas. This is similar to separating rivers and lakes from adjoining fields, so that the people can grow crops, yet still travel by boat to a neighbouring village – ensuring that life can proceed.

Su Wen describes the importance of having the appropriate amount of body fluids in the right location as Larre and Rochat de la Vallée describe below.

It is important to underline that the Bladder, which seems so unimportant, has in reality an action of control which is very great. It controls, by eliminating or re-injecting into the body, the quantity and quality of liquids from below.

(Larre and Rochat de la Vallée, 1992b, pp. 133–138)

The Bladder has an important role in maintaining body fluids in their natural quantity and quality. It was stated in the previous chapter that up to 60% of the body is made of water. The Bladder has a crucial role to do with many functions associated with the body fluids. These include creating:

* moist eyes to see
* saliva in the mouth to digest
* nasal fluids when breathing
* a moist throat and vocal chords to speak
* sufficient synovial fluid in all the joints to move smoothly
* a moist large intestine to pass stools with ease
* a moist vagina for pleasurable sex
* flexible, moist skin to protect and maintain beauty

Mind, emotions and spirit as well as body

The correct amount and quality of fluids also affects people on the levels of body, mind and spirit. For example, just as physically the fluid in the joints helps people to throw a ball, the fluids of the mind and spirit help them to flow and manifest smoothly.

When a person is frightened, their whole body can tighten up as they think about what might happen in the future. The perceived 'threat' can stop them from moving forward in their lives as they become scared of what lies ahead. Fear prevents them from thinking in a fluid way. An example of this is when a person 'dries up' when speaking in public. In this situation some people say that their mind is racing and they cannot formulate a coherent speech. Others report that their mind has gone blank.

When this pattern is chronic, people become limited in their thoughts and only see a small proportion of what is possible. They find it hard to move their minds from subject to subject and they may protect themselves from a threat by keeping still, inhibiting movement. The result can be an unmoving mind-set from where they resist change. Alternatively their minds can become agitated. They find it hard to still their minds sufficiently to formulate effective strategies as their thinking becomes panicky and scattered. The mind and spirit require appropriate fluids to manifest smoothly.

Patient Example

A patient explained: 'When I'm scared my movements are more jerky or at the extreme I'm trembling, especially if I'm concerned that I'm under someone's eye and I'm also more shaky, but I cannot move.'

A vicious cycle can ensue from the situation described above. Being chronically afraid can lead to static fluids and less ability to respond to any threatening situations. The subsequent threats increase the fear and reduce the flow even further. On the other hand, good flow with adequate fluids enables people to deal with a threat. This stops the chronic build up of fear and thus makes people better able to deal with any new fears.

Observation of Water CFs reveals that they often demonstrate both physical and mental jerkiness. This is different from the 'lack of smooth flow' described under the Wood Element. The former situation is due to a lack of fluidity that creates physical and mental 'stiffness' in the Water CF. The latter situation that affects the Wood CF results from the Blood not nourishing tendons and ligaments as well as the Liver's tendency to allow the *qi* to stagnate.

The time of day for the Organs

The 2-hour period for the Kidneys is 3–5 p.m. and for the Bladder is 5–7 p.m. Many people who have an imbalance in their Water Element feel most vital at these times. Others are tired and lacking in energy at these times but find their vitality returns later in the evening. For many people, however, this time coincides with the end of their working day and they feel very differently as they switch activities. This makes reporting tiredness at this time unreliable as a diagnostic indicator.

Patient Example

A Water CF patient whose practitioner had explained about the time of day said: 'Even before I knew about the time and the organ, I was aware of a time that I needed to switch off in the afternoon. I called it the "4 o'clock wall". You couldn't get anything out of me at that time.'

Many Water CFs and people with weak Water Elements find that they wake in the night to urinate between 3 and 5 a.m. This is the lowest time for the Kidneys and Bladder and when Water *qi* is at its lowest. If people wake around this time of night it is also often because of anxiety or heat. Fretting is a common reason why people struggle to get back to sleep again. This is often most marked in people whose Kidneys are becoming agitated due to becoming 'burnt out' from over-work. When the Kidney *yin* is deficient the tendency to be too hot at this time of night is marked. It is striking how often people who struggle to sleep during these hours report that they can sleep really well after about 7 a.m. Virtually nobody reports night sweats after this time, even if they sleep late into the morning.

When collecting information and hearing about atypical behaviour, it is always useful to ask at what time it occurs. When people are vague or say it is random, then there may be no significance. If they are exact about the time and credit the symptoms with regularity, it is worth comparing it with horary time. A symptom of this sort can support the case for a CF, but it is definitely not sufficient on its own.

How the Kidney and Bladder relate

The functions of these two Organs overlap. Both deal with fluids, one as the Controller of Water and the other as the Controller of the Storage of Water. The difference in terms of a patient's symptoms or experience may be subtle.

The Kidneys are more concerned with the quality of the fluids and the Bladder with their distribution, but this also is a subtle distinction, hard to translate into specific symptoms. The major difference is the Kidney's function of storing the *jing* and therefore being the source of strength to fuel the long-term cycles of growth, development and reproduction. The capacity to develop sexually, to endure, to reproduce and to grow old gracefully come from the Kidney and not the Bladder.

Summary

1 *Su Wen* Chapter 8 says that 'The Kidneys are responsible for the creation of power. Skill and ability stem from them.'

2 The Kidneys store the *jing* which is responsible for birth, growth, reproduction and development.

3 The *zhi* is the spirit of the Kidneys. It has been translated as will, willpower, ambition, drive or motivation.

4 *Su Wen* Chapter 8 says that 'The Bladder is responsible for regions and cities. It stores the body fluids. The transformations of *qi* then give out their power.'

5 The Kidneys are sometimes known as the Controller of Water. The Bladder is sometimes referred to as the Controller of the Storage of Water.

6 The 2-hour period for the Kidneys is 3–5 p.m. and that for the Bladder is 5–7 p.m.

Patterns of behaviour of Water Constitutional Factors

22

CHAPTER CONTENTS

Introduction

This chapter describes some of the most important behavioural characteristics that are typical of a Water CF. Some aspects of a person's behaviour can be observed in the treatment room. Others can only be discerned from the patient's description of themselves and their life. As stated in the previous chapters, behaviour can be an indicator of a patient's diagnosis but it can only be used to *confirm* the CF. It should always be used in conjunction with colour, sound, emotion and odour, which are the four primary methods of diagnosis. Once the CF is confirmed the patterns of behaviour may, however, support the practitioner's diagnosis.

The origin of the behaviours was described in Chapter 7. The imbalance of the Element of the CF creates instability or impairment of the associated emotion. Thus specific negative emotional experiences are more likely to occur to one CF as opposed to another. The behavioural traits described in this chapter are often the responses to these negative experiences. In the case of Water the person experiences a feeling of fear and she or he is responding to this.

Patterns of behaviour of a Water CF

The balanced Element

Patients with a healthy Water Element are able to assess risks and know the appropriate degree of a 'threat'. People are continually assessing 'threats' in their daily lives. These can vary from dealing with cars when crossing a road, the threat of a potential burglary or the threat of physical, or verbal, attack.

People with a healthy Water Element notice danger and assess the extent of the risk it presents. They then take action to protect themselves from it. If a threat has been averted they reassure themselves that they are safe. If it has not been averted they take further action to deal with it. This whole activity is usually carried out in a matter of split seconds, but it is extremely important as it ensures their physical and emotional survival.

Formative events for a Water CF

A Water CF usually has significant difficulties when faced with threats but all people, whether they are Water CFs or not, experience fear at some time during their childhood. Sometimes these fears are appropriate. For example, children who are bullied become scared because they have been threatened or children who have hurt themselves are extra vigilant for a time while they learn how to cope with the situation.

Sometimes children have inexplicable fears. The lines between reality and fantasy get blurred and the child fantasises horrific situations. They may imagine, for example, that the large dog next door will eat them up, or that the toilet will overflow and drown them. If a child tells these fears to an adult, hopefully the adult will reassure them that they are safe. The reassurance of an adult will usually make the child feel less anxious.

Most children who are given enough reassurance learn to reassure themselves. They will be able to anticipate real danger and deal with it and steady themselves when their fears are unfounded. Some children, however, never stop feeling afraid. These children are often Water CFs. Because their imbalance is constitutional they are less able to assess and deal with potentially dangerous situations. They often notice potential threats that people with healthy Water Elements don't see. They may also ask for reassurance but then find it difficult or even impossible to take in.

Although it is likely that people are born with their CF, many of their experiences, especially emotional ones, are also coloured by it. Many Water CFs didn't feel reassured as children. Maybe their parents didn't appreciate the extent of their fear and they were laughed at for being fearful. Sometimes the children may never have spoken of their fears, so they never received the feelings of safety that they needed in order for their Water Element not to be further imbalanced.

Patient Example

A patient who is a Water CF described how she was always extremely nervous as a young child. She was especially afraid of learning any new physical activity such as swimming or riding a bike, and she reported that her father often told her, 'You're so nervous you'll never be able to learn.' 'It took "an act of will" for me to overcome my fear and consequently I learned things much more slowly than other children, but I learned to be very determined.'

The main issues for a Water CF

For the Water CF certain needs remain unmet. This situation creates issues which centre on these areas:

* needing to be safe
* trusting
* drive

* being reassured
* excitation in danger

The extent to which someone is affected in these areas varies according to the person's physical, mental and spiritual health. Relatively healthy Water CFs will have less disturbance with these aspects of life, whilst those with greater problems end up with their personalities being strongly influenced by this imbalance.

Because of these issues they may consciously or unconsciously ask themselves various questions such as:

* How can I deal with danger?
* Who can I trust?
* Where will I be safe?
* How can I be reassured?

Responses to the issues

So far we have described how a weakness in the Water Element leads to a lesser capacity to assess risks and know the appropriate degree of a threat. The issues that subsequently arise lead to a spectrum of typical ways of responding to the world. These are common, but not exclusive, to Water CFs. If other CFs have patterns of behaviour that seem similar it may indicate that there is a different set of motivations underlying them or that the Water Element is also imbalanced but is not the CF. Noticing these responses is therefore useful but does not replace colour, sound, emotion and odour as the principal way of diagnosing the Constitutional Factor.

The behavioural patterns are along a spectrum and can go between these extremes:

1	risk-taking	_____	fearing the worst/over-cautiousness
2	distrusting	_____	trusting
3	intimidating	_____	reassuring
4	driven	_____	no drive
5	agitation	_____	paralysis

Risk-taking – fearing the worst and over-cautiousness

Risk-taking or bravado

People take risks on a daily basis, usually without much thought. Driving a car, crossing a road, operating a power tool and climbing a ladder are all potentially risky everyday events. The risk potential of an activity depends on the individual. Running downstairs is dangerous if people are unstable on their feet. Jumping into a swimming pool is risky if a person can't swim. Most people avoid taking these kinds of risks. Many Water CFs, however, like to push themselves beyond 'ordinary' risks to give themselves much greater challenges. As it says in *Ling Shu* Chapter 64 'The Water type of man has no respect for fear' (Wu, 1993).

Why do they need to do this? There are a variety of reasons. Often Water CFs of this kind present a rather still exterior. They may suppress their fear and try not to feel it or they perceive that they never experience fear at all. Often they like to feel challenged or they just enjoy the release of adrenaline which accompanies the risk-taking. They may have suppressed their fear and sense of excitement so effectively that life often feels lack-lustre. Participating in activities that adrenalise them is often the only time they feel any sense of vitality or exhilaration at all.

Evel Knievel, America's legendary daredevil, is an example of someone who took many risks and showed an extreme lack of fear. He finally retired in 1981 having broken 35 bones, been operated on 15 times and spent three years of his life in hospital. When asked about this, he is reported to have shrugged and said, 'Hey, you have to pay the price for success.'

Not everyone takes such high-profile risks as Evel Knievel. Others take risks by undertaking activities such as deep sea diving, riding motor bikes, hang gliding, rock climbing, parachuting or snowboarding in order to give themselves an adrenaline rush. Sometimes when questioned, however, these people admit that the risks are not carried out recklessly. They often calculate exactly how 'safe' the risk is and know how close to the edge they can go.

Patient Example

A patient who was a Water CF worked as a tree surgeon, which involved a certain amount of danger. In order to 'relax' in his spare time he loved to go rock climbing. He told his practitioner, 'When I climb a rock face I know the dangers. I check and I double check. It's a calculated risk because I know my equipment and I know the people I climb with and so I know it's a safe activity.'

Others take needless risks in their day-to-day lives. They may knowingly drive too fast or overtake when it is not safe. One Water CF told his practitioner that he was known for a 'devil may care' attitude when it came to crossing the road. He described launching himself in front of a car and expecting it to stop. It always did! He said, 'I know how big the gap is and I know I can make it. I know exactly how far I have gone and what the situation is. One of these days I might come unstuck but it's a calculated risk.'

The need to cover up fear can also lead people to do risky things to prove to themselves that they are not afraid. Unlike those who calculate the risks, they love the buzz of taking needless risks. Examples of people who are driven to do this are rich people who shoplift, or people who take recreational drugs when they do not know what constitutes a safe dose. The poet Percy Shelley met his death after insisting on setting sail when all the locals warned him not to.

Patient Example

An acupuncture student who is a Water CF described how, when she worked as a lighting technician, she would focus the lights for large concerts. In order to do this she might be 100 feet above the ground. To move across the ceiling of the large hall she would jump from beam to beam. 'I'd lean out and get one hand on the next diagonal beam. Once I'd put both hands out I was committed and had to leap across and catch it with my legs. If I'd missed I probably would have fallen to my death.' She admitted she was terrified of the jump but said, 'I think I was more scared of not being seen as "one of the boys" than falling to my death, so I carried on doing the job for two years!'

Fearing the worst

At the opposite end of the spectrum to the risk-takers are Water CFs who fantasise about potential threats. The thought of what *might* happen can grow large in their minds until it becomes almost a reality. They constantly anticipate an impending disaster. They may describe themselves as constantly on the alert, always having their 'antennae' out and taking in all the 'vibes' around them to ensure there is no danger. If this tendency becomes too strong then the person may start to get 'panic attacks', especially if the imbalance in the Water Element starts to affect the Heart across the *ke* cycle.

To compensate for any impending crisis some Water CFs plan for emergencies. They prepare themselves by learning first aid, knowing the exits in buildings or becoming skilled in martial arts. 'You never know what might happen.'

Patient Example

A Water CF told his practitioner about his constant paranoia, saying that if people were late by ten minutes he wouldn't suspect that they'd got stuck in traffic but would imagine they were in a serious road accident. 'I laugh about it but it's such a real feeling of paranoia and I feel it several times a day. Paranoia is such a big thing for me but it's quite hard to admit it. I know the rationale and intellectually I know I'm being stupid but I can't stop myself having those feelings.'

Because of their ability to think of the worst possibilities Water CFs can be very imaginative. Unfortunately their imagination sometimes gets the better of them and they easily think of worse catastrophes and more horrifying disasters than most people. As one Water CF put it, 'I imagine very dramatic, huge, dreadful things or somebody will say something to really hurt me and it's like I will dramatise it in my mind and turn it into something much bigger than it really is.'

Over-caution

Some Water CFs are very careful. For example, they may be financially cautious and ensure that they are properly insured, 'just in case'. Others may drive slowly or even walk everywhere for fear of accidents (the opposite of the risk-takers who drive too fast). Others may be full of trepidation about going out of the house, travelling for long journeys or some may find it hard to embark on new projects, in case things go wrong.

Patient Example

Some Water CFs are so cautious that they refrain from participating in events that other CFs might think were exciting opportunities. One Water CF missed out on the chance to travel to the United States when she was a teenager. At first she thought it would be exciting to go but as the time to depart drew closer her forebodings grew. Finally she decided to not go after all. 'I was scared and I wasn't interested in pushing myself to do something new,' she told her practitioner.

Being over-cautious can also ensure that Water CFs are vigilant and meticulous in their work and life. For example, a nurse who described herself as a cautious person said that she went through all of the possible difficulties before doing anything. 'Everything has to be gone through in great detail. For instance, my sterile technique. I think of what could happen if I didn't do it. So I do it very correctly, almost obsessively.' The nurse said she did it for herself. 'I admit I'm scared of what might happen to me, rather than the patients, if things went wrong.'

Water CFs often check things that others wouldn't notice. This can make them extremely skilled in certain areas of their life. For instance, some people who are good businessmen may be Water CFs who *appear* to take risks when negotiating a business deal. In reality, however, they may have taken their time to weigh up what might go wrong and have looked at every possible dire consequence that could happen before proceeding to close the deal.

Distrusting – trusting

Distrustfulness

Water CFs may react to people or situations with suspicion and one common characteristic in the treatment room can be their wariness. However reassuring, friendly or sympathetic the practitioner is, the patient never really lets down their guard. They may ask questions to gain reassurance and to ensure that the practitioner is trustworthy. The answers Water CFs receive are no guarantee, however, that they will be reassured. Although they often search for reassurance, when it is forthcoming it often fails to make more than a momentary impact on their fearfulness.

People often have to prove their trustworthiness to a Water CF. Trust is not automatically given because the person has a title or honour, job status or because they have received certain qualifications. The questions the Water CF asks will be designed to get below the surface to find out the true ability or integrity of a person or the real state of a situation.

Double-checking

Questioning may lead a person to find out important facts and information. For example, some Water CFs may ring up 'expert' friends whenever they need advice. Often they will not accept the advice of only one person but will double-check by looking through books, by finding out more information from the internet or by asking more than one 'expert'. Only when they have gone to a variety of sources will they put together the results of their research and decide on the action they will take.

Sometimes this double-checking is more frightening than reassuring for Water CFs. For example, if a Water CF has a health problem she or he may look at all the worst possible reasons for a symptom. A minor symptom can be blown up to seem life threatening or at least much worse than it really is. The fear may then prevent the person from getting further help as she or he is too frightened of 'hearing the worst' to ask for help.

Trust

Other Water CFs can be overly trusting. One Water CF, for example, described how she had a strong sense of trust and assumed that everything would go right in her life. She very rarely prepared for holidays and would go abroad by herself with just a few clothes in a rucksack and would trust that everything would work out. On reflection she admitted that this was really a denial that something could go wrong. 'I can't bear to think of what might go wrong because it would build in my mind and become overwhelming, so I don't think about it at all.'

Other Water CFs who are trusting will project magical properties on to certain people. They may think the person is all-knowing instead of having a balanced view of their imperfections as well as their good qualities. Rather than double-checking an 'expert's' advice (see the example above) they may trust it implicitly. They may then project immense power onto the person. A meditation teacher, for example, may be raised up in the Water CF's mind to being a mystic. A doctor may be trusted so implicitly that it blinds the Water CF from being discerning about treatments. A psychic may be relied on to give 'true' advice about the future.

Imagining that another person can do no wrong allows Water CFs to feel safe and stop feeling frightened whilst under the expert's 'protection'. This *modus operandi* works well as long as nothing goes wrong. If something goes wrong, however, and the expert is shown to be 'human', the Water CF may turn full circle and lose all trust, never giving the person another chance.

Trust is an important part of any practitioner–patient relationship and one way for a practitioner to gain a patient's trust may be to give them a safe space to talk. Many Water CFs find it difficult to talk to other people about their distress. In fact they often become adept at covering up their suffering so that no one can see how bad they really

Patient Example

A Water CF described how her son was bullied at school. 'I used to be a very trusting person and had been told that the headmaster of the school was exceptionally good. I had taken this on trust. My son wasn't given the help he needed and the headmaster did nothing to stop the bullying.' After that she never automatically trusted other people's word again. 'I learned from my experience to always ask lots of questions and check things out to ensure that what I heard was accurate.'

feel inside. Because of this if they find someone they can really trust it can be a great relief. Even then it may take time for them to open up about their most personal issues.

Patient Example

A Water CF described how being given permission to say 'I'm frightened' and to talk about his fears was important. 'It doesn't matter how small or silly it may seem, if I can tell my practitioner I'm feeling scared or worried about something it's a great relief not to be told, "Don't be silly that won't happen". Then I can start to look at the fear and put it in perspective.'

Another Water CF who was a nurse pricked himself with a needle and went completely off the 'deep end'. 'For that month I was sure I'd got hepatitis. I couldn't focus on anything else. Finally I was in such a state that I talked about it to my wife. As soon as I talked to her I felt much better. I realised that my patient was a health worker and I could easily check her hepatitis B status. My fear was quickly dispelled.'

Knowing who to trust

Knowing who to trust can be a question that preoccupies many Water CFs, even if most of the thinking about it goes on at an unconscious level. So what does a Water CF look for if they are deciding if someone is trustworthy? Steadiness seems to be one of the most important qualities. As one Water CF said, 'It's an intuitive feeling as to whether a person is OK or not. One attribute of the person I talk to the most is that she's not shaken or shocked by anything I say so I know I can tell her anything.'

For many Water CFs the bottom line is less about whether they trust other people and more about whether they trust themselves. For most Water CFs their own judgement is the main issue. As one Water CF said, 'If I feel someone is trying to reassure me, I think, "If you think you've considered every possibility then you're wrong and that's because I've already done that and I know I'm right!"'

Intimidating – reassuring

Reassuring

As was stated earlier in the chapter, reassurance is a common antidote to fear. Most people who are not Water CFs will accept reassurance, as long as they trust the source of the knowledge. For instance, if we feel ill we wouldn't trust our car mechanic to tell us we had nothing to worry about. We would want to go to a trusted medical practitioner. Many Water CFs are not easy to reassure. Their fear is so deep that many say that no one can reassure them.

Patient Example

A practitioner became frustrated because whenever he tried to give his patient reassurance she said, 'Yes, but …' and gave another reason to be scared. They talked about her inability to take any reassurance. The patient told him that on reflection she thought it would be impossible to reassure her and that she couldn't remember when she was last reassured by anybody. The patient told him that having her fears listened to and understood was important. 'But I think the only person who can reassure me is myself.'

Because they value reassurance, many Water CFs are particularly good at giving it to others. They are often the 'rocks' that others turn to when they are afraid. In fact, when Water CFs have amassed large amounts of reassuring information (see above) they can then pass the material on to others who are in need. All of the information gained from books, talks, the internet and from those with expert knowledge is used not only for themselves but for all others who need help. Deep inside, in spite of this reassuring quality, many Water CFs are still aware that they

are feeling fearful inside even when they are at their most reassuring. One Water CF described himself as more reassuring than most people because he knew where someone who's scared was coming from. But he was really 'jelly-legged' inside. 'I sometimes feel that there's a chink in how I look when I'm giving reassurance and someone who knows me would see a doubt in me as I gave it.'

Threats and intimidation

Not all Water CFs like to reassure. Some prefer to make threats. Some Water CFs feel so scared that they use intimidating behaviour to defend themselves, even if the threat has not yet arisen. Their motto could be, 'The best form of defence is attack.' They may create a climate of fear in those around them, and this may be an important diagnostic indicator. The practitioner may feel unsettled and edgy as a reflection of the patient's subtly intimidating manner.

When people are afraid they may start to imagine all sorts of catastrophes arising in the future, and earlier in the chapter it was described how Water CFs might exaggerate them. Some Water CFs attempt to motivate others by using fear to illustrate the dire consequences resulting from any 'unwanted' behaviour. For example, a mother might warn her child of murder or a serious accident if the child does not come straight home after going out. A teacher may vividly outline the consequences of not working hard at school in terms of failure and misery. A vicar might warn of hell and damnation for committing misdeeds. If these scenarios are told in graphic detail and with sufficient intensity, the Water CF hopes that they will instil fear and dread in the other person. Although it is a negative form of motivation, the hope is that it will keep others safe from harm.

Some Water CFs use the threat of physical violence in order to feel safe. They learn fighting skills such as martial arts, boxing or wrestling. For example, one Water CF who came for acupuncture treatment for a knee injury explained that he was so afraid of his father when he was young that he learnt martial arts to defend himself if necessary. He is now a very skilled karate teacher with many students.

Other Water CFs may intimidate by being prone to anger. Although the Element associated with anger is the Wood Element, a person expressing anger might really be fearful underneath. The anger they are showing can be a show of bravado that is being used in self-defence.

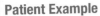

Patient Example

A Water CF described getting very angry when he felt intimidated. He told his practitioner that he knew that he was seeing fear where it didn't exist – especially physical intimidation. This made him extremely defensive and brought up his own anger and desire to intimidate. 'I feel like I'm flailing in the dark – it's mental panic – I say things that are not logical and can seem extremely angry to other people.'

Another more subtle way of threatening others is the use of shock. For example, a patient described being a punk in his past and that he thought, 'This is who I am. You can take me or leave me. If you can't get beyond it, it's too bad.' People often found him very intimidating when they saw him in the street and he secretly enjoyed it when people crossed over the road because they thought he looked scary. He recently said, 'I still have a need to shock and it comes out when I feel under threat. When I'm arguing with someone and I know I'm right, they don't have a leg to stand on. I'll say something shocking and it feels fantastic!'

Driven – no drive

The *zhi* is the spirit of the Kidneys. *Zhi* has variously been translated as drive, will, willpower, ambition, or the 'tendency towards something'. It has been called, 'that which pushes the organism into actualising it's potential' (Larre *et al.*, 1986, p. 176). People who have healthy Kidney *qi* naturally have this drive or will. They have an ability to move forward through changes and obstacles in their lives. They have little need to push themselves. The Kidneys help them to do the work in hand and take them forward through all the necessary cycles and changes that affect the person's body, mind and spirit.

Water CFs on the other hand often don't have this natural and flowing will or drive and can be either extremely driven or have very little drive or will at all.

Strong will

Many Water CFs describe themselves as having stronger will than others and may take pride in their powerful drive or determination. Once they have decided on a course of action they follow it through,

no matter how hard or how much of a grind it is, and they often carry on with activities well beyond the endurance of other people. They may override their emotional responses in order to prove, often to themselves, how long and hard they can work. By doing this they are pushing through life rather than trusting that life will naturally take them through. For example, a Water CF described how when he first took up running he ran for 10 miles on his first run and 15 on the second. Another said that when she worked she would often go on for 12 to 14 hours without a break 'just because I could'.

Although the people described above may not have experienced what they were doing as extreme, over time they are likely to pay a price for this lifestyle and their reserves become drained. Sometimes the resulting depletion causes the *zhi* to compensate still more by giving them even more forward push. A vicious circle begins. The more drained they feel the more drive they have. They may finally end up swinging to the other extreme and being left exhausted.

Patient Example

A Water CF described how he used to override his emotional responses in order to carry on working. 'I would work really hard and hated stopping. I used to be driven all of the time but now I'm the lazy one. I don't have any energy left and find it hard to become motivated to do things.'

No drive

Some Water CFs have the experience of never having much drive or will. They feel tired at the thought of doing anything and find it hard to get moving to carry out even everyday tasks. Sometimes this is because they are too afraid to act. For instance, one Water CF described how she felt powerless and inadequate if faced with a new challenge at work. 'I feel terrified and sure I won't be able to do it. I seem to sit around with no energy feeling too depleted to move. Once I start to act I have an iron will and go under and over any obstacle until my task is completed.'

Other Water CFs feel too tired to move or gather the motivation to do things. For example, a person may sit and watch TV even if the programme is not interesting to them. It may seem too difficult to get up and do something else. Sometimes they may have a good idea but when they check in with their body it says, 'Oh no! I'm much too tired', so they don't act. Sometimes a person eats dinner in front of the TV and then falls asleep while watching. Of course people of all CFs can have this pattern of behaviour for periods of time. Combined with other signs that suggest that the person is a Water CF it can, however, be an indication. Sometimes a person swings between the two states, sometimes feeling unable to rest and at other times feeling totally depleted.

Patient Example

A patient was brought for a consultation. Her main complaint was extreme tiredness. The patient and practitioner had driven to the clinic together and chatted on the way. The practitioner found out that the lady, who was immaculately dressed, took 40 minutes to put her eye make-up on, had a spotless, four-bedroomed house, looked after three children and a quadraplegic husband and had two lovers. She also worked part-time for four days a week.

Agitation – paralysis

Fear is often the most hidden emotion, so it can be difficult to be sure that it is the patient's underlying predominant emotion. Practitioners, however, can often realise that the patient's Water Element is out of balance by noticing their behaviour on a spectrum between agitation and paralysis.

Agitation

Continual agitation will result in sudden bursts of energy. These ultimately deplete the adrenal glands and lead to exhaustion. When people feel agitated they can sometimes become so restless that they find it difficult to sit still. This also affects their ability to concentrate. Fearful thoughts and catastrophic fantasies race through their minds at such a rate that it is impossible for them to think of any sensible or reassuring thoughts to calm themselves. Other signs and symptoms may be shaking and trembling, sweating, shortness of breath and/or rapid breathing. People may also complain of palpitations, a dry mouth and the inability to sleep.

In a situation of extreme fear, people may find it difficult *not* to talk about their symptoms. They literally babble with nerves. They may talk to all and sundry about their fears, but never seem to be reassured. At first glance it would be easy for the

Patient Example

A Water CF started getting panic attacks after her mother died. She couldn't rest or settle and talked incessantly about her feelings to anyone who would care to listen. Her father had died suddenly when she was 10 and at that time she had been bewildered and shocked by his sudden disappearance. Although she had dealt with her grief, she had never got over the fear that others close to her might die. The death of her mother triggered this fear and she then also became afraid for her husband and children. It took many months of intense treatment for the patient to come to terms with her loss and to deal with the underlying reasons for it.

acupuncturist to think that these patients are seeking sympathy, as all they want to do is talk about their problems. However, it should become clear that sympathy does not evoke much response and the patient really is looking for steadiness and reassurance from the practitioner.

Agitation can be catching. When a person can't be calmed it easily passes on to others who also feel the fear. Practitioners also need to be aware of the way anxiety can spread. Sometimes practitioners only realise how fearful their patients are by recognising how anxious the patient is making them feel. In general it is important that an acupuncturist is calm and solid on the outside. If she or he shows anxiety when carrying out a treatment the patient will quickly pick this up and become fearful too. This will dramatically reduce the efficacy of the treatment.

Paralysis

At the other end of the spectrum people can become 'paralysed' or 'freeze up' when afraid. On the inside they may be a quivering mass of fear. Their mouth may be dry, they may be in a cold sweat and their heart may be thumping loudly. On the surface, however, they may pretend that everything is all right and appear cool, calm and collected. The practitioner needs to look for an unnatural stillness in the body as the patient attempts to lessen the intensity of sensations caused by the descending movements of *qi* that accompany fear.

Because some Water CFs appear still or calm on the outside it can be difficult for the practitioner to see their fear. Water CFs may learn to be extremely competent and capable in everything they do in order to compensate for their internal sense of paralysis. For this reason some Water CFs can be difficult to diagnose.

> I have always thought it rather interesting to follow the involuntary movements of fear in clever people. Fools display their cowardice in all its nakedness, but the others are able to cover it with a veil so delicate, so daintily woven with small plausible lies, that there is some pleasure to be found in contemplating this ingenious work of the human intelligence.
>
> (De Tocqueville; in Auden and Kronenberger, 1962)

Hesitancy

A state of paralysis can also manifest in the way a person speaks. This is a less extreme form of what happens when a public speaker 'dries up'. Under the effect of fear, the person's mind jams and they find it difficult to maintain fluency.

Some people may be hesitant or faltering when they speak or take time to give an opinion. If they admitted what is going on inside they might say that they need to stop and calculate what they want to say because they are fearful of giving an untrue or inappropriate answer. After deliberating, they will give

---

Patient Example

A Water CF described his fear by saying that it was either all-pervading or non-existent. He said it sometimes rendered him 'frozen' and he then felt unable to speak in a normal way. In fact it changed the tone of his voice to weak and quiet and he also spoke from higher in his chest. He also felt more tense and his movements felt 'paralysed'. Alternatively they could become more jerky in which case he felt like 'a poor quality mechanical toy'.

---

their considered opinion. This is sometimes more thoughtful and insightful than an opinion given by

others who have taken less time to reflect on an answer.

People who 'freeze up' in the face of fear may restrict what they do in order to compensate. Sometimes people may find it difficult to go out and are labelled 'agoraphobic'. Others may just find that they are extremely nervous when they go out and have their antennae out waiting for an 'attack' from the outside even if logically they know they are safe. A Water CF walking in her local town said, 'It's like I'm waiting for something to happen. I'm on my guard all the time. In fact I can only relax when I'm tense!'

Not acting or reacting

Water CFs can become frozen when unscripted events 'jump out' at them. They may then have difficulty knowing how to respond in such a situation, wanting to change things but being scared to do so. They may feel 'damned if they do and damned if they don't'. The result may be that they do nothing. This was the case with a social worker who was charged with the care of a vulnerable child. On trying to visit the child she was terrorised and threatened by indignant parents. Yet she had been told that the child was at risk. She became paralysed and

---

Patient Example

A Water CF described how much she hated breaking minor rules. When out walking with her boyfriend she found that she was in a field with a 'private' sign on it. 'I was frozen to the spot – I thought the owners were going to shoot me.' She said she couldn't assess the true risk of what she was doing. 'Breaking minor rules is hard for me.'

---

deliberated for far too long about the situation. She was rightly accused of not acting competently and realised that her good intentions were not enough. She later resigned from the job.

The inability to make changes easily can have a positive side. When this kind of Water CF does act she may have made a very careful 'risk' assessment first. This means that any venture she embarks on will tend to be well planned. It might take a long time to be put in motion, but it will be so carefully anticipated that success is almost certain in the end.

Summary

1 A diagnosis of a Water CF is made primarily by observation of a blue colour on the face, a groaning voice, a putrid odour and an imbalance in the emotion fear.

2 Water CFs tend to have issues and difficulties with:
- needing to be safe
- trusting
- drive
- being reassured
- excitation in danger

3 Because of these issues Water CFs' behaviour and responses to situations tend to be along a spectrum and can go between these extremes:

- risk-taking   _____ fearing the worst/over-cautiousness
- distrusting   _____ trusting
- intimidating _____ reassuring
- driven   _____ no drive
- agitation   _____ paralysis

Some common confusions between different CFs

23

CHAPTER CONTENTS

Introduction

The most common reason why a patient doesn't immediately respond to treatment is because the practitioner has not yet discovered the patient's CF. Below are the most common reason why CFs can be confused.

Wood and Fire

Some Wood CFs cover up their anger with sociability and laughter. If this is the case they are more likely to stay 'up' and laughing for a prolonged period of time. The laughter is likely to be more loud and raucous than that of the Fire CF. Some Wood CFs also love poking fun at others as their humour often has an aggressive edge.

When Wood CFs are depressed they can also descend into deep gloom. This could be mistaken for a lack of joy. The depression of a Wood CF is caused by internalised anger that is unexpressed. Because of this Wood CFs often feel somewhat better when the source of frustration has been removed whilst a Fire CF is more likely to brighten up when given warmth or a compliment by someone else.

Wood and Earth

When Earth CFs want sympathy but feel that no one is giving it to them they may feel angry. This can give a practitioner the impression that they are Wood CFs. However, when Earth CFs are then given the support and consideration that they want, they change and feel better (see Shifrin, Chapter 15, p. 169, in MacPherson and Kaptchuk, 1997).

When Earth CFs tend to reject sympathy they may appear to be hard and angry and can also be mistaken for Wood CFs. This is because they find the sympathy difficult to deal with and harden themselves in order to keep it away.

The *qi* of many Wood CFs naturally travels outwards. As a result they may be very giving and benevolent by nature. This may make it easy to mistake them for sympathetic Earth CFs. The object of their sympathy is frequently a cause they are supporting and their motivation is seeking justice. It is important to assess their colour, sound, emotion and odour to ascertain whether their behaviour is pathological or not.

Wood and Metal

Wood CFs and Metal CFs may both have a slightly impenetrable exterior and pretend that they don't care about what others think of them. They may both also have a strong sense of their boundaries. Metal CFs have strong boundaries because they feel fragile and wish to protect themselves from 'attack'. They can have a cutting anger, especially when they feel that their boundaries have been invaded or they have not been treated respectfully. In this case they could be mistaken for an angry Wood CF. Many Wood CFs hold back on fully expressing their anger. Instead they express it indirectly, causing them to make cutting remarks. In this case they resemble a critical Metal CF.

Both Wood and Metal CFs may also have quiet voices – the Wood CF's voice may be lacking in a shout and the Metal CF may have a weak voice because their lungs and throat are not strong.

Wood and Water

Water CFs' fear may cause them to become threatening. Rather than being intimidated they may react to these 'threats' by intimidating others and 'getting their retaliation in first'. In this situation it is common for them to be mistaken for a Wood CF. In this case if Wood, the 'child' Element, is treated it may be effective for a short time but the treatment will 'run out'. This may indicate that the practitioner should then test the mother, Water, as the CF.

A Wood CF who is lacking in anger can also be mistaken for a Water CF. The person is likely to be timid and this is often mistaken for the fear of a Water CF. Colour, sound, emotion and odour are obviously crucial but, in terms of behaviour, it is the lack of assertion that is mistaken for fearfulness and suggests Water.

Fire and Earth

Earth and Fire CFs are both often 'people persons'. Both can be upbeat and can put a lot of their energy into others. Both are often hungry for more contact with people. It is important to observe exactly what they are trying to obtain from others as Fire CFs' need to give or receive love and warmth can be mistaken for Earth CFs' need to give or receive emotional support. This is a very common mistake (especially in patients who, in the viewpoint of TCM, suffer from Spleen *qi xu* and Heart Blood *xu*; the key is to discern which syndrome is primary).

Worry can also be mistaken for anxiety. The worry from the Stomach and Spleen may be centred around the abdomen whilst the anxiety from the Heart will usually be felt in the chest.

Fire and Metal

Confusing Fire and Metal CFs is a common mistake made by many practitioners. The white facial colour can be mistaken for 'lack of red' and at the same time the unhappiness of the Fire CF is often confused with the grief of the Metal CF.

Sadness (*bei*) affects both the Fire and Metal Elements and grief (*you*) is also held in the chest area. It is important to assess the emotions carefully. Fire CFs are more likely to become joyful then drop into sadness. Metal CFs are less likely to go up and down but will have difficulty taking in respect. In general, Metal CFs are less volatile and more brittle. They are also less inclined to be driven to make intimate contact with the practitioner.

Fire and Water

Water CFs can easily be mistaken for Fire CFs because a common way for them to cover up their fear is by smiling and laughing. Laughter is a person's most sociable emotion so it is often used to hide fear and give the appearance of ease and comfort. These are qualities many Water CFs would love to project. The practitioner may notice that the patient never goes into a state of lack of joy. They may then wonder what other emotion lies behind the joy and may see that the joy covers up fear. Often the laughter of a Water CF is more of a nervous laugh or titter or a phoney raucous laugh. It probably fails to elicit joy in others.

Fire CFs can also be mistaken for Water CFs if they are extremely anxious. Shock or fright affects both the Heart and the Kidneys. For many people who have had rather traumatic lives both these Organs can be extremely imbalanced. If the *shen* is disturbed, it can cause the person to feel panicky or have difficulty sleeping. If the Fire and Water are out of harmony, it can make the diagnosis more confusing and it can be difficult to tell which Element of the two is the primary imbalance. Colour, sound, emotion and odour, as ever, are essential in finding the primary imbalance.

Earth and Metal

Earth CFs may cut themselves off from others in order to push away sympathy. In this case they may appear distanced and hard and may be mistaken for Metal CFs who are cut off for other reasons. Earth CFs may also be desperately unhappy and this can be confused with the sadness evident in many Metal CFs.

Earth is the mother of Metal and when the Earth Element is the underlying cause of a person's problem signs and symptoms may initially appear to be coming from the Metal Element. If the Metal Element is treated it may have some effect but treatments will tend not to hold until the underlying cause, which is in the Earth Element, is treated.

Earth and Water

Earth CFs can become very agitated and fearful if they feel that their security is under threat. This is especially true for Earth CFs who lack strong feelings of internal security. This may give the appearance that they are Water CFs. The Earth CFs need support, however, and sympathy and support will tend to settle their agitation.

In comparison, Water CFs who don't get reassured can keep asking for more and more reassurance. The need for reassurance can be mistaken for the need for sympathy. In this case it is the opposite way around. No amount of empathy and support will appease them. Worry, anxiety and fear are words that are used interchangeably by some people, and these two emotions can easily be mistaken for each other.

Metal and Water

Commonly both Metal and Water CFs have more internal and *yin* emotions. They show their feelings less than Wood, Earth and Fire CFs whose emotions are more *yang*. Metal and Water CFs may therefore be more difficult to understand. They are often more hidden and enigmatic. This can cause these two CFs to become confused.

Section 3

Diagnosis

Diagnosis – the purpose and process

24

Introduction to the diagnosis chapters

'To see', 'to hear', 'to ask' and 'to feel/smell' are the four traditional methods of diagnosis used in Chinese medicine. To use these diagnostic tools, practitioners both employ their senses as well as ask questions. Some styles of diagnosis pay more attention to one or the other of these methods. For example, contemporary Chinese herbalists emphasise asking questions about the complaint and the patient's general condition. Although they also use hearing, looking and feeling, these are generally considered less important than questioning. In contrast, practitioners of Five Element Constitutional Acupuncture ask fewer questions and are more reliant on seeing, hearing, smelling and feeling. For this reason the five chapters on diagnosis pay special attention to how practitioners can use and develop their senses in order to make an accurate Five Element diagnosis.

In this first chapter on diagnosis two main aspects are described. The first is how to record the case history and make a diagnosis, and the second is the importance of developing rapport and how to achieve it.

The second chapter (Chapter 25) covers the essential methods used when diagnosing the CF. These are the observation of colour, odour, sound and emotion.

The following chapter (Chapter 26) is about body language and observing a patient's posture, gestures and facial expression. It illustrates how much assessment of a patient is carried out by simple observation.

The next chapter (Chapter 27) on diagnosis covers two important areas. One is reading 'golden keys'. Golden keys are unusual aspects of a patient's behaviour or values that may support a CF diagnosis. The other is determining the appropriate level of treatment the patient requires. This may be the body, mind and/or the spirit.

Finally, the fifth chapter of the diagnosis section (Chapter 28) covers much of what comes under the area of 'to feel' and the physical examination of the patient. The specific areas covered are pulse diagnosis, the Akabane test, feeling the three *jiao* and the palpation of the abdomen. These methods of diagnosis can indicate that an Element is significantly out of balance and they can also support the diagnosis of the CF. However, they are less important in actually determining the CF.

The purpose of making a diagnosis

The main goals of making a Five Element Constitutional diagnosis are:

• to diagnose the patient's CF

- to determine if any other Elements require treatment
- to establish whether the patient has any blocks to treatment
- to ascertain the level of treatment required – body, mind or spirit

Diagnosing the patient's CF

The main goal of diagnosis is to find the patient's CF. Once the CF has been confirmed, it will be the basis of much of the treatment. This is because using points associated with the Organs of the CF are likely to have the most significant effect on the patient's overall health. Having said this, there are situations when this is not the case. For example, acute problems such as infections usually respond better to points chosen to clear the symptoms directly. Also, patients with acute traumatic injuries have better changes from points that move *qi* in the area of the trauma than from treatment centred on the CF.

Diagnosing the other Elements

Determining the patient's CF involves an assessment of all of the Elements. Whilst making the diagnosis the practitioner forms an opinion about the balance of each one. The basis for diagnosing an imbalance in any Element is the same as determining the CF. The main difference is the intensity and number of the diagnostic indicators. Knowing that an Element other than the CF Element is weak is crucial.

A person may be a Water CF, for example, but in the aftermath of an unhappy love affair the Fire Element may be devastated for a considerable period of time. Alternatively this person's Metal Element could be shattered by a recent bereavement.

In many cases treatment on the CF greatly improves the balance of all of the other Elements. Sometimes, however, one Element does not respond and treatment also needs to be directed to that Element. In these situations the practitioner may decide to treat the affected Element as well as influencing it indirectly by treating the CF. This will re-establish harmony within the Five Elements, which will in turn help the person to overcome heartbreak or endure loss with greater internal strength and fortitude.

Diagnosing possible blocks

Next the practitioner needs to establish whether the patient has any blocks to treatment. If blocks are present, they have to be cleared first. They are:

- Aggressive Energy
- Possession
- Husband–Wife imbalance
- Exit–Entry blocks

The blocks and their diagnosis will be described in Chapters 29–33.

Diagnosing the level of treatment

During the course of the diagnosis the practitioner assesses whether treatment should be directed more towards the patient's body, mind or spirit. Determining which level most requires treatment is important as it affects point selection. More is written about this area of diagnosis in Chapter 27.

The process of making a diagnosis

Recording the main complaint, systems and other information

A Five Element Constitutional Acupuncturist always takes a full case history. This involves asking about many areas including:

- the patient's main complaint
- the health of the 'systems', such as the digestion, cardiovascular, urinary and reproductive system
- the general health of the patient's parents and family
- the patient's medical history and educational, work and personal history
- the patient's current living and relationship situation, work, interests, etc.

A Five Element Constitutional Acupuncturist does not use the actual content of this information in order to make a diagnosis of the CF, but it is still important in three ways.

- Firstly, many opportunities for emotion testing will arise whilst collecting this information. Emotion testing will be described in the next chapter. The practitioner can also notice the patient's colour, voice tone and odour during this time. Rapport is also established.

- Secondly, it helps to set a benchmark for the patient's current health. Patients are often most concerned about their *main* complaint when they first come for treatment. Consequently they may not mention other systems that are not functioning well. For example, some patient's bowels may be too frequent or their sleep patterns less than optimum. Patients may also tell the practitioner about other areas of their lives where they are experiencing difficulties, for example in work situations, friendships or close relationships. When practitioners know about all of these areas they can monitor the patient's progress. Many aspects of a patient's health improve when the root is treated. Monitoring this information often tells a practitioner that the patient is getting better even when the main complaint has not yet responded. As well as helping to monitor treatment, patients will also benefit from a wider notion of what constitutes health.

- Thirdly, this information can, in spite of what was said previously, help to confirm the diagnosis. For example, the history of the complaint may reveal that it began shortly after leaving home, the break-up of a relationship or after a frightening experience. The emotional response to these situations may reveal which Element has become imbalanced. This information is never the basis of a diagnosis, but it can confirm and support it. People's health and welfare depends on them being able to receive nourishment from all of the Elements on a regular basis. External changes to their ability to receive this nourishment may reflect on their health. The patient who developed multiple sclerosis after her child ran away or the patient who became ill after his one constant source of love and affection walked out, can be telling us something significant. Patients' non-verbal expressions can be as significant as their words.

What a diagnosis does not involve

A Five Element Constitutional Acupuncturist makes a diagnosis based upon the *person* who has the illness rather than the nature of the illness itself. Therefore the main complaint or symptoms suffered by the patient are important, but are not used to make the diagnosis. The fact that the patient is constipated, paralysed or suffering from migraines is *not* a basis for the CF diagnosis. The patient's Western diagnosis, for example, rheumatoid arthritis, manic depression or diabetes, is also never the basis of a diagnosis. Symptoms often reveal that an Organ is dysfunctional but do not indicate whether that Organ is the primary or secondary cause of the problem.

The stages of making a diagnosis

The context of treatment

Throughout this book, when we refer to practitioners making a diagnosis, we assume they are working in a professional context. This means that the practitioner diagnoses, then treats a patient, and that this is carried out in the practitioner's acupuncture practice.

Most practitioners sometimes find themselves making a diagnosis in other contexts. For example, a friend may call to consult on the telephone or someone at a party might talk about a problem she or he is having. It is useful for practitioners to apply their diagnostic skills in many different situations if they wish to develop them. It is not appropriate, however, to treat in these situations. We recommend that, if a diagnosis is to lead to treatment, the practitioner should carry out a complete diagnosis and have appropriate conditions under which to administer the treatment.

The two levels of activity during a diagnosis

While taking a case history, practitioners are frequently operating on two levels at once. Whilst doing the 'business' of taking the case history, they may also be making significant interventions and observations. Although there are various stages to the process of making a diagnosis, many of them can be done at almost any time. For example, looking at colour, smelling an odour, observing the person's emotional state, recording childhood diseases or taking pulses can be done in any sequence.

Often more than one activity is carried out at any one time. For example, while practitioners are discussing and recording the patient's main complaint, they may also be attempting to discern the facial colour, odour and sound in the voice. Alternatively, when a patient is describing a pain, as well as recording its nature, location and intensity, it may also be a perfect moment for the practitioner to give sympathy and assess the emotion of the Earth Element. There are more examples of ways that practitioners operate on two levels in the next chapter.

The stages of taking a case history

The following are the main stages of taking a case history. This is only one sequence and case histories can be taken in many different ways. Newly qualified practitioners or those just starting to use this system of acupuncture are recommended to more or less follow the sequence laid out below. At the same time, as long as the practitioner gains the essential outcomes of a Five Element Constitutional diagnosis (see above), then they can work in any order.

The stages of the case history are:

1 establishing rapport
2 taking the main complaint
3 questioning the systems
4 finding out about personal health history, family health history, relationships and present situation
5 'to feel'
6 'to see'

Establishing rapport

Establishing rapport is the first priority when making a diagnosis. Without rapport practitioners are operating without the patient's trust. As a result patients are less likely to co-operate and disclose themselves freely. Instead they will wonder if they have chosen the right practitioner and will hold themselves back until they are sure. Although rapport-making is an activity that can be carried out on its own, it is also something that is done at the same time as taking the case history.

At various times when taking the case history, especially early on, the practitioner will focus almost exclusively on the development of rapport. At other moments it will be a background consideration. Although in one sense rapport comes first, it also continues throughout the case history. Rapport-making is discussed in more detail later in this chapter.

Taking the main complaint

Earlier it was stated that a traditional diagnosis is made up of four aspects. These are 'to see', 'to hear', 'to ask' and 'to feel'. Taking the main complaint is mostly associated with the aspect of the diagnosis associated with 'to hear'. Most patients come to treatment with one or more complaints and they expect the practitioner to listen to them carefully.

Early on in the interview, the practitioner may ask the patient 'What would you like acupuncture to help you with?' or 'What is your problem, how long have you had it and what have you had done about it?' The patient can then talk about the complaint in depth. Once the patient has described the problem, the practitioner asks further questions in order to gain a complete picture of the patient's problem. It is essential for the practitioner to record the complaint in detail and in the patient's own words. The patient may have more than one complaint and each should be dealt with in a similar way. The purpose of recording the complaint is to:

- help make a diagnosis of the patient's CF as well as the state of the other Organs
- form an accurate assessment of the complaint in order to monitor progress
- discover and explore what happened around the time the complaint began
- create and maintain rapport by meeting the patient's expectations and providing opportunities for compassion to be communicated

Patients do not necessarily remember how they were at the start of treatment. Keeping the information gained at the start can be useful later on so that patient and practitioner can evaluate the impact of treatment.

A well-recorded complaint will:

- be recorded in the patient's own words
- record when it started and what was happening around that time
- describe where it is located
- describe its quality and the intensity, for instance, of the pain or sensations involved
- describe whether it is continuous or intermittent and, if intermittent, its frequency
- say what makes it worse or better
- record what the person can or cannot do as a result of the problem
- include any associated symptoms
- record what other treatments the patient has tried and any medication she or he has taken

Questioning the systems, or the 'Ten Questions'

This stage covers what Western physiology describes as a patient's 'systems'. In Chinese medicine, questions about these areas are known as the 'Ten Questions'. This section of the diagnosis is especially concerned with the 'to ask' aspect of the traditional diagnosis. Each area of questioning may involve a great amount of detail.

- *Sleep*. Quality – depth of sleep; how the patient feels in the morning on waking; restlessness or agitation at night. Quantity – time the patient goes to bed; when goes off to sleep; when wakes up. Insomnia – waking in the night; trouble getting off to sleep; waking early, reason for waking. Drugs – sleeping tablets. Dreams – dream disturbed sleep; recurring or frequent dreams; nightmares.

- *Appetite, food and taste*. Appetite – good, bad, 'too good'; hungry but can't eat. Digestion – good, bloating/distending when eats, indigestion, nausea, vomiting. Likes/dislikes – hot, cold, any taste preference or craving. Taste – bitter, sweet, salty, etc. Diet – when patient eats and what they eat on a normal day. How healthy is the patient's 'relationship' with food?

- *Thirst and drink*. Quantity of fluid per day. Thirst – how thirsty. Type of fluid – hot/cold, tea, coffee, etc. Alcohol – how much, when, what, any history of drink problems.

- *Bowels*. When – are they regular, every day. Consistency – diarrhoea: how often, smell, colour, undigested food, watery; constipation: how often, dry, soft. Mucus, blood. Pain – strong/weak, when better/worse.

- *Urine*. Quantity – amount, frequency. Colour – light, dark, cloudy, blood. Odour – strong smell, no smell. Pain/distension – when better/worse. Enuresis.

- *Sweating and temperature preference*. Sweating – how much, e.g. normal, heavy, light; when, e.g. on exertion, day, night. Temperature – hot or cold; which area, for example, all over, deep inside or extremities.

- *Women's health*. (i) Menstruation: regularity, length of period. Blood – colour, quality, quantity, clots, flow. Pain – type, time, frequency. Emotional changes. Age when started period. (ii) Discharges – colour, smell, amount. (iii) Pregnancy and childbirth: how many, any problems, e.g. miscarriages, infertility, type of birth, post birth. (iv) Menopause (if appropriate): what age; any problems, for example, flushes, emotional changes, lack of energy, etc. (v) Contraception (if appropriate) – pill, coil, etc.

- *Head and body*. Headaches – onset, time of day, location, type of pain, better/worse. Dizziness – onset, acute/chronic, strong/slight, better/worse, accompanying symptoms.

- *Eyes and ears*. Eyes: vision – normal/short/long sight; blurred vision; irritations, for example, red or blood-shot eyes; dryness; floaters; pain. Ears: quality of hearing; tinnitus – onset, character of noise. Numbness – where, when comes on.

- *Thorax and abdomen*. How are the chest; flanks; epigastrium; hypochondrium; abdomen – any pain or distension.

- *Pain*. Where; when comes on; full/empty (Maciocia, 2005, pp. 323-324); fixed/moving; better/worse with activity; heat or cold.

- *Climate and season*. Feel better/worse in any climate or season, e.g. cold, heat, damp, wind, dryness, etc.

There are other questions that the practitioner can also ask. These can include questions about a patient's allergies, resistance to infections and changes in well-being and vitality at different times of day.

The main categories listed above are best described as 'areas to question', as each of them can involve many specific questions. The practitioner may wish to first ask an open question about each system such as 'How are your bowels?' or 'How is your sleep?' Once this has been answered, the practitioner may then ask the patient other more specific questions about that area.

For example, if the first question is 'How is your sleep?', then depending upon the answer, subsequent questions could be: 'What time do you go to bed?', 'What time do you get up?', 'Do you wake in the night?', 'How many times?', 'How is your temperature when you wake?', 'Do you feel rested in the morning?' and so on. The relevance of some of these questions is a basis for judging the patient's progress and, depending upon the other Chinese medicine patterns the practitioner uses, the answers may also have diagnostic relevance.

The list of questions above is useful as a checklist and it enables practitioners to decide whether they have questioned all aspects of the patient's health. Experience and sensitivity tell the practitioner when to go further and ask more questions and when to leave a topic. For example, after questioning menstruation many times, the practitioner is better able to evaluate whether the patient has a significant problem in the area or not.

For the Five Element Constitutional Acupuncturist this information is used to determine in which respects a person's body, mind and spirit is not working well. People often have a symptom or symptoms, which they think are unimportant so they do not include them with their main or subsidiary complaint(s). For example, a patient may be complaining of migraines and period pains, but they may also have night sweats and digestive problems. As these may well respond to the CF treatment, it is important that they are acknowledged and can be used to monitor progress. The migraines may be irregular, making progress difficult to assess. The improved digestion and the absence of night sweats may, however, confirm that treatment is being at least partially successful.

Personal health history, family health history, relationships and present situation

The information collected here concerns four broad areas: the patient's health history; the family health history; relationships; and the patient's present situation.

Questioning a patient's personal history is often the most diagnostically important part of the taking of the case history. Patients may exhibit no obvious emotions when they recount their health problems and history. While discussing family and intimate relationships or difficult phases in their lives, however, they often reveal more of their emotions.

Rapport is crucial. Superficial rapport limits the patient's willingness to disclose painful emotional areas. Patients give different answers to the same question depending on the trust they feel in the person asking the question. Excellent rapport allows the patient to reveal in which Elements the most intensely felt emotions are to be found.

Personal health history

It is important to see the patient's current health problems in the context of their past health. The current complaint may be just one more instance of the same thing occurring over time or it may be the first time they have ever been seriously ill. The following are some guidelines topics to ask about:

- birth – premature, health at birth, wanted or otherwise
- early childhood rashes, digestion, illnesses (mumps, scarlet fever, rheumatic fever, whooping cough, etc.)
- other past illnesses
- accidents, injuries or visits to hospital
- medication – it is obviously important to ascertain which medications are being taken. Some symptoms may be the effect or side-effect of a drug
- recreational drugs, including alcohol
- smoking
- difficult periods in the patient's life
- schooling
- career

Family health history

Some families have hereditary diseases and other are known for being 'long livers'. This information can explain the occurrence of some illness and it can also create false expectations on the part of some family members. The practitioner needs to find out about:

- health of parents
- family diseases
- siblings and their health

Relationships

As friendship and close relationships are an essential part of our welfare, an understanding of these is useful. The pattern of relationships, for example, the ability to maintain or not maintain them, can give supportive evidence for a CF. Discussion of these kinds of topics also often reveals emotions that were not evident while discussing the patient's physical health. The practitioner should aim to cover the following areas:

- relationship with parents and siblings and other significant relatives
- friends at primary and secondary school
- significant friends
- significant teachers, mentors or authority figures
- marriages and sexual relationships
- children

Present situation

This term covers the patient's present living situation:

- married or living with partner
- housing
- jobs, friendships, children
- religious or spiritual beliefs
- hobbies and interests
- hopes for the future

'To feel'

The traditional notion of 'to feel' covers several things:

- pulse diagnosis (see Chapter 28)
- three *jiao* (see Chapter 28)
- palpating front *mu* points and back *shu* points (see Chapter 28)
- abdominal diagnosis (see Chapter 28)
- palpation of (and visually inspecting) the channels
- palpation of musculo-skeletal symptom areas for swelling, pain, temperature
- joint flexibility and range of motion
- skin temperature, moisture, texture
- nail strength

'To see'

The 'to see' part of the diagnosis goes on throughout the case history, for example, when asking questions or during palpation of the abdomen. It includes such things as the following:

- the colour on the face
- the spirit as reflected in the sparkle of the eyes
- scars
- observation of emotional responses

Pulling it all together

Having collected the above information, the practitioner needs to sift through it and bring it together. Both inexperienced and experienced practitioners can end up with some degree of uncertainty. For example, a practitioner may be able to make a strong case for Wood but also a strong case for Metal. During the process of pulling the case history together, it is useful for practitioners to keep a list of any information they did not collect and any signs that they have doubts about. For instance, they may be unsure of the facial colour and wonder if it was yellow or green. They can then go back and concentrate on this aspect at a later treatment.

A beginner takes considerable time over this phase – sifting the information, separating primary from supportive evidence and trying to determine whether or not the symptoms, pulses or touch of the person are genuinely supportive of the CF diagnosis or simply insignificant. New practitioners may take more time pulling the information together than they took collecting it. More experienced practitioners start to pull information together as it gets collected.

So far we have concentrated on the content and sequence of collecting information. We turn now to rapport.

Rapport

What is rapport?

Rapport occurs when the patient feels close to the practitioner. It is not something that is either on or off, but is a question of degree. Rapport allows the patient to trust the practitioner. The level of trust achieved may not extend to other areas of the patient's life, but is specific to the matters relevant in the practitioner/patient context.

Practitioners are concerned about rapport because it facilitates the following:

- It helps the practitioner to 'emotion-test' more effectively – good rapport encourages a patient to reveal more of their emotional self to the practitioner.
- It helps the practitioner elicit more accurate information and better understanding – the deeper the rapport, the more the patient can open up and reveal their inner world.
- It enables the practitioner to carry out treatments that affect deeper aspects of a person – without rapport the patient's spirit is not accessible to the practitioner.

How does a practitioner make rapport?

Rapport often comes easily. There are, however, times when it doesn't occur naturally and the practitioner needs to know how to generate it. In some cases rapport can also be improved. There is a big difference between 'getting along OK' and achieving a deep level of trust. Deep trust allows patients to feel sufficiently safe to reveal the intensity of their emotional world.

A mechanism for gaining rapport

People tend to trust those they have something in common with or who they perceive are like them. In Britain, for example, two people in a railway carriage, wearing the same football team's scarf already have a bridge between them. In the USA, supporting the same baseball team can be a natural link. A person might meet someone who has a similar taste in music. They love the music and think, 'A man who loves that music as much as I do can't be all bad.' Opposites may attract, but *'similars' gain rapport*. A method for gaining rapport, therefore, is to create and draw attention to similarities.

In what respects can people become more similar?

In Box 24.1 is a list of areas for which similarity helps to generate closeness. Take, for example, the tempo at which a person operates. Tempo will manifest in the rate of a person's speech, gestures and body movements. Someone who is slow will speak slowly, gesture slowly and move slowly. Someone who is fast will speak quickly, gesture quickly and move quickly. Tempo is a fundamental characteristic of a person. A fast person has difficulty feeling comfortable with a slow one, and vice versa. Fast practitioners with slow patients will create more rapport as they slow down. Slow practitioners with fast patients will create more rapport as they quicken their tempo.

To improve rapport, the practitioner can match each of the aspects in Box 24.1. (For further reading, see Brooks (1989) and Richardson (2000). These are detailed and enthusiastic. See also O'Connor and Seymour (2003) and Young (2004), both of which have sections on rapport.)

How does a practitioner learn to do this?

The best way to learn how to match is to take one area at a time and to match it. For example, when learning to match someone else's tempo, practitioners can devote time (in daily life or in specially arranged sessions) to adjusting their tempo so that it is similar to other people's. People have a range of tempos, but if overall the practitioner is faster than the patient, he or she needs to slow the tempo down a notch – to close the gap. To do this, the practitioner thinks, gestures, breathes and speaks more slowly.

Sometimes it is easy to match but sometimes it is not. For example, speaking more slowly, to some degree, is easy. However, a slightly greater shift can tip the balance and learners may say that they no longer feel like themselves. People have said they feel 'odd', 'not myself' and even 'weird' when moving outside their normal comfort zone. It is important that practitioners remain comfortable whilst matching and realise that they are in control and can decide the degree to which they match. In order to gain rapport with another person it is not necessary for the practitioner to be *exactly* the same. It is much more important to make *similar* movements or gestures. A small shift towards similarity can create a large amount of rapport.

It is often useful to learn to match in a class with a teacher or observer present. In this situation, unlike real life, the person learning can make mistakes and be given feedback from a peer acting as a 'patient'. People's perception of how much change they have created is not always easy to determine and an outside observer can also be helpful.

Learning to match another person is also best done in small stages. For example, practitioners may learn to adjust the tempo of their speech until they can do it without thinking. They may then learn to match the variation in the pitch of the voice until they can also do this without thinking. Practitioners' skill in matching soon increases and they can rapidly gain the ability to match without thinking. Sometimes saying the word 'match' to themselves can act as a trigger so that they automatically start to match the patient.

Which areas are essential to match?

With reference to Box 24.1, the following areas are the most important ones to match to gain rapport:

Box 24.1

Areas practitioners can learn to match

Body posture	**Gestures (especially repetitive key gestures)**
Tempo (voice/body/mind)	Voice tone and volume
Values	Breathing
Use of language and metaphors	Words and phrases

- body posture
- gestures generally
- voice tone and volume
- tempo (voice/body/mind)

The following can make a big increase in the capacity to gain rapport:

- the most repetitive or 'key' gestures
- values

The remaining areas to match can be important, but are difficult to learn:

- breathing
- words and phrases
- the use of language and metaphors

Matching and diagnosis

As well as enabling practitioners to gain rapport, matching can also increase their ability to make a diagnosis. When practitioners are matching a patient's tempo, voice tone, posture and key gestures, they are not just observing passively. In order to carry out the matching the practitioner is both observing and at the same time taking on these other aspects of the patient. The act of matching automatically makes the practitioner feel more like the patient. The more matching is carried out, the more this increases. Thus the practitioner's understanding of the patient increases too. Hence, matching is in part a diagnostic method.

The practitioner might also ask if there a danger of becoming too like the patient. When practitioners have learned to match and do it consciously, it is relatively easy to stop. They have clear control over 'getting the feel of the patient' and returning back to be themselves. However, if practitioners naturally match and do it unconsciously, then they need to be careful. Some practitioners complain that they feel 'drained' by patients or even take on their patients' symptoms. This can be an extreme form of unconscious matching. If this is done momentarily, it can be useful for diagnosis. Otherwise, it is dangerous and practitioners risk becoming ill. Learning to match consciously helps a practitioner to gain better control over this unconscious and harmful matching.

How much rapport do we need?

Developing trust

It can be tempting for practitioners to believe that they only need to ask the right questions and the patient will answer correctly. However, gaining deep rapport involves far more than the practitioner just turning up, being pleasant and asking the right questions. It involves inner development and the engagement of the practitioner's full compassion.

Matching is an excellent way for the practitioner to be in harmony with the patient. It also encourages the patient to develop trust and confidence in the practitioner. For many patients to reveal their emotional world to the practitioner a very deep level of rapport is required. Some patients easily show their anger, fear, need for sympathy or sadness to their practitioner. Others do not. These patients need to feel a great deal of trust in the practitioner and this places more demands on her or him.

Acceptance and compassion

Above all it is necessary for practitioners to give patients their full attention. The practitioner needs to see the patient's internal pain and suffering. As well as matching, acceptance and compassion are essential requirements. These are not possible unless the practitioner is prepared to be touched and affected by the patient's story and feelings. Patients can find it especially difficult to reveal grief and sadness unless the practitioner is able to resonate with and respect those feelings.

Being fully present

When making rapport practitioners also need to use their intention (*yi*). Guo Yu described a situation when his intention was not 'fully there' and how it hindered his ability to bring about a cure (see Chapter 6, this volume, for more on the inner development of the practitioner and the situation Guo Yu was describing). If the practitioner's intention is not fully present, then the patient's spirit will not be wholly available for the treatment. If rapport is limited, the practitioner's ability to diagnose may be affected as the practitioner is unable to observe aspects of the patient's spirit. In consequence treatments will be less effective.

Developing deep rapport improves the quality of information collected, makes emotion testing more effective and enables the patient to become more open and ready to change when the practitioner carries out the treatment. There is no exact answer to the question 'How much rapport do you need?' Practitioners who have virtuosity (*linghuo*) have developed their rapport-making skills and these are an enormous benefit to them in their practice.

Summary

1 'To see', 'to hear', 'to ask' and 'to feel/smell' are the four traditional methods of diagnosis used in Chinese medicine.

2 The main goals of making a Five Element Constitutional diagnosis are:
- to diagnose the patient's CF
- to determine if any other Elements require treatment
- to establish whether the patient has any blocks to treatment
- to ascertain the level of treatment required – body, mind or spirit

3 Making a diagnosis involves both using the senses to discern colour, sound, emotion and odour and also listening to the content of what the patient is saying.

4 A Five Element Constitutional Acupuncturist always takes a full case history. This involves asking about many areas including:
- the patient's main complaint
- the health of the 'systems', such as the digestion, cardiovascular, urinary and reproductive system
- the general health of the patient's parents and family
- the patient's medical history and educational, work and personal history
- the patient's current living and relationship situation, work, interests, etc.

5 Rapport is vital to a Five Element Constitutional Acupuncturist as good rapport facilitates a deeper level of diagnosis and treatment.

Diagnosis – the key methods

25

Introduction

This chapter covers the key methods of diagnosis used in Five Element Constitutional Acupuncture. These are:

• colour
• odour
• sound
• emotion

Colour

The background

The colours associated with each Element are:

• Wood – green
• Fire – red/lack of red
• Earth – yellow
• Metal – white
• Water – blue

There are four significant places for a Five Element Constitutional Acupuncturist to observe colour. These are by the side of the eye, under the eye, in the laugh lines and around the mouth. Some people's colour shows in broad swathes on the sides of the face. The colour at the side of the eye is the most important area to notice when diagnosing the CF.

Sometimes at least two colours appear on the face. For example, there may be a green colour around the mouth and a different colour next to the eye. In this case the colour by the eye normally takes precedence.[1]

One anomaly about facial colour is that Fire CFs, rather than showing a red colour, normally have a dull pale facial colour, especially at the sides of the eyes. This colour is called 'lack of red'.

The difference between seeing and labelling

There are two distinct steps for the practitioner to take when learning to observe colour. Firstly, practitioners need to *see* the colour. Secondly, they need to be able to *label* it. Seeing is not the same as labelling.

Seeing colour

Some practitioners try to label colour before they have seen it properly. In this case they have left out the first step. They need to learn to see colour

---

[1]Facial colour is used in different ways by different traditions of acupuncture. It may be useful to read the description of the use of facial colour in TCM given by Kaptchuk (2000, pp. 180–181). The overlap is obvious and the differences are significant.

first. This can be an important part of the training when learning Five Element Constitutional Acupuncture. More is written about this below.

Labelling colour

Other practitioners see a distinct colour but then do not know what to call it. Some people have a wider range of labels for colour than others. For example, a person who mixes colour for a paint manufacturer or a person who paints landscapes is likely to have more labels for different colours than solicitors or linguists who use their visual acuity less. It can be helpful if practitioners take the time to observe a wide range of colours, especially those seen in nature, in order to increase their colour 'vocabulary'. Being able to label colour is essential as it links what practitioners observe with their Five Element diagnosis.

Seeing facial colour

In order to increase their ability to see colours, practitioners can set themselves certain tasks. For example, one task may be to spend 15 minutes sitting at the window of a café or restaurant observing the facial colour of those passing by. Another option may be to observe the colour of 10 different people during the course of a day. It may also be useful for practitioners to observe colour with a fellow learner and compare what they see. In order to fine-tune their skills, practitioners need to look at the facial colour of almost everyone they meet.

When observing colour, it is important that practitioners relax their eyes. Squinting, moving the head forward or getting anxious make it less likely that the practitioner will be able to discern the colour. Below we discuss how practitioners can develop their sensory acuity by:

- comparing colour
- observing in different lights
- being aware of how light is reflected
- softening their eyes

Comparing colour

Comparing colour increases sensory acuity. For example, looking at two faces simultaneously (or at least quickly moving back and forth) heightens practitioners' visual awareness. Acupuncturists who are working on their own, looking at only one patient, can easily cross the habituation threshold. To focus their minds on the sensory input it can be useful for them to compare different areas of the patient's face. This gives them several colours to observe. To help them to do this they can ask themselves a question, such as, 'How do the colours on either side of the face compare?' or 'Which colour is paler?' The landscape painter does this naturally as his or her eye travels back and forth from field to canvas and back again.

In a group, when people are learning to see colour, it can be useful to line up two to five people to compare their different colours.

Observing in different lights

Natural light is important when observing colour, so practitioners may sometimes need to ask patients to step outside or over to the window of the treatment room in order to find the best light. It is often useful to ask patients to face the light and to then turn their heads slowly from one side to the other. This will enable the practitioner to observe the facial colour on all areas of the face.

Observing in different lights can be useful as this helps the practitioner to understand the benefits of good light. Mid-winter in Britain is not a good time for natural light. The skies are greyer and the days are shorter. Many treatment rooms have little natural light and artificial light subtly distorts the true colour. Making comparisons between artificial and natural light, one side of the room and another, bright sunlight and soft northern exposure, enables a practitioner to get used to the effects of different lights. A change in colour will easily convince the practitioner that bringing the patient to the best source of light is a good idea.

Awareness of how facial colour can be distorted

Light is reflected off walls, blankets and clothes. A patient with a green shirt or pink blanket may appear different when wearing a brown shirt or using a blue blanket. It is useful for the practitioner to experiment and notice any differences caused by different lights.

It can also be useful to remember that make-up distorts colours and the practitioner may need to ask some patients not to wear make-up on the day of treatment. Figure 25.1 describes an exercise to help develop the practitioner's awareness of facial colour.

Sit in a place where you have natural light and observe a person near you. Ensure that this person is facing the light. Compare the person's colour on the following areas (indicated in Figure 25.1): 1 and 2, 3 and 4, and 5 and 6. Then compare other areas such as areas 1 and 4, 2 and 5, 7 and 3. Notice any similarities or differences between the different areas. This will help you to build your awareness of facial colour.

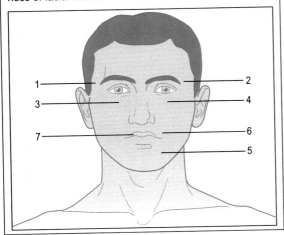

Figure 25.1 • An exercise to aid seeing colour

Softening the eyes

Hard eyes limit the range of our vision and make it difficult to see colour. The more we relax and soften the eyes the wider our vision and the better we can see the patient's colour (Box 25.1).

Box 25.1

An exercise to soften the eyes

The following is an exercise to soften the eyes:
Two practitioners, A and B, work together and sit opposite each other.

A closes her or his eyes and then relaxes them as far as possible.

He or she then concentrates on the eye itself and just behind it.

When the eye feels somewhat different, A opens the eyes just for a second or two and looks at B's colour.

A then closes her or his eyes and repeats the softening.

A then once more opens the eyes, this time for slightly longer and repeats until she or he experiences seeing the colour better and at the same time seeing 'more'.

Labelling colour

Sometimes labelling is easy. The colour is obviously blue or obviously green. On occasions, however, there is a dispute as to whether that colour, which two people are both looking at, is yellow or green, or is it both or a mixture of the two? When there is disagreement, it is best to revert to observing the colour again and looking at it in the best light conditions possible. Confusion decreases over time, but some uncertainty may remain.

When practitioners are unsure of the correct label, the following method can help them to learn to identify colour. If, for instance, a practitioner can't decide whether the patient's colour is yellow or green, she or he can still make a diagnosis based on other factors such as the emotion, odour or voice tone. If that diagnosis is then confirmed by a positive response to treatment, then the practitioner might make an inference about the colour, based on the confirmed diagnosis. For example, if the treatment response confirms that the patient is a Wood CF, then in spite of the earlier confusion between yellow and green, the practitioner might conclude that the predominant colour was green. Learning in this way is probably the easiest way for practitioners to improve their ability to recognise colours. (The ability to recognise odour and voice tone can also be partly learnt in this way.)

Once the practitioner becomes aware that reflected colour can change the patient's colour, it is inevitable on many occasions to ask the patient to stand in front of a window where the light is optimum. The practitioner can then ask the patient to turn their head slowly from side to side which presents the best conditions for viewing colour. It seems that shyness stops practitioners from doing this, but getting the colour right is far more important. This is also the best position in which to examine the tongue.

Odour

The background

The odours for each of the Elements are:

- Wood – rancid
- Fire – scorched
- Earth – fragrant
- Metal – rotten
- Water – putrid

As soon as there is an imbalance in a person's *qi*, their odour will change. During the diagnosis the practitioner will endeavour to smell the patient's predominant odour.

Smelling and labelling odours

Smelling odours

As with colour, smelling more keenly is an essential stage to go through before learning to apply the correct odour labels. After taking a case history, a common complaint from practitioners is that they didn't smell an odour. The reason for this is simple. Most people do not need to be able to smell to get through their day. Apart from smelling smoke (indicating a fire), a gas leak or perhaps food to determine whether it has gone off, most people do not regularly use their ability to smell. Compared to a cat or dog, both of which will constantly be checking their environment for odour information, humans barely use their sense of smell. Thus to use odour regularly with patients requires some development.

Labelling odours

When practitioners learn to hone their sense of smell, they still have the problem of identifying the smells correctly. The labels for the odours listed above are not particularly helpful, as many people do not have clear ideas about, for example, the smell of rotten as opposed to the smell of rancid.

Increasing the ability to smell

One problem when smelling odour as opposed to looking at colour is that a colour is more constant and objective. If practitioners look at the colour by the eye, then look away again, they expect to look back and see the same colour again. This is especially true if they do it quickly and they or the patient do not change position or alter the light. This is less true with odour because people habituate to smells very quickly. This habituation is similar to what happens if we repeat a word endlessly and it seems to lose its usual meaning. We may initially smell something strongly, but then the smell quickly fades. The fragile nature of an odour is a matter of degree, but it is less constant and substantial than colour. Box 25.2 describes an exercise to help develop the ability to smell odours.

When to smell the odour

Because people habituate quickly, it becomes important to 'catch' odours by surprise. One of the best times for practitioners to smell a patient's odour is

when they have just entered the treatment room. If a patient has removed some clothing, the odour seems to fill a room and build up, especially if the patient has been in the room for several minutes. The practitioner can smell the hallway and then smell the room, in a matter of one to two seconds. In this way they can use contrast and comparison to accentuate the odour. After the practitioner has been in the room for more than a minute or two, the chances of detecting the odour become considerably less.

If a patient is lying under a blanket in a warm room this may also provide the practitioner with an opportunity to smell the odour. When the blanket is lifted in order to check the temperature of the three *jiao* or to carry out abdominal diagnosis a smell may be detected.

It can also be useful for practitioners to notice the odour in the area between a patient's shoulder blades. The odour is often more distinct here as this is a difficult area for people to clean.

How to smell the odour

The more the practitioner is relaxed the easier it is to smell the odour. 'Trying hard' to smell is especially ineffective. Sometimes the odour becomes stronger and clearer when it is least expected. When a practitioner is deeply relaxed, for example, when taking pulses, the odour may suddenly become more apparent.

It is important for practitioners not to obviously sniff or show that they looking for an odour or rapport can easily be lost. The patient may wrongly conclude that the practitioner thinks she or he has an offensive smell!

Artificial smells

Another point the practitioner needs to remember is that patients are often wearing a number of artificial and acquired smells that cover up the underlying odour. These range from perfumes, hairsprays, what the patient last ate, deodorants, toothpaste, whatever is clinging to clothes (freshly dry cleaned or not) to flatulence. It is often appropriate for the practitioner to ask patients not to wear perfumes and other artificial smells on the day they come for treatment.

The labels of the smells

Most practitioners' 'smell vocabulary' is less developed than their colour vocabulary. The vocabulary they do have often includes many judgmental words like 'awful', 'yucky' or 'gorgeous'. These do not help a person to improve their ability to label odours. In Table 25.1 an attempt is made to describe the various odours.

As with colour, one way practitioners can enhance their ability to recognise odours is to make a diagnosis using the other three key methods of diagnosis and then link the odour to that Element. Some practitioners are naturally gifted in the ability to smell odours, but for many it is their least developed sense. The challenge for them is to develop their ability to use it effectively. Box 25.3 suggests a practical way to improve the ability to distinguish smells.

Sound

The background and principles

The voice tones associated with each Element are:
- Wood – shouting/lack of shout
- Fire – laughing/lack of laugh

Box 25.3

Increasing our ability to smell using 'smell' bottles

'Smell-bottles' are a useful device when learning to smell odours. Their purpose is to enable practitioners to:
- Increase the amount they consciously smell
- Refine their ability to make smell distinctions
- Increase their ability to remember smells
- Assist them in labelling smells

Smell bottles are not high-tech. All that is needed is to:
- Acquire five small, identical, opaque, containers that have tight-fitting tops to keep any material and its odour inside. These may be bought specially, but many foods and medicines come in these kinds of containers.
- Mark distinct numbers on the bottom, for example from one to five, and place something that is natural and has a distinct odour in each one.
- Open each bottle one at a time and get used to the smell. At this stage look at the number on the bottom.
- Mix the bottles up and open them one by one. Smell the contents and try to put them in the order of one to five.

This game enhances the practitioner's ability to smell, discriminate, remember and possibly label the smells in order to remember them. There are many variations to the game above. For example, the practitioner can start with just two bottles and work up to five, or, to make the exercise more difficult, the contents of the bottles can be made more similar. This game can also be played with a partner.

Table 25.1 A description of the odours

Element	Conventional label	Description
Wood	Rancid	Like rancid butter or cut grass. Slightly prickly inside the nose and a bit musty at the same time
Fire	Scorched	Like clothes coming out of the tumble dryer or the smell of ironing or like burnt toast
Earth	Fragrant	Unlike 'fragrant' flowers. Heavy, cloying and sweet. A smell that hangs around the nostrils
Metal	Rotten	Like rotting meat or a rubbish bin or garbage truck where many different substances are decomposing. Grabs the inside of the nose with tiny prickles
Water	Putrid	Like a mixture of a urinal and chloride of lime. Can also be like stale wine, a tom cat's spray or bleach. A sharp smell

- Earth – singing
- Metal – weeping
- Water – groaning

A normal voice tone contains each of the five sounds when they are appropriate. When an Element is out of balance, one sound predominates or becomes absent. When there is reasonable balance these voice tones are appropriate to the emotion being expressed. When there is imbalance they are inappropriate. The Five Element Constitutional Acupuncturist listens to the voice tone in order to determine which sound is most out of balance.

When learning to listen to voice tones, practitioners first need to be able to distinguish between a congruent or incongruent voice tone and emotion. They can then evaluate the voice tone in conjunction with the emotion the patient is expressing and the content of the discussion.

Voice tone and emotion

When people are relatively whole and balanced, their channels of emotional expression are also relatively balanced. For example, a shouting tone denotes anger or an attempt to assert oneself. To hear this sound when someone is actually angry is appropriate. To hear the same sound when a person is expressing love or warmth is inappropriate. Box 25.4 describes an experiment to help practitioners distinguish between congruent and incongruent sounds.

Once people are alert to inconsistencies between the voice tone and emotion they often notice them more and find that they sound strange. What is even stranger, however, is that people often hear incongruency in everyday life and do not register it as unusual.

Box 25.4

Experimenting with incongruent sounds

To understand the difference between congruent and incongruent sounds and emotions, try this experiment. Feel friendly and say 'hello' in an angry tone. Feel sympathetic and express this in a frightened tone of voice. Try using other incongruent voice tones and emotions. Notice how often you hear these inconsistencies as you go about your daily activities. Often, without training, practitioners just accept these blatant incongruencies as 'just how someone is'. They are, however, important diagnostically.

Throughout the treatment practitioners need to maintain a heightened state of awareness and alertness as to whether the patient's voice tone is appropriate or not. Paying attention to the nuances in the voice makes demands on the practitioner, but diagnosis by voice tone is often a key part of the diagnosis of the CF. Time spent honing the ability 'to hear' is time well spent. The focused awareness required can also intensify the rapport between patient and practitioner.

Descriptions of the sounds

When learning to recognise an imbalance in patients' voice tones, the first stage is to recognise the difference between each sound. In order to clarify these differences, a more detailed description of each voice tone is listed below.

Fire is 'laughing'

The 'laughing' sound is not an actual laugh, but is more like a pre-laugh. It is as if a person is being given a little tickle and might break into real laughter. The sound itself tends to move upward in the body.

Some people have a voice tone that is lacking in laughter. This voice tone has no sparkle or animation to it. It can easily be mistaken for a groaning voice. A distinguishing feature is that it often has a croaky quality, as though it comes from deep in the person's throat or chest.

Earth is 'singing'

The 'singing' voice is used by a mother when she is soothing her upset child. It can also be compared to the voice of a rider calming an agitated horse. It is the voice tone often used by someone being ingratiating. The sing, as compared with other voices, has more frequent and more extreme variations in pitch.

Metal is 'weeping'

The weeping voice is not actually weeping, but more as if the person is *about* to weep. It often tails off in volume near the end of sentences, as if the lungs are too weak to sustain their power for a whole sentence. It is often a bit thin, quavers or sounds fragile. To use a photographic analogy, the density of the weeping voice often has a lower resolution and fewer pixels. The underlying grief can create a 'catch' or slight choke in the voice.

Water is 'groaning'

A groaning voice lacks the variations in pitch of a singing voice and is often recognised for being flat or expressionless. It is as if a normal voice has a flat upper and lower governor that squashes any upward and downward variation in pitch. It is easy to imagine its connection with fear. If a person is in a dangerous situation, say, in a room where there is reported to be a poisonous snake, then in order not to create panic or frighten the snake, she or he might easily put a clamp on variations in pitch, keeping the voice level and constant. The voice can often 'drag' towards the end of the sentence.

Wood is 'shouting'

'Shouting' usually implies an increase in loudness and, while often true, loudness is not the essential quality of this voice tone. Another way of describing this sound is that it contains an 'emphasis'. Emphasis means that one syllable, for example, of a three-syllable word, is louder. For instance, if a person says the word 'exactly' and emphasises the middle syllable – ex*act*ly. Another description of this sound is that it is clipped, implying an abruptness or sharpness. Such a voice can be quiet but assertive.

Some people have a voice tone that lacks any strength to it. This voice is unnaturally quiet or becomes so when the person is challenged or uncertain. It does not have the power or force that would be expected from that particular person. The practitioner often needs to strain slightly to catch what is being said. It is as though the voice cannot be projected sufficiently to easily travel across the intervening distance between the two people.

Box 25.5 suggests an exercise to develop the ability to discriminate sounds.

The content and emotional context

The next stage is the comparison of the voice tone with content of the person's speech and their emotional expression. A person may be speaking about the family coming to stay for Christmas and may also be smiling. At the same time, the voice tone may contain more than an appropriate amount of emphasis. She or he is talking in a friendly way, but the voice tone is angry.

Another person may speak about having physical or emotional pain with a laugh in the voice. Another person speaks about an enjoyable time with the

---

Box 25.5

An exercise to aid learning the sounds

This is a useful way to learn the different voice tones:
1. Ask two members of a group to carry on a conversation.
2. Take the components of sounds – emphasis, variation in pitch or lack of it, the direction of movement of the voice in the body and the density of the voice – and listen to the two people speaking.
3. One by one, ask, 'Which of the two people has more emphasis in the voice?' 'Which of the two has more variation in pitch?' and so on.

This exercise uses comparison to assist sensory discrimination. It also encourages the listener to pay attention solely to the sound. The latter can be difficult. Practitioners get attracted to the content of people's conversation and are afraid they will miss something important while listening to the voice tone. It can be helpful to close one's eyes, but perseverance may also be necessary. Once it becomes second nature to hear the voice tones, then the listener also loses the fear of not absorbing the content of what the person is saying.

---

family and looks happy, but the voice is groaning. Another person is saying they are angry about an incident when they were ignored, but their voice is singing.

In all of these cases, the practitioner of Five Element Constitutional Acupuncture will be observing the imbalance or incongruency – the lack of resonance between the content of the mind, the verbal and non-verbal expressions and the sound in the voice. It is less easy to hear an imbalance in the voice tone when a person is comfortable and chatting. The practitioner is much more likely to notice incongruous sounds in the voice when the patient is talking about something that carries emotional charge.

Training to recognise the least appropriate sound

There are three important stages to recognising the inappropriate voice tone.

The first stage to remember is that the practitioner is aiming to identify the Element that is most out of balance. If the sound that resonates with Wood is the least appropriate voice tone, then this is evidence for the Wood Element being the CF.

The second stage is to learn to identify the sounds normally associated with anger, joy, sympathy, grief and fear and to be able to sort them out from other sounds and characteristics of the voice. When learning Five Element Constitutional Acupuncture people start with different talents. Some can only make some rough distinctions at first while others immediately have a much more conscious appreciation of the different voice tones and can imitate and recognise them with ease. It is useful for beginners to practise, perhaps using the exercises suggested above.

The third stage is to monitor three things simultaneously:

- the contents of the person's mind, for example, are they thinking about or talking about something that would make most people angry?
- the non-verbal expression of the emotion, such as the person's posture, gestures and facial expression
- the sound in the voice

While monitoring these three areas, the practitioner needs to pick out which sound is most out of balance. This may sound easy, but it is a bit like patting the head, drawing circles on the stomach and making circles with the elbows, all at the same time. It requires practice to do each part separately before they can be successfully combined.

Emotion

Background

The emotions associated with each Element are:

- Wood – anger
- Fire – joy
- Earth – sympathy
- Metal – grief
- Water – fear

When people are in good health the five emotions are expressed appropriately. For example, people laugh at a joke or shout when they are angry. When their *qi* is imbalanced they feel and show emotions inappropriately. For example, they may show joy even when discussing something painful, or experience no fear in a situation that is dangerous. People may have a lack of or an excess of an emotion when their *qi* is imbalanced and some patients may swing between the two, especially if it is the emotion connected to their CF.

The practitioner assesses which emotions are being expressed inappropriately. These are sometimes assessed simply by observation and sometimes by interacting with the patient and observing the patient's response. It is often difficult to draw a distinct line and say that a certain response is definitely inappropriate. For example, how long is it appropriate to be devastated by the death of one's child?

Sometimes it is easy to diagnose an emotional imbalance. A person may exhibit a particular emotion that jars and which makes the practitioner think, 'that is strange!' Sometimes it is the intensity of an emotion that is striking. It may be understandable that somebody is angry with the person that made her or him redundant, but surely not *that* cross, not *that* bitter.

Sometimes what is striking about a particular patient is that whatever situation arises and whichever emotions could be regarded as appropriate, one emotion always seems to predominate. The practitioner understands, for example, that a patient might be cross with her parents for various events that have happened. The patient might also be angry with her first boyfriend for leaving her and with her husband for how he is with the children, etc., etc. What is most noticeable is that whatever event occurs, anger is the predominant emotional response.

The importance of the emotion

Of the four key diagnostic criteria used by Five Element Constitutional Acupuncturists, emotion is the most complex and any judgements about normality or appropriateness can have important moral and cultural implications. At the same time the inappropriate emotion provides one of the most accurate keys to a patient's CF. By observing a patient's least fluent emotion, practitioners can also increase their understanding of how this same emotional pattern appears in many other aspects of a patient's life.

Emotional language

What is meant by an emotion?

The English language distinguishes at least three descriptions of different types of emotions. These are an 'incident', a 'mood' and the 'feeling capacity of a temperament'.

An *incident* creates a one-off emotion. For example, a person becomes very angry when insulted.

In contrast, a *mood* goes on for some time. For example, a patient may say they have been depressed on and off for several weeks. The statement about mood does not mean that the person has been having the emotion continuously. It suggests that the feeling comes and goes or surfaces from the background and becomes more foreground.

In further contrast, a *temperament* may predispose someone to incidents of emotion that are typical of that temperament. For example a person may describe her or himself by saying 'I am a fairly happy person. I generally feel happy and always have been' or 'I tend to be an anxious person. I get frightened over the smallest things.' A temperament is like a mood but one that is more entrenched in the person's character.

The Element–emotion association is one of temperament. A person who has a particular CF is prone to experiencing certain emotions because the *qi* of that Element is constitutionally weaker. When the *qi* of an Element is healthy this permits the emotions associated with that Element to be expressed in a balanced way. When the *qi* of an Element is out of balance it means that the emotions resonating with that Element become less resourceful.

Because the CF is constitutional, people's personalities, at least in part, develop around the imbalanced emotion. A Fire CF, for example, will have less resourceful emotions around joy, a Water CF around fear, and so on. Thus assessing emotions is really observing the *qi* of an Element.

Assessing a patient's emotions

The patient's most inappropriate emotion can be assessed in two ways. Sometimes it is possible for the practitioner to observe it by just watching the patient. At other times it is less obvious and the practitioner must 'test' the patient's emotion.

Observing emotions

When people's most inappropriate emotion is on the surface it can easily be observed. For example, when people seem frightened about almost everything, they may be judged to have excessive fear that might, therefore, be used to support a diagnosis of Water.

Emotional expression is conveyed by observing different aspects of a person, for example, eyes, facial expression generally, the words a person uses, the tone of voice, the body posture and specific gestures. Sometimes the label for a person's emotion may be obvious. At other times, it is less clear and different

observers may disagree about what they observe. (See Ekman, 2007, Chapter 1, for the scientific case that the emotional expression of the face exists across cultures.)

The difference between observing and testing emotions

Often patients will exhibit some of their emotions to the practitioner and there is no need to deliberately 'test' them. When practitioners just observe, however, they may not get information about all of the Elements. People are often happy to reveal some emotions, but not others. Also, a patient who is shy and withdrawn may avoid being expressive. The practitioner may have no idea that a particular emotion is so inappropriate or intense unless she or he evokes it. Emotion testing attempts to overcome these problems.

Emotion testing

In contrast to observing a patient, a practitioner may 'test' a patient's emotional response. 'Emotion testing' involves the practitioner consciously attempting to evoke emotions in the patient (see Box 25.6). The practitioner then observes the response. Does the patient respond at all? Does she or he respond more

---

> ### Box 25.6
>
> #### Emotion testing – the theatre stage in the patient's mind
>
> The patient's mind being like a theatre stage is a metaphor that can be used to explain the process of testing an emotion. The practitioner is a theatre director whose job it is to create the right dramatic moment – using props, other actors, etc. – on the stage of the patient's mind. 'The right moment' means the moment that would naturally produce the emotion the practitioner is attempting to induce. For instance, a patient mentions a loss of a pet. The practitioner asks what the patient especially liked about the pet. In order to answer, the patient remembers moments of pleasure with the pet. The stage is now set to gently remind the person of the loss and to invite a feeling of grief. The practitioner's non-verbal expression of grief – through facial expression, body posture and tone of voice – is a key part of the 'props' on the stage of the patient's mind. How the patient responds will be an outward show of the flow of the *qi* of the Metal Element.

intensely than seems appropriate to the context? Does the voice, facial expression or body language change, and does this change indicate disharmony in the patient's *qi*? The practitioner assesses whether the emotions resonant with each Element are in balance or out of balance.[2]

At the crucial moment of testing the emotion, practitioners must be able to access the emotion inside themselves. No patient will respond to sympathy, joy, grief or any of the emotions if the practitioner is not authentic in its expression. Saying sympathetic words to someone will not touch them if it does not come from the heart. This is why practitioners must be able to access each of the emotions in themselves and why this is one of the most important goals in the inner development of the practitioner of Five Element Constitutional Acupuncture.

The limitations of the practitioner in the skill of emotion testing form one of the greatest obstacles to becoming an excellent diagnostician. It is the cause of many mistaken diagnoses. The practitioner tries to induce an emotion in a patient but because the feeling was not truly present, the patient does not respond as they would if the feeling had been authentic. In the example of testing grief given in Box 25.6, the patient will respond totally differently to two different practitioners. An acupuncturist who has good rapport and genuinely accesses grief about the death of the pet, will receive a different response from another practitioner who really thought grieving about a pet a bit pathetic. The ability to test grief, and all the other emotions, effectively depends upon such differences.

Emotion testing during the practitioner– patient interaction

Emotion testing is like talking with a friend and from the outside it should be indistinguishable. The patient will be unaware that the practitioner is doing anything other than taking a case history and making rapport. An emotion test that is overt or is obvious to an observer has not been skilfully carried out.

Conversing with a friend does not require a high level of concentration. Emotion testing, however,

does require focused awareness and while carrying out a test practitioners also need to:

- monitor what is happening – one part of the practitioner's attention is acting as an observer and is monitoring what information has been collected so far and what to do next
- pay attention to the more subtle non-verbal changes in the patient
- use all of their knowledge of the Element and people in general to make an assessment of the appropriateness of the emotional response

The use of the expression 'emotion testing'

The phrase 'emotion testing' is not an ideal one, particularly because the word 'test' is used in conjunction with emotions. It does, however, accurately describe what practitioners do. The 'test' evokes an emotional response resonant with an Element. The emotion is a movement of *qi* and this gives the practitioner a chance to observe the movement of *qi* resonant with a particular Element. There is no better way of prompting an Element to reveal its nature to the practitioner.

Emotions and culture

It is important for practitioners to be aware of the range of emotional responses of people from different cultures. (See Kaptchuk, 2000, footnote 16 on pp. 168–169, for a discussion about how people in one culture speak differently about their emotions from those in another culture.) It is much easier to have a sense of the appropriateness of emotional response if the patient is from a similar culture to the practitioner. It would be very hard, for example, for a practitioner born and brought up in the Midwest of the USA to have a great understanding of the emotional responses of an Australian Aborigine. Even among people from the same country there can be significant differences in emotional expression dependent upon age, gender, ethnic background, social class, subculture, etc. For example, grieving processes vary in different cultures. Different cultures tolerate very different levels of aggression amongst members. Men tend to accept sympathy from male practitioners less readily than from female practitioners. The practitioner must have a broad vision of these factors and make appropriate allowances.

---

[2]There are stories in the classics of practitioners evoking emotions for therapeutic, rather than diagnostic, reasons. For example, in Larre and Rochat de la Vallée (1996, p. 68), Rochat discusses the tragic story of Hua Tuo in the third century. Hua Tuo made a prince angry in order to move the *qi* to clear a blood clot. The treatment was successful, but during the angry state the prince killed Hua Tuo. The treatment was successful, but the doctor died.

The stages of emotion testing

Why stages are useful

In order to learn the process of emotion testing it is useful to break it down into stages. This enables the practitioner to understand the order of the different parts of the test, which activities need to be carried out at different times and the purpose of these different activities.

Having stages to this process might suggest a mechanical and laborious process, but this is far from the truth. In fact the 'stages' help practitioners who are learning how to test emotions and also enable more experienced practitioners to improve what they are already doing.

Emotion tests can take minutes, but equally they can occur in seconds, simply because the mind can recognise patterns in an instant and respond in a second. Testing an emotion can be compared to the process of telling a joke. Joke-telling also occurs in stages, like getting people's attention, introducing the characters, right down to the punch-line. Yet a witty remark can be delivered in a second.

The stages of emotion testing

The stages of emotion testing are:

- rapport
- creating or recognising opportunities to test
- choosing the emotion
- setting up the test
- delivering the test
- evaluating the response
- notating the response

Rapport

A good level of rapport is essential when testing emotions. The degree to which a patient will reveal her or himself to the practitioner is in direct proportion to the level of rapport achieved. Patients are being asked to respond genuinely from the inside and to do this it is essential that they trust the practitioner. Without this trust patients will not normally show themselves, especially any of their painful emotions.

Creating or recognising opportunities to test

Sometimes opportunities present themselves. At other times practitioners need to generate them. For example, in order to determine if a patient has reasonably balanced anger, it is useful to be discussing some event where the patient was frustrated. Frustration tests the ability of a person's Wood Element to make new plans when previous ones have been thwarted. For each emotion, there are some events that can easily lead to a 'test' situation. These are referred to in Tables 25.2–25.8, listing the testing process for each Element under the heading 'Opportunity'.

At first, students think that opportunities to test occur only rarely and are difficult to create. With experience and by establishing a deep level of rapport with patients, they realise that more opportunities arise than they thought. They also realise that an opportunity to test grief may also be an opportunity to test sympathy, anger or another emotion. They can use the same event and simply nudge it in one direction or another, in order to elicit the emotion they feel they need to understand more. Once students understand what constitutes an opportunity, they can begin to create them (see Box 25.7).

Choosing the emotion

Practitioners are frequently presented with a situation in which more than one emotion could be tested. For example, a complaint by the patient may generate a choice of testing either anger or sympathy. After this has become apparent, there is a moment when the practitioner has to make a choice. The practitioner will then need to decide if all of the criteria for the test are in place. These are referred to in Tables 25.2–25.8 under the heading 'Criteria for a workable test'.

Setting up the test

Once the practitioner has chosen an emotion, she or he needs to ensure that certain factors are present so that the patient can naturally experience the emotion. These are referred to in Tables 25.2–25.8 under the heading 'When to test'.

Delivering the test

This is the verbal or non-verbal 'request' to experience the emotion, to get angry, feel respected, etc. In order to understand another person's emotions

Table 25.2 A testing process for Wood and anger

Opportunity	Practitioners can test anger if patients raise an issue where they have been 'abused' in some way. They may have been frustrated, or feel themselves to have been treated badly by someone else or by some organisation. This does not need to be anything extreme.
Criteria for a workable test	1. There is an abuse. 2. The abuse must be recent or ongoing. 3. There must be someone who committed the abuse – a person is best, an organisation is not so good, God or nature cannot be used. 4. There is some 'wrongness' to the abuse. This may be to do with things such as social norms, fairness or an agreement. For example, someone reneged on a promise.
When to test	When the person is talking about the abuse, but is not manifesting much anger about it. The practitioner may notice some signs of minor discomfort but no overt anger or annoyance. If the person is already angry, do not test the anger – observe only.
How to test	Having listened to the patient talking about the abuse, the practitioner expresses a feeling of anger on the patient's behalf by making a statement such as 'You must have been angry at X.' The words are accompanied by the practitioner's non-verbal expression of an appropriate level of annoyance.
Emotion	Practitioners should express their own feelings with an appropriate amount of anger through emphasis in the voice and facial tightening.
Evaluation	A patient with a reasonably balanced Wood Element will show some anger. This may be evidenced by a shift in posture or a more clipped tone of voice. The expression of the emotion will be appropriate in intensity and smooth in flow. A person who has a chronically imbalanced Wood Element will often deny the anger – possibly by changing the information or by saying that there's no point in doing anything about the 'abuse'. Alternatively the expression of anger will be more than expected or it may be jerky and/or held in and it will not flow smoothly.

Table 25.3 A testing process for Fire and joy

Opportunity	Practitioners can give patients a compliment or personal warmth when they arrive. Alternatively the practitioner can test joy when patients are remembering recent events normally associated with pleasure and joy or are anticipating joyful events in the future.
Criteria for a workable test	The patient is emotionally available, not taken up with other feelings.
When to test	At almost any time that the patient is not already experiencing joy or pleasure. It is important to take the person from a relatively neutral state.
How to test	The practitioner expresses congruent and sincere warmth and admiration for the patient, for example, by saying, 'You look well today' or 'That's a lovely jumper.' Alternatively the practitioner may ask the patient about something pleasurable she or he has done recently or may do in the future. The practitioner may encourage this with appropriate joy and by saying for example, 'Mmmm, that sounds great!' Once the warmth has been given, the practitioner's expression of the emotion must stop and the practitioner then observes the patient's response.
Emotion	When practitioners share in the joy, they are feeling joy themselves and show this through their facial expression, posture and gestures.
Evaluation	With a healthy Fire Element, the patient can 'hold' the feeling of joy when the practitioner stops expressing it. The joy can rise and fall away again smoothly. If the Fire Element is chronically imbalanced the joy will drop suddenly (and not smoothly). Alternatively it may rise up into excessive joyfulness that doesn't drop away. If the patient fails to become joyful this is also a sign of an imbalanced Fire Element.

Table 25.4 A testing process for Earth and sympathy

Opportunity	Practitioners can test sympathy if the patient has run into difficulties, encountered frustrations or is having a difficult time. This can be when a patient is describing her or his main or secondary complaint.
Criteria for a workable test	1. The patient should have a complaint that is recent or ongoing. 2. It should be something the patient cannot easily change or, at least, the patient should be clear that if they do anything about the problem, it will create even more problems. 3. In order to be authentic, the practitioner must accept that the complaint is in some sense justified.
When to test	Whenever a complaint or difficulty is being discussed.
How to test	The patient tells the practitioner of the problem or complaint and the practitioner then gives the patient some support or understanding by making a statement like, 'Oh, I am sorry to hear that. That must have been very difficult.'
Emotion	The sympathy must be appropriate and empathetic, not babyish or patronising.
Evaluation	When the patient accepts the practitioner's sympathy, it may evoke a feeling of acknowledgement and being supported. A patient with a healthy Earth Element will take in and accept the sympathy but will not dwell on it or keep asking for more. If the Earth Element is imbalanced the patient may not seem to have really taken in or digested the understanding and may take it in and ask for more sympathy. Alternatively the patient may simply reject the sympathy/understanding and may even change the information the practitioner has given by saying, for example, that the problem isn't really so bad.

Table 25.5 A testing process for Metal and grief

Opportunity	Practitioners can test grief if the patient has recently lost something. This may be physical (a possession), emotional (a person) or mental (an ambition or belief). Alternatively the practitioner can use phrases which direct the patient's mind back in time. For example, 'When you look back over. . .', or 'When you think about how things used to be . . . .'
Criteria for a workable test	The practitioner takes the patient back to remembering the good aspects of what they once had before the loss. The practitioner gets the patient to re-experience the previous good feelings and why what was lost was important.
When to test	When the patient is remembering how good it was to have whatever is now lost.
How to test	The practitioner 'asks' the patient to feel the loss using a statement like 'It is sad that you don't have that any more.' At the same time the practitioner's non-verbal expression – face, touch, tone, words and gestures – must be congruently coming from an inner state of loss. This 'test' puts the 'previous satisfaction' and 'the awareness that it is gone' side by side in the stage of the patient's mind.
Emotion	It is important that the practitioner accesses grief internally, and, for example, is not obviously sympathetic.
Evaluation	If the Metal Element is healthy the patient will move into an appropriate intensity of grief and come out again. If the Metal Element is out of balance the patient is likely to choke or tighten in the chest/throat area to stop the feeling. Alternatively, although rarely, the patient may sometimes become temporarily overwhelmed by the intensity of the feeling.

Table 25.6 A testing process for Metal and respect

Opportunity	Practitioners can check out the patient's ability to receive respect by asking them about a time when they had a struggle. This could be anything from adolescence, a divorce, financial problems, etc. The practitioner can then label a genuine positive inner quality, such as generosity, compassion or perseverance, that the patient has demonstrated, that enabled her or him to get through this situation.
Criteria for a workable test	The positive inner quality can be supported by what the patient has said. Ideally, the patient is not aware she or he has this quality.
When to test	Just after the moment the patient has described the difficulty.
How to test	The practitioner listens carefully to the person's description of a struggle and formulates the patient's positive inner quality. She or he then attributes the inner quality to the patient, for example, 'It sounds as if, especially in those circumstances, you displayed great generosity of spirit'. If the patient appears not to take this in, or indeed they deny having this quality, the practitioner can attract the patient's attention again (possibly by touching) and repeat back to the patient the factual things they said that support them having the positive inner quality.
Evaluation	If a patient has a healthy Metal Element, she or he can take the compliment in and feel pleasure in it. If the Metal Element is out of balance the patient may love receiving the compliment but may deny having the positive inner quality. They may change the information to diminish the quality or clench up or hold themselves tightly in the chest or throat area.

Although respect is not in itself an emotion, giving respect can elicit unresolved grief (see Chapters 17 and 19, this volume).

Table 25.7 A testing process for Water and fear

Opportunity	Practitioners can test fear when a patient describes a situation that would normally induce a degree of concern or fear for his or her welfare but she or he is demonstrating no fear at all.
Criteria for a workable test	1. The practitioner has detected a possible *threat* or area that is of concern to the patient. 2. The patient thinks that there may be undesirable consequences that might occur as a result of the threat. 3. The patient believes that she or he has no control or limited control over whether the undesirable consequences occur or not.
When to test	When the patient is discussing the threat, but showing very little indication of fear in their facial expression, voice tone or posture or gestures.
How to test	The practitioner listens to the patient's account of the threat and then expresses some concern or fear. For example by saying, 'Goodness, you must be nervous/frightened that X will occur.' The practitioner may show most of the concern non-verbally.
Emotion	The practitioner's internal state should be that of concern/fear. Her or his non-verbal expression of fear is very important: for example, there may be a slight pulling back of the upper body and a ponderous nodding of the head.
Evaluation	A normal response is for the patient to express some fear. An abnormal response is to express no fear. A common abnormal response is for the practitioner to see a flash of intense fear in the patient's eyes that quickly disappears.

Table 25.8 A testing process for Water and reassurance

Opportunity	Practitioners can check out the patient's ability to receive reassurance when she or he has some concerns about the future or is afraid.
Criteria for a workable test	The practitioner needs to know: 1. The *threat*. 2. What undesirable consequences the patient expects to happen as a result of the threat. 3. Some genuine *information* about the likelihood of these undesirable consequences really occurring or not occurring. This information can arise from many different sources such as medical tests, rumours, the fact the doctor *didn't* say anything, old wives' tales, superstition, articles in journals/magazines, what someone in the health food shop said, etc.
When to test	When the patient has expressed what appears to be fear.
How to test	It is important that the practitioner listens to and then acknowledges the patient's fear and does not belittle it. She or he then lists each 'reason' why the threat will *not* occur and lets the patient know about any other reassuring information.
Emotion	The reassurance should be given to the patient in a calm, thoughtful way. Frequently the opportunity to reassure is lost because the practitioner goes straight to, 'Oh don't worry, I'm sure it will be all right', which seriously mismatches how the patient is feeling.
Evaluation	If patients have a healthy Water Element they show signs that they can hear and take in what was said and feel reassured. A patient with an imbalanced Water Element may show signs that they are unwilling to take the information in, for example, by turning away, shaking the head or speaking over what is being said. Or the patient may appear to take the information in, seem reassured, but return with another similar fear.

Box 25.7

Creating opportunities for testing

The following are some examples of how opportunities may be created by practitioners.

- When a patient comes in describing an experience they've had recently, such as a car accident, the practitioner can test a number of different emotions. For example, sympathy for the person's bad luck, anger at another careless driver, fear that it could happen again. This requires some questioning on the part of the practitioner to elicit which aspect of the event that it is appropriate to test.
- Practitioners can refer to another person's experience, for example, 'I saw someone yesterday who always seems to be having bad luck (losing things, being threatened, generally having a hard time, etc.). Have you ever had a phase like that?'
- Another alternative is for the practitioner to rely on some people's natural inclination to deny that things are good. For example, if the practitioner asks, slightly in jest, whether they have been having a perfect, totally blissful time, many people will deny this. It is then easy to elicit a few complaints that can lead to 'tests' for sympathy or anger.

it is important for practitioners to understand their own emotions and be able to access them. The delivery of the test requires that the practitioner carrying out the test expresses genuine and congruent emotion. The delivery must be short and then stop. Examples of how such requests might be made are given in Tables 25.2–25.8 under the heading 'How to test'.

Evaluating the response

Practitioners are evaluating the patient's response (especially non-verbal) in the first few seconds after the 'request'. Hence alertness and concentration are essential. Making the judgement accurately requires a level of experience and wisdom about how people respond in different situations.

In order to have a balanced viewpoint it is also necessary for practitioners to be aware of their own emotions and which situations evoke intense or inappropriate emotions in themselves. This will allow them to judge whether the patient's response is 'normal', 'inappropriate' or, as is sometimes the case, hiding another emotion which is close to the surface, but not easy to observe.

The aspects to observe during an emotion test are the fluency and the intensity of the change evoked when the emotion is felt. Examples of how these observations are made are in Tables 25.2–25.8 under the heading 'Evaluation'.

Notating the response

As testing is carried out several times, it is important that the practitioner has a quick way to notate the type of test and the judgement about the patient's response. Stopping at that moment to write for thirty seconds will appear odd to the patient and rapport can be lost.

One way to notate the emotion tests is for the practitioner to use abbreviations for the emotions, for example, 'J' for joy. If the patient seemed unable to express anger about a noisy neighbour, even when it was obviously appropriate, then the practitioner might record 'A → no A'. Ideally the practitioner will add a few words which remind the practitioner of the incident, for instance, writing 'noisy neighbour' might be a sufficient reminder.

The overall judgement about a test can be complex. The practitioner is looking for which of the patient's responses to the emotion tests are the *least* fluent and most disturbed. Most patients have one emotion that is markedly more imbalanced than the others. In others several emotions are inappropriately intense or frequently expressed and it can be hard to decide which one indicates the CF. These judgements require the practitioner to review several of the patient's responses and compare them to what is a normal response. The practitioner also needs to compare the 'lack of fluency' from one Element to another. Good recording helps to develop the practitioner's ability to make this judgement. These judgements are usually made intuitively and in milliseconds, so when the practitioner is learning, it is useful to carry out the process consciously and slowly.

The testing process for each Element

Tables 25.2–25.8 outline the basic processes for testing emotions. After a period of practice and experience and as the process becomes more automatic and unconscious, the practitioner will no longer need to follow this routine, but to begin with this outline may be useful.

Summary

1 Colour, sound, emotion and odour are the four key methods of diagnosis used in Five Element Constitutional Acupuncture. If the practitioner finds at least three of these key areas pointing to an imbalance in an Element, then this is a strong pointer to the patient's CF.

2 The emotion is the most important of these four key areas and the practitioner needs to take special care to assess the balance of patients' emotions. The emotions are the internal causes of disease and the ability to detect the emotions that produce or inhibit movements of *qi* is crucial.

3 The practitioner may need to deliberately evoke a person's emotions in order to gain a full understanding of how they are balanced within a person.

The body language of the different CFs

26

Introduction

Emotion testing, as described in the previous chapter, involves the practitioner interacting with the patient to evoke an emotional response. Much assessment of the patient, however, is done by simple observation. This observation is important and involves three areas:

- facial expression
- posture
- gestures

People in China, Japan and other East Asian countries are especially known for the skill of keeping 'face' and showing little in public of what is really going on inside them. Everyone does this to some degree, however, and most people literally have a 'public face' they tend to show the world as well as a 'private face'. The remnants of people's true emotional state can still be detected on the face, however, as these chronic emotional patterns become etched into people's facial lines and reflected in the chronic holding of their facial muscles.

An example of this is someone who experiences significant degrees of frustration over a period of time. They can appear to have their eyebrows drawn together and develop what are called 'Liver lines'. Liver lines are vertical lines on the forehead that have developed from holding an 'angry' face for long periods of time.

> If we could read it, every human being carries his life in his face ... On our features the fine chisels of thought and emotion are eternally at work.
>
> (Alexander Smith, quoted in Auden and Kronenberger, 1962)

Sometimes, and especially if patients are trying to hide their emotions, the facial expression may appear on the face as a 'micro' emotion for only about a fifth of a second or less (see Eckman, 2007, p. 220). Micro-emotions can also occur when the emotion is being inhibited and is outside the person's consciousness. It is important for Five Element Constitutional Acupuncturists to learn to spot them on patients before they settle back to showing their 'public face'.

Posture can also provide the practitioner with insights into the state of a person's body, mind and spirit. Whilst people may try to hide their facial expression, their posture and gestures are harder to disguise and tend to indicate what is going on below the surface. Over time patients also develop chronic physical holding patterns. For example, a Fire CF may have an underdeveloped chest or an Earth CF may slump in the area of the middle *jiao*.

It is important for practitioners to learn to recognise these postures and gestures and the fleeting or more long lasting facial expressions. They may be key methods of discovering people's primary emotional imbalance and their CF.

The following descriptions of these indications are arranged Element by Element and by the facial expression, posture and gestures within each Element.

The Wood Element: facial expression, posture and gestures

Facial expression

An angry facial expression is shown in Figure 26.1 below. Frequent feelings of frustration and anger may become etched in the lines between the eyebrows, the look in the eyes or the set of the mouth and jaw. The brows, eyes and jaw are all especially involved in the facial expression of anger.

- The brows are drawn together and lowered, creating two vertical lines between the eyes. As was stated above, a person who is habitually angry may have these 'Liver lines' deeply engraved onto the forehead.

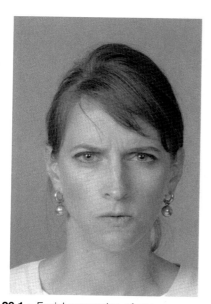

Figure 26.1 • Facial expression of anger

Table 26.1 Facial expression, posture and gestures – anger

Face	Brows	Lowered and drawn together, vertical lines appear between the brows
	Lids	Lower lid tense, may or may not be raised. Upper lid tense, may be lowered by brow
	Eyes	Hard stare
	Lips	Pressed together firmly
	Jaw	Tense, may jut out
Posture		Body may be erect, muscles tighten. May be a slight move forward
Gestures		Emphasised. Can be jerky. May point or make a fist
Breathing		Loud, rapid, shallow, irregular

- The area around the eyes may be affected. The lower lid will be tense, causing the area under the eye to rise upwards. At the same time the upper lid moves down following the movement of the brows. This pushes against the upper part of the eyes, causing them to narrow. As a result of these movements the eyes look intense: fixed, hard and staring. Holding this expression may result in a tight aching feeling behind or around the eyes. Anger is the only emotion where the lower eyelid tenses.
- The jaw and mouth may take on a number of positions. People who are angry may purse their lips or pull in their lips and hold them firmly together. This 'tight-lipped' expression usually indicates that a person wants to hold back their expression of anger. It is as if by keeping their mouths firmly closed they don't let out what they really want to say. It is interesting to note that the deep pathway of the Liver circles the mouth on the inside of the lips in the orbicularis oris muscle. This is the muscle that pulls in the mouth.

Suppressed anger may also cause a person's jaw to become tense and people who are habitually angry will often be locked or tight in this area. People who grind their teeth at night usually do so because their jaw is tense. Their tense jaw becomes even tighter while they sleep. Sometimes tension in the jaw causes it to jut out and be held slightly upwards. This gives the person an appearance of slight defiance.

Although the colour on the face of a Wood CF is green, people who are angry may also redden as they feel the heat of their anger and frustration welling up inside. (For more on the facial expression of anger, see Ekman and Friesen, 2003, p. 78.)

Posture

The posture of someone who is angry is likely to be erect. The *qi* rises and people can appear to expand in size. In addition, there is often a very slight movement forward. Although not necessarily overtly attacking, there is an underlying sense of aggression and pushing forwards towards the other person.

When a person has been chronically angry for long periods of time, the ligaments and tendons often lose elasticity and become tight. An extreme example is a soldier on parade, standing stiffly to attention, expanding his chest, thrusting his face forward and giving a jerky salute. As well as the jaw, which was discussed above, the neck, shoulders, hips and lower back can also be tense and possibly the musculature of the whole body. A practitioner may notice that when holding the patient's arm to take pulses that the arm is left somewhat stuck in space when released. It remains tense and does not easily move back to its previous position. Tight ligaments in the feet may cause the toes to pull up and back.

Often a Wood CF's body may appear 'packed' and solid and tightly held together or squashed down as if not allowed to push upwards and to grow to its full size. The packed quality is the opposite of the expansion described above and will develop when anger has been suppressed.

Gestures

The gestures of someone who has long-term problems with anger tend to be aggressive and jerky. The person may point aggressively at people, make a fist or gesture with their hands in an abrupt and jerky manner.

Breathing

Anger will immediately change a person's breathing. It may become louder, more rapid and more irregular as well as shallower. Anger can cause a person to have

difficulty breathing in and out smoothly. As a result, Wood CFs often sigh a lot, the sigh being a way of releasing the tension felt in the chest.

The Fire Element: facial expression, posture and gestures

Facial expression

Typically the facial expression of a Fire CF either lights up with joy and happiness or drops into sadness and misery. For example, joy may reveal itself in subtle ways, such as the lines at the sides of the eyes or sadness by the set of the mouth. The most significant expressions are the changing from joy to sadness, excessive joyfulness or an absence of joy.

Joy

When a person smiles with joy the whole face moves upwards (see Figure 26.2). This causes the naso-labial folds to deepen, the cheeks to rise up and the lower eyelids to wrinkle and rise. 'Crows feet' then appear at the side of the eyes. A person with a truly joyous expression will have a sparkle in the eyes as the joy wells up (Ekman, 2007, pp. 190–212).

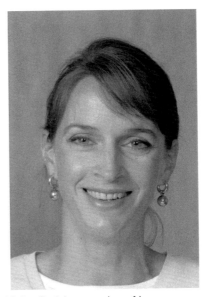

Figure 26.2 • Facial expression of joy

Table 26.2 Facial expression, posture and gestures – joy

Face	Mouth	Corners drawn back and up. Lips may or may not be parted
	Naso-labial fold	Deepens
	Cheeks	Raised
	Lower eyelids	Wrinkled and raised. Not tense
	Eyes	Crows feet at corners. Eyes sparkle. Orbicularis oris muscle around eye is activated
Posture		Upwards and expansive
Gestures		Tend to be upward movements

Table 26.3 Facial expression, posture and gestures – sadness

Face	Brows	Inner corners drawn up and sometimes in
	Lids	Upper corner of eyelid is raised
	Lips	Corners of the lips are down
	Cheeks	Raised as if squinting
	Eyes	Tend to look down
Posture		Slumped, chest caved in
Gestures		May be a withdrawal of movement

Sadness

The facial expression of sadness usually shows itself in three main areas in the face (see Figure 26.3). Firstly, the mouth is dropped open and the corners of the lips are turned down. Secondly, while holding the lips down the cheeks are raised as if squinting. Thirdly, the inner corners of the brows are raised up and are at the same time drawn together. They may also be pulled together in the middle. In general the eyes also tend to look downwards. Some Fire CFs can have a smile on their faces but a sad look in their eyes at the same time (Ekman, 2003, pp. 82–109).

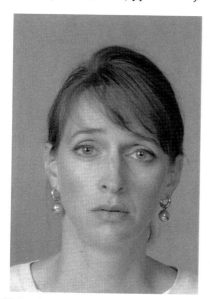

Figure 26.3 • Facial expression of sadness

It is interesting to note that when people are truly smiling they activate the orbicularis oculi muscle that circles the eye. This muscle can only be activated voluntarily by 10% of the population. The rest of the population can only activate it when they are smiling and expressing joy. It has been said that this muscle 'unmasks the false friend'. A person who is pretending to laugh at their friend's jokes or who is not truly expressing joy will not be using this muscle.

Many Fire CFs have volatile faces that can easily move between joy and sadness. Some Fire CFs' faces look rather serious until they smile. When they do smile, however, their face often lights up and becomes radiant. It is as though they come alive. This transformation can be an excellent diagnostic indication.

Posture

Bearing in mind that the main *yin* Organs associated with the Fire Element are the Heart and Heart-Protector, it is not surprising that the chest area is affected in many Fire CFs. Sometimes there is a lack of physical development in this area. The chest may look weak and underdeveloped or sometimes it may be a more concave shape.

In order to protect this vulnerable area, many Fire CFs habitually fold their arms across their chest. Sometimes there is habitual tension in the upper body. This has formed as the person has endeavoured to defend the chest area. It is a bit like a door with iron bars across it to prevent burglars from entering. The problem, however, is that the barricaded door also keeps the person inside from getting out.

Gestures

Joy is *yang* in nature and the gestures of someone who is happy reflect this by tending to be expansive, quick moving and upwards in direction. In *Su Wen* Chapter 39, it is said that joy makes the *qi* 'loose'.

On the other hand, the nature of sadness is more *yin*, and a person who is feeling miserable is likely to be more withdrawn with slower movements or, if extremely sad, very little movement at all.

The Earth Element: facial expression, posture and gestures

Facial expression

The typical facial expression of someone who is wanting or giving sympathy is shown in Figure 26.4. A practitioner watching Earth CFs going about their daily activities wouldn't necessarily notice a sympathetic expression on their faces.

Because Earth CFs often go into states where sympathy is an issue, some aspects of the expressions becomes etched into their facial features. For example, the look of sympathy may reveal itself in subtle ways such as a tilt of the head, the slight wrinkling of the forehead or the look in the eyes.

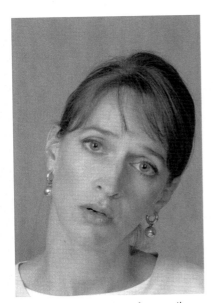

Figure 26.4 • Facial expression of sympathy

Table 26.4 Facial expression, posture and gestures – sympathy

Face	Eyes	Soften and open wider
	Brows	Raised. Small lines may appear on the forehead
	Cheeks	Loosen
	Mouth	May open, soften and relax
Posture		Head tilts to one side. Middle of torso may be collapsed
Gestures		May like to touch or be touched

This expression will be apparent for some, but not all of the time.

Typically the facial expression of a person giving or receiving sympathy is a soft caring look on the face (see Figure 26.4). The expression in the eyes has been compared to that of a 'puppy dog' and the cheeks and mouth may be open, soft and relaxed. There is also a distinctive tilt to the head when someone is being understanding and caring and the forehead may have a few small lines of concern on it.

The look on the Madonna's face that painters have usually attempted to portray is a good example of this quality. She is nearly always depicted as the embodiment of maternal love and empathy. The devotion paid to her by Catholics, as it is to Kuan Yin by the Chinese, is testament to people's need to feel loved and cared for by mother figures. Gentleness, tenderness, acceptance and forgiveness are regarded as the predominant qualities in such archetypes.

When people reject sympathy they may show their discomfort by pulling back in the neck, tightening in the abdomen and slightly tightening and pulling down the lower lip. The muscles of a person's face may appear to be impassive or may harden to brace against the sympathy. This can often be mistaken for anger. Beneath this hard exterior, however, can be a softness and need for support that is being covered

Table 26.5 Facial expression, posture and gestures – rejecting sympathy

Face	General	May appear impassive or may harden
	Lower lip	Slightly tightened and pulling down
	Eyes	Soft expression
Posture		Neck pulled back. Abdomen tightened

over. In this case the eyes may retain the soft expression described above, indicating that an underlying need for support is still there.

Body and posture

Although a practitioner can never classify the body shape, posture, gestures, etc., of each CF, it is still possible to notice certain physical tendencies that are characteristic of some Earth CFs.

Earth CFs can tend to be overweight. Their digestive system may be sluggish due to the weakness of the Stomach and Spleen. This makes it difficult for them to rot and ripen food and move fluid. This 'slow metabolism' causes the food and fluids to stagnate and in consequence weight problems arise.

Alternatively some Earth CFs may not be getting nourished physically, causing them to become thin and undernourished rather than overweight. The extreme of this could be severe anorexia but more often a person will just be slightly thin and bony. The legs may also be skinny and underdeveloped.

Some Earth CFs have a weakness in their middle abdomen. This can cause them to easily bloat in the abdomen or have a large belly. They can appear to collapse around the waist area and lose their waistline and take on an 'apple' shape.

The pear shape can also be characteristic of an Earth CF, especially when the Spleen doesn't move fluids. In this case their legs may be somewhat large and they have an excess of body fat collecting around the hips and thighs.

Sometimes an Earth CF may habitually place their hands over the abdomen for protection as this area may feel slightly weak and vulnerable.

Gestures and touch

Touch is important when people are giving or receiving sympathy. Earth CFs who enjoy receiving sympathy may also like to both touch other people and be touched by them. When children or adults are distressed, one of the most effective ways to care for them is to give them a hug or cuddle. Touch is evocative of early contact with the mother and for many people it is much more supportive than words. The quality of touch must be soft and caring in nature and express 'I understand'. When distressed people happily disengage from physical contact it is a sign that they have received sufficient support.

The Metal Element: facial expression, posture and gestures

Facial expression

The typical facial expression of someone who is grieving is shown in Figure 26.5. Grief may reveal itself in subtle ways such as the look in the eyes, the relaxation or tension in the facial muscles or the set of the mouth. This expression will be apparent for some, but not all of the time.

A person's eyes, cheeks and mouth are all involved in the expression of grief. When a person is grieving the

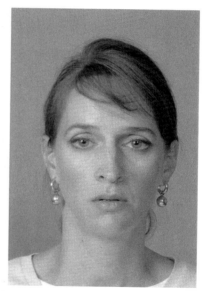

Figure 26.5 • Facial expression of grief

Table 26.6 Facial expression, posture and gestures – grief

Face	General	Downward movement of face
	Mouth	Corners turned down. May be slightly open
	Cheeks	Pulled down
	Lower lids	Loose
Posture		Chest caved in
Gestures		May be very little movement
Breathing		May be shallow

face tends to have a downward movement and appear slack. The lower lids will be loose and the cheeks will hang down. The mouth will also tend to be slightly turned down. Often when a person has been unable to express grief the sad facial expression is replaced by a dead or blank look. Others try to hide the feelings of grief behind a bright expression. If this is the case a degree of emptiness and loss usually remains in the eyes.

If feelings of grief are expressed rather than held in, then people's faces will crumple as they weep and let their feelings out. In some people this crumpled expression becomes chronic.

Posture and breathing

A Metal CF's chest area is often inert or tight. The area may have very little movement, giving the appearance of a 'shield' over the chest. This lack of vitality may have accumulated gradually from chronically tensing the chest to avoid strong feelings of sadness or loss. The chest is sometimes weak and underdeveloped and in extreme cases, can even be concave. This is because the underlying Lung *qi* is constitutionally weak.

The posture associated with the Metal type of chest is stooped. Sitting hunched over a desk compresses the Lung and the breathing. This habitual posture can both cause and be a consequence of weak Lung *qi*.

The breathing of a Metal CF may be shallow and weak. Some Metal CFs have difficulty breathing deeply unless they have consciously worked on strengthening their lungs by doing breathing exercises.

Gestures

Someone who is holding in grief tends not to make many gestures. Some people may hide away and silently grieve, in which case they may have very little movement at all.

The Water Element: facial expression, posture and gestures

Facial expression

The typical facial expression of someone who is feeling scared is shown in Figure 26.6. Water CFs often go into states where fear is an issue. The look of fear may reveal itself in subtle ways such as the lines on

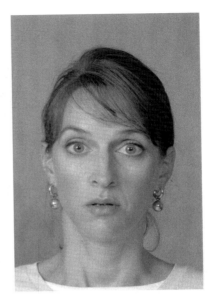

Figure 26.6 • Facial expression of fear

Table 26.7 Facial expression, posture and gestures – fear

Face	Brows	Raised and drawn together
	Forehead	Wrinkles at centre
	Upper lid	Raised, exposing the sclera
	Lower lid	Tense and drawn up
	Eyes	Fixed and pulled back or move from side to side
	Mouth	Open and lips slightly tensed or stretched and drawn back
Posture		Slight backward movement
Gestures		Tentative. May shake or may be very still
Breathing		May breathe high up or hold breath. May be shallow and rapid

the forehead, the look in the eyes or the set of the mouth. This expression is only apparent some of the time.

Fear can often be seen in the eyes. Because Water CFs may try to hide their fear, the expression in the eyes is often the most overt manifestation of the underlying fear. Fear usually creates agitation and often it is rapid movement of the eyes that indicates its presence. Eye contact is often avoided by looking downwards, with quick flashes upwards to maintain intermittent contact. This agitation is common to all sorts of animals when they feel threatened.

Some people attempt to still themselves when they are afraid. This is reflected in eyes that can appear fixed and as if they are pulled to the back of the head. Although there is little movement, they are in a state of high alertness. The eyes may also open wider and the upper eyelid rise up exposing the sclera. The area below the eye is then tensed and drawn up. As the eyes widen the eyebrows rise up and the brows knit together. This causes a horizontal wrinkle to appear in the forehead.

Fear can vary in intensity from slight apprehension to pure terror. The upper lid rises more and the tension in the lower lid increases according to the intensity of the fear. The lips also become more drawn back if the fear is intense.

It is important that the acupuncturist can recognise the facial expression of fear as this is often the most hidden of the emotions. Reading the face and body can be an important 'way in' so that the practitioner can understand the patient's emotional state.

When Water CFs strive to cover up their fear, the emotion may first have manifested fleetingly, only to be quickly modified into another expression. This interference can be minor. For example, Water CFs may change their expression a little so that it becomes an expression of slight worry. Alternatively it can be a major change. For example, fear may be covered up either by a deadpan expression or a laugh or aggression. No matter how covered up the fear is, a trace of the original expression usually remains, if only the practitioner can see it. Often the fear remains in the eyes. If the practitioner can see the fleeting original expression or the remains of the covered up fear, this can be an important means of corroborating the CF along with the other signs of colour, sound and odour.

Posture

A person who is afraid will have a tendency to move the whole torso backwards. This is usually a subtle shift rather than a large movement. The practitioner may notice that some people seem to be stuck in this stance and appear to be permanently shifting backwards as if to avoid an unseen threat or being 'hit' by something or someone.

The spine is the central pillar of the body and holds us erect. Some Water CFs appear to have a collapsed spine. It is interesting to note that the word 'spineless' is an expression used for a person who is overly fearful.

Of especial note on the spine is the lower back, which is the home of the Kidneys. This is often the weakest area of a Water CF's torso. Because of this weakness, many Water CFs may compensate by holding this area rigid and there may be tight musculature around it. It can also be weak and collapsed and patients may experience frequent aching in the lower back.

Gestures

A person who is afraid can sometimes shake and tremble with fear. This is something that they will usually try to cover up. Unfortunately, the more they try to forcibly stop the shaking the more tense they often become and this only exacerbates the problem. Alternatively a person may be rendered 'frozen' to the spot and they may have difficulty making many movements at all.

Breathing

When people are scared, the fear affects their breathing. For example, breathing may become shallow and rapid, as happens in a panic attack. Alternatively people may hold their breath or slow it down as they try to suppress their agitation.

Summary

1 Much assessment of the patient is done by simple observation.

2 Over time, frequent emotions become etched on the face. Emotions also create changes to a patient's posture and gestures.

3 Each Element has typical associated facial expressions, postures and gestures.

4 All patients are individuals and each expresses their CF in their own unique way, so the connections are not always consistent.

Diagnosis – levels and golden keys

27

CHAPTER CONTENTS

Introduction

This chapter covers two important methods of diagnosis. The first is based on the notion that a person functions on three levels: a physical level, a mental level and a spirit level. (We have described in Chapter 3 how Traditional Chinese Medicine spoke somewhat differently about levels. *Shen* encompasses both mind and spirit. In this chapter we will discuss the mind and spirit separately.)

The second method is called 'Golden Keys'. This involves noting particular aspects of a patient's behaviour that are so strikingly individual to that person that they are indicative of a profound level of imbalance in one of the Elements.

Diagnosing level – body, mind or spirit

The purpose of determining the level

Determining the correct level of treatment affects both the selection of points and the practitioner's intention (*yi*). Patients who are primarily imbalanced at the level of their 'spirit' may require practitioners to use points that predominantly affect this level. Points have many overlapping uses and can often affect more than one level, so this emphasis is a matter of degree. In many cases the *yuan*-source points and/or the Element points are sufficiently broad ranging to have the required effect. At other times, however, focusing on spirit points can be crucial. Point selection is discussed in Chapter 45 on treatment planning.

Clarifying the terms body, mind and spirit

Although the terms 'body', 'mind' and 'spirit' are not used in the common translations of Chinese medical texts, Chinese medicine has always been concerned with the patient's spirit. Indeed, much of acupuncture's appeal in the West has been because Chinese medicine pays attention to a patient's spirit as well their body.

It is desirable to classify which of a patient's symptoms stem from imbalance of which level. For example, a person with a sprained ankle has a physical problem. A person who is unable to think clearly or remember things has a mental problem. A person who is well qualified and wanting to get work when it is available, but who somehow cannot manage to get that work, probably has a spirit problem. In this case the body is not complaining, the mind seems to function well, but it might be said that the spirit is not willing.

Some classifications are less easy to make, however. For example, nightmares that arise from eating cheese late at night or skin problems apparently due to an allergy are more difficult to classify. J. R. Worsley partially explained this issue when he wrote:

> If the body is sick, the mind worries and the spirit grieves. If the mind is sick, the body and spirit will suffer from its confusion; if the spirit is sick, there will be no will to care for body or mind ... imbalances, and the illnesses arising from them, are always experienced at all levels.
>
> (Worsley, 1990, p. 185)

There are some circumstances when a patient is sick on one level only and the other levels are healthy. As the quote above explains, however, illness on one level will generally affect the others so all levels are usually affected to some degree. In spite of this, a practitioner still needs to decide on the level that is *primarily* out of balance. Treatment is then directed towards that level.

> However, we make a decision about the primary level of illness and that will determine our selection of points and the type of treatment required. We decide which of the three levels is in the most trouble and needs to be the focus of our help at this time.
>
> (Worsley, 1990, p. 186)

Although practitioners can be guided by their patient's signs and symptoms, they should not be misled by them. Whatever the patient presents, whether this is a sprained ankle or a reluctance to get out of bed in the morning, practitioners still need to make a decision about the 'primary level of illness'. The primary level is the one that will most improve the patient's functioning as a whole.

A patient's imbalance is not diagnosed by simply adding up the symptoms or other signs manifesting from the body, mind and spirit and arriving at a result. Although signs and symptoms matter and a practitioner should notice their balance, it is still important to remember that a disturbance on one level causes a subsequent disturbance on another.

So how *do* we decide?

Making the diagnosis of the level

In order to diagnose the level of a patient's imbalance, the practitioner needs to look deeper than the symptoms and observe how well a person's body, mind or spirit is working. The following sections are designed to help the practitioner to focus attention on these different levels.

The physical level

Because the body is frequently affected by dysfunction of the mind or spirit, it is essential to discover how a patient's physical problems arose. The more obvious the physical or environmental cause, the more likely it is that a symptom is a genuinely physical problem. A sports injury, sunstroke, being caught in a snow storm and suffering from cold, food poisoning, living in a damp area and having stiff joints are all predominantly physical problems because their origin appears to be physical. At the same time, however, a person may also have underlying deficiencies, which have resulted from problems at a deeper level and these must still be taken into account.

Practitioners can make a further check by discovering what affects the symptom, for example, whether further activity makes the injury worse, whether exposure to the sun is debilitating or whether wearing wet clothes after a rain storm makes the joints even stiffer. Physical symptoms can, however, also be radically affected by the state of the patient's mind or spirit. For example, a patient's pain in the neck may get worse when she or he is anxious or frustrated but the cause is still physical.

The mental level

People's ability to think is a reflection of their mental level. Practitioners can therefore evaluate the mental level by assessing a patient's mental clarity, memory and by noticing their ability to solve problems. For example, when people's minds are clear they can solve problems by:

- staying focused
- clearly defining what their goals are
- knowing what resources they already have and what they need to obtain
- drawing on the expertise of others who have already solved such a problem
- balancing costs (of all sorts) against benefits
- assessing whether the solutions are achievable
- considering the effect of each solution on the rest of their life
- making a good choice

While taking a case history the practitioner can observe how well the patient's mind has worked when dealing with past problems. It also provides opportunities to ask patients how they will deal with current situations.

Another common sign of a mental level problem is an unrealistic attitude to what causes events to occur. People have widely differing notions of what makes things happen, so it is useful for the practitioner to explore this area generally when using it to make an assessment of the patient's mental level. If a patient says that in order to get a larger house, they are going to buy more lottery tickets, the practitioner may wonder if the patient's imbalance is primarily at this level.

The spirit level

Because the spirit is more subtle than the mind and body, it can be more difficult to diagnose. In order to diagnose this level accurately, it is often important for practitioners to be aware of the context of the patient's life situation. For example, some patients may seem to be very healthy until a difficulty arises. The fragility of their spirit then manifests as they crumble under the strain of what appears to others to be a relatively minor problem. In contrast, even a very healthy person may have difficulty coping with an emotional shock if it is severe enough.

The health of the spirit manifests in various ways. Listed below are some areas that the practitioner can observe:

- *The look in the eyes and eye contact*. The sparkle in a patient's eyes and the patient's ability to make eye contact are two of the most reliable ways of assessing the spirit. The eyes of a healthy person are shiny, clear and bright and the person is able to make good eye contact. If the spirit is not healthy the eyes may be dull and lifeless and eye contact is less direct. In some cases the eyes may reveal something of the agitation in the patient's spirit.

- *Posture*. A person whose spirit is healthy has an upright posture. A person with a less healthy spirit is often more slumped. The posture may be slumped in the head, chest or abdomen or the person may not stand upright but instead tilts to one side. Agitation in the spirit may make it hard for patients to keep their body still.

- *Clothing and hygiene*. People with a healthy spirit are likely to take some pride in their appearance and personal cleanliness. When people are either over-obsessive or at the other extreme are unkempt and no longer care about their appearance and hygiene, this may indicate that they are unwell at this level.

- *Communication*. People with a healthy spirit will tend to have relatively clear verbal and non-verbal communication with others. People who are unwell in their spirit are more likely to avoid or be evasive and indirect in their contact with others.

- *Language*. People who have a healthy spirit are likely to use clearer and more positive language than those with a less healthy spirit. People with problems at the spirit level are more likely to use language peppered with words like 'I can't', 'I won't', 'It all seems hopeless', 'I feel helpless'. Although they may be physically and mentally capable, they may feel powerless and unable to do certain activities because of their fragile spirit.

- *Relationships*. People with a healthy spirit will be able to give love to others and enjoy receiving others' love. Those with less healthy spirits will have more difficulties giving love to others and knowing that they are loveable.

- *Dealing with difficulties*. People with healthy spirits are likely to attempt to work through problems that arise in their lives or to move on when a problem is irresolvable. People with a less healthy spirit may easily give up and resign in the face of adversity. Alternatively they may hold on and try to prevent change at all costs rather than let go when problems are irresolvable.

- *Purpose and meaning*. People with a healthy spirit have a sense of their life being meaningful and are endeavouring to fulfil their potential. Those with a less healthy spirit are more likely to feel that their life has no meaning or purpose.

- *Emotional reactions*. Patients with a healthy spirit are more likely to experience their various emotions as they arise and to work through their emotional distress. Those with a less healthy spirit are more likely to become overwhelmed by their emotions when they are distressed or to suppress their feelings and have very little outward emotional reaction. People's emotional reactions may also appear to be out of context to the severity of the external situation.

Diagnosing the inner capacities of a patient

It can help practitioners to deepen their understanding of their patients' spirits if they focus on the inner capacity of each Element. For example, looking at each Element, people should have the ability to:

- love and enjoy themselves
- care and nourish others and allow themselves to be cared for

- feel grief appropriately, receive inspiration and let go of what is no longer required
- protect themselves and feel safe
- grow and develop and assert themselves appropriately

Practitioners can use their knowledge of the Five Elements to consider which of these aspects are healthy, which are deficient and where the patient's potential is not yet manifested. The practitioner can focus on any aspect from the above list and make an assessment. For example, the practitioner may decide that a patient has an imbalance in the area of caring and nourishing. When practitioners are planning future treatment they can consider including spirit level points that have an effect on this function. This area of diagnosis will usually dovetail with that of the CF.

The practitioner could also go further by gently questioning whether the patient is happy with that area of their life and whether they have hopes or wishes for being better cared for and to care better for others. It is important for practitioners to be sensitive at this stage as they may be entering an area where a difficulty in the spirit will manifest. The response may be unpredictable. These aspects of a person's spirit are often highly defended and full of ambivalence, awkwardness and pain. Three things are essential: high-quality rapport, complete acceptance of the patient whatever they say, and accessing the appropriate inner state.

Box 27.1 outlines a way of developing the ability to assess patients' spirits from their eyes.

Diagnosing through response to treatment

The results of treatment often reveal the level of treatment the patient requires. In general, a person will show pleasure if they have relief from pain, regain the ability to walk freely or are able to sleep again. Sometimes patients surprise us and continue to complain even though their physical symptoms have disappeared. This may indicate that the problem is at a deeper level and treatment has not yet reached this level. Practitioners can use the patient's response to changes from treatment to refine their diagnosis of the level.

It is also interesting to observe how the patient responds when asked how she or he has been since the previous treatment. It can be indicative of the

---

Box 27.1

Assessing a patient's spirit by their eyes

Look at the eyes of all the people you contact over a period of a week. If looking at everyone is too difficult, decide when you will do this. For example, it may be with friends, people on the street and in shops or with people at work. Using a small notebook write down what you saw, for example, 'eyes looked hard' or 'sad-looking eyes' or 'sparkling and clear'. When you have notated about 30 observations, decide on a method of notation for a spectrum of qualities that interest you. These may be, for example:

- sparkling to dead
- worn out to energetic
- soft to hard
- clear to dull
- jittery to steady

Devise a scoring system such as from 1 to 10 and rate the next 30 people using the two qualities you have chosen. For the next stage, decide on two different qualities and continue to use a notebook to record them.

---

state of the person's spirit if they reply in terms of their mood or how they have felt in themselves rather than their main complaint. Their physical symptoms may be distressing for them but are relatively unimportant compared to how they feel in themselves.

Patient Example

A patient came for treatment complaining of almost daily migraines. The woman was expressionless, seemed reluctant to be in the treatment room and reticent to say much about herself, other than having migraines. She gave very little feedback, but when pressed at the beginning of the fourth treatment, she reluctantly told the practitioner in a very flat voice, that she had not had a migraine for two weeks. The practitioner was very confused and took some time to conclude, and several treatments more to verify, that the treatment was in some sense correct, but was definitely not getting to the correct level. Change in the patient's physical condition was not leading to a change in her spirit.

The ability of the practitioner to direct treatment to the appropriate level of body, mind or spirit is one of the most important keys to successful treatment. For more on this, see Chapters 37 and 46. Sometimes it is necessary to treat a physical problem with a very 'physical' approach. At other times it is appropriate for practitioners to connect with a deeper level. In order for patients to benefit at the level required and return to health, practitioners must focus their intention and take great care in the quality of rapport and in their choice of points.

The golden key approach to discovering CFs

The golden key method of diagnosis is an approach that is often intuitive and was developed by experienced practitioners. It is described in this chapter as a supplementary approach to diagnosing the CF. Its use partly depends upon developing an understanding of non-traditional Five Element resonances.

One of the drawbacks of this form of diagnosis is that practitioners may use it when they are uncertain about the patient's colour, sound, odour and emotion. This is not a viable option for practitioners who truly wish to grow and develop their skills. This is because it is the cultivation of the senses and the ability to see, hear, feel and smell that eventually allows practitioners to improve their levels of expertise.

Traditional and non-traditional resonances

The difference between a traditional and non-traditional resonance

Colours, sounds, emotions and odours are traditional Five Element resonances that are laid down in the *Nei Jing*. Non-traditional resonances have never been written down in the Chinese classics. Instead they have been developed recently by practitioners and have been drawn from the observation of thousands of patients. Using their understanding of the Element and the associated Officials, the practitioner decides that certain behaviour or attitudes are resonant with a particular Element. Much of the material for this form of diagnosis is set out in chapters associated with each CF.

The nature of golden keys

Golden keys are usually significant moments that strike a practitioner as odd, quirky or unusual. They are often expressed via the patient's words or behaviours and they often carry a sense of being an unhealthy rather than healthy expression of the patient.

To begin with practitioners might notice something unusual about the patient and their curiosity is aroused, but at the same time they may not associate golden keys with any particular Element. The practitioner may wonder what could cause the patient to behave or think in this way and she or he strives to understand the underlying cause of this particular behaviour. *It is this cause, rather than the behaviour itself, that informs the diagnosis*. For example, noticing that a person has withdrawn from others does not help the diagnosis. Realising what has driven them to withdraw, however, could be the key to a correct diagnosis.

An example of a golden key

A patient, Mr Green, was a secondary school teacher. He was threatened by a possible thrombosis in his leg and wondered whether acupuncture could help. Throughout the case history, Mr Green mentioned several accidents that had occurred to him. The first was when he was 6 and he lost an eye when he and a friend were going fishing and climbed over a farm gate. His friend's fishing rod entered his left eye, with the result that his sight was severely impaired. He said that this accident happened on 5 August 1931 in the early morning. There were another five such 'accidents' and for each the date and time were given, without prompting. By the third account, the practitioner was thinking, 'This is odd. So many severe accidents and such precise times and places.'

The incident immediately preceding the threatened thrombosis was not presented as one of these incidents, but it had a similar flavour. A student in Mr Green's school had mischievously set off the fire alarm knowing that, because of regulations, the whole school would be required to assemble in the playground with all students being accounted for. Classes were severely disrupted. Mr Green thought he knew the culprit and was inwardly furious. The weather in the playground was very windy, which Mr Green commented upon, and said he found annoying. The swelling of his leg occurred that evening.

What are the golden keys? There were several accidents and the patient knew the date and time of each one. They all *seemed* to be accidents, but after one or two the practitioner became suspicious.

Yet no one deliberately arranges for his or her eye to be poked. The practitioner might ask, 'What might tie all these incidents together?'

At this point, those who are new to the Five Elements may be puzzled, but most experienced practitioners, whatever style they practise, would probably have the Element or the Organ in mind, especially as there are some helpful associated clues – the anger and the wind.

What is the method?

The process

Assuming that the golden key represents a more generalised pattern and truly is a pathological manifestation of the patient's underlying imbalance, the method of diagnosis is as follows:

* The practitioner is struck by some odd behaviour or statement
* It is useful for the practitioner to describe what exactly it is that is odd. For example, is it just the accidents, the number of them or the exact dates and times?
* The practitioner can check that it really is a pattern and notice if it is repeated
* All Organs and Officials have different capacities (see the section 'Diagnosing the inner capacities of a patient' above). The practitioner asks her or himself what capacity is missing or impaired that could cause the event(s) to happen

By now it is probably easy to guess that Mr Green is a Wood CF. The Gall Bladder is the Organ responsible for judgement and the Liver is responsible for planning. His pattern was to both put himself in places of danger, evidencing poor judgement, and to also remember and communicate vast amounts of detail, implying over-planning. Both of these behaviours are significant golden keys and should be used to support the use of colour, sound, emotion and odour but not to replace it.

When processing golden keys, other resonances, such as wind and anger, may also come up and these should also support the diagnosis. The use of colour, sound, emotion and odour alongside the golden keys confirms the power of the Five Element approach when assessing the overall pattern.

It is with trifles, and when he is off guard, that a man best reveals his character.

(Schopenhauer; Auden and Kronenberger, 1962)

Using the method

The method for using golden keys that is written down in the above section is rarely carried out in its entirety. Under normal circumstances practitioners are struck by the behaviour or information and attribute it to an Organ or Element.

By treating patients, establishing their CFs and seeing them change as a result of treatment, practitioners build up a repertoire of patterns or 'resonances' that are non-traditional, but are nevertheless based on clinical experience. The greater the practitioner's experience, the more solid and reliable is their repertoire of unconscious patterns. Intuition builds faster when it is encouraged. New practitioners who consciously ask the three questions listed below will be more inclined to develop intuition and discover more 'golden keys'.

* What does this person do or say that is odd and possibly pathological?
* What capacity of which Organ, were it diminished, could explain this pattern?
* What aspect of this patient's potential is not being realised?

Patient Example

A patient was a primary school teacher aged 29. She was suffering from great exhaustion and regular illnesses and complained bitterly as she was so passionate about her teaching. She loved her students (7 to 8-year-olds) and the craftwork that she taught. Her energy and passion about her complaints was as strong as her passion about teaching. She explained, with great displays of energy, how much effort she had to put into her work in order to keep going. The practitioner was struck both by her exhaustion and the emotion and effort expended in describing it. It became clear that it was desperate willpower that was keeping her going. Other signs corroborated that she was a Water CF. Treatment on Water changed her presentation and exhaustion.

Over time, some of these golden keys become part of the practitioner's diagnostic framework and the practitioner begins to notice that certain behaviours correlate with certain CFs. These are written about in greater depth in the chapters on the patterns of behaviour of the CF.

It is important for practitioners not to rely solely on golden keys when identifying a patient's CF. To prevent incorrect generalisations and explanations from being made they must always then be checked against colour, sound, emotion and odour and subsequently against the results of treatment. An ongoing verification process is essential as only then can valid generalisations be made.

Summary

1 Treatment may need to be directed at the level of the body, mind or the spirit.
2 Determining the correct level of treatment affects both the selection of points and the practitioner's intention.
3 The health of the spirit can be observed by the practitioner in a number of ways, including:

- the look and sparkle in a person's eyes and their eye contact
- their posture, clothing and hygiene
- their communication and language
- their relationships
- how they deal with difficulties
- the purpose and meaning in their life
- their emotional reactions

4 Practitioners may supplement their diagnosis of colour, sound, emotion and odour by using 'golden keys'. Golden keys are usually significant moments that strike a practitioner as odd, quirky or unusual. They are often expressed via the patient's words or behaviours. They often carry a sense of being an unhealthy rather than healthy expression of the patient.

Diagnosis by touch

28

Introduction

Most of the methods of diagnosis discussed in this chapter involve touch. They are:

- pulse diagnosis
- palpating the three *jiao* or burners
- palpating the abdomen
- palpating the front *mu* points
- the Akabane test

These methods of diagnosis cover much of the 'to feel' aspects of diagnosis. This is the part of the diagnosis covered in the physical examination of a patient. Of these five areas, pulse diagnosis is by far the most important. Assessing the way the pulses respond during a treatment can be especially useful when diagnosing the CF. All of the other methods of diagnosis can indicate that an Element or Organ is significantly out of balance and can also support the CF diagnosis. They are, however, far less important in determining the CF.

Pulse diagnosis

The purpose and value of taking the pulses

Taking pulses by feeling the radial artery on the wrist is of one the most important diagnostic practices of Chinese medicine and practitioners of Five Element Constitutional Acupuncture place enormous importance on it.

The main goals of pulse diagnosis are to:

- assess the level of *qi* of an Organ and Element
- determine whether the *qi* of an Organ or Element is excessive or deficient, thus governing the needle technique used
- help to diagnose any blocks to treatment (see Section 4, this volume)
- assess changes in the patient's *qi* during and after treatment

How to take the pulses

The position of the pulses

The pulses are felt on both wrists in three positions along the radial artery. The styloid process of the radius (shown in Figure 28.1) lies opposite the middle pulse position.

© 2011, Elsevier Ltd.
DOI: 10.1016/B978-0-7020-3175-5.00028-0

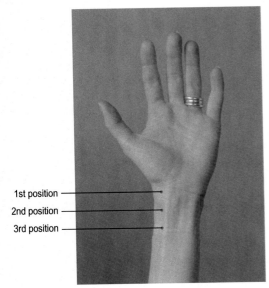

1st position —

2nd position —

3rd position —

Figure 28.1 • Pulse positions along the radial artery

Position of the patient

When having their pulses taken the patient should:

- be relaxed, sitting or lying down
- have the arm free of obstructions such as watches, bracelets or tight sleeves
- have the arm level with, but no higher than, the patient's heart

Position of the practitioner

When taking pulses the practitioner should:

- start by taking the pulses on the patient's left-hand side, then the right
- stand at right angles to the patient and hold the patient's left hand in their left hand as if shaking hands
- stand comfortably with a relaxed posture, weight evenly distributed and head held upright

Taking the pulses

When taking the patient's pulses the practitioner goes through these stages:

- First, place the middle finger over the radial styloid until the tip reaches the radial artery.[1]

---

[1] The use of the tip of the finger is probably a Japanese influence (see Eckman, 1996, pp. 206–207). Other traditions locate the pulse positions in the same place. They may, however, not hold the hand with the one that is not feeling the pulse and they may use the pads of the finger rather than the tips

At the same time use the thumb as a fulcrum at the back of the wrist.

- Next, let the middle finger drop on to the pulse of the middle pulse position.
- Having located the middle position, feel the first, second and third positions in turn. The first pulse position is distal to the middle position and is felt under the tip of the index finger. The third position is proximal to the middle position and is felt under the tip of the ring finger. When feeling each position, the practitioner should place only one finger on the artery at a time.

The two levels and the position of the Organs

The pulse is felt at two levels, superficial and deep. The superficial level is at the top part of the artery and is felt using light pressure. The deep level is lower down and is felt by using slightly heavier pressure. These two depths reveal the *qi* of the twelve *yin* and *yang* Organs. Table 28.1 shows the Organs in relation to the twelve positions.

At different times in the history of Chinese medicine, slightly different pulse positions have been used (for a discussion of these, see Birch, 1992, pp. 2–13; Hammer, 2001, pp. 17–29; Maciocia, 2005, pp. 354–355 and Scott, 1984, pp. 2–7). Practitioners of Five Element Constitutional Acupuncture use the positions laid down in the *Nan Jing*. Classical Chinese texts from the traditions of herbal medicine generally place the Kidneys at the third position on the right hand. Contemporary Chinese acupuncture texts usually place Kidney *yang* in the rear right-hand position, but this is a more modern (post 1949) development (see Birch, 1992, for a fascinating piece of research into the history of the placing of pulse positions in 101 different texts drawn from different periods in history).

Table 28.1 The pulse positions and Organs

| | Left arm | | Right arm | |
	Light	Deep	Deep	Light
Distal	Small Intestine	Heart	Lung	Large Intestine
Middle	Gall Bladder	Liver	Spleen	Stomach
Proximal	Bladder	Kidney	Pericardium	Triple Burner

Notating the quantity

Traditionally pulse diagnosis has determined the presence of up to 28 different qualities. Five Element Constitutional Acupuncturists focus on two, which are excess (full) and deficiency (empty). (Again, see Eckman, 1996. This emphasis on deficiency and excess is also a Japanese influence.) The overall fullness or emptiness is notated by using a numbering system ranging from −3 to +3 against the individual positions. Table 28.2 is an example of notating the pulses in this way.

Feeling the quantity

When taking pulses the practitioner learns to discern the differences in strength between the different positions. At first the student concentrates on feeling the main differences, for example, the left middle position may feel stronger than the right middle position or the right first position may feel weaker than the right third position. After some experience has been gained by measuring this comparative strength, the practitioner attempts to find a 'norm' for the person.

The 'norm' in pulse taking

In order to find the patient's 'norm', the practitioner considers the patient's age, sex, physique and physical activity and decides on the level of strength that is a '✓' or 'just right' for that individual. The norm for a young and strong person will be higher than that of an older and less strong person.

Having decided on the norm, the practitioner then records the pulses in relation to it. Some of the patient's pulses may be stronger or weaker than the norm, so it is important that the practitioner bears in mind the level of the norm throughout pulse taking. Although this process is subjective, it has a sound basis in most practitioners' experience. Almost all practitioners using any style of acupuncture will have experienced feeling a patient's pulses and being surprised by their weakness or strength. This indicates that the practitioner has unconsciously decided on a norm. This is an important part of the diagnosis as most practitioners then look for an explanation for any apparent discrepancy.

Pulse changes during treatment and the overall change

So far the description of pulse diagnosis has outlined how practitioners can read the strength of individual pulse positions. Pulse taking in this way is crucially important because it reveals the strength of the *qi* in the Organs. There is also another reason for taking pulses, however. This is to consider the *overall* change that takes place in the pulses. This method is invaluable for both diagnosis and the evaluation of a treatment.

The overall view of the pulses

In order to feel this overall change in the pulses, the practitioner concentrates on how the different positions relate to each other. In this case the ideal is that the pulses are harmonious. Balance and harmony are more important than increasing the strength of an individual pulse position or even all the pulses.

When considering the notion of 'harmony', the practitioner will look for:

* the different pulse positions being similar in strength
* the different pulse positions being similar in quality
* similarity on one side of the pulses to those on the other
* clarity of the pulses or easy readability

Feeling for this overall harmony suggests that although Five Element Constitutional Acupuncturists are not directly taught to recognise pulse qualities, they are still indirectly feeling them when making these comparisons.

'Clarity' arises as an issue when practitioners find it difficult to specify that a pulse is − or + in quantity or the boundaries of a pulse seem 'fuzzy' and less precise than usual. After treatment, the pulse or pulses should change and become clearer.

Thus defined, harmony is a complex overall quality. With experience practitioners recognise it and make a judgement that the treatment has brought

Table 28.2 Recording a pulse picture

Left arm		Right arm	
Light	**Deep**	**Deep**	**Light**
−1	−1	−1½	−1½
+1	+1½	✓	✓
−2	−2	−3	−3

about greater or lesser harmony. It is a common experience for a Five Element Constitutional Acupuncturist to treat a patient on the CF and then return to the pulses to find that they have become overall much more harmonious.

When practising Five Element Constitutional Acupuncture, the practitioner needs to recognise this feeling of greater harmony and use it as a standard for having carried out an effective treatment.

There is another important aspect to feeling pulse changes. When practitioners feel the pulses change to become more harmonious and a better quality, they may look back to remember what the pulses were like before the change. Making this before-and-after comparison enables practitioners to recognise pulse qualities that are not quite right more quickly, rather than noticing them only in retrospect, after a pulse change.

The CF pulse change

During the first few treatments, the practitioner concentrates on confirming the patient's CF. For instance, the practitioner may have diagnosed the patient as a Fire CF. The diagnosis is only confirmed, however, when the patient is showing clear signs of improvement. Ideally, the diagnosis is confirmed by the beginning of the second treatment, but it often takes longer. An intermediate stage, which suggests that the diagnosis is correct, is achieving a 'CF pulse change'.

The pulse change that is felt when the patient is treated on the correct Element of the CF has two characteristics.

- Firstly, all of the pulses change by becoming more harmonious, a better quality and often stronger. This overall change is crucial as it indicates that the condition of the other Elements is dependent on the health of the Element being treated.

- Secondly, the pulse positions associated with the CF may hardly respond at all or may even feel weaker.

At first these changes seem counter-intuitive, but they can be explained. The explanation is that the chronic imbalance of the CF is keeping the other Organs from performing well. As soon as the CF is treated, the other Organs can immediately respond. In the case of a Fire CF, the Earth pulses may feel very deficient because Earth has not been adequately nourished by Fire along the *sheng* cycle. Nothing is wrong with the Stomach and Spleen that treating the long-term imbalance, caused by the Fire CF, will not cure.

The CF pulse change is a valuable indicator when confirming the CF and evaluating whether treatment has been sufficient. During the course of treatment it is important to monitor the pulses to see which Elements respond well to treatment on the CF and which do not. For example, a patient may be a Metal CF and the Water and Wood Elements are also extremely imbalanced. The pulses of the Water Element may respond well to treatment on the Metal CF. Due to the patient's excessive alcohol consumption, however, the pulses of the Wood Element do not respond so well. This may indicate that the Wood Element needs to be treated directly.

Pulse diagnosis can also be important when diagnosing and treating blocks to treatment especially a Husband–Wife imbalance or an Entry–Exit block. For more on this, see Chapters 32 and 33.

Feeling the chest and abdomen

Introduction

There are three methods of diagnosis that involve feeling the torso. The first is the assessment of the three *jiao* (or burners). The three *jiao* were discussed in the section on the Fire Element and the Triple Burner. The second is abdominal diagnosis involving palpation of various locations on the abdomen. The third is the palpation of the front 'mu' or 'alarm' points. To some degree these methods overlap and can be carried out in one process.

The three *jiao*

The torso is divided into three 'burning spaces' (see Figure 28.2). These are:

- the Upper Burner – which is situated in the chest and lies above the diaphragm. It contains the Heart, Pericardium and Lung.
- the Middle Burner – which lies between the diaphragm and the navel. It contains the Stomach, Spleen, Liver and Gall Bladder, and joins the Lower Burner at the navel.

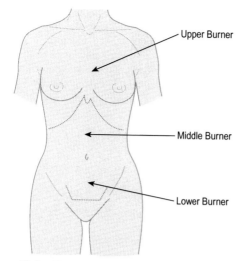

Upper Burner

Middle Burner

Lower Burner

Figure 28.2 • The Three Burners

* the Lower Burner – which lies below the navel. It contains the Small and Large Intestines, Bladder and Kidney.

The purpose of assessing the *jiao*

The three burners are assessed visually and by touch in order to:

* assess the warmth and strength of the *qi* in each burner
* determine if moxibustion or warming needs to be a significant part of treatment
* assess the progress of treatment
* assess how the patient reacts to physical contact

Feeling the three *jiao*

In order to feel the three *jiao*, the patient should lie down on the treatment couch. She or he is covered with a sheet or blanket in such a way that the areas can easily be exposed.

The practitioner stands to one side of the treatment couch and uncovers each *jiao*. The practitioner then places the flat of the hand across each burner, paying attention to its temperature. When feeling the Upper Burner, the middle of the hand should lie over *Ren* 17 to 18. For the Middle Burner it should lie over *Ren* 12 and for the Lower Burner *Ren* 5 to 6. On the Upper Burner the hand should be placed

lengthways between the breasts on a woman and horizontally across the chest on a man. The locations are approximate.

Patient Example

A woman in her early fifties came for treatment because she coughed up copious amounts of phlegm every morning and occasionally vomited phlegm. She was an Earth CF and her middle *jiao* was very cold to the touch. On the first treatment, moxibustion as well as needles were used on Sp 3 and St 42, the source points of the Earth channels, and also on *Ren* 12. The middle *jiao* was immediately warmer. Over the next six treatments the practitioner used moxibustion consistently. The symptoms improved and the temperature of the middle *jiao* came much closer to the others.

Assessing the three *jiao*

When starting to feel the *jiao* it is useful for the practitioner to rank them from cool to warm or hot in relation to each other. With more experience, in a similar way to pulse diagnosis, the practitioner develops the idea of a 'norm' and can rate the burners as cold, cool, normal, warm and hot. Practitioners can use the method illustrated in the example below to record the temperature.

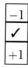

$$\begin{array}{|c|}\hline -1 \\\hline \checkmark \\\hline +1 \\\hline\end{array}$$

The above record says that the middle burner is a normal temperature, the upper burner is cool and the lower burner is warm. 'Warm' implies that the *jiao* is warmer than it should be, as normal is the desirable temperature. The case study above illustrates how temperature can be used to assess a patient's improvement.

Observing the *jiao*

When looking at the three *jiao* together, the practitioner may also touch the skin and flesh. This is not to feel the temperature, but to verify and support what she or he sees. The practitioner is assessing several aspects:

1 the colour of the different areas, for example, redness, darkness or paleness

2 the appearance of vitality or lack of vitality in different areas, for example, a water-logged lower abdomen

3 the structure of the area, for example, a tight and pinched rib cage

The observations should be recorded alongside the temperature findings

Relating findings to the CF

Sometimes the assessment of the three *jiao* is unhelpful but at other times it is crucial. The Organs for Metal and Fire CFs lie in the Upper Burner. The Organs of Earth CFs relate to the Middle Burner and Water CFs to the Lower Burner. Wood CFs are more difficult to connect via the *jiao*. This is because the Liver Organ is clearly in the middle *jiao*, but some texts have attributed the Liver to the lower *jiao*.

Where there are abnormalities in the temperature, look or feel of the three *jiao*, these can sometimes be connected to the Organs of the CF. Abnormalities can also be useful when the practitioner is deciding whether to use moxibustion and helpful when assessing longer-term changes.

Abdominal diagnosis

The purpose

Practitioners carry out abdominal diagnosis by palpating various areas on the abdomen. By discerning the sensitivity and feel of these locations they then make inferences about the balance of the various Organs. This method of diagnosis originated in Japan and practitioners of Five Element Constitutional Acupuncture give it considerably less emphasis than it is given by many Japanese acupuncturists. Five Element Constitutional Acupuncturists use this method of diagnosis only as a supplementary approach to other forms of diagnosis.

The locations on the abdomen

Figure 28.3 shows the locations to palpate. The relevant Organ is also indicated.

Carrying out the diagnosis

- The practitioner clearly explains the test to the patient. The practitioner should also reassure the patient that when palpating he/she will release the pressure if the patient indicates that the area is tender.
- The patient lies on the treatment couch with the abdomen exposed and the legs extended. The knees should not be bent.
- The practitioner stands beside the couch and initially observes the overall symmetry or lack of symmetry of the patient's abdomen and the breathing.
- To palpate the areas, the practitioner uses the pads of the three middle fingers and presses down

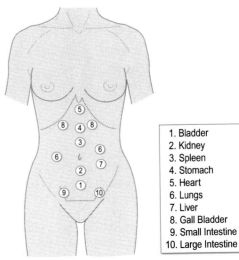

1. Bladder
2. Kidney
3. Spleen
4. Stomach
5. Heart
6. Lungs
7. Liver
8. Gall Bladder
9. Small Intestine
10. Large Intestine

Figure 28.3 • Palpation locations for abdominal diagnosis

while the patient is exhaling. Pressure should be made firmly and slowly to a maximum of two inches or five centimetres.

- The patient gives the practitioner feedback by describing any abnormal, painful or just uncomfortable feelings.
- The practitioner records the patient's response.

Responses to the palpation

The kind of responses the patient will give are that:

1 the area is painful and palpation should be stopped

2 there is some discomfort – which the patient can describe

3 the location is normal and is not tender

Although the patient's feedback is important, with experience practitioners will also begin to notice other feelings of abnormality under their hand as they palpate. This will include feelings such as tension, flaccidity or lumps. The practitioner should also record these feelings. Ideally a patient has a pain-free response. Where there are abnormalities, this indicates that there is imbalance of some sort in the associated Organ. (It is useful to consult other texts about abdominal diagnosis, for example Denmei, 1990, and Matsumoto and Birch, 1993b, as the locations associated with the different Organs vary.)

Palpating the front *mu* or alarm points

Description and purpose

The front *mu* points are located on the chest or abdomen. There is one point associated with each Organ, although the points are not necessarily located on the channel of the associated Organ. These points have been called the 'alarm' points, suggesting that they are indicators of disease or imbalance. The translation of '*mu*' is given as to 'collect', suggesting that the *qi* of the relevant Organ 'collects' at this point. (Maciocia gives alternative translations of 'raise, collect, enlist, recruit'; Maciocia, 1989, p. 351.)

The points, unlike the areas used in abdominal diagnosis, are palpated as points, that is with one finger and using less pressure. When palpating these points the practitioner makes a note of any areas of tenderness.

The points

The points and their associated Organ are listed in Table 28.3. These points are not used for treatment in their capacity as front *mu* points, although many of these points may be used due to other indications (see Chapters 38–44 for more information on the use of the points).

The assessment of the three burners, abdomen and alarm points can best be done as one process.

The Akabane test

Introduction

The origin and purpose

A Japanese practitioner, Akabane Kobe, devised this test sometime in the 1950s or 1960s. Its value lies in measuring the balance of the *qi* in the channels on one side of the body compared with the other. Practitioners usually assume that although the channels are bilateral, the *qi* of a channel overall is balanced. Akabane perceived that this is not always the case and his test was designed to measure the balance between the channels on the right and left sides. The test assumes that a channel with less *qi* is less sensitive to heat applied to a point on the channel.

Table 28.3 Organs and their associated alarm points

Organ	Alarm point
Lung	Lu 1
Large Intestine	St 25
Stomach	*Ren* 12
Spleen	Liver 13
Heart	*Ren* 14
Small Intestine	*Ren* 4
Bladder	*Ren* 3
Kidney	GB 25
Pericardium	*Ren* 15
Triple Burner	*Ren* 7
Gall Bladder	GB 24 or 23
Liver	Liv 14

Carrying out the test

To carry out the test:

- The practitioner locates the nail points of all the channels of the hands and feet. In the case of the Kidney, the point on the medial side of the little toe is used. This is opposite Bl 67.
- The practitioner lights a taper or Japanese incense stick. This is passed back and forth over the point on both the right and left sides.
- When carrying out the test, the patient's finger or toe is held firmly by the practitioner with the hand not holding the stick. The hand that is holding the stick is stabilised close to the patient (see Figure 28.4).
- The practitioner moves the lighted end of the incense stick over the acupuncture point towards the nail and then away from it. The stick travels over a distance of approximately 0.7 centimetres, with the acupuncture point in the middle. The stick is moved at a constant speed as well as at an even distance (approximately 0.4–0.5 centimetres) from the skin. The even distance and speed is a crucial part of the test.
- The patient is asked to tell the practitioner as soon as they feel the heat. It is important that the patient says 'hot', having felt the same amount of heat on either limb.
- As the practitioner passes the lighted stick over the point she or he counts each pass as the stick travels back and forth. The practitioner must find a distance from the point so that the patient does not feel the heat immediately, but does feel it after five or more passes. The practitioner counts and records the number of passes needed on the channels of each side before they become hot.

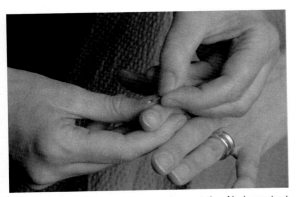

Figure 28.4 • A practitioner carrying out the Akabane test

Interpretation of the test

A significantly higher count on one side indicates that that side of the channel is relatively deficient in *qi*. For example, if the patient allows 12 passes over LI 1 on the right and only six on the left, then the right-hand side of the channel can be judged to be deficient.

A further test should be carried out on the channel or channels that are out of balance to check the result. If the result is consistent, then the imbalance can be corrected.

Correcting the imbalance

To correct this imbalance, the practitioner tonifies the *luo*-junction point on the deficient side (the side with the highest number). The test is then repeated and the ideal result is that the sensitivity to the heat is more closely balanced. If this treatment does not bring about the desired change, the *yuan*-source point of the deficient side is tonified.

If more than one channel is out of balance practitioners should notice if the imbalance follows the Organs of the *sheng* cycle. When correcting the imbalance, the first channel on the *sheng* cycle should be corrected first. The other imbalances may then correct by themselves.

Practising the Akabane test

This test and the subsequent treatment follow in the Five Element tradition of concentrating on balancing the patient's *qi*. The test is only accurate, however, if it is carried out carefully and it requires much practice to ensure reliable results. When learning to do the test, it is important for several practitioners to test one person. This enables them to check that their findings are accurate. Practitioners do not need to count the same number of passes, but they should come to agreement about which channels are out of balance. Only when practitioners get consistent results should the test be used on patients.

Summary

1 Pulse diagnosis is carried out by feeling the radial artery on the wrist. It is of one the most important diagnostic practices of Five Element Constitutional Acupuncture.

2 The main goals of pulse diagnosis are to:
- assess the level of *qi* of an Organ and Element
- determine whether the *qi* of an Organ or Element is excessive or deficient, thus governing the needle technique used
- help to diagnose any blocks to treatment
- assess changes in the patient's *qi* during and after treatment, thereby evaluating the effect of the treatment

3 The three methods of diagnosis that involve feeling the torso are palpating the three *jiao* or burners, abdominal diagnosis and palpating the front *mu* points.

4 The Akabane test measures the balance of the *qi* in a channel on one side of the body compared to the other in order to ensure that the *qi* is balanced.

Section 4

Blocks to Treatment

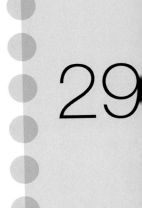

The Five Element blocks to treatment

Introduction

When treating a new patient, a practitioner usually begins by testing for the patient's Constitutional Factor. If a practitioner is treating a patient on the correct CF, the patient is likely to feel healthier because the most underlying imbalance is being treated. Sometimes the patient does not experience an improvement in well-being. The patient feels no change or on rare occasions experiences a worsening of symptoms. There are many potential reasons for this lack of progress. For a practitioner of Five Element Constitutional Acupuncture, one of the main reasons is a block to treatment.

An alternative situation occurs when the practitioner anticipates that there is a block and treatment begins with removing the block.

The four blocks

The four blocks are:
- Aggressive Energy
- Possession
- Husband–Wife imbalance
- Entry–Exit blocks

Each block takes a very different form and will be described in the following chapters. All have one thing in common – they can have a profoundly negative effect on the patient's physical or psychological health unless they are cleared. This is especially true of the first three blocks. The fourth, the Entry–Exit block, is usually less damaging. It can, however, still cause a major impediment to the patient's flow of qi and therefore inhibit a patient's progress towards better health.

Treating the blocks

Because of the importance of these blocks, a practitioner will endeavour to clear them before treatment on the CF begins. This is not always possible, however, and sometimes a block arises during the course of treatment. For example, although it is rare, a severe emotional shock or a serious illness can injure the Organs and lead to Aggressive Energy.

If the blocks are not cleared the patient is likely to deteriorate in her or his health. In some cases these blocks can be so injurious to the person's health that they threaten the person's spiritual, mental or physical stability and can even be life-threatening.

Results of treatment

Treatment to clear these blocks will often cause significant positive shifts in the patient's health. Sometimes there is a dramatic transformation and a person immediately feels better in body, mind and/or spirit.

At other times the changes can occur less dramatically, although with no less efficacy. The effect of these treatments may not seem possible until the practitioner has repeatedly observed them on numerous patients.

Once these blocks have been cleared, normal treatment can commence and the patient is likely to progress as the practitioner expected.

Order of treating the four blocks

Although it is rare, there are occasions when a patient needs to be checked for more than one of these blocks. For instance, a practitioner may suspect that a patient is possessed but also want to check to see if Aggressive Energy is present. In the case of more than one block the order of treatment should normally be:

1 Possession
2 Aggressive Energy
3 Husband–Wife imbalance[1]
4 Entry–Exit block

There is one further block that is less frequently found that comes from a scar; for more on this, see Appendix D.

---

[1] Husband–Wife imbalances should not be treated before Aggressive Energy is cleared, as there is a possibility of transferring it from one Organ to another.

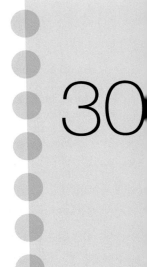

Aggressive Energy

What is Aggressive Energy?

Its nature

Aggressive Energy is described as *qi* 'which has become contaminated or polluted' (Lavier 1966; Worsley, 1990, Chapter 6, p. 175). Aggressive Energy can also be described as evil or unhealthy (*xie*) *qi* as opposed to upright or healthy (*zheng*) *qi*. (This was first suggested by Flaws, 1989.)

The contamination caused by Aggressive Energy can severely affect a person's health and well-being. Physically it may cause life-threatening or debilitating illnesses. Aggressive Energy can affect a person's mind and spirit and can cause symptoms such as instability, depression, despair or fluctuating emotional states. The treatment of Aggressive Energy can have a dramatic effect on the patient's body, mind and spirit, enabling them to be restored to better health.

How Aggressive Energy develops

Once Aggressive Energy is present in one or more of the Organs, it is hard to expel without treatment. Healthy (*zheng*) *qi* naturally flows from Organ to Organ along the *sheng* cycle – the nurturing cycle of *qi* (see Chapter 2, this volume). Aggressive Energy is not healthy so it does not travel along this cycle. Instead it travels along the *ke* cycle. The *ke* cycle is usually translated as the 'control cycle' but when Aggressive Energy is present in the system the *ke* cycle becomes a destructive cycle. The *yin* Organs are connected across the *ke* cycle and this *qi* travels across it from *yin* Organ to *yin* Organ. Aggressive Energy is not usually found in the *yang* Organs.

Su Wen Chapter 65 describes how disease travels across the *ke* cycle:

> If a disease first develops in the Heart, there will be cardiac pain. One day later it reaches the Lung, causing dyspnoea and cough. Three days later, it reaches the Liver, causing propping fullness in the (free) rib region. Five days later, it reaches the Spleen, causing blockage and stoppage, generalised pain and heaviness. If it is not cured within three days, the condition is fatal.
>
> (Huang Fu Mi, translated by Yang and Chace, 1994)

If two Organs across the *ke* cycle have Aggressive Energy present, it is said that one 'leg' of the *ke* cycle is affected (see Figure 30.1). For example, if a person has Aggressive Energy on the Pericardium, this Organ may pass it on to the next Organ along the *ke cycle* – the Lung. If both the Pericardium and the Lung are affected this forms one 'leg' of the cycle.

The Lung will then attempt to throw off this unhealthy or evil (*xie*) *qi* but it may be transmitted to the Liver. If the Pericardium, Lung and Liver all have Aggressive Energy, then two 'legs' are affected (see Figure 30.2). The more Organs that are affected the more serious the condition for the patient (see Figure 30.3).

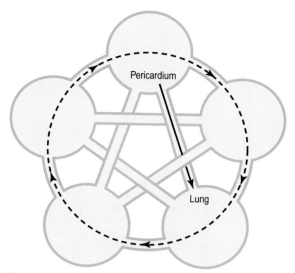

Figure 30.1 • One leg of the *ke* cycle affected

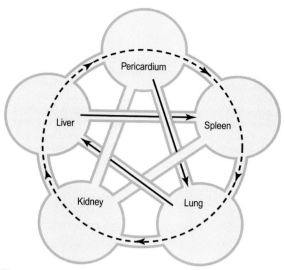

Figure 30.3 • Three legs of the *ke* cycle affected

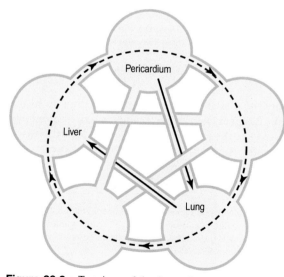

Figure 30.2 • Two legs of the *ke* cycle affected

The aetiology and pathology of Aggressive Energy

Aggressive Energy can arise from an internal or an external cause.

Aggressive Energy from an internal cause

If Aggressive Energy comes from an internal cause, an emotional trauma is usually the initial trigger. This can be anything from relationship problems, financial worries, work difficulties, family concerns or shocks. Under normal circumstances people recover from the effects of these stresses. When patients have had intense and repetitive emotions over a long period of time, however, this tends to cause disease, especially if the emotion is not expressed and has created stagnation.

In Chinese medicine emotions are called the internal causes of disease because they arise from inside us. Emotions that are not resolved eventually stagnate. As with all stagnation, this may eventually turn to toxic heat or fire. This may accumulate within an Organ as Aggressive Energy.

Mantak Chia, a *qi gong* teacher, describes heat in the Organs in the following way:

> . . . each organ is surrounded by a sac or membrane, called fascia, which regulates its temperature. Ideally the membrane releases excess heat out through the skin, where it is exchanged for cool life force energy from nature. An overload of physical or emotional tension causes the membrane, or fascia, to stick to the organ so that it cannot properly release heat to the skin nor absorb cool energy from the skin. The skin becomes clogged with toxins and the organ overheats.

(Chia, 1985, p. 71)

Aggressive Energy from an external cause

Evil or unhealthy (*xie*) *qi* derives from the external pathogenic factors of Wind, Cold, Damp, Dryness, Fire or Heat and can arise from inside or outside the body. The cause of a pathogen entering the body from the outside is often a climatic condition which 'invades' the body. It can also arise internally after an Organ becomes weakened or a drug or a vaccination has been administered. This causes a pathogen such as Heat to form in the body. (For more about 'latent Heat' and 'residual pathogenic factors', see Maciocia, 2008, pp. 1133–1139.)

If the patient's healthy (*zheng*) *qi* is strong, then the pathogen is normally thrown off or dealt with. Having evil or unhealthy (*xie*) *qi* inside the body will not in itself be a cause of Aggressive Energy. Over time, however, if a pathogen is not thrown off by the body's healthy (*zheng*) *qi*, it may penetrate deeper into the body. Finally it will reach the *yin* Organs. This is the deepest place that it can reach, so it stays there and stagnates. Over time, accumulation or stagnation turns to Heat and this unhealthy or evil (*xie*) *qi* may become toxic heat or fire in the *yin* Organs. It has now become Aggressive Energy.

Su Wen alludes to this when it describes disease penetrating deeper and deeper into the body in Chapter 5:

> It is best to treat diseases at the level of the skin and hair; the next best is to treat them at the level of the muscles and flesh; the next best is to treat them at the level of the sinews and vessels; the next best is to treat them at the level of the six *yang* organs; the next best is to treat them at the level of the five *yin* organs. When treating the level of the five *yin* organs half the patients die and the other half survive.
>
> (*Su Wen* Chapter 5; translation from Bensky and Barolet, 2009, p. 4)

Aggressive Energy and the CF

Pathogens can only invade the system if the upright (*zheng*) *qi* is weak. If a person's *qi* becomes weakened, it is usually the Organ of the CF that is the first to be affected. Correspondingly, the first Organ to be affected by Aggressive Energy is likely to be the

yin Organ related to the Element of the CF. In the Fire Element, Aggressive Energy is more commonly found on the Pericardium than the Heart. This is because the Pericardium normally protects the Heart from Heat and Fire. As it says in *Ling Shu* Chapter 71:

> If the Heart is attacked by a pathogenic factor, the *shen* suffers, which can lead to death. If a pathogenic factor does attack the Heart, it will be deviated to attack the Pericardium instead.
>
> (quoted in Maciocia, 2005, p. 165)

Diagnosis of Aggressive Energy

Aggressive Energy can be a difficult pattern to diagnose, as there may not always be specific signs and symptoms manifesting. Certain general predisposing circumstances can, however, lead the practitioner to suspect its presence.

Factors that may indicate the presence of Aggressive Energy

The main indications of Aggressive Energy are:

- a serious or life-threatening physical illness
- severe mental or spiritual problems
- unexpected or unusual aggravations to treatment
- a history of intensive drug therapy or addictions to alcohol or recreational drugs
- signs of colour, sound, emotion or odour which resonate with two Elements across the *ke* cycle
- chaotic or unstable pulses

Life-threatening or serious physical illness

If a patient has a long-term chronic illness, Aggressive Energy may have either developed from the disease or it may itself have caused the severe debilitation. A practitioner should test for Aggressive Energy if a patient has any severe illness or degenerative condition, or any signs and symptoms that seem extreme or in any way strange or bizarre.

Severe mental or spiritual problems

People with Aggressive Energy may describe having feelings such as desperation, hopelessness, despair or resignation. Some patients have a sense that they are unwell but feel unable to verbalise what is wrong. This level of internal distress may seem disproportionate to the person's description of their health.

> **Patient Example**
>
> A patient came for treatment complaining of a backache. During the course of the consultation she said that she inexplicably felt that she was going to die soon. Aggressive Energy was found and drained and at the next treatment she reported this feeling had left her.

Unexpected or unusual aggravations to treatment

On some occasions a patient has extraordinary reactions to treatment and feels worse rather than better. Obviously an aggravation can occur if the patient has

> **Patient Example**
>
> A patient was transferred to the student clinic from another practitioner. She was not checked for Aggressive Energy. The patient was diagnosed as a Fire CF and her Pericardium and Triple Burner were treated. She had an aggravation after this treatment, describing feeling tired and depressed as well as having a headache. The practitioner checked for Aggressive Energy and found it on the Kidneys and Pericardium. After it had been cleared the treatment progressed as expected.

been incorrectly diagnosed and treated, but if it happens for no obvious reason it may suggest that the practitioner should test for Aggressive Energy.

A history of intensive drug therapy or addictions to alcohol or recreational drugs

Any kind of drugs (prescribed or non-prescribed) that are used consistently eventually cause toxicity in the system. This is especially the case if medicines are used to suppress or alleviate a symptom without treating the underlying cause. Many recreational drugs, such as cocaine, amphetamines, ecstasy, LSD or the opiates, easily give rise to Aggressive Energy. Drugs given over long periods of time may eventually stagnate in the Organs and turn to toxic heat.

> **Patient Example**
>
> A patient with long-standing asthma was given large doses of corticosteroids after an asthma attack. The patient's asthma improved but he felt as if all of his enjoyment of life had disappeared. Aggressive Energy was found on the Kidneys. After it had been drained his spirits returned to normal.

Signs of colour, sound, emotion and odour resonating with two Elements across the *ke* cycle

A patient may be yellow and singing, fearful and putrid – indicating that both the Water and Earth Elements are out of balance. Alternatively, the patient may express grief and weeping whilst looking green and smelling rancid, indicating that Metal and Wood are both imbalanced. If two Organs across the *ke* cycle are affected, the practitioner should always consider that Aggressive Energy may be present.

Patient Example

A patient told his practitioner, 'When I look into the future, I can't see my life continuing. It's like pulling a roller blind down.' The patient looked green and his inability to see any future also alerted the practitioner to the fact that the Liver was out of balance. The patient was also weeping and displaying signs of grief. The practitioner found Aggressive Energy on the Lung and Liver.

Chaotic or unstable pulses

Although there are no special pulse qualities associated with Aggressive Energy, some pulse qualities may be more indicative than others. Someone with Aggressive Energy may have 'erratic' or 'unstable' pulses. Pulses have also been described as having 'significant signs of pulse unrest' and 'which strike us as far more serious than only a mere inconsistency' (Worsley, 1990, p. 176). These pulse qualities may sometimes be felt on the Organs across the *ke* cycle that are affected by the Aggressive Energy, for example, on the pulses of the Spleen and Kidney or the Liver and Lung.

Testing and treating Aggressive Energy

When to check for Aggressive Energy

The practitioner can test for Aggressive Energy whenever several of the conditions listed in the diagnosis section above are present. It is often tested for at two stages of treatment:

1 at the beginning of treatment
2 during treatment if there is a failure to respond to treatment or a downturn in the patient's condition

At the beginning of treatment

Aggressive Energy may be present without obvious signs and symptoms manifesting, so a practical option is to always test for it during the first treatment. If Aggressive Energy is present and is not cleared at this stage, then it could be spread to different Organs or be driven deeper into the body. This is most likely to happen when *qi* is transferred via the *sheng* and *ke* cycles, during subsequent acupuncture treatments.

During the course of treatment

Aggressive Energy should always be checked if a patient doesn't respond to treatment or has an unexpected decline in health during the course of treatment. In this case the patient may already have had Aggressive Energy that had not been found at the start of treatment. Alternatively she or he may have had some stress or trauma which caused the Aggressive Energy to form during the course of treatment.

The testing process

Position of the patient

Patients are usually sitting with a relaxed yet straight back. Their arms are supported in their lap. It is important that the patient is upright. In this position the back is opened up and the points are accessible. If the patient slouches forward, then the rib spaces move up in relation to the intervertebral gaps. In this case the anatomical descriptions of the point locations need to be adjusted.

When inserting needles it is preferable to have the patient supported because of a slight possibility of needle shock causing the patient to faint. This is rare but can happen when Aggressive Energy is checked, as needle shock is most likely to occur during the first treatment (for more on needle shock, see Chapter 34). To support the patient, place a chair sideways against a treatment couch. Patients can either fold their arms loosely in their lap or rest their hands on the couch.

On the rare occasions that a patient faints while Aggressive Energy is being checked, it is best to test again at the next treatment but with the patient lying down in a prone position. In this case the practitioner should ensure their arms are stretched out to the sides to open up the space between scapula and the spine. The upper thoracic rib spaces are located slightly higher in this position than when the patient is sitting up.

The testing process

To check for the presence of Aggressive Energy, needles are placed in the back *shu* points. Aggressive Energy is found in the *yin* Organs of the body. These *shu* points connect directly to the *yin* Organs and are used for 'draining' the Aggressive Energy. 'Draining' is the term used when the practitioner finds that Aggressive Energy is present and treats it by leaving the needles in. To test for Aggressive Energy:

* insert needles into the back *shu* points of the *yin* Organs, i.e. Lung, Pericardium, Liver, Spleen and Kidney (not the Heart). Leave the needles in place
* place a unilateral 'check' or 'dummy' needle about an inch away from each level of back *shu* points and at the same level and depth. Leave these needles in place

Figure 30.4 shows the needles in place on a patient who is being tested for Aggressive Energy (Table 30.1).

Needle depth

When testing for Aggressive Energy the needles are inserted just under the surface of the skin to a depth of approximately 0.1 *cun*. This superficial insertion helps to draw the Aggressive Energy from the Organs at the same time as ensuring that it is not driven deeper into the body. If the needles are inserted more deeply they are likely to have a slight sedating effect on the Organs, which is not the intention of the treatment.

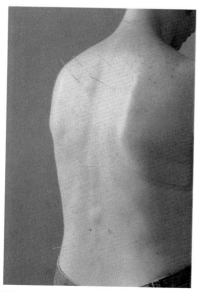

Figure 30.4 • Needles used for Aggressive Energy

Table 30.1 Points used to treat Aggressive Energy

Point	Back *Shu* point of which Organ
Bl 13	Lung
Bl 14	Pericardium
Bl 15	Heart (only if necessary)
Bl 18	Liver
Bl 20	Spleen
Bl 23	Kidney

Testing the Heart

It is best not to place needles in the back *shu* point of the Heart unnecessarily for two reasons. Firstly, the Pericardium is the protector of the Heart, so if the Fire Element has Aggressive Energy the Pericardium will usually be affected rather than the Heart. Secondly, long-term retention of needles could unnecessarily drain the Heart *qi*.

The practitioner should test the Heart if:

* Aggressive Energy is present on the Pericardium – in this case it may also be present in the Heart.
* Aggressive Energy is present on the Kidney and Lung but not on the Pericardium. In this case the Aggressive Energy is on two legs of the *ke* cycle and may have travelled through the Heart rather than the Pericardium.
* The Heart pulse or Heart signs and symptoms show disturbance as on rare occasions sometimes Aggressive Energy can be present on the Heart alone.

Signs of the presence of Aggressive Energy

Aggressive Energy is present if:

* an erythema (reddening of the skin) appears around the main needle and *not* the check needle. This indicates the presence of Aggressive Energy in the Organs. The erythema may be present for anything from 30 seconds to one hour
* there are significant changes in the patient's pulses or colour, sound, emotion and/or odour.

Aggressive Energy is not present if:

- no erythema appears round any of the needles
- the erythema is the same or more on the check needles than on the needles in the back *shu* points
- there are few or no changes in the pulses or colour, sound, odour and emotion

Procedure if Aggressive Energy is present

If Aggressive Energy is suspected, leave the needles in place until all of the erythema disappears in order to fully clear the Aggressive Energy from the Organs.

Sometimes Aggressive Energy may be cleared in 10 or 20 minutes or less, but there are other times when it can take up to an hour for the erythema to disappear. It is important that the needles are not removed until all the erythema has cleared or some of the toxicity will be left in the body.

Aggressive Energy is not a common condition and is found in approximately 1% of patients.

Possible causes of erythema that are not Aggressive Energy

Sometimes an erythema arises on the skin but it is not Aggressive Energy. There are several reasons for this.

Sensitive skin

Pale-skinned people are likely to have more reactive skin than people with darker skin or hair. The presence of a dummy needle which is not in an acupuncture point ensures that a reddening due to skin sensitivity is not mistaken for Aggressive Energy.

Too many needle insertions in a small area

If a needle seems to be slightly misplaced on the first insertion the practitioner may wish to remove it and place it in a new position or insert another needle close to it. Inserting additional needles ensures that the correct point has been needled so that all Aggressive Energy is removed. At the same time, the additional insertions may cause the skin to react and become redder and give a false indication of Aggressive Energy.

Other congestion or toxicity

Erythema can appear around a needle if there is tightness, spasm or heat in the underlying muscles rather than in the organs.

Reactions to treatment

After Aggressive Energy has been removed from the patient's system she or he will generally report feeling different. Sometimes this can be dramatic. Often the patient reports feeling 'better in myself' as well as a significant improvement in symptoms at the next treatment session. Sometimes a patient feels very tired immediately after treatment followed by a feeling of being re-energised. Signs and symptoms vary according to each individual patient.

Patient Example

A patient was being tested for Aggressive Energy in a student clinic. His face looked puffy and red and he was so angry he looked ready to explode. Fifteen minutes later, on opening the door of the treatment room, the supervisor momentarily thought he was in the wrong room. He had failed to recognise the patient, who had changed dramatically. He now looked somehow smaller and paler, calm and quiet.

Subsequent treatment

If a patient has Aggressive Energy it is best to re-check at the next treatment to ensure that it has all been cleared. Sometimes more Aggressive Energy comes up after the first draining. This is unlikely to happen more than once or twice provided that it has been fully cleared at each treatment.

As long as no other blocks are present, regular treatment can continue after all Aggressive Energy has been cleared.

Summary

1 Aggressive Energy is a form of unhealthy (*xie*) *qi*. Its cause can be external or internal and the resulting stagnation usually turns to heat and is then trapped in the *yin* Organs.

2 Aggressive Energy travels between the *yin* Organs connected along the *ke* cycle.

3 The presence of Aggressive Energy can cause severe and possibly life-threatening illnesses.

4 Aggressive Energy is checked by placing needles in the back *shu* points of the *yin* Organs. It is present if an erythema appears around the needles (but not the 'dummy' needles). The needles are then left in place to drain the Aggressive Energy.

When the erythema disappears the Aggressive Energy has been cleared.

5 If Aggressive Energy has been present the patient experiences significant improvement in health and the pulses and/or colour, sound, emotion and odour often change as a result of the treatment.

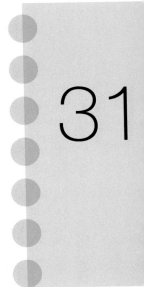

Possession

31

CHAPTER CONTENTS

What is possession?

The nature of possession

Clearing possession is one of the oldest forms of healing known to civilisation. In fact, there are many indications that clearing possession in early China was a more prevalent system of healing than acupuncture.[1] People in the Western world might describe it as being out of date and perhaps even rather over-dramatic, but the term is one that has been used in every culture in the world, including the modern-day Western culture.

In most ancient cultures the concept of possession described someone being fully or partially taken over by an entity of some kind. This caused people to no longer be fully in control of a part of themselves. The entity was usually thought to be the spirit of a dead person who was trying to find another body to inhabit.

---

[1]There are many indications in ancient Chinese texts that 'demonological' healing was prevalent in China from the earliest of times and continued to be used alongside other forms of Chinese medicine until the present day. Many serious works of Chinese medicine by renowned Chinese doctors had sections in them with suggestions for demonological treatments of certain ailments (see Unschuld, 1992, p. 216).

In China this spirit was called a *gui*. Interestingly, the radical for a *gui* is embedded in the character for both the *hun* (spirit of the Liver) and the *po* (spirit of the Lungs), two of the five *shen*. This indicates the level of belief in the world of spirits that was prevalent amongst the physicians during the Han and preceding dynasties. The idea that part of the human spirit inhabited the same realm as ghosts was enshrined in Chinese thought.

The use of the term 'possession' by a Five Element Constitutional Acupuncturist has been broadened. It is used to include many other ways that a person may be out of control of their mind and spirit. Signs and symptoms can manifest along a spectrum from obsessive thoughts or behaviour to the kind of possession by spirits described above.

Historically there have been many powerful methods that have been used to clear possessions. These have included magic and ritual as well as talisman and herbal prescriptions (Unschuld, 1992, pp. 29–50). The method used by Five Element Constitutional Acupuncturists to clear possession is to call on the 'Seven Dragons to overpower the Seven Demons'. The treatment uses seven acupuncture points that 'wake' the Dragons.

Possession in ancient China

The belief in possession as a cause of illness is widely documented as far back as the early Chou period, around −1100. At this time a person was typically described as being 'assaulted by demons' or 'possessed by the hostile' (Unschuld, 1992, p. 36).

The existence of evil spirits was not just a superstition but was a widely held belief amongst all classes of Chinese people for many centuries. Han Fei, who died in −233, stated: 'When a person falls ill he has been injured by a demon' (Unschuld, 1992, p. 37).

Later texts, especially many written from the sixteenth century onwards, described treatments in detail. For example, in the eighteenth century a physician called Xu Dachun cited 'irrefutable evidence' for the influence of demons on the well-being of man. He compared evil spirits to wind, cold, summer heat and other similar phenomena. Just as an underlying deficiency can allow a climatic pathogen to enter the body, so can an 'emotional fatigue' allow demons to gain entrance (Unschuld, 1992, p. 222).

The famous physician Sun Si-miao (581–682) also described various methods of treatment against demons (Unschuld, 1992, p. 42). One method described was the use of 13 *gui* or 'ghost' points. These are still in use today, especially in the treatment of the *dian-kuan* category of disease, which includes illnesses such as schizophrenia or bipolar disorder.

Since the Communist government came into power in 1949 the treatment of possession was cast out of Chinese medicine. At that time anything connected with popular religious belief was termed 'superstition' (*mixin*). It is still to be found in Chinese communities around the world, however, but a 'great deal of administrative effort has gone into eradicating belief in spirit possession' (see Sivin, 1987, pp. 102–106). Bob Flaws (1991) states that:

> The expurgation of ghosts as an etiological factor is part and parcel of modern TCM's attempt to conform to Western materialist science and the Chinese communist regime's rejection of anything spiritual.

Certainly the use of the 'Seven Dragons for Seven Demons' is not mentioned in any currently translated Chinese texts. It was, however, identified as a Tang dynasty prescription for 'mania' by a veteran Chinese medicine physician at the Yunnan College of TCM in Kunming in 1982 (verbal communication from members of China Study Trip, 1982). Bob Flaws concurs that there is 'nothing un-Chinese about the treatment'. Such a treatment is in fact 'characteristic of the Chinese people's pluralism and enduring embrace of spiritualism and magic' (Flaws, 1989).

Vulnerability to possession

Conditions leading to possession

The causes of possession can be external or internal and it can result from a physical, but more usually, a mental or spiritual cause. However, it is extremely rare for something to 'invade' from the outside or to disturb the person from the inside if the person is in good physical, mental and spiritual health.

> If a person's essence and spirit are firmly established, no evil outside of the body will venture an assault. But whenever that which protects the essence and spirit fails, the harmful agents will collect in its place.
>
> (Hsu Ling-t'ai I; quoted by Unschuld, 1992, p. 337)

The topics, images, feelings and themes that disturb people are usually the ones that may later possess her or him. A mind preoccupied by certain thoughts can start to become obsessed. If the obsession is not contained and dealt with it may later turn into a 'possession' that takes control of the person's every thought and action.

> Minds occupied with fortune and misfortune may be invaded and controlled by devils. Minds occupied with love affairs may be attacked by lustful ghosts. Minds worried about deep waters may be subjected to the ghosts of the drowned. Minds worried by unrestrained activity may be attacked by mad ghosts. Minds occupied with oaths may be attacked by magical ghosts. Minds concentrated on drugs and tempting food may be attacked by the ghosts of material things.
>
> (Quan Yin Tzu, quoted in Needham, 1956, p. 67)

A person's vulnerability to possession is increased by:

- underlying poor physical or psychological health
- emotional shocks or instability
- physical shocks or accidents
- drug or alcohol abuse
- engaging with the occult
- opening the self up to others, without protection
- exposure to intense climatic factors

Underlying poor physical or psychological health

The underlying health of a person is extremely important when considering who is vulnerable to possession. The pathologies below illustrate this, but a weakness in *any* Organ may cause a person to become more susceptible.

The Blood of the Heart allows the *shen* to be housed in the body. When the Heart Blood is deficient, the *shen* will 'float' rather than be settled inside the Heart (see Maciocia, 2005, pp. 109-112). If this becomes severe it can leave a void. In this case the Supreme Controller is no longer fully in control and the person may lose full control of their mind and spirit.

Obstruction to the Heart orifices may leave a person more easily affected by possession. If there is too much Heat and Phlegm affecting the Heart, a person may also have difficulty being settled in their *shen*. This condition can result in mania followed by a swing into depression. In this situation the person's health is already chaotic and the vacuum left by the unsettled *shen* may leave the person even more susceptible to possession. The same is true when Phlegm 'mists' the Heart, causing mental confusion or unconsciousness. (For a discussion of Phlegm Fire harassing the Heart, see Maciocia, 2005, pp. 474–477.)

If the Lungs are healthy this can also protect a person from becoming possessed. Just as the Lungs are responsible for the *wei qi*, which protects us from invasion by climatic forces, the Corporeal Soul or *po* protects us from invasion affecting the spirit (Maciocia, 1993, pp. 10–18). A person whose Metal Element is thus affected may feel extremely fragile in some circumstances. They may feel unable to protect themselves when, for example, they are grieving after a death or in any situation where sadness or a sense of loss is intense.

Emotional shocks or instability

Emotional shocks can be caused by sudden grief, sadness, disappointment, anger, fear, terror or even sudden and extreme happiness. Often, although not always, an emotional shock involves another person – an intimate relationship breaks up, a friend badly disappoints us, a family member dies or a work colleague suddenly turns on us. An emotional shock of any kind can leave people feeling traumatised and temporarily out of control. The *qi* is 'scattered'. In most circumstances people recover their equilibrium following the initial shock. On some occasions, however, they do not recover their former control and the intensity of the emotions overwhelms the mind and spirit.

People have varying degrees of emotional stability. Those with a damaged sense of identity may be anxious, lonely, depressed and in general have a low level of self-esteem. This may lead to obsessive or addictive behaviour directed towards areas such as work, sex, cleanliness, food, gambling or alcohol.

Patient Example

A patient was being treated for a sinus problem. At every treatment she talked about her ex-boyfriend. She couldn't get over this relationship, which had ended suddenly. In her experience, one minute he was with her, the next he was gone. She was now thinking about him constantly. She seemed obsessed by him. Following the Internal Dragons treatment she reported feeling 'separate from him' for the first time since the relationship ended.

Physical shocks or accidents

These can include a huge range of possibilities such as road traffic accidents, surgical operations, electric shocks including ECT (electro-convulsive therapy) or physical injuries such as those brought about by being beaten up or physically abused. The *shen* is usually affected when a person has a severe physical shock or accident. In these circumstances the *shen* may be temporarily 'separated' from the body so that it is no longer housed in the Heart. This leaves the person more vulnerable to possession.

Patient Example

A patient had three car accidents in quick succession. This left her extremely shaken, feeling 'cut off from reality' and a feeling that she described as 'being half out of my body'. When CF treatment didn't help, the possession treatment was carried out enabling the patient to feel more in control again. She immediately felt more stable and 'in her body'.

Drug or alcohol abuse

Alcohol and drug abusers are often susceptible to possession. They suffer from the reasons that led them to substance abuse and the abuse further weakens their healthy or upright (*zheng*) qi. When

A patient came for treatment having had a 14-year history of taking many drugs, including amphetamines, LSD and cocaine. Possession treatments, using both the Internal and External Dragons were used, as well as treatment on his CF. The treatment helped him to recover from the effects of the drugs. Although he did not know about the nature of the points being used, the patient commented that treatment 'had seemed like an "exorcism".' (For more on this case history, see Hicks, Chapter 38, p. 425, in MacPherson and Kaptchuk, 1997.)

under the influence of drugs, their minds are sometimes open and susceptible. The five *shen* become disturbed and the mind then becomes open to invasion. Sometimes after a time on drugs and/or alcohol, the person's mind may be inert and empty, as if no one is at home. This void predisposes them to 'possession'.

Engaging with the occult

This includes playing with magic, 'doing' automatic writing, holding seances or using an ouija board. All of these activities can involve calling on 'spirits' for 'help'. It has been known that a person who is spiritually vulnerable may experience being taken over by a 'malevolent' spirit who subsequently seems to plague them with negative thoughts and feelings.

Patient Example

A 25-year-old patient came for treatment having held seances using an ouija board when she was 14 years old. Since that time she had been terrified of being alone in the dark and said she continually felt strange 'presences' around her. She felt the need to wear a crucifix around her neck to protect herself. Treatment using the Internal Dragons helped to rid her of these 'presences'.

Opening the self up to others, without protection

Followers of cults or people who are under the influence of charismatic leaders, witch doctors or anyone who uses hypnotic power in a negative way can come into this category. Although most meditation or spiritual work is safe, in the wrong hands it can become

harmful. If people obey others without question and follow spiritual 'rules' without understanding what they are doing, they can end up being controlled by the cult or the leader of the cult.

Patient Example

Followers of the Reverend Jim Jones in Jonestown, Guyana, appear to have given over parts of themselves to him. In 1978 the whole group of 910 people took their own lives in an orderly fashion when ordered to do so by their leader. (For more analysis about this event see Cialdini, 2001, pp. 131–133.)

Exposure to intense climatic factors

The external climatic factors may cause conditions such as Heat-stroke or an extreme attack of Dampness, Wind or any other external pathogenic factor. When a climatic factor causes possession the patient is likely to have been subjected to a long-term or extreme pathogen which has penetrated deeply and thus taken over the patient's system. The External Dragons are often used first in these cases.

Patient Example

During World War II a patient had worked in the engine room of a ship travelling from East Africa to India. It was in the hottest part of the year. During the trip he went 'mad' and became manic and paranoid. Forty years later he visited an acupuncturist because he was unable to hold down a job, had behavioural obsessions and paranoid fantasies. Treatment using the External Dragons was carried out. He became able to retain a job; the behavioural obsessions were dramatically reduced; and he no longer had the paranoid fantasies.

The diagnosis of possession

Signs and symptoms of possession

Practitioners may be alerted to the possibility of patients being possessed if they have been in one of the situations or internal states outlined above. Not all patients who are possessed have been subject to these circumstances, however, and sometimes it is hard for the practitioner to be sure that possession is present. In this case the practitioner will make the diagnosis on the patient's presentation. One key sign is that something about the patient is extremely unusual.

Every patient who is possessed is possessed in their own unique way. If possession is suspected it is best to use the Seven Dragons treatment immediately. If possession is not present, the treatment will tend to have no effect. If possession is present, however, it can transform the patient and make subsequent treatment effective. Although none of the signs and symptoms below is in itself a sure diagnostic sign of possession, the following are some areas that can strongly indicate that possession is a possibility.

- The eyes are veiled and the practitioner can't get 'into' the person.
- Abnormal mental patterns are revealed in speech or behaviour.
- The patient experiences intense dreams or fantasies that are terrifying or evil.
- The patient hears voices in the mind.
- The patient exhibits obsessions or addictive behaviour.
- Patients say they 'feel' possessed or out of control.
- Treatment doesn't progress or the patient keeps relapsing.
- Pulses are unusual or lacking harmony.

Eyes are veiled and the practitioner can't 'reach' the person

People's eyes often give the clearest indication that they are possessed. When making eye contact people usually feel some connection with another person. When a person is possessed, this connection is hard to make. It may seem as 'though the lights are on but no one is at home', or that the eyes have a veil in front of them or a glazed look. Sometimes patients can't hold someone else's gaze and their eyes slide away or become shifty. There may be a crazed expression in the person's eyes.

Other descriptions of the eyes of possessed patients are a 'staring quality', a 'deadness' in the eyes, 'an inability to look in other people's eyes' or, at the extreme, 'someone else is staring out from the eyes'.

None of these descriptions is in itself a diagnosis of possession. For instance, a dead look in the eyes or an inability to look into another person's eyes could also indicate that the Heart is seriously out of balance. A staring quality could indicate a problem with the Liver.

Abnormal mind patterns as revealed in speech or behaviour

In some circumstances it is virtually impossible to take a case history from a patient. This can happen, for example, if patients are incapable of answering questions, virtually catatonic or extremely agitated. The practitioner may find that it is impossible to make any significant rapport with them and their spirit may seem to barely be present in the room. In this case the practitioner may conclude that the patient's behaviour or the workings of their mind are so unusual that they may well be possessed.

Intense dreams or fantasies that are terrifying or evil

Recurrent terrifying or evil dreams can indicate possession. Examples of dreams that have indicated possession have been dreams of monsters, of small scaly creatures, of ghosts or of being taken over by another person. In one case a child who continually had dreams of evil monsters had this treatment, after which she never had the dream again.

Images that haunt a person while they are awake can also indicate possession. These might either be of a particular memory, or in some cases can be of a particular symbol. For example, one patient almost constantly had an image of swastikas in his mind.

Voices in the mind

These might be controlling, obsessive or out of character with the person's normal personality. The voices may say things that are negative or taunting or they may predict negative things. They may make the person feel guilty or tell the person to do things they don't feel they should do. They may be clear or indistinct. If they are clear and intense, the person may have already been diagnosed as having a mental illness such as schizophrenia. At this level of disharmony it can be difficult to restore the patient to a relatively healthy state. Sometimes, however, this treatment may have a significant effect, and can be repeated over a course of treatment with further benefits.

Obsessions or addictive behaviour

This category can overlap with the previous one above but differs in that the patient feels that the thoughts are their own. Everyone at some time has had thoughts that become stuck in their head. For example, most people have experienced having the words of a catchy song going around their heads, and this is obviously not possession. Possession is more likely to be indicated by thoughts that take over the functioning of the mind. For example, if a patient has negative thoughts such as ones of wanting to do harm to another or themselves or feeling constantly negative about themselves, then this might indicate possession. The key is to discover whether the person has any control over the thoughts or whether the person cannot stop or change them.

Some people become fixated with some aspect of their life. They might constantly perform some obsessive action such as washing their hands, cleaning the house or locking the door. Other people feel they have to carry out some ritual, such as touching something a certain number of times before being able to go about their daily lives. Some people's lives are taken over by a particular phobia. They may be unable to stop themselves swearing, eating, talking or having bizarre bodily movements. All of these and many other extraordinary behaviours can be indicative of possession.

Patients say they 'feel' possessed or out of control

Patients may describe being out of control of their feelings. They may have outbursts of anger or rage for no clear reason or excessive fear that takes them over. Alternatively, it has been known for patients to confide to the practitioner that they feel possessed or as if they have been taken over by some kind of force. They may also make comments like, 'I feel I've got the devil in me' or 'I don't feel in control of what I do.' Some patients also say that they feel the presence of spirits around them.

Treatment doesn't progress or the patient keeps relapsing

Sometimes it is hard for the practitioner to notice any of the above signs and symptoms of possession, but at the same time they may know that acupuncture treatment is not having any significant effect. Alternatively the treatment might have some effect, but doesn't hold and the patient relapses. Either of these situations may indicate that the person needs the Dragons treatment as there is something preventing the treatment from helping the patient to progress.

Pulses not in harmony

Very rarely a patient can become possessed while under treatment. In this case the practitioner might notice that the quality of the pulses becomes much less harmonious. If the patient is possessed at the start of treatment, then a similar presentation may occur. In this situation the practitioner is unable to compare the pulses with any previous pulse pictures and the lack of harmony may not be so obvious. Because of this the practitioner will sometimes explain away this disharmony by other aspects of the diagnosis.

Choosing the Internal or External Dragons

After diagnosing that the patient is possessed, the next decision is whether the External or Internal Dragons are required. If the cause of the patient's problem is obviously from an internal cause (such as emotional shocks, instability or poor psychological health), then the Internal Dragons should be used. If the cause is obviously from an external cause (such as drinking, drugs or overexposure to the elements), then the External Dragons should be used. Having said this, it is not always clear to the practitioner if the cause is internal or external.

If this is the case it tends to be best to use the Internal Dragons first, as these are usually the most effective. If this does not make a change, the External Dragons are then used.

The treatment of possession

(Table 31.1)

The Seven Dragons treatment

Traditionally in China dragons have been regarded as having a benevolent influence. They symbolise power and justice and are thought to bring good fortune and wealth. Their image was worn on the robes of the imperial family and nobility indicating their great authority.

The Seven Dragons treatment uses combinations of seven points. Each point wakens and rouses a Dragon and the seven chase the Devils out. Practitioners sometimes ask why these particular points are used. Although there is no definitive answer to this, the following may be some explanation. The Internal Dragons are on the front or *yin* side of the body and *yin* is resonant with the most internal areas of us. The first point lies on the *Ren* channel that is the most *yin* channel of the body and the others lie on the Stomach channel close to the *Ren*.

The External Dragons are on the back or most *yang* side of the body and *yang* is resonant with the most external areas of us. The first point lies on the *Du* channel that is the most *yang* channel of the body and all the other points lie on the Bladder channel which lies next to the *Du* channel.

The points used for the Internal Dragons

For the Internal Dragons, the points used are:

- the extra point 0.25 *cun* below *Ren* 15
- St 25
- St 32
- St 41

(An alternative combination of points was taught during the 1970s and early 1980s which can be used if a patient is depressed. They are: the extra point 0.25 *cun* below *Ren* 15, St 25, a point halfway between St 36 and St 37 and St 41.)

The points used for the External Dragons

For the External Dragons, the points used are:

- *Du* 20
- Bl 11
- Bl 23
- Bl 61

Position of the patient

Internal Dragons

The patient should be lying comfortably on the back, with their arms by their sides and their legs extended.

External Dragons

When using the External Dragons it is easiest to have the patient sitting up on a stool facing the treatment table. This means that the practitioner needs to locate Bl 61 while the feet are on the floor. If the practitioner seats the patient on a chair, then it should be placed sideways on to the table so that

Table 31.1 Points used for the Seven Internal or External Dragons

Internal Dragons	External Dragons
Extra point 0.25 *cun* below *Ren* 15	*Du* 20
St 25	Bl 11
St 32	Bl 23
St 41	Bl 61

the practitioner can locate the points on the patient's back. Once the needles have been inserted, patients can then support themselves by folding their arms and putting them up on the table. Tall patients might need a pillow under their arms.

Alternatively, it is possible to mark the External Dragons with the patient lying face down on the treatment table. This may be preferable if the patient is large or if the practitioner thinks they may be difficult to support if there is a strong reaction to the treatment.

Carrying out the treatment

The needles should be inserted into the points from top to bottom using sedation technique. (For clarification of this technique, see Chapter 33, this volume.) The needles should then be left in position until the pulses have harmonised or a change can be detected in the patient. This will usually take approximately 20–30 minutes. Special attention should always be paid to the patient's eyes, as they are likely to be clearer, steadier or less veiled when the treatment is completed. The patient's colour, sound, emotion and odour may also change during the course of the treatment. The needles are then removed from top to bottom.

Reactions at the time of treatment

A few patients have immediate and dramatic reactions at the time of treatment. For example, some patients have shaken, shivered, made strange noises, taken on unusual facial expressions or felt sick during the course of the treatment. Some patients can have a reaction after treatment, for example, one patient had a dream of a 'spirit' being in the room with her and then leaving. Others may feel tired after the treatment or alternatively they may feel energised.

At the other extreme, most patients have no reaction at the time of the treatment at all. Often they feel extremely relaxed as the treatment is carried out, only to notice a change sometime afterwards.

Changes from treatment

Patients often undergo a fundamental transformation and release from this treatment. The signs or symptoms of possession should recede if the treatment has been successful. Sometimes patients will describe feeling lighter, freer or more in control of their life. Others have known that they feel better but find it hard to describe what has changed.

Repetition of the treatment

Often only one treatment is necessary, but some patients may need more than one treatment. In some cases, the patient is better for a period and normal treatment has good effects. However, the possession can return with similar signs and symptoms, but less intense. In this case the treatment should be repeated. In unusual cases, the practitioner may end up doing several repeat possession treatments, interspersed by non-possession treatments.

Summary

1 Possession is a cause of disease that is widely documented in many Chinese texts.

2 There are many signs and symptoms of possession. For example, it can manifest as obsessive behaviour or the person feeling that he or she has been taken over by spirits. The person may have veiled eyes, terrifying or evil dreams, voices in the mind, stuck thoughts or treatment which keeps relapsing.

3 A range of other situations increases a person's vulnerability to possession, but often when a person becomes possessed they have underlying poor psychological health or are under severe emotional strain.

4 The Seven Dragons for Seven Demons are points used to clear possession. These can be internal or external.

5 If the possession is cleared, a patient may experience a fundamental transformation and release following the treatment.

Husband–Wife imbalance

What is a Husband–Wife imbalance?

A Husband–Wife imbalance arises when the Organs associated with the pulses on the left wrist, the 'husband' side, have lost harmony with the Organs associated with the pulses on the right wrist. The overall quality and quantity of the pulses on the left side should normally be slightly stronger than the ones on the right side. If instead the right side is stronger, a Husband–Wife imbalance may be present.

A Husband–Wife imbalance indicates a severe and deep imbalance which, if left untreated, can be life-threatening in some cases. It has been said that it is the most dangerous of the four blocks to treatment as it is a sign that 'Nature is giving up and the inner healing resources of the person are becoming power-less' (Worsley, 1990, p. 180). Patients nearing the end of their lives may manifest this imbalance – although it may be difficult to correct at this stage. If it is corrected, however, it can have the effect of prolonging the patient's life.

The use of the term 'Husband–Wife'

When we use the term 'Husband–Wife' we need to bear in mind that China has always been a predomi-nantly patriarchal society and this metaphor would have seemed more apt to a practitioner in ancient China. A Chinese saying about this imbalance states:

> Weak husband, robust wife; then there is destruction,
> Strong husband, weak wife; then there is security.
>
> (Soulié de Morant, 1994, p. 122)

In this context the left-hand pulses (the Heart and Small Intestine, Liver and Gall Bladder, Kidney and Bladder) are connected with the husband. In general men are more *yang* in body type and are physically larger and more powerful than women. In ancient societies they would be the hunters and gatherers who went out searching for food. We would expect the pulses to reflect this and be stronger.

The right-hand pulses (the Lung and Large Intes-tine, Spleen and Stomach, Pericardium and Triple Burner) are associated with the wife. In general women are physically smaller and more *yin* in body type than men. Women are more often the home-makers. This was certainly true in ancient China, although it is less true today. The pulses of the wife would therefore be expected to reflect this situation by being slightly weaker.

The term 'Husband–Wife' reflects the Chinese culture. Today this imbalance would doubtless be labelled differently.

We can also think of the Husband–Wife in terms of *yin* and *yang* (this was also suggested in Worsley, 1990, p. 180). In this case we can define it by stating that the *yin* and *yang* energies are severely out of harmony, which the Chinese thought was a forewarning of death. The separation of the *yin* and *yang* creates an alienation from the person's true self at a fundamental level. This following quotation demonstrates the importance of the two qualities of fire (*yang*) and water (*yin*) in the relationship between husband and wife:

> When the 'wife' follows the husband, water and fire balance each other.

(Liu Yiming; quoted in Cleary, 2001, p. 34)

(Using the term 'fire' to represent *yang* and 'water' to represent *yin* is not using these terms in a Five Element context, but more a *yin/yang* context.)

Diagnosis of a Husband–Wife imbalance

Pulse diagnosis of a Husband–Wife imbalance

The main method of diagnosing a Husband–Wife imbalance is by pulse diagnosis. The pulses on the left-hand side should be slightly stronger in quality and quantity than those on the right. When this imbalance is present, the right side may be felt as hard, tight and aggressive in nature and the ones on the left weak, feeble and flaccid. There will usually be a difference in strength as well as in the qualities on the pulses. Care must be taken not to make a diagnosis purely based upon pulse diagnosis. Some people have abnormal radial arteries on one of their wrists. Diagnosis should be based on a combination of pulse diagnosis and at least one of the following signs or symptoms.

Other signs and symptoms of a Husband–Wife imbalance

Pulse diagnosis always needs to be confirmed by other signs and symptoms that are affecting the person's health. Severe and uncontrolled disharmony of the patient's *qi* is the distinguishing feature of a Husband–Wife imbalance. It may be primarily affecting the body, mind or spirit. Signs and symptoms include:

- The patient has a serious or life-threatening illness.
- The patient has extreme internal conflicts, often involving their sexuality or relationship issues.
- The patient is resigned or fearful at a deep level.
- The patient's mind is disturbed or in turmoil.
- The patient may have aggravations if treated on channels of the right-hand pulse side or the patient may relapse or not change from normal treatments.

The patient has a serious or life-threatening illness

As stated above, many people have this imbalance when their life is coming to an end. Their minds and spirits might still be strong and vital, but their body is dying. The condition may be too advanced to reverse by this stage. Even if it is reversed, this may be only temporary and the imbalance reappears. However, if it can be reversed, continued treatment can bring about a remission and renewed health.

Patient Example

A patient came to treatment having been diagnosed with an aggressive form of ovarian cancer. She attributed the onset of the cancer to a combination of overwork and intense feelings of resentment towards her husband for his withdrawn behaviour. After chemotherapy she was given a maximum of 12 months to live. Her CA 125 count was over 4000 (normal is 20). Continued treatment of a Husband–Wife imbalance brought about a radical change in her pulses. At the time of writing, six years after the start of treatment, she is alive and well. Her CA 125 count is 18. She leads a much more independent life from her husband than previously and no longer resents him.

The patient has extreme internal conflicts involving their sexuality or relationship issues

Sometimes patients with this imbalance have had sexual or relationship problems that they are unable to resolve. Unlike the example above, in most of these cases the patient does not have a terminal illness. The Husband–Wife imbalance is affecting their spirit rather than their body. The patient often feels that she or he is caught in an unresolvable situation. For example, there may be a history of sexual abuse or a severe conflict when young with an older family member. Sometimes a patient may describe insurmountable difficulties in a personal relationship that they feel unable to resolve. A common pattern is a history of relationships that flourish for a period and then go wrong, for no apparent reason.

Patient Example

A patient came for treatment saying that she didn't know whether to leave her husband. She was thinking of it constantly and obsessively, but was unable to act. Her pulses indicated that she had a Husband–Wife imbalance that the practitioner treated. The patient came to the next treatment saying that she now felt much happier in her relationship and there was no longer an issue about leaving. The practitioner continued to treat the patient as a Metal CF and yet the patient relapsed a few sessions later and again felt conflict about the relationship. What emerged at this point was her memory of early sexual abuse. The eventual successful result involved treatment that strengthened the CF, periodically addressed the tendency to a Husband–Wife imbalance and psychotherapy that addressed the early sexual abuse.

The patient is resigned or fearful at a deep level

This imbalance is often accompanied by a deep sense of resignation or fear. For example, a patient may describe feeling numb or desperate or give the impression of having given up or of feeling hopeless inside. In these cases desperate fear often precedes the resignation. This fear can be all pervasive but the person is often unable to relate it to any particular threat. It sometimes manifests as an excessive fear of their own death, which they may feel is approaching rapidly. When people lose the will to live, a Husband–Wife imbalance is often present.

One characteristic of this condition is that some issues that were once fundamental certainties are called into question. For example, patients may become confused about whether they want to live or die, which gender they are or how to relate to others.

Patient Example

A male patient, in his mid-twenties, was suffering from 'panic attacks' and depression. After sufficient rapport had been established, he revealed that he was tormented by guilt and confusion over whether he was homosexual or not. Pulse diagnosis, coupled with the intense nature of his internal conflict, indicated a Husband–Wife imbalance. Treatment yielded no improvement for four treatments but with repeated Husband–Wife treatments he suddenly started to respond. After six treatments he was feeling much less troubled. Very soon afterwards he decided that he definitely was homosexual and has been in no doubt or regret about his sexuality ever since.

The patient's mind is disturbed or in turmoil

In young and middle-aged people the Husband–Wife imbalance usually affects the mind or spirit rather than the body. We are not describing patients who are suffering from 'common unhappiness', some confusion or anxiety. If a Husband–Wife imbalance is present the patient's mind or spirit is in profound turmoil or distress. Being 'in turmoil' can take many different forms and it is impossible to describe them all. Each time a practitioner sees a patient with this condition, they see it manifesting in a different way. To misquote Tolstoy, 'All happy people resemble one another, each unhappy person is unhappy in his or her own way.'

Patient Example

A patient in her mid-thirties had been a senior psychiatric nurse, with some responsibility for money. She had succumbed to temptation, had stolen some of the money and had subsequently been sacked. This had been very difficult for her to deal with but she was bearing up. Some months later the disciplinary hearing finally took place and the verdict was printed in the local paper. This threw her into a complete state of panic and her feelings of shame overwhelmed her. She became extremely depressed and suffered panic attacks when she went out, fearing that people would recognise and confront her. Pulse diagnosis, coupled with the intense fear and internal conflict, indicated a Husband–Wife imbalance. Treatment of this imbalance and strengthening her CF helped her to rediscover a level of happiness and confidence.

The patient may have aggravations if treated on channels of the right-hand pulse side or the patient may relapse or not change from normal treatments

If the Husband–Wife imbalance is not diagnosed, there is a danger that the practitioner may unwittingly strengthen the imbalance by tonifying the

---

Patient Example

A practitioner treated a patient on his Stomach and Spleen. He returned to the pulses and expected to find increased harmony. Instead the practitioner found the pulses on the right-hand side surprisingly wiry and hard whilst those on the left became weaker. Along with other symptoms this indicated a Husband–Wife imbalance, which the practitioner then treated.

Organs represented by the right-hand pulses. If this happens the practitioner may find that the pulse picture changes to one of even greater imbalance between the left and right sides. Although not ideal, this can be a reliable method of diagnosis.

Treatment of a Husband–Wife imbalance (Table 32.1)

Treatment of a Husband–Wife imbalance aims to re-establish harmony between the pulses on the two sides by pulling *qi* over from the right side to

Table 32.1 Points used to rebalance a Husband–Wife imbalance

Point	Type of point	Action
Bl 67	Tonification point	Transfers *qi* from Large Intestine to Bladder
Kid 7	Tonification point	Transfers *qi* from Lung to Kidney
Kid 3	Earth point	Transfers *qi* from Spleen to Kidney
Liv 4	Metal point	Transfers *qi* from Lung to Liver
Can also use:		
Ht 7	Source point	Balances the Heart
SI 4	Source point	Balances the Small Intestine

the left side. The pulses of the right side represent the Fire (PC/TB), Earth and Metal Elements, while those on the left side represent the Water, Wood and Fire (Ht/SI) Elements. Figure 32.1 shows their connection on the *sheng* and *ke* cycles.

The balance between the left and right sides can be restored by transferring *qi* across the *sheng* and *ke* cycles (see Chapter 36 for more details). This can be done in the following way:

- via the *sheng* cycle from Metal to Water using Bl 67 and Kid 7, the tonification points
- via the *ke* cycle from Earth to Water using Kid 3
- via the *ke* cycle from Metal to Wood using Liv 4

This is illustrated in Figure 32.2. The points should all be tonified bilaterally without retention. The transfer of *qi* from the right to the left side enables the side of the husband to become stronger and to once again take control.

Points along the channels of the right side (i.e. Lu/LI, St/Sp and PC/TB) should not be tonified, as this can strengthen the imbalance.

It can be useful as part of the treatment to balance the Heart and the Small Intestine. When a patient has a Husband–Wife imbalance, the overall control usually enjoyed by the Heart has been taken away and the Heart can suffer as a result. Patients can also lose the ability to 'sort out' priorities in their lives. The use of Ht 7 and SI 4, the source points of the Heart and Small Intestine, helps the Supreme Controller to resume its position and also enables the person to gain clarity and perspective.

Frequency of treatment

An extraordinary imbalance in the person's *qi* is present. Some patients may need only one treatment in order to 'break' the Husband–Wife imbalance. For other patients this imbalance is harder to correct. In this case the patient may need to be treated every 2–3 days in order to 'force' the *qi* back into balance. After this block has been broken it may still be necessary to avoid treating the Organs of the right side for a while, or at least use extreme care if treating this side to ensure that the imbalance does not reassert itself and cause a relapse in the patient's symptoms. If there is any suggestion of the Husband–Wife imbalance returning, the practitioner should transfer *qi* over from the right to the left side immediately.

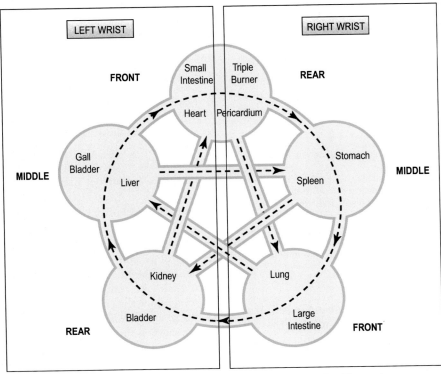

Figure 32.1 • Pulses of the left and right wrist in relation to the Five Elements

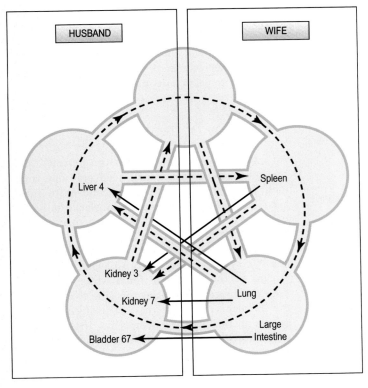

Figure 32.2 • Balancing a Husband–Wife imbalance

Reactions to treatment

People whose *qi* is relatively harmonious do not usually suffer from Husband–Wife imbalances, unless they have an intense trauma that they completely fail to come to terms with. After the Husband–Wife imbalance has been 'broken' patients usually experience fundamental changes in their health and well-being. They no longer experience the internal conflict that caused this imbalance to develop with the same intensity. This is manifested by an improvement in their signs and symptoms. For many patients, however, when the imbalance is cleared the profound disharmony of *qi* from before it developed is still present. If the patient is still in the situation that initially brought on the Husband–Wife imbalance, there is a danger of a relapse. For this reason, continued treatment to help restore balance is recommended.

Summary

1 A Husband–Wife imbalance arises when the Organs represented by the left-hand side pulses (husband) are no longer in harmony with the Organs represented by the right-hand side pulses (wife).

2 This may be life-threatening and is a sign that the inner healing resources of the patient are compromised.

3 Sometimes patients with a Husband–Wife imbalance have extreme internal conflict about gender or sexuality or patients are resigned, fearful or disturbed at a deep level.

4 When treating the Husband–Wife imbalance, the practitioner aims to re-establish harmony between the left and right side of the pulses by transferring *qi* over from the right-side Elements to the left via the *sheng* and *ke* cycles.

5 After the Husband–Wife imbalance has been 'broken' a patient will experience fundamental changes in health and well-being.

Entry–Exit blocks

Introduction

Aggressive Energy, Possession and Husband–Wife imbalances are major blocks to treatment because they can cause extensive deterioration to a patient's health. An Entry–Exit block will not be as damaging, although if untreated it can still reduce or even stop the patient's normal progress towards health.[1]

What are Entry and Exit points?

(Table 33.1)

The Entry and Exit points are specific points close to the beginning and end of each channel. The 12 main channels are connected to each other and form a complete circuit. This circuit is outlined in the *Ling Shu* Chapter 16. It is the same as the *qi* flow between the Organs described in the 24-hour clock which is discussed in the Law of Midday–Midnight in Chapter 2. The points where the channels connect are called the Exit and Entry points.

What is an Entry–Exit block?

Sometimes the connection between the Entry and Exit point becomes blocked. This may be at the Exit point of one channel, which can no longer connect with the Entry point of the following channel. There may be either a complete or a partial blockage of the *qi* flow between the channels. Alternatively, the whole channel can be blocked. In this case the Entry point and Exit point of the same channel may be treated.

An Entry–Exit block may be treated by the practitioner at the initial diagnosis. More commonly it becomes evident during the course of treatment.

The Entry–Exit points

The circuit of Entry–Exit points takes *qi* through the channels in the following order:

Lung – Large Intestine – Stomach – Spleen – Heart – Small Intestine – Bladder – Kidneys – Pericardium – Triple Burner – Gall Bladder – Liver and back to the Lung.

The Entry points are

Lu 1	LI 4	St 1	Sp 1	Ht 1	SI 1
Bl 1	Kid 1	PC 1	TB 1	GB 1	Liv 1

---

[1]It is not clear from where this treatment originated, although Eckman states that it was taught in a Shanghai TCM College in the 1960s (see Eckman, 1996, p. 204). It is mentioned by Felix Mann in his book *Acupuncture: the Ancient Chinese Art of Healing* (Mann, 1971). In his article 'Four LA blocks to treatment' (Flaws, 1989), Bob Flaws stated that Entry and Exit points were taught to him by his teacher, Dr Tao Xi-Yu. Dr Tao learned it from his uncle in Beijing. Interestingly, Dr Tao was an associate of Wu Wei-Ping and translated for J. R. Worsley when he learnt from Wu Wei-Ping in Taiwan.

Table 33.1 The Entry-Exit points

Entry	Exit
Lu 1	Lu 7
LI 4	LI 20
St 1	St 42
Sp 1	Sp 21
Ht 1	Ht 9
SI 1	SI 19
Bl 1	Bl 67
Kid 1	Kid 22
PC 1 (PC 2 on a woman)	PC 8
TB 1	TB 22
GB 1	GB 41
Liv 1	Liv 14

All Entry points except for one (LI 4) are the same as the first point on the channel. In women PC 2 is used in place of PC 1 due to its location on the breast.

The Exit points are

Lu 7   LI 20   St 42   Sp 21   Ht 9   SI 19
Bl 67   Kid 22   PC 8   TB 22   GB 41   Liv 14
Some of the Exit points are also the last points on the channel. The others (Lu 7, St 42, Kid 22, PC 8, TB 22 and GB 41) are not the last point, although they are close to the end of the channels.

Diagnosis of an Entry–Exit block

Pulse diagnosis to detect an Entry–Exit block

An Entry–Exit block is usually detected by pulse diagnosis. A blockage is usually indicated in one of these three ways:

* a relatively full pulse is followed by a deficient pulse

* pulses on consecutive Organs/channels don't change during treatment
* a similar quality pulse appears on the pulses of consecutive channels

A full pulse is followed by a deficient pulse

There may be a relatively full pulse on one Organ/channel followed by a very deficient pulse on the next. This fullness does not change with normal treatments. This is most often felt between the Liver and Lung or the Spleen and Heart, but it can also

Patient Example

A patient who was treated as a Fire CF usually felt better after treatment. Over time, however, her progress slowed and she stopped feeling the benefits. The practitioner noticed that the Spleen pulse felt full and did not change following treatment. An Entry–Exit block between the Spleen and Heart was diagnosed. After treatment to clear the block the patient's progress resumed.

occur when there is a block between the Triple Burner and Gall Bladder or the Large Intestine and the Stomach.

Pulses on consecutive Organs/channels don't change

Treatment does not change the pulses of a number of Organs/channels along the circuit.

Patient Example

A patient who was a Fire CF was mainly treated on the Small Intestine. After some time treatment did not change the pulses as expected. The practitioner also noticed that there was no change on the Bladder and Kidney pulses and the patient had a twitch around the inside corner of her right eye. Treatment was given to clear through the Small Intestine, Bladder and Kidney channels using Ht 9, SI 1, SI 19, Bl 1, Bl 67 and Kid 1. This cleared the block. The patient felt an immediate improvement at the time of treatment and the eye symptom also improved.

Similar pulse qualities appear on consecutive Organs/channels

There may be a similar quality on the pulses of two consecutive Organs/channels or the pulses of two consecutive Organs/channels are extraordinarily deficient compared with the other pulses.

Patient Example

A patient who was diagnosed as a Water CF complained that he was getting easily upset by his girlfriend. The practitioner noted the similar soft quality on the Kidney and Pericardium and treated Kid 22 and PC 1. This, along with further treatment on the CF, helped the patient to feel stronger in himself emotionally.

Other signs and symptoms of an Entry–Exit Block

Along with the pulse diagnosis, certain signs and symptoms might indicate the presence of an Entry–Exit block. These are:

- treatment stops working
- signs and symptoms appear around the area of the blockage
- signs or symptoms appear in two Organs or Elements that follow each other along the circuit of *qi*
- the patient who was improving has an unexpected treatment reaction

Treatment stops working

Treatment might become less effective or it might stop working entirely. The above example of the patient with the Spleen/Heart block is an example of this. There may, of course, be many reasons why treatment is not as effective as hoped, but Entry–Exit blocks are an example of this.

Signs and symptoms around the area of the blockage

There may be symptoms around the area of the Exit and Entry points or along the channel, such as pain, discomfort or swellings.

Patient Example

A patient in her late twenties suffered from extremely blocked sinuses. The condition had started when she was 17, soon after the death of her beloved grandmother. She still missed her grandmother intensely and she felt that this was because her grieving had been repressed by her family. After the Entry–Exit block between the Large Intestine and Stomach had been cleared by stimulating LI 20 and St 1, the patient experienced a huge improvement in her sinuses. When asked some weeks later and subsequently, she said that she no longer felt the loss of her grandmother anything like as intensely as she had. The suppression of her grief had caused imbalance in her Large Intestine which had led to the Entry–Exit block.

Signs or symptoms indicate imbalance of two Organs or Elements that follow each other along the circuit of *qi*

A patient with a significant Entry–Exit block may manifest diagnostic signs from different Elements. For example, a block between the Triple Burner and Gall Bladder channels could be suspected if the patient was both green and showed lack of red, lack of shout, lack of joy and scorched. If a significant block is subsequently cleared practitioners should re-assess their CF diagnosis, as the key diagnostic signs can change dramatically.

Patient who was improving has an unexpected treatment reaction

Occasionally an Entry–Exit block is diagnosed when a patient who has been making good progress has a reaction following treatment. In this case the patient may feel extremely unwell for no obvious reason. The practitioner may feel confused by this sudden downturn in the patient's health. This kind of block is ironically caused by the extra *qi* that has been generated from treatment. The Exit or Entry point of the channel involved may have been partially blocked for a long period of time, but the patient had no symptoms as a limited amount of *qi* was flowing through the channel. As treatment progresses and the patient's health improves, a greater amount of *qi* begins to travel through the channel. As the *qi* builds, the area where the *qi* enters or leaves the channels comes under increasing strain.

Treatment of an Entry–Exit block

Points

Entry–Exit blocks are most commonly treated by using the Exit point of one channel and the Entry point of the next, for example Liv 14 and Lu 1. The practitioner may choose to use Exit and Entry points along more than one channel. For example, GB 41, Liv 1, Liv 14, Lu 1, Lu 7, LI 4.

Less commonly the Entry and Exit points can be used to clear through one channel only. To do this the practitioner treats the Entry point first, then the following Exit point. For example, if a patient has symptoms along the Liver channel and a block is suspected, use Liv 1 followed by Liv 14.

Patient Example

A patient who had been prescribed large quantities of antidepressant drugs in the past would often point to the area around her Liver saying that it felt congested. Command points on the Liver channel had very little effect. After the Entry and Exit points of the Liver were treated, the patient returned the next week to say that the congestion had disappeared.

Needle technique

Needle technique depends on the fullness or deficiency of the channel being treated. If the pulse of one channel is full whilst the following channel is deficient, sedate the Exit point and tonify the Entry point. For example, if the Liver pulse is full and the Lung pulse deficient, sedate Liv 14 for 5–10 minutes then tonify Lu 1. Then remove needles from both points.

If the pulses of two consecutive channels are both deficient, tonify both points – usually without retention of the needle. For example, if a block is suspected between Small Intestine and Bladder, tonify SI 19 bilaterally and remove the needle, then tonify Bl 1 and remove the needle.

Entry–Exit blocks can be found between consecutive channels of the same Element but are most often found between two channels of different Elements. These may be the Spleen and Heart, Liver and Lung, Small Intestine and Bladder, Triple Burner and Gall Bladder, Large Intestine and Stomach, or Kidney and Pericardium.

It is important to treat the Entry and Exit points bilaterally although the block is often only present on one side of the body. It is common for the patient to feel more intense sensation at the point where the block is present. Also one point often produces a much more significant pulse change than the others.

Reactions from clearing Entry–Exit blocks

As with any block, the patient's signs and symptoms will change after the block is cleared. After the block has been broken normal Five Element treatments can be resumed. The practitioner can expect the patient to progress and the pulses to change more readily.

Ren and *Du* channel blocks

The *Ren* and *Du* channels can sometimes be blocked although it is rare. A *Ren* and *Du* block may be diagnosed if:

- all of the pulses are extremely deficient and do not respond to any other treatment that would normally tonify the patient
- there are symptoms around the area of the Exit and Entry points or along the *Ren* and *Du* channels

If this block is diagnosed the Entry and Exit points are *Ren* 1, *Ren* 24, *Du* 1, *Du* 28 and needles are inserted in this order using tonifying technique.

Patient Example

A patient had an episiotomy when giving birth to her first child. Some years later she still felt numb around the area and also said her health had never recovered from the birth. The practitioner diagnosed and treated a *Ren* and *Du* block, after which her health slowly began to improve.

Needling the points

Because of the positions of these points, especially *Ren* 1 which lies in the centre of the perineum, extreme care and sensitivity is required on the part of the practitioner when carrying out this treatment. It is important for the practitioner to be aware of a patient's potential embarrassment about having these points treated and to keep the patient covered as much possible in order to preserve their privacy. If a male practitioner is treating a female patient he should ask a female practitioner to carry out the treatment. If this is difficult he should discuss this with the patient and ask her to bring in a companion while the treatment is carried out.

Summary

1 The 12 main channels form a circuit of *qi* and are connected via Entry and Exit points that are close to the beginning and end of each channel.

2 Sometimes the connection between two channels becomes blocked. The Exit point of one channel and the Entry point of the other channel are normally treated.

3 The whole channel can be blocked. In this case the Entry and Exit point of the same channel is treated.

4 The *Ren* and *Du* channels can also become blocked but this is rare.

5 An Entry–Exit block is diagnosed by the pulses and by signs and symptoms around the area of the blockage.

6 After an Entry–Exit block has been cleared, a patient's signs and symptoms will improve and the subsequent treatments will progress more easily.

Section 5

Treatment Techniques

Needle technique

34

> If you should want to heal disease there is nothing so
> good as the needle! Its skill lies in the mystery of its
> working – one's labour exposes its sacred principles.
>
> (*Da Cheng*; Bertschinger, 1991, p. 81)

The art and the mechanics of needle technique

'Tonification' and 'sedation' are the two needle techniques used by practitioners of Five Element Constitutional Acupuncture. This chapter will describe these techniques taking into account both the 'mechanics' and the 'art' of needle technique.

The section on the 'mechanics' of needle technique will outline how each needle technique is carried out. The section on the 'art' of needling discusses how the practitioner can develop internally so that treatment can be aimed at healing a person at the level of body, mind and spirit. A great concert pianist must have impeccable technique but also needs to integrate that expertise by accessing her or his inner expression. A practitioner with experience (*jingyan*) and virtuosity (*linghuo*) is capable of similar levels of excellence.

When to use each technique

The predominant needle technique used in Five Element Constitutional Acupuncture is tonification. There are occasions when the *qi* of an Organ appears full, in which case sedation is used. Pulse diagnosis is the main method used to decide which technique to use (see Chapter 28, this volume, for more on pulse diagnosis). In some cases because of the difficulty in establishing a 'norm', this can require experience on the part of the practitioner.

Because Five Element Constitutional Acupuncture is treating a person's underlying constitutional imbalance, it is not surprising that tonification is used more often than sedation. Occasionally at the start of treatment a pulse feels full and later becomes deficient. When the pulses begin to change, a different needle technique becomes appropriate.

Less commonly, a sedation needle technique needs to be carried out for a longer period, although an underlying deficiency may still emerge later on.

Needle technique for physical versus spirit level

The needle gauge, number of points used, retention time and amount of needle sensation vary according to the level of treatment a patient requires. In general, the subtler spirit levels are reflected by more refined and subtle needle techniques. Table 34.1 summarises the use of needle technique when treating the physical level versus a more spirit level.

Table 34.1 Needle technique when treating physical versus spirit level

	Physical level	Spirit level
Needle gauge	Thicker	Finer
Number of points	More points	Fewer points
Retention time	Longer retention	Less or no retention
Obtaining *deqi*	More sensation	Less sensation

The mechanics of needle technique

Tonification technique

Tonification is used to strengthen a patient's *qi* when it is deficient. This technique involves inserting a needle to contact the patient's *qi*, then immediately removing it. The whole technique usually lasts for only 2–3 seconds. (The equivalent technique used by practitioners of TCM is different. It is usually called 'reinforcing' and the needle is left in place for up to 20 minutes.) The *Ling Shu* Chapter 1 states:

> Once *qi* has arrived there is no further need to retain the needle in the patient's body as the aim of the manipulation has now been achieved.
>
> (Auteroche *et al.*, 1992, p. 47)

In the *Ling Shu* Chapter 3 it states:

> A good physician withdraws the needle as soon as *qi* has arrived.
>
> (Auteroche *et al.*, 1992, p. 47)

A practitioner of Five Element Constitutional Acupuncture who finds that a patient's pulses are deficient uses this needle technique. For example, if the Metal Element is deficient, the practitioner may choose to use any of the points on the Lung and Large Intestine channels. In this case the needle action will be tonification.

The procedure for tonification needle technique

The following instructions assume that the reader is already trained in appropriate sterile procedure.

- Hold the needle angled 10° off the perpendicular and towards the flow of *qi*.

- Needle the left side of the body first then the right.
- Insert the needle slowly to the required depth, as the patient breathes out.
- Contact the patient's *qi* (*deqi*).
- Turn the needle 180° clockwise.
- Remove the needle immediately.
- Close the hole by pressing a clean swab over the point.

Tonification is the most common needle technique used by practitioners of Five Element Constitutional Acupuncture. This is because it is primarily concerned with strengthening long-standing deficiencies in the Organs and Elements.

Sedation technique

Sedation needle technique is used to calm a person's *qi* when there is an excess or full condition. This technique involves contacting the patient's *qi* then leaving the needle in place for 20–30 minutes until the pulses have changed sufficiently.

A practitioner who finds that a patient's pulses are hyperactive may decide to soothe an Organ using this needle technique. For example, if the Wood Element is hyper-functioning this may be reflected in the patient's pulses feeling full or agitated. In this situation the practitioner may choose to use Liver and Gall Bladder points such as the source points (Liv 3 and GB 40) or the sedation points (Liv 2 and GB 38) with a needle action of sedation technique. (Sedation is most similar to the technique known to practitioners of TCM as 'even' technique rather than 'reducing' technique.)

The analogy about sedation given below has been used by J. R. Worsley (1990, p. 190):

> If we imagine a swollen river threatening to flood, there are several ways in which its flow returns to normal. Water can be drawn away or barriers impeding its course can be removed. This is how we should visualise sedation.

The procedure for sedation needle technique

- Hold the needle angled 10° against the flow of the *qi*.
- Needle the right side of the body first then the left.
- Insert the needle quickly, to the required depth, as the patient breathes in.

- Turn the needle 360° anticlockwise.
- Contact with the patient's *qi* (*deqi*) is usually made while turning the needle.
- Retain the needle for between 5 and 30 minutes, until the desired pulse change has occurred.
- Remove the needle slowly.
- When removing the needle, do not close the hole.

Breakdown of stages of needle technique (Table 34.2)

1. Needle angles

> The method is quick to grasp and clear – simply understand facing up or following on and you can work.
>
> (*Da Cheng*; Bertschinger, 1991, p. 85)

The above quotation describes the need to angle the needle with or away from the flow of *qi* when either strengthening a deficient Organ or calming an Organ that is hyper-functioning (see Figure 34.1). In general, the needle is angled towards or against the flow of *qi* but only a few degrees away from the perpendicular. Large angles are rarely used unless the point is situated on a bone, for example LI 6. In this case it is necessary to use a more oblique angle in order to insert it to the required depth.

2. Depth of insertion of needles

Five Element Constitutional Acupuncturists do not use extremely deep needle insertions. The depth of insertion varies according to which point is being used but 0.5 *cun* is common on an arm or leg. In this

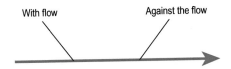

Figure 34.1 • Needle angles with and against the flow

case a one-inch long needle is most often used (approximately 2.5 cm). Half-inch needles are used for nail points when the insertion is very shallow. Needles one-and-a-half inches long are used for deeper insertions such as Ren points on the lower abdomen. (This is in contrast to practitioners primarily trained in TCM, who may use longer needles.) For a list of the most common depths, see the individual needle depths in the chapters on the different points in Section 6.

3. Needle manipulation

A practitioner usually inserts a needle to the required depth, then gently turns it in order to make contact with the patient's *qi*. As the turn is slight – 180° for tonification and 360° for sedation – this requires a continuous movement and clear intention on the part of the practitioner.

4. Needle sensation

The patient usually experiences the *qi* by feeling a dull ache, soreness, heaviness, a pulling sensation, heat or numbness. This sensation should not be extreme. At the same time the practitioner will usually feel a pulling sensation. This feels as if the needle is being held firmly by someone's fingers or it is described as like 'catching a fish'.

Table 34.2 Stages of needle technique

	Tonification	**Sedation**
Angle	10 degree angle towards the flow	10 degree angle against the flow
Needle order	Needle left side first, then right	Needle right side first, then left
Insertion	Insert slowly as patient breathes out	Insert quickly as patient breathes in
Needle manipulation	Turn the needle 180 degrees clockwise	Turn needle 360 degrees anti-clockwise
Length of retention	Do not retain needle	Retain needles until desired pulse change has occurred (from 5 to 30 minutes)
Removal	Immediately remove needle. Remove needle quickly	Remove needle slowly
Closing hole	Close hole using clean swab on removal	Do not close hole on removal

Practitioners will generally ask their patients to let them know when they have felt the *qi*. The aim of practitioners is to become more sensitive to feeling the *qi* so that they no longer need to rely on the patient for feedback as to whether they have 'hit' the point. This is only possible if the practitioner maintains a calm mind and spirit when needling.

Compared to some of the more robust needle techniques used in China, especially for the treatment of acute conditions, the needle technique used by Five Element Constitutional Acupuncturists is relatively gentle. This is partly a consequence of its roots in Japanese acupuncture, where practitioners tend to use gentler needle techniques than in China. It is also because when the subtler levels are treated, more delicate needle techniques are required.

5. Length of retention

As stated above, needles are not usually left in place when a patient's *qi* is being strengthened.

When using sedation technique, however, needles are retained. In this case, the changes felt on the patient's pulses are the key factor helping the practitioner to decide when to remove the needles. Practitioners monitor the patients' pulses over a period of 5–30 minutes, although the usual period of retention is around 20 minutes. The practitioner only removes the needles when the pulses have changed sufficiently (see Chapter 28 for more on what a practitioner looks for in a pulse change). The practitioner expects the change on the pulses to move towards becoming more settled, harmonious and even.[1]

6. Closing the hole

If a point has been tonified, the hole is closed with a cotton wool swab after the needle has been removed. If a point has been sedated, the hole is left open after the needle has been removed.

7. Needle gauge

The usual gauge of a needle used by a Five Element Constitutional Acupuncturist is very fine – usually 36 gauge (0.20 mm). This reflects the fact that practitioners often concentrate their treatments on contacting the patient's *qi* on a 'spirit' level. The subtler the levels treated, the finer the needle that is used.

---

[1] In contrast, a TCM practitioner usually judges when to remove the needles by the length of time they have been left in and will usually remove them when 20 minutes have passed.

8. Breathing

Some practitioners ask their patients to breathe in or out while inserting the needle to the required depth, but this is optional. Breathing with needling is used in the following way:

- Tonification – the needle is inserted to the required depth on the patient's exhalation and withdrawn on inhalation.
- Sedation – the needle is inserted to the required depth on the patient's inhalation and withdrawn on exhalation.

9. Number of needles used per treatment

A practitioner of Five Element Constitutional Acupuncture usually uses only a small number of needles in one treatment – two to four points is not unusual. This is in keeping with the principle of minimum intervention. When contacting the patient's mind or spirit, only a few carefully chosen points are required in order to have a large effect.

Hua Tuo (+110–207), the renowned physician, was famous for using only one or two points per treatment and would tell his patients what they should expect to feel – as soon as they felt the sensations he would remove the needles and they would be cured.

> As for moxa, he applied it to no more than two places and not more than seven or eight times in one place. In needling two places were sufficient and often only one.
>
> (*Yi Xue Ru Men* by Li Chan, 1575; quoted in Soulié de Morant, 1994, p. 10)

In the *Ode to the Streamer out of the Dark* there is the comment:

> What these doctors (who used what is known as spiritual healing) in all sincerity thought most highly of was a single needle inserted into a hole, the disease responding to the hand and it lifting.
>
> (Bertschinger, 1991, p. 17)

Needle sensation when contacting the patient's *qi*

Deqi if the *qi* is deficient

If a patient has very deficient *qi* it can be more difficult to contact it. Because the *qi* inside the Organs is weak, it moves less easily. In this case it may take time for the patient to feel a needle sensation. The practitioner needs to maintain his or her intention and patiently wait for the *qi* to come to the needle rather than assuming that she or he has missed the point.

It is better for the practitioner not to constantly reinsert the needle as this can cause unnecessary shock to the patient's system. In some cases it may be preferable for a practitioner to hold the needle, adjust his or her posture and wait. In time the *qi* may arrive at the needle without the need for new insertions.

Needle technique for transfers of *qi*

Transfers of *qi* are carried out in order to move *qi* from where there is an excess in one Organ to another Organ where there is a deficiency (see Chapter 36). The *qi* can be moved in different ways.

- Along the *sheng* cycle. An example of this is when *qi* is moved using a tonification point or a sedation point.

Figure 34.2 shows the route of a tonification or sedation point, in this case Bl 67 and Kid 7 (Metal points) along the *sheng* cycle.

- Between *yin* Organs across the *ke* cycle, for example, using Kid 3 (Earth point) and Liv 4 (Metal point) when re-balancing a Husband–Wife imbalance (see Chapter 32, this volume, for more on this).

Figure 34.3 shows the route for taking energy across the *ke* cycle (in this case using Kid 3, an Earth Point).

- To redistribute *qi* within an Element using a Junction point, for example, using Kid 4 (*luo* junction point) to pull *qi* from the Bladder to the Kidneys or Stomach 40 (*luo* junction point) to pull energy from the Spleen to the Stomach.

Figure 34.4 shows the route for moving *qi* using a junction point (in this case using Spl 4, a *luo* junction point).

The transfers described above are very simple and usually involve the use of only one or two needles. More complicated transfers of *qi* can also be used in order to rebalance the *qi* from a relatively hyperactive Organ to a deficient Organ. As these are more complicated, the route must be carefully planned, as they are likely to travel across more than one Organ.

How to plan a transfer

Draw on a diagram where the full (+) *qi* is felt and where it is deficient (−). Then mark out a route from the + to the −, making sure that the flow travels in a clockwise direction.

The next step is to work out which needles should be used, remembering always to insert the first needle into the deficient Organ and to work backwards along the pathway. The needles between

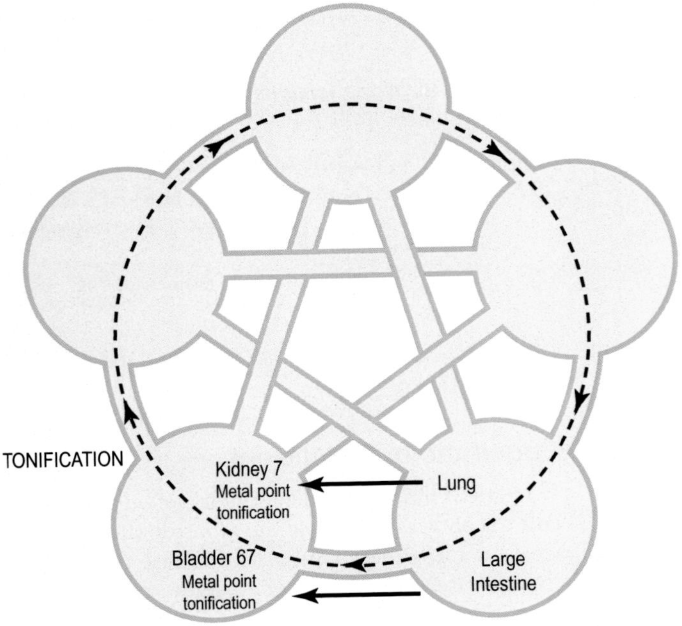

Figure 34.2 • Movement of *qi* along the *sheng* cycle using a tonification point

TONIFICATION

Kidney 7
Metal point
tonification

Lung

Bladder 67
Metal point
tonification

Large
Intestine

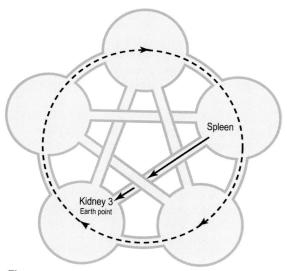

Figure 34.3 • Route of *qi* transfer across the *ke* cycle

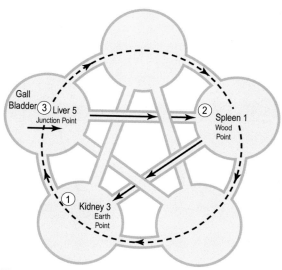

Figure 34.5 • The Five Elements showing a pathway for transferring *qi* from the Gall Bladder to the Kidney

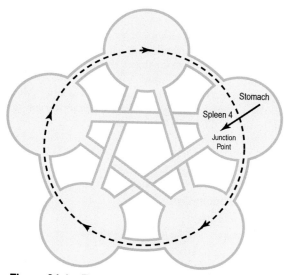

Figure 34.4 • Transfer of *qi* using a *luo* junction point

the + and the − are called 'carrier' needles and allow the *qi* to transfer along the pathway. There is no needle in the excess Organ.

Example 1: Moving the *qi* from the Gall Bladder to the Kidney

In this situation the energy in the Gall Bladder is full and the Kidneys are deficient. Figure 34.5 show the route needed to transfer *qi* from the Gall Bladder to the Kidney.

First point	Kid 3 (Earth point)	Pulls the *qi* from the Spleen to the Kidney
Second point	Sp 1 (Wood point)	Pulls the *qi* from the Liver to the Spleen
Third point	Liv 5 (Junction point)	Pulls the *qi* from the GB to the Liver

Example 2: Moving the *qi* from the Spleen to the Gall Bladder

In this situation the *qi* in the Spleen is too full and the Gall Bladder is deficient. Figure 34.6 shows a pathway from the Spleen to the Gall Bladder.

First point	GB 37 (Junction point)	Pulls *qi* from the Liver to the Gall Bladder
Second point	Liv 4 (Metal point)	Pulls *qi* from the Lung to the Liver
Third point	Lu 9 (Earth point)	Pulls *qi* from the Spleen to the Lung

Factors to consider when carrying out a transfer

• All points must be accurately needled in order for the transfer to be successful.

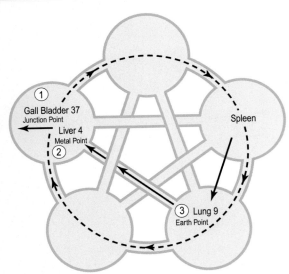

Figure 34.6 • The Five Elements showing a pathway from the Spleen to the Gall Bladder

- It is best to choose the shortest route to decrease the chances of missing a point.

Needle order for carrying out a transfer

The needle order for a transfer is as follows:

1 The first needle is placed in the point of the deficient Organ using a 'hint' of a tonification, i.e. a slight turn but not to the full 180°. Place needle in the left side then the right.

2 The second needle is placed in the point of the next Organ working back along the pathway – also using a hint of a tonification. Needle the left side then the right.

3 All further needles use the same procedures working backwards along the pathway until all needles are in position.

4 Fully tonify the needle in the deficient Organ, first on the left side then the right side.

5 Remove all remaining needles in the same order as they were inserted, first the left side and then the right side.

Needle shock

On some rare occasions a patient can faint during a treatment. This 'needle shock' can occur if a large amount of *qi* is moved. Some predisposing factors are that a patient is extremely nervous, hungry or exhausted or is sitting up when being needled.

If needle shock occurs the needles should be removed immediately and first aid treatment for shock applied. Some practitioners also treat using LI 4 if needles were in the lower part of the body or St 36 if the needles were in the upper part of the body. If the needles are in both areas of the body, both points are treated.

The art of needle technique

The 'art' of needle technique involves the development of practitioners' *qi*. This is especially important when treating a patient's mind and spirit. The greater the practitioners' awareness of their own spirit when treating at this level, the deeper is their connection with the spirit of the patient. This in turn increases the depth of the effect attained from treatment.

This section on the 'art' of needle technique gives some general signposts that may enable practitioners to hone their ability to contact the patient's spirit with a needle. These are a culmination of the experiences of many Five Element practitioners but they are not the only methods that can be used. A combination of experiences gained from practising acupuncture and one's inner development are also necessary and these build over a period of time. More on the internal development of the practitioner can be found in Chapter 6, this volume.

The practitioner's internal state

Some qualities a practitioner can develop to improve needle technique are:

- clear intention
- relaxation
- focusing the attention
- good posture
- good rapport and sensitivity to the patient

Clear intention

Firstly, clear intention is of utmost importance when a practitioner is needling a point. If the practitioner is certain that the point to be used is the best possible choice, it is likely to have a more positive effect on the outcome of treatment. If a practitioner is unfocused and places the needles into points without fully considering the implications for their use, a less significant effect is likely to be gained from the treatment.

The difference our minds and spirits make to treatment has been clearly understood by practitioners of Chinese medicine for thousands of years as this quote from the *Ling Shu* Chapter 9 suggests:

> Prior to needling a practitioner should retire to a quiet place and commune with his spirit with doors and windows shut. The doctor's *Hun* and *Po* must not be scattered, his mind must be focused, and his essence undivided. Undistracted by human sounds, he must marshal his essence, concentrate his mind and direct his will entirely towards needling.
>
> *Ling Shu*, Chapter 9; (Huang Fu Mi) translated by Yang and Chace, 1994

A 'good heart'

A strong desire for the patient to be made well will help a practitioner to gain clear intention when needling. This desire to heal can in itself help the practitioner to reach the correct level of body, mind and spirit. At the same time, practitioners can do more to develop their sensitivity to the patient and increase the flow of their own *qi* when manipulating a needle.

Relaxation

Physical tension and tight muscles block the flow of *qi* through the body, whilst relaxation encourages the flow of *qi*. The ability of the practitioner to relax both mentally and physically is especially important to encourage this free flow from practitioner to patient. It is also important that the atmosphere in the treatment room is comfortable and relaxed – a patient who is tense is less likely to gain benefit from treatment than one who is relaxed.

Cultivating a relaxed attitude

Mental tension is often at the root of physical tension and it is important for the practitioner to cultivate a relaxed attitude while treating.

> In the mind of the physician there should be no desires, only a receptive and accepting attitude. Then the mind can become *shen*. The mind of the physician and the mind of the patient should be level, in harmony following the movements of the needle.
>
> (Zhen, 1996)

As this text suggests, our mind should be alert at the same time as being relaxed. If we are too relaxed we will become unresponsive to our patients. The relaxation needed when needling is a vital and dynamic state that comes from having a clear focus at the same time as letting the mind become calm and peaceful.

Relaxing the body

A relaxed body will create a relaxed mind, and vice versa. All areas of the body including the feet, legs, hands, arms, spine, shoulders and head should be relaxed.

For a practitioner, the shoulders, shoulder blades, arms and hands should be *particularly* relaxed. This allows the *qi* to travel down the arms when inserting and manipulating the needle. Tension in these areas can cause a damming up of *qi* and over time can contribute to the practitioner becoming exhausted and burnt out.

Each practitioner develops their own specific way of relaxing themselves before treating – simple exercises such as shaking or massaging the hands, arms and shoulders can be helpful. Gentle breathing, especially breathing into the lower *dan tian*, will also encourage the practitioner to relax. (The *dan tian* is an area about 1½ inches below the navel and known by practitioners of *qi gong* as the centre of gravity and a place from where people can preserve their health. For more on this, see Housheng and Peiyu, 1994, pp. 301–309.)

Focusing the attention

There is a saying that 'where the mind goes *qi* follows' (for more on this, refer to *qi gong* books such as Frantzis, 2006, p. 23). The practitioner's attention needs to be clear and focused in order to maximise the effect of needling. When needling a patient the practitioner's attention should be focused on the tip of the needle rather than the handle. Focusing on the tip will allow the practitioner's *qi* to extend to the patient, ensuring the practitioner can connect more deeply with the patient's *qi*. Concentration on the handle of the needle will lessen the flow of the practitioner's *qi*.

Whilst concentrating on the tip of the needle it can be useful for the practitioner to simultaneously focus on her or his own *dan tian*. This allows practitioners to monitor their own internal state as they remain centred in the body. *Su Wen* says this about our concentration when needling:

> In the course of needling, the acupuncturist should remain as alert as if being at the point of an abyss and his hand should hold the needle as persistently as if holding a tiger; and he should concentrate on what he is doing without distraction.
>
> (Lu, 1972, p. 173)

The practitioner also needs to be able to focus on any changes that occur in the patient during and after the needling. *Su Wen* Chapter 25 also states:

> Applying acupuncture is like treading the edge of a precipice; the hands should be firm and strong. The twisting of the needles must be done in an even and regular way, quietly and attentively watching the patient to observe any minute changes that occur when the *qi* arrives; such changes are so obscure that they can be hardly seen. When the *qi* arrives it is like a flock of birds, or a breeze in the waving millet – only too easily can one miss the fleeting moment.
>
> (Lu and Needham, 1980, p. 91)

When the *qi* arrives at the needle, the changes to the patient may be subtle as the text above suggests. The practitioner can nevertheless strive to tune in to changes that occur to the colour, sound, emotion and odour of the patient. These, along with the pulse changes and differences occurring to the sparkle in the patient's eyes and the general demeanour, will indicate that the treatment has touched the required level.

Good posture

Poor body alignment when using a needle will cut off the flow of the practitioner's *qi* – rather like a badly constructed plumbing system that gets blocked up. Good posture, on the other hand, will allow the *qi* to flow smoothly when using a needle. This increases the practitioner's ability to make contact with the patient.

A *qi gong* teacher would suggest that a practitioner stands with the legs at shoulder width apart, the joints relaxed, the spine straight, the head upright and the armpits open, whilst at the same time centring the consciousness in the *dan tian*.

The practitioner's self-development

Some practitioners will decide to regularly practise internal exercises that encourage relaxation, good posture and a focused mind. Finding a teacher who gives clear feedback can also be helpful. Classes in *qi gong*, *tai ji*, yoga or a soft martial art such as *aikido*, as well as meditation practice, can all be helpful.

Summary

1 'Tonification' and 'sedation' are the two needle techniques used by practitioners of Five Element Constitutional Acupuncture.

2 Tonification is used to strengthen a patient's *qi* when it is deficient. The technique involves inserting a needle to contact the patient's *qi*, then immediately removing it.

3 Sedation needle technique is used to calm a person's *qi* when there is an excess or full condition. This technique involves contacting the patient's *qi*, then leaving the needle in place for 20–30 minutes until the pulses have changed sufficiently.

4 The needle gauge, number of points used, retention time and amount of needle sensation vary according to the level of treatment a patient requires.

5 Transfers of *qi* are carried out in order to move *qi* from where there is an excess in one Organ to another Organ where there is a deficiency.

6 Some qualities a practitioner can develop to improve needle technique are clear intention, relaxation, focusing the attention, good posture, and good rapport and sensitivity to the patient.

The use of moxibustion

35

CHAPTER CONTENTS

Moxa

What is moxa?

Moxa is a downy material prepared from the leaves of the herb *Artemesia vulgaris latiflora*. This is similar to the common mugwort plant that is grown in the UK and USA. To prepare the artemesia, the veins of the leaves are stripped, then ground, aired and dried before it becomes what is commonly called moxa 'punk' or 'wool'.

When is moxa used?

An acupuncturist uses moxa during a treatment in order to warm a patient. Whether to use moxa or not is an important issue. In some cases it can be essential in order for patients to make progress. For example, patients who are cold will not improve, or will take much longer to get better, if they do not have moxa. On the other hand, it can be dangerous to heat a patient who is already too hot.

How is moxa used?

Most commonly a Five Element Constitutional Acupuncturist rolls the moxa into small cones that are then placed on the acupuncture points and lit. Sometimes a moxa stick is used instead of cones, especially if a large area needs to be warmed. Moxa cones can be used alone and have a stimulating effect on a patient's *qi*. More often they are used before the needles are inserted and in this case they warm a point and the needles take the heat to the point.

Deciding whether to use moxa

As a result of the diagnosis, the practitioner should be able to decide whether to use moxa. The patient will fall into one of three categories:

- The patient definitely needs moxa and is unlikely to get better or will not get better as quickly without it.
- Moxa may be used to tonify the patient but is not essential. In this case the patient may not be abnormally cold, but the warmth will prepare the point before a needle is inserted.
- Moxa should definitely not be used. It will not help and it may make the patient worse.

A patient may change categories as treatment progresses, and this should be noted during the ongoing process of diagnosis.

DOI: 10.1016/B978-0-7020-3175-5.00035-8

Moxa is used more frequently in cold weather and during the winter, or when there is a cold and damp climate.

Keys to deciding if moxa is appropriate

Touch, visual observation, questioning and smelling give the practitioner the relevant information needed in order to decide whether moxa will be of benefit.[1]

Touch

When palpating the patient during the physical examination, the practitioner may notice that certain areas of the body are cold. For example, one or more of the three *jiao* may be cold. This indicates that moxa might be beneficial when treating the Organs situated in the cold *jiao*. Additionally, if the patient's feet, hands, legs and arms or lower back are cold to the touch, there is also a case for using moxa.

If a patient's pulse is particularly slow, for example 60 beats per minute, this may indicate a need for warming the *qi*. Some exceptions to this are if the patient is undergoing strenuous physical training or is taking medications such as beta-blockers, both of which cause the pulse to slow.

Observation

A very pale face (pale and bright even more so) suggests the patient is cold and would benefit from moxa. There may be more obvious signs such as a person wearing a jumper when others are in T-shirts or the person huddling close to heaters and shivering.

Questions

It is important for the practitioner to question several areas when deciding if the patient needs moxa:

- Does the patient feel cold?
- Is one or more parts of the body cold or hot?
- Does the patient notice any difference between their own and others' temperature? For example, do they wear thermal underwear even in the summer, or always turn the central heating down while others want it turned up?
- Does the patient have symptoms that are better for cold or heat?
- Does the patient prefer one season to another and is this to do with the temperature?
- Does the patient like hot or cold drinks or hot or cold food? For example, preferring drinks that come straight from the refrigerator suggests that the patient is hot and the practitioner should take care with moxa.
- Does the patient have a bitter taste in the mouth? This can be an indication of heat.
- Is there any area of the body where there is inflammation?

Indications that the patient is dry can also be relevant because moxa is drying as well as warming. Care should be taken if moxa is used on a patient who is frequently thirsty and has dry skin and hair as it could possibly increase the symptoms of dryness.

Smelling

Strong odours tend to indicate heat. For example, a strongly smelling vaginal discharge, diarrhoea which has a strong odour or urine which is yellow and strong smelling all indicate that there is some excess heat. These may be local as opposed to systemic indications and should be recognised as such when integrating all the other indications for using moxa or not.

Integration of information

Many patients are straightforward and it is easy for the practitioner to discern whether they tend towards being cold, hot or more or less in the middle. Thus they place themselves in one of the categories suggested above.

Contradictions, where some observations indicate cold and some indicate heat, are more difficult to resolve. Even if patients have some signs of cold, but several of their major indicators point to heat, the practitioner would be advised to avoid moxa. Using moxa when a person is already hot can be damaging. Thus, if in doubt, the practitioner should avoid using moxa.[2]

---

[1]The concept of *yin* and *yang* is useful here. *Yang* energy is warming and moving. *Yin* energy is nourishing and cooling. *Yang* deficiency requires the use of moxa, *Yin* deficiency may or may not require moxa and Full Heat definitely indicates that moxa is forbidden. For these distinctions, see a good TCM textbook, such as Maciocia, 2005.

[2]Five Element practitioners do not use the tongue in diagnosis. If the tongue is used, a pale, swollen tongue is more indicative of cold and a red, dry tongue of heat. The tongue can be a key indicator as to the advisability of moxa.

Testing using moxa

When a patient has a mixture of cold and heat signs, the practitioner may be in doubt as to whether to use moxa or not. In this case, the practitioner can select an appropriate point and use one moxa cone on it and then check whether the pulses feel any better or any worse. If the pulses feel slightly better, then the practitioner can use a few more moxa cones, continuing to check for improvement. After the minimum number of moxa cones have been used the practitioner should wait for the patient's feedback at the next treatment in order to decide whether using moxa is suitable or not.

If the pulses tighten or feel less harmonious as a result of treatment, no further moxa should be used and the conclusion drawn would be that moxa is not appropriate.

Moxa cones and sticks

Making moxa cones

Grades of moxa may be rough, intermediate or fine. The intermediate grade is most commonly used for making moxa cones. The rougher moxa is often too coarse to roll into cones. Some practitioners prefer to use the fine-grade moxa but this is thought by others to burn too rapidly. The fine moxa is often used by Japanese acupuncturists.

To make a moxa cone a small amount of moxa punk is rolled between the thumb, index and middle fingers until it becomes a cone shape. This is slightly larger than a grain of wheat – about 0.75 cm in height and 0.5 cm in diameter. At first the practitioner may prefer to prepare all of the cones before starting to use moxa on the patient. In time she or he will become adept at creating the cones more rapidly and is then able to make them while the moxa treatment is in progress.

Using moxa cones

The use of moxa cones is called direct moxa as the cone is placed directly on the skin (Figure 35.1).

- The cone is placed on the acupuncture point then lit with an incense stick.
- As the cones burn down the patient feels a warm sensation on the points as heat is generated directly to the *qi* in the channels.

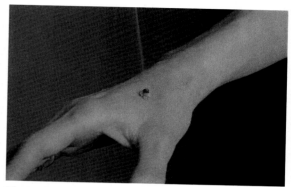

Figure 35.1 • A burning moxa cone

- The moxa cone is removed when the patient indicates that it feels hot. The practitioner removes the moxa with the thumb and little finger (the fingers not used for pulse taking) or with tweezers.
- The left side is treated first, followed by the right.
- Usually three to seven moxa cones are applied to each point, depending on which point is used. Some points can take more moxa cones than others, for example up to 100 cones can be used on Bl 43, although this is unusual. (For suggested numbers of moxa per point, see the chapters on the different points in Section 6, this volume.)

Before applying moxa for the first time, it is vital that the patient understands what the practitioner is about to do and knows the importance of saying when the moxa cone is hot. If a cone is left on for too long this could burn the patient and cause scarring.

If moxa is used on the umbilicus (*Ren* 8) it is placed on a bed of salt to protect this sensitive area. Moxa can also be placed on ginger; in this case it is more warming as well as providing protection for the skin.

Moxa sticks

Five Element practitioners use moxa sticks less frequently than moxa cones, although they may use one to warm a large area, for example, the lower abdomen after childbirth. A moxa stick can be:

- held in one place for 5–10 minutes
- moved in a circular motion to spread heat and cover a large area
- pecked at a point without touching the skin – this is used for quick stimulation of a point

Contraindications

Moxa is contraindicated when there are signs of heat. In this case a patient may:

- feel hot
- like the cold
- be hot to touch
- have red, hot skin
- have a florid appearance
- have hot flushes
- have a fever
- have high blood pressure, if caused by heat

In addition, moxa should not be used on the following areas:

- the face or sensitive areas
- on the lower back or abdomen of pregnant women
- on large blood vessels

Summary

1 Moxa is prepared from the herb *Artemesia vulgaris latiflora*.

2 It is used during a treatment to warm a patient and in some cases can be important in order for a patient to progress.

3 It is most often used as small cones or in the form of a moxa stick.

4 It is important to use moxa when a patient is cold. Sometimes it is not essential to use moxa but it will help to tonify a patient. Moxa is contraindicated if a patient is already hot.

5 Touch, observation, questioning and smelling inform the practitioner as to whether moxa will be beneficial.

Section 6

The Use of Points

The use of acupuncture points in Five Element Constitutional Acupuncture

36

Overview of the use of points

Practitioners of Five Element Constitutional Acupuncture use points in three different ways.

1 According to the **type of point**. These uses were first laid down in the early classics. For example, different types of points are back *shu* points, *yuan* source points, Element points, tonification points, etc.

2 According to the qualities implied by the **names** given to them in antiquity, for example, using points such as Ht 7, Spirit Gate or Kid 25 Spirit Storehouse to treat a person at the level of the spirit. In some instances the location of the point is also considered.

3 Using a **combination of points**. Some points are used together to create a specific effect. For example, using *Ren* 15, St 25, St 32 and St 41 to clear possession or Exit and Entry points, such as Liv 14 and Lu 1, to clear a block.

This chapter will concentrate on how the different types of points described in the Chinese classics are used by a Five Element Constitutional Acupuncturist. Chapter 37 will discuss using points according to the qualities implied by the names, especially when they are used to treat a person's spirit.

The use of points according to traditional usage

Command points

The *Nei Jing* and the *Nan Jing* outline several different classifications of points and give some indications as to how these points should be used. Much emphasis is placed on the use of 'command' points, the points situated below the elbow and knee.

> The 360 points of the whole body have their command in the sixty-six points of the feet and hands.
>
> (*Yi Xue Ru Men* by Li Chan, +157; quoted in Soulié de Morant, 1994, p. 145)

(In this quotation the number 66 comprises the five *shu* points of the 12 channels and the *yuan* source points of the *yang* channels, which are *shu* points.)

The command points are considered to be especially effective at enhancing the *qi* of the Organs. Giovanni Maciocia (1989, p. 335) describes them as being more 'dynamic' than points on other parts of the body for two reasons. Firstly, because they are more superficial in nature (for more on this see the Element points below), and secondly, because of the rapidly changing and relatively volatile *yin/yang* dynamics present at the beginning and end of the channel.

These points are commonly used to direct, enrich and 'command' the *qi*. The types of points discussed in this chapter are:

- Element points – especially the tonification and sedation points
- *yuan* source points
- horary points
- *luo* junction points
- *xi* cleft points

Other points with specific uses

Besides command points, there are a number of other points that are discussed in this chapter that are commonly used by Five Element Constitutional Acupuncturists. They are:

- back *shu* points
- Exit–Entry points
- points on the *Ren* and *Du* channels
- front *mu* points (these points are palpated for diagnosis only)

Although practitioners frequently use points on various parts of the body, they tend to complement them with command points. This usually enhances their effect. If a significant change has been effected in the patient's colour, sound, odour, emotion or pulses by using only the body point then it may be unnecessary to use a command point as well.

Command points

Element points

Ling Shu Chapter 1 compares the channels to rivers, starting with a 'well' at the tips of the toes or fingers and flowing into a 'spring', 'stream' and 'river' until it reaches a 'sea' at the knee or elbow. Here the *qi* travels deeper inside the body. This transformation is associated with particular points on the channel which are usually called the 'Five *Shu* points'.[1]

In the *Nan Jing* these points are linked with each of the Elements. These points are frequently used by Five Element Constitutional Acupuncturists.[2]

Uses of Element points

1 They are most often used in the form of tonification or sedation points that are used to transfer *qi* around the *sheng* cycle.

2 They can be used to transfer *qi* between Organs across the *ke* cycle.

3 They can be used to treat a patient's 'Element within the Element' (see Chapter 4, this volume). Element points are rarely used in this way and describing this use is not within the scope of this book.

The Element points are listed in Table 36.1.

Position of Element points

The Element points are sited on the limbs. All nail points on the *yin* channels are Wood points, the second points are Fire points and the third points are Earth points. Points at the elbows or knees are Water points. Metal points vary slightly in their position but naturally lie between the Earth and Water points.

All nail points on the *yang* channels are Metal points, the second points are Water points and the third points (except GB) are Wood points. Points at the elbows or knees are Earth points. Fire points lie between the Wood and Earth points and can vary in their positions.

The concept of 'transferring' *qi* between Organs

The idea of transferring *qi* from an Organ that is in excess relative to another Organ is extremely old in Chinese medicine. The *Maishu*, recently excavated at the Zhangjiashan burial site, and probably the earliest extant treatise on acupuncture states:

> Those who treat illness take the surplus and supplement the insufficiency.

(quoted in Lo, 2001, p. 29)

---

[1] In the 1970s J. R. Worsley described these points and called them 'Antique' points. He recommended that they were used according to the season.

[2] Different passages in the *Nei Jing* and *Nan Jing* give different and even contradictory usages for these points. The use of these points in Five Element Constitutional Acupuncture is based, like much else, upon the *Nan Jing*.

Table 36.1 The Element points

Organ	Wood point	Fire point	Earth point	Metal point	Water point
Lung	11	10	9	8	5
Large Intestine	3	5	11	1	2
Stomach	43	41	36	45	44
Spleen	1	2	3	5	9
Heart	9	8	7	4	3
Small Intestine	3	5	8	1	2
Bladder	65	60	40[a]	67	66
Kidneys	1	2	3	7	10
Pericardium	9	8	7	5	3
Triple Burner	3	6	10	1	2
Gall Bladder	41	38	34	44	43
Liver	1	2	3	4	8

[a] J. R. Worsley used a slightly different numbering system for some points on the Bladder channel to the one used by the Chinese. In that system it is Bladder 54.

It is mentioned in *Su Wen* Chapter 5, that:

> If there is a *qi* deficiency in a particular location or channel, the *qi* can be conducted or guided from other channels to supplement the weakness.
>
> (Ni, 1995)

Su Wen, however, gives no specific treatment protocols for the process of 'transferring' *qi*. In the Ming dynasty, Xu Feng (+1439) and Gao Wu (+1529) set out the use of 'tonification' and 'sedation' points. This led to these treatment protocols becoming widely used, especially amongst Korean and Japanese acupuncturists.[3]

The importance of harmonising the *qi* of the 12 Organs is fundamental in this style of acupuncture. This means that it is common practice to transfer *qi* between Organs even if the relatively stronger Organ is somewhat deficient in absolute terms. Pulse diagnosis is crucial in making this judgement.

Tonification points

The tonification point on a channel is the point associated with the preceding Element on the *sheng* cycle, the 'mother' of the Organ involved. Tonifying these points transfers *qi* from the mother Organ to the child. *Qi* can only be transferred from a *yin* Organ to another *yin* Organ or from a *yang* Organ to another *yang* Organ. For example, Bladder 67, the Metal point of the Bladder channel, can be used to pull *qi* from the Large Intestine into the Bladder or Kidney 7, the Metal point of the Kidney, to transfer *qi* from the Lung to the Kidney.

The tonification points are:

- Lung 9
- Large Intestine 11
- Stomach 41
- Spleen 2
- Heart 9
- Small Intestine 3
- Bladder 67
- Kidney 7
- Pericardium 9
- Triple Burner 3
- Gall Bladder 43
- Liver 8

[3]These treatment protocols are not used in contemporary TCM. It is interesting, however, to note that they were being taught at the Shanghai Military Medical College between 1964 and 1970. Entry/Exit protocols were also being taught; Eckman, 1996, p. 160.

Sedation points

The sedation point on a channel is the point associated with the following Element on the *sheng* cycle or the 'child' of the Organ involved. The sedation point on the channel is sedated if the *qi* in an Organ is in relative excess compared to that of the Organ that follows it on the *sheng* cycle. For example, St 45, the Metal point, can be sedated if the practitioner wishes to transfer *qi* to the Large Intestine.

The sedation points are:

- Lung 5
- Large Intestine 2
- Stomach 45
- Spleen 5
- Heart 7
- Small Intestine 8
- Bladder 65
- Kidney 1
- Pericardium 7
- Triple Burner 10
- Gall Bladder 38
- Liver 2

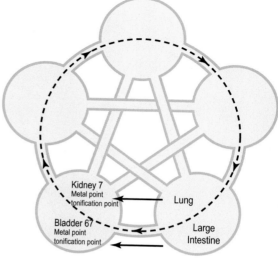

Figure 36.1 • Use of the tonification points

The use of tonification and sedation points

Tonification points are more frequently used than sedation points. This is because more emphasis is placed on tonifying underlying deficiencies than on sedating excess. Sometimes, both points can be used together. If, for example, the Liver pulse is full or in excess, and the Pericardium pulse is deficient, then the sedation point of the Liver channel (Liv 2, the Fire point) can be sedated at the same time as reinforcing the tonification point on the Pericardium channel (PC 9, the Wood point). This is most commonly carried out when an excess pulse is felt on the mother Organ. The tonification point is used in preference to the sedation point when the mother Organ is only relatively fuller than the child but pulse diagnosis still shows it to be deficient overall.

The use of these points is largely determined by which Element the practitioner is focusing on in the treatment. If, for example, the practitioner is treating a Water CF whose Metal Element is stronger than the Water, it would be usual to use the tonification points of Water (Bl 67 and Kid 7) several times during the course of the patient's treatment (see Figure 36.1). It would be unusual to use the sedation points of Metal (LI 2 and Lu 5) unless the Organs of the Metal Element had an excess of *qi*, which is unlikely.

On the other hand, if a practitioner is treating a Wood CF, with a full Liver, it would be usual to use the sedation points of this Organ (Liv 2), especially if the Heart or Pericardium is deficient. It should be noted, however, that if the Heart and Pericardium were deficient in absolute terms, then it would be quite common to stimulate the tonification points of the Fire Organs (Ht 9 or PC 9). If the Stomach Organ is full and the Large Intestine is deficient, then the sedation point of the Stomach (St 45) might be used. Again, if the Large Intestine is deficient in absolute terms, then it would be quite common to stimulate the tonification point (LI 11). Figure 36.2 shows transfers of *qi* with emphasis on the sedation points – but tonification points can also be used.

The principle is put succinctly in the *Ode to the Streamer out of the Dark* (+1234):

> As to needling the original channel, there is also the Mother and Child. Supposing the Heart is weak, select Little Rushing In (Ht 9) from the original channel and reinforce it; Little Rushing In is the Well Wood point, and Wood can produce Fire. When it is strong then select the Sprit Gate (Ht 7) and drain it; Spirit Gate is the *shu* Earth point, and Fire can produce Earth.

(Bertschinger, 1991, p. 21)

Transferring *qi* across the *ke* cycle

Another method of transferring *qi* between Organs is to transfer between *yin* Organs that are linked on the *ke* or control cycle. For example, a practitioner can

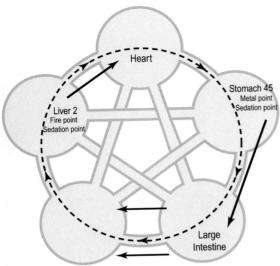

Figure 36.2 • Use of the sedation points, but tonification points can also be used

transfer *qi* from a relatively excess Liver to a relatively deficient Spleen by stimulating Sp 1, the Wood point on the Spleen channel. This is less commonly used than tonification points and sedation points while treating the person's CF, but these points

can be very valuable for some patients and in some specific circumstances.

Transferring *qi* in specific treatment protocols

This method of transferring *qi* across the *ke* cycle is most frequently used in the following circumstances.

1 When treating a Husband–Wife imbalance (see Figure 36.3 and Chapter 28). The four points that have the ability to transfer *qi* from the Organs on the wife's side over to the husband's side are Bl 67, Kid 7, Kid 3 and Liv 4.

2 When using the 'Four Needle Technique'. This was first described in the 1600s by the Korean monk, Sa Am (Eckman, 1996, p. 154). It is also used by many Japanese, Korean and other practitioners for 'root' treatments. Practitioners of Five Element Constitutional Acupuncture use it extremely rarely. Its main use is to exert more force when transferring *qi* between two Organs linked on the *sheng* cycle. This kind of force is most commonly needed when a patient has a Husband–Wife imbalance and the *qi* fails to transfer sufficiently from the right to the left side.

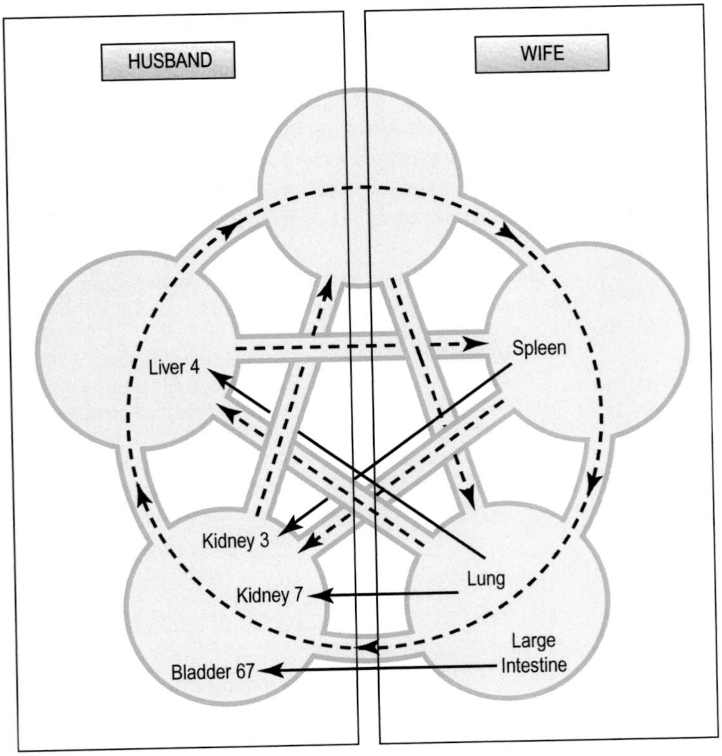

Figure 36.3 • Points used for Husband–Wife imbalance

(See Appendix C for a description of Four Needle Technique.)

3 It is also rarely used in a system of transfers between Organs not directly connected to each other on the *sheng* or *ke* cycles. (See Chapter 34 for a description of these transfers.)

Yuan source points

Uses of *yuan* source points

These are the most commonly used points in this style of acupuncture. This is for several reasons:

- They are regarded as the best points to use to 'test' for the CF. This is because they are both reliable and powerful.
- They are regarded as reliable points to support the use of other points on the same channel. For example, they may be used if the practitioner has needled other points and wishes to support and enhance the treatment.

The effect on the *yuan qi*

These points have a particular effect upon the *yuan qi*, 'the most basic motive force within the body' (Rose and Zhang, 2001). *Yuan qi* is 'nothing but *jing* in the form of *qi* ..... It is the foundation of vitality and stamina' (Maciocia, 1989, pp. 41–42). This is especially important to Five Element Constitutional Acupuncturists as so much of their work focuses on enhancing the patient's constitutional health.

The *Nan Jing* describes the *yuan qi* as 'the root and foundation of all the twelve conduits (channels)' (Unschuld, 1986, Chapter 8). As the *yuan qi* is specifically described as *jing* in *qi* form, it is the most important form of *qi* to stimulate if the practitioner wishes to influence the patient's constitutional health, the *jing*.

The importance of the source points is expressed in the *Nei Jing* in the following passage:

> When any of the five viscera are diseased, the most appropriate point among the twelve source points should be chosen. The twelve source points are the places by which the five viscera irrigate the three hundred and sixty five joints with the *qi* and flavours they have received.

> (*Ling Shu*, Chapter 1; Yang and Chace, 1994)

Nan Jing Chapter 66 also discusses source points. It places particular emphasis on the use of the source point of Triple Burner, TB 4. This is because one of the main functions of the Triple Burner is as the 'avenue for the *yuan qi*' (Maciocia, 1989, p. 118), responsible for distributing *yuan qi* to all the channels and Organs of the body. The *Nan Jing* says that: '"Origin" (*yuan*) is an honourable designation for the Triple Burner' (Unschuld, 1986, Chapter 66) with reference to its ability to nourish the *yuan qi* and distribute it to the other Organs.

The *yuan* source points are:

- Lung 9
- Large Intestine 4
- Stomach 42
- Spleen 3
- Heart 7
- Small Intestine 4
- Bladder 64
- Kidney 3
- Pericardium 7
- Triple Burner 4
- Gall Bladder 40
- Liver 3

Luo junction points

The *luo* junction points are commonly used in several different contexts.

1 They connect the *yin* and *yang* Organs within an Element. If the practitioner determines that the pulse of an Organ is more deficient than its partner, then the junction point on the relatively deficient Organ is tonified in order to bring about greater harmony between the Organs. For example, if the pulse of the Spleen is weaker than that of the Stomach, Sp 4, the *luo* junction point can be tonified (see Figure 36.4). If both Organs are full, the practitioner can reduce the junction point on the fuller of the two Organs, but this is done much less commonly. (In the Fire Element, the traditional pairings of Heart/Small Intestine and Pericardium/Triple Burner are used.)

2 The *luo* junction points are often used in combination, in order to generally tonify or reduce an Element. This is particularly true if the practitioner perceives some difference, in quality or quantity, between the two Organs, although this is not essential. PC 6 (*Nei Guan*, Inner Frontier Gate) and TB 5 (*Wai Guan*, Outer Frontier Gate), for example, can both be tonified even when no difference is detected between the pulses of the Pericardium and Triple Burner. GB 37 (*Guang Ming*, Bright and Clear) and Liv 5 (*Li Gou*, Insect Ditch) can be reduced together when the Wood Element is full, or tonified together when the Wood Element is deficient.

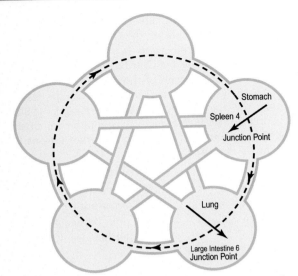

Figure 36.4 • The *luo* junction point is used to balance the disharmony between these paired organs

3 They can be paired with the *yuan* source point of the opposite organ. The *luo* junction point and the *yuan* source point are connected via an internal pathway. Using these points together is known as combining the 'host' and the 'guest'. The host is the Organ primarily affected and the 'guest' is the paired Organ.[4] For example, the junction point of the Lung can be tonified with the source point of the Large Intestine. This will connect the two Organs and enhance the Metal Element generally.

4 They are used in complex transfer protocols. (See Chapter 34 and Appendix C.)

5 They are used to correct Akabane imbalances. (See Chapter 28.)

The *luo* junction points are:

- Lung 7
- Large Intestine 6
- Stomach 40
- Spleen 4
- Heart 5
- Small Intestine 7
- Bladder 58
- Kidney 4
- Pericardium 6
- Triple Burner 5
- Gall Bladder 37
- Liver 5

---

[4]Different methods have been used over history to determine which Organ is the 'host'. *Ling Shu* Chapter 10 and the *Great Compendium of Acupuncture and Moxibustion* propose diagnosis based upon physical symptomatology. In Five Element Constitutional Acupuncture, the decision would be made based upon a wider picture of the 'Officials', or because the practitioner has previously discovered which Organ produces the more significant pulse change when treated.

Horary points

Horary points are the points on the channel whose Element is the same as the channel itself. It is a horary point only during the channel's 2-hour period of maximum activity. For example, PC 8, the Fire point, is the horary point on the Pericardium channel (the Pericardium being an Organ of the Fire Element) between 7 and 9 p.m. Table 36.2 gives the time of day for the different horary points.

The concept of 2-hour periods when the *qi* of an Organ is at its strongest comes from the school of biorhythmic methodology known as *zi wu liu zhu fa* and goes back to at least the Tang dynasty (+618–906). (Soulié de Morant, 1994, p. 121, claims it goes back to −104 in the Han dynasty, but gives no reference.)

The 2-hour horary times are based on the passage of the sun, i.e. midday is when the sun at its zenith, and the practitioner must make allowances for variances from sun time, such as Summer Time. It is very difficult to be sure of the exact time by the sun in any particular place and in practice these points are used fairly liberally in this respect. To use some of the horary points at the right time of day would involve working extremely unsocial hours, so in practice it is the Stomach and Spleen, Heart and Small Intestine, and Bladder and Kidney horary points that are used most commonly. These

Table 36.2 Horary points

Horary point	Time of day
Lung 8	3–5 a.m.
Large Intestine 1	5–7 a.m.
Stomach 36	7–9 a.m.
Spleen 3	9–11 a.m.
Heart 8	11 a.m.–1 p.m.
Small Intestine 5	1–3 p.m.
Bladder 66	3–5 p.m.
Kidney 10	5–7 p.m.
Pericardium 8	7–9 p.m.
Triple Burner 6	9–11 p.m.
Gall Bladder 41	11 p.m.–1 a.m.
Liver 1	1–3 a.m.

points can also be sedated when an Organ is full at the lowest time of day but this is not their main use.

Uses of horary points

1 During their 2-hour period, horary points give powerful enhancement to the *qi* of the Organ on which they are used.

2 Used outside horary time, the Element points will also have a strengthening effect, although this is less powerful than when used as a horary point.

3 Element points (or seasonal horary points) are occasionally used when the practitioner wishes to treat an Organ during the season resonant with the associated Element. For example, the 'seasonal horary' points in the spring are GB 41 and Liv 1. These might be tonified if these Organs are deficient.

4 Element points are also used in a particular way in the Four Needle Technique (see Appendix C).

Xi cleft or accumulation points

Xi cleft points are points where *qi* 'accumulates'. They are usually used to back up other points or to generally tonify or reduce an Organ. They have the advantage of being situated amongst the 'command' points (with the exception of St 34, which lies above the knee), so they are often dynamic and powerful points. None of these points is an Element point so they also have the advantage over some other points of not affecting the balance of the Element 'within' the Element.

Other points with specific uses

The back *shu* or 'associated effect points'[5]

These are points on the back which lie along the Bladder Channel and directly affect the related Organ (see Table 36.3). The use of these points goes back

Table 36.3 Back *shu* points

Organ	Back *shu* point
Lung	Bl 13
Large Intestine	Bl 25
Stomach	Bl 21
Spleen	Bl 20
Heart	Bl 15
Small Intestine	Bl 27
Bladder	Bl 28
Kidneys	Bl 23
Pericardium	Bl 14
Triple Burner	Bl 22
Gall Bladder	Bl 19
Liver	Bl 18

to the *Ling Shu*, Chapter 51. They are very commonly used to either stimulate or sedate the *qi* of an Organ. They are especially effective when the *qi* of the patient is extremely depleted. Their effect is thought to be directly upon the Organ itself, rather than being mediated by the channel associated with the Organ as are other points. They are also used in the diagnosis and treatment of Aggressive Energy (see Chapter 30).

Entry and Exit points

These points are situated on or near the beginning or the end of the channels. They connect the channels together to form a complete circuit of *qi*. (See Chapter 33 for more on the use of these points.)

Entry and Exit points are used when the practitioner determines that the *qi* is not flowing freely between two channels that are linked in the circulation of *qi*. This circulation follows the traditional usage, set down in *Ling Shu* Chapter 10, starting with the Lung and ending with the Liver. It is the same circulation that is found in the Chinese clock (see Horary points above).

In general, the point of Entry is the first point on the channel and the point of Exit is the last point, but there are exceptions to this rule. The exceptions are given in bold in Table 36.4.

[5]J. R. Worsley used the term 'Associated Effect Points', a term which was also used by Felix Mann, an influential writer and teacher of acupuncture. The term is now unfamiliar to almost everyone apart from practitioners of Five Element Constitutional Acupuncture.

Table 36.4 Entry and Exit points

Organ	Entry point	Exit point
Lung	1	7
Large Intestine	4	20
Stomach	1	42
Spleen	1	21
Heart	1	9
Small Intestine	1	19
Bladder	1	67
Kidney	1	22
Pericardium	1[a]	8
Triple Burner	1	22
Gall Bladder	1	41
Liver	1	14
Ren	1	24
Du	1	28

[a]On most women it is impossible to needle PC 1, so PC 2 is needled instead.

Sometimes the Entry points on a channel are tonified in order to give a general boost to the *qi* of the channel.

Ren mai and *Du mai* points

The 12 main channels are compared to rivers but these two vessels are likened to seas. The *Ren mai* is known as the 'sea of *yin* channels' and the *Du mai* as the 'sea of *yang* channels'. Points on these channels are used to support treatment on the CF and other Elements. This is particularly the case when there is severe depletion of *qi* and the practitioner is struggling to initiate sufficient improvement in the patient. (See Chapter 44 for usage of specific points on these vessels.)

Front *mu* or alarm points

These are points on the torso that directly affect a related Organ. These points can be used diagnostically. If they are found to be tender on palpation,

it may indicate imbalance in the associated Organ. Tenderness on palpation is not regarded as a reliable indicator, however, as some people's acupuncture points are much more sensitive than other's. For this reason, and because they give no help in diagnosing the CF, few practitioners place much emphasis upon their use. Practitioners of Five Element Constitutional Acupuncture never use front *mu* points therapeutically, although many of the points are frequently treated for other characteristics that they have. (See Chapter 29 for more on front *mu* points.)

In common with many practitioners who learned from Japanese sources, J. R. Worsley's listing of front *mu* points is slightly different from that taught in China (Worsley, 1982, p. 285). This is indicated in the listing given in Table 36.5 by showing the points where there is a difference in bold.

The use of the points given in this chapter forms the basis for much of the patient's treatment. If the practitioner wishes to affect the patient's mind and spirit more specifically, the use of points as described in the next chapter is indicated.

Table 36.5 Front *mu* or alarm points

Organ	Front *mu* or alarm point
Lung	Lu 1
Large Intestine	St 25
Stomach	*Ren* 12
Spleen	Liv 13
Heart	*Ren* 14
Small Intestine	*Ren* 4
Bladder	*Ren* 3
Kidney	GB 25
Pericardium	**Ren 15**
Triple Burner	*Ren* 5
Upper *jiao*	*Ren* 17
Middle *jiao*	*Ren* 12
Lower *jiao*	*Ren* 7
Gall Bladder	**GB 23 and 24**
Liver	Liv 14

Summary

1 Practitioners of Five Element Constitutional Acupuncture regularly use points based upon uses set out in the *Nei Jing* and *Nan Jing*.

2 'Command' points, which lie below the elbows and knees, are frequently used.

3 Transfers of *qi* from relatively full Organs to more deficient Organs are carried out using Element points in the form of tonification and sedation points. Transfers can also be made across the *ke* cycle between the *yin* Organs. These are more commonly used when patients' pulses indicate marked imbalances between the Elements.

4 *Yuan* source points are very commonly used. They affect the *yuan qi*, the *jing* in *qi* form, and thereby directly influence the person's constitutional health. They are the main points used to test the CF and the response to treating an Organ or Element.

5 When the *qi* of a person is especially deficient, the back *shu* points, horary points and points on the *Ren mai* and *Du mai* are commonly used.

Using points to treat the spirit

37

Treating the spirit in Five Element Constitutional Acupuncture

Practitioners of Five Element Constitutional Acupuncture place a high value on generating change at the level of a person's spirit in order to alleviate many chronic health problems.

> To have the spirits (*de shen*) is the splendour of life.
> To lose the spirits (*shi shen*) is annihilation.
>
> (*Su Wen*, Chapter 13; Larre and Rochat de la Vallée, 1995, p. 33)

When discussing the use of points to treat the person's spirit, the word 'spirit' is used in the same sense as it is used in Chapters 3 and 27. When practitioners attempt to bring about a change in a person's 'spirit' through treatment they are endeavouring to initiate deep and fundamental changes. These changes manifest in how patients feel in themselves and thereby how they interact with the world.

Treating at the appropriate level

Choosing the correct level of treatment is of prime importance. Some patients, for example, have purely physical symptoms that are causing pain, impaired function and/or lowered vitality. In this case a few simple treatments may bring about sufficient balance so that the physical symptoms are cleared. However, even simple symptoms like these may be arising from a deeper level.

For example, a person with pain, impaired function and/or lowered vitality may also have had an anxious disposition throughout his or her life. In this case it is important to ensure that treatment addresses the anxious disposition. If the patient is a Water CF the practitioner may start by re-balancing the 'descending' movements of the Kidney *qi* to allow him or her to feel more settled inside. If this can be achieved by using simple treatments such as 'command' points, transfers of *qi*, back *shu* points, etc., on the Water Element, there is no need to use points that treat the spirit specifically. Some patients can experience a radical transformation in their state of health in body, mind and spirit from very simple treatments.

If, on the other hand, simple treatment does not generate significant improvement in the patient's spirit, then the practitioner may need to choose points that affect the spirit more directly. Practitioners know that the spirit level has been affected if patients report feeling better in themselves. There should also be an improvement in the colour, sound, emotion and odour as well as the symptoms.

Health and the spirit

What constitutes 'health' is different from patient to patient. Increased relaxation, vitality, happiness, strength, creativity, spontaneity, decisiveness, clarity, purpose, hope or many other aspects of the human condition are all possible changes that patients need to experience in order to have a sense of well-being. If the root of the problem lies in the spirit but only the physical symptoms respond, they will continue to live a diminished life. Their physical problems may also return or new ones emerge.

Choosing spirit points

It is usual to choose spirit points that are on the channels of the CF. Spirit points are usually only used on Elements other than the CF when a person's spirit has been especially affected by traumatic and difficult situations involving intense emotions. For example, an Earth CF who has just suffered a bereavement may be unable to return to her or his previous level of well-being and happiness. In this case it might be necessary to treat points on the Metal Element whose main effect is on the spirit. Without supporting the Metal Element, the patient may be unable to return to their previous level of balance.

Reaching the spirit level

> For every needling, the method above all is not to miss the rooting in the Spirits.
>
> (*Ling Shu*, Chapter 8; Larre and Rochat de la Vallée, 1995, p. 81)

It is all too easy to say that it is important to treat the patient at the spirit level, but reaching the level of the spirit is not always possible.

How does a practitioner initiate improvement in a person's spirit? There are no easy answers and all practitioners are familiar with the experience of frustration at seemingly being unable to generate the changes that they feel are required. Two main factors interrelate with each other when treating the spirit: the inner development of the practitioner and the choice of points.

The inner development of the practitioner

This is the subject of Chapter 6, this volume, but its importance can hardly be overstated. The key factor in the practitioner–patient relationship is the trust and depth of rapport established. Practitioners will often be unable to evoke changes in the spirit if they fail to establish sufficiently deep rapport with the patient. This is especially true when patients are suffering intensely from sadness, frustration, anxiety, grief and other emotional states. If rapport is limited

to just 'getting along fine', patients continue to hide away the parts of their spirits that suffer. They are never revealed or touched in the therapeutic encounter.

That is not to say that practitioners should spend their whole time dragging up patients' unhappiness and suffering. It is more that the practitioner has contacted those aspects at some stage. Patients then know that those parts of themselves have been seen and acknowledged. When patients come for treatment knowing that their inner struggles are recognised they can allow themselves to discard much of the mask they wear during their daily life.

Only practitioners who have an awareness of these areas of suffering in themselves and genuinely care for the suffering of others are capable of this level of rapport. That is why practitioners must strive to hone their skills and refine their spirits. Patients can then bring the level of suffering that most needs to be healed to the treatment room.

Intention

The intention of the practitioner is crucial to the practice of acupuncture. The response in the patient is hugely affected by whether the practitioner needles Kid 25, believing its effect to be limited to the physical indications of cough, asthma and chest pain (see Cheng, 1987, p. 187), or if they use it in the context of its time-honoured name as *Shen Cang*, the storehouse of the *shen*. As Sun Si-miao wrote, 'Medicine is intention (*yi*). Those who are proficient at using intention are good doctors' (quoted in Scheid and Bensky, 1998).

Many pianists can play the notes of a piece of music, but only those who are capable of allowing their own spirit to be present in the playing can touch the spirits and feelings of their listeners.

In order to reach the patient's spirit the practitioner needs to be fully present. Otherwise the level of rapport between practitioner and patient may not facilitate sufficient change in the patient's spirit. Acupuncture, relying as it does only on inserting fine needles into a person's *qi*, is a powerful but extremely subtle form of medicine. It is an art as much as it is a science. If the practitioner fails to realise this, the value of the points referred to in the following section will forever remain a mystery.

The choice of points

Before discussing the choice of points it must be said again that, in the right circumstances, change can be initiated in a person's spirit from any point on the body. Although some points tend to influence the spirit more readily than others, there are many patients who can change profoundly in themselves just from treating 'command' points. It is only when patients do not change in themselves that the practitioner uses points that primarily affect the spirit.

One of the underlying principles of point selection in Five Element Constitutional Acupuncture is that each point on a channel has a different effect on the Organ, rather like each hole on a flute produces a different note.

Frequency of using points

Just as patients can acquire a tolerance to some medications that, over a period of time, makes them less effective, they can also fail to reap the same level of benefit from some points if they are used too often. Constant repetition of the same points is therefore discouraged. In order to use these points with precision and elegance, practitioners need to explore the repertoire of points on a channel. They can then assess what changes different points can initiate. It may sometimes be necessary to use the same points frequently, especially on channels with few points or on patients who require long-term or frequent treatment. In this case the points are often used in different combinations.

Using points according to their names

The names of many of the points go back to the Han dynasty. The names of 160 of the points are found in the *Nei Jing* and therefore, not surprisingly, the influence of Daoism and Confucianism can be clearly seen in many of their names. The Daoist view of man and the human body as a microcosm of, and a link between, Heaven and Earth is especially evident in many point names.

The body as a landscape

There is a Daoist saying that, 'The human body is the image of a country' (Schipper, 1993, p. 100) and this is reflected in the point names – streams, marshes, mounds, valleys, mountains and seas. The names of stars and planets are found as well. Burial grounds, treasuries, palaces and city gates, some of the constructions and institutions of the dynamic and creative Han dynasty are also present.

The great physician Sun Si-miao wrote, 'The names of the points are not nominal; each has a profound meaning' (quoted in Ellis *et al.*, 1989). The use of points based on the name of the point became a major aspect of the point selection of many Daoist practitioners and is described in the Yellow Court Classic (+ second century), a component of the Daoist Canon or *Dao Zang* (Eckman, 1996, p. 213). There are still Daoist practitioners who have maintained the tradition of using point names extensively in their treatments.[1]

The use of points by anatomical terms

The *Jia Yi Jing* (+282), based on the *Nei Jing* and the *Ming Tang* (a Han dynasty classic of acupuncture and moxibustion lost in antiquity), added another 189 points, which accounts for the names of 349 of the points. Many of these names are topographical in nature, describing the anatomy to be found at or near the point. These names offer little or no help to contemporary practitioners as to the particular characteristics of a point.[2]

The use of spirit points

Each channel also has points where the name carries some meaning that links the point either with Heaven or with some aspect of a person's spirit. It is important, however, to also bear in mind the Organ and Element on which the point is located. A point such as Liv 14, the Gate of Hope, may be effective if the patient's lack of optimism and inspiration is predominantly due to an imbalance of the Liver. If it comes from dysfunction of another Organ or Element, then the Gate of Hope will not be effective. Some points, such as the Windows of the Sky, Kidney chest points or the outer back *shu* points are grouped together. Some points have the word 'spirit' in their name, translations of either *shen* or *ling*. These groupings are discussed below. (See Appendix A for more on the different terms used in Chinese medicine to mean 'spirit'.)

---

[1] J. R. Worsley probably learnt the concept of using the point names and interpretations of some points from J. Lavier, who studied extensively with many practitioners throughout the Orient.

[2] No versions of the original publication of *Jia Yi Jing* survive. The earliest extant version dates from +1601, so it is impossible to know how many of the point names originate from later eras. Joseph Needham thought that the naming of all the points was completed by +300; see Lu and Needham, 1980, p. 101.

Interpreting point names

The major problem of relying on the name of the point for information about its characteristics lies in its interpretation. What was meant in antiquity when the point was named is not always clear. Practitioners need to be careful to not just place their own interpretation on the name of the point in such a way that they end up with a mistaken view of its characteristics. For more on the interpretation of point names, see Ellis *et al.*, 1988; Hicks, 1999; College of Traditional Acupuncture, 2000; Willmont, 2001.[3]

The use of points by location

Although many of the most powerful points are situated distal to the elbow and knee, there are also other areas of the body that have a large number of powerful points.

These areas are especially centred on the three *dan tian* of the body (see Figure 37.1). More emphasis has historically been placed on these three foci in *tai ji quan*, *qi gong* and Daoist meditation practices than in medicine. (There are similarities to, but also key differences from, the Indian concept of *chakras*.) There are, however, considerable overlaps that can be most clearly seen in the names and use of acupuncture points. These centres of *qi* are resonant with the Heaven–Humanity–Earth paradigm.

The lower *dan tian*

This is located just below the umbilicus. This connects with the area between the Kidneys called the *ming men*. These two areas have special significance in Oriental medicine and also in many Oriental spiritual disciplines. The *qi* in these areas 'constitute man's life' and are 'the source and basis of the 12 conduits' (channels or meridians) (Unschuld, 1986, Chapter 66). In Japan this area is known as the *Hara*, and is the focus of many Japanese meditative practices. Palpation of the *Hara* constitutes a major

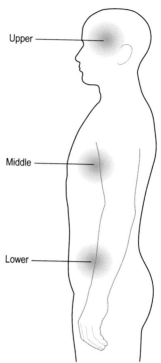

Figure 37.1 • The three *dan tian* of the body

Upper

Middle

Lower

diagnostic component of many styles of Japanese acupuncture. (In the Indian tradition the area of the *dan tian* is the site of the second *chakra*.) In the model of Heaven–Humanity–Earth, it is the main energetic centre of the body that links us to the *qi* of the Earth. The Han dynasty classic, the *Book of the Centre*, describes it as:

> The *dan tian* is the root of a human being. This is the place where the vital power is kept. The five *qi* (of the Five Elements) have their origin here.
>
> (Schipper, 1993, p. 106)

When the lower *dan tian* is deficient the person usually lacks physical and sexual vitality and is prone to feelings of insecurity and anxiety. The spirit is not 'rooted'.

The middle *dan tian*

This is centred in the chest and governs our connection with Humanity. Our ability to create intimate relationships and engage creatively and productively with the world of people and the '10,000 things' is dependent upon the condition of the middle

---

[3]The modern Chinese emphasis on expelling all Daoist or superstitious (*mixin*) influences from Chinese medicine has meant that the importance of point names has been all but expunged from TCM acupuncture. This is a great shame. Modern practitioners who are interested in sometimes using points based upon their names need to reflect upon the names, study the various books that discuss this aspect of acupuncture, and above all be prepared to explore a wide repertoire of points and assess their characteristics for themselves. In this book we draw upon the name of the point for insight into its characteristics as well as relying heavily upon our own clinical experience and that of other practitioners of this style of acupuncture.

dan tian. Many points linked to the Heart and Heart-Protector are sited around the middle *dan tian.*

The upper *dan tian*

This is sited in the brain between the eyes and is responsible for our connection to Heaven. It was known as 'the cavity of *shen*' and the 'upper crucible' by Daoist adepts.

Inspiration, a sense of purpose and a sense of connection to nature are dependent upon the vitality of the upper *dan tian.* Many of the points in this area, for example, GB 13 *Ben Shen,* Root of the Spirit; *Du 24 Shen Ting,* Spirit Hall; and *Yin Tang* (located above the upper *dan tian* between the eyebrows) have long been used to strengthen and calm the spirit.

The practitioner's repertoire of points

Different practitioners use different repertoires of points and the points listed in Table 37.1 are the points that the authors and their peers and colleagues commonly use. This is not to say that other points cannot be used to generate change specifically in a patient's spirit. Similarly one practitioner may find that a point is powerful but when another colleague uses it, it does not seem to have the same powerful effect. On this topic there is no substitute for treating a large number of patients and using a wide variety of points. The practitioner can then maintain a vigilant awareness of the changes evoked in the pulses and in the person. Over the years, practitioners need to reflect on their use of individual points and the changes they have facilitated in their patients.

It must not be forgotten that any point on a channel will have some, albeit in some cases very little, effect. In the hands of a *sheng ren,* a practitioner who 'through his power awakens and develops people's higher nature' (see Chapter 6, this volume), profound change can be effected through any point on the body.

Specific groups of spirit points

The 'Windows of the Sky'

This grouping of points comes from the *Ling Shu.* They are referred to in Chapters 2, 5 and 21, but the different passages give slightly different listings and indications. There are in fact no psychological

Table 37.1 Points used specifically to treat the spirit

Element	Points used specifically to treat the spirit
Wood	Gall Bladder 9 *Tian Chong,* Heavenly Surge Gall Bladder 13 *Ben Shen,* Root of the Spirit Gall Bladder 15 *Tou Lin Qi,* Head Above Tears Gall Bladder 16 *Mu Chuang,* Eye Window Gall Bladder 18 *Cheng Ling,* Receiving Spirit Gall Bladder 24 *Ri Yue,* Sun and Moon Gall Bladder 37 *Guang Ming,* Bright and Clear Gall Bladder 40 *Qiu Xu,* Wilderness Mound Bladder 48 *Yang Gang,* Yang Net Liver 2 *Xing Jian,* Moving Between Liver 13 *Zhang Men,* Chapter Gate Liver 14 *Qi Men,* Gate of Hope Bladder 47 *Hun Men,* Gate of the *Hun*
Fire	Heart 1 *Ji Quan,* Supreme Spring Heart 2 *Qing Ling,* Blue-Green Spirit Heart 4 *Ling Dao,* Spirit Path Heart 7 *Shen Men,* Spirit Gate Bladder 44 *Shen Tang,* Spirit Hall Small Intestine 11 *Tian Zong,* Heavenly Ancestor Small Intestine 16 *Tian Chuang,* Heavenly Window Small Intestine 17 *Tian Rong,* Heavenly Appearance Pericardium 1 *Tian Chi,* Heavenly Pond Pericardium 2 *Tian Quan,* Heavenly Spring Bladder 43 *Gao Huang Shu,* Vitals Back *Shu* Point Triple Burner 10 *Tian Jing,* Heavenly Well Triple Burner 15 *Tian Liao,* Heavenly Foramen Triple Burner 16 *Tian You,* Heavenly Window Triple Burner 23 *Si Zhu Kong,* Silk Bamboo Hollow
Earth	Stomach 8 *Tou Wei,* Corner of the Head Stomach 9 *Ren Ying,* People Welcome Stomach 23 *Tai Yi,* Supreme Unity Stomach 25 *Tian Shu,* Heavenly Pivot Stomach 40 *Feng Long,* Abundant Prosperity Spleen 4 *Gong Sun,* Grandfather and Grandson Spleen 15 *Da Heng,* Great Horizontal Spleen 18 *Tian Xi,* Heavenly Stream Spleen 20 *Zhou Rong,* Encircling Glory Spleen 21 *Da Bao,* Great Enveloping Bladder 49 *Yi She, Yi* Dwelling

Table 37.1 Points used specifically to treat the spirit—cont'd

Element	Points used specifically to treat the spirit
Metal	Lung 1 *Zhong Fu*, Central Treasury Lung 2 *Yun Men*, Cloud Gate Lung 3 *Tian Fu*, Heavenly Treasury Bladder 42 *Po Hu*, Door of *Po* Large Intestine 17 *Tian Ding*, Heavenly Vessel Large Intestine 18 *Fu Tu*, Support the Prominence
Water	Bladder 1 *Jing Ming*, Bright Eyes Bladder 7 *Tong Tian*, Heavenly Connection Bladder 10 *Tian Zhu*, Heavenly Pillar Bladder 52 *Zhi Shi*, *Zhi* Dwelling Kidney 1 *Yong Quan*, Bubbling Spring Kidney 21 *You Men*, Dark Gate Kidney 23 *Shen Feng*, *Shen* Seal Kidney 24 *Ling Xu*, Spirit Burial Ground Kidney 25 *Shen Cang*, Spirit Storehouse Kidney 26 *Yu Zhong*, Elegant Centre Kidney 27 *Shu Fu*, Empty Treasury
Ren mai and *Du mai* and extra points	Ren 1 *Hui Yin*, Meeting of *Yin* Ren 4 *Guan Yuan*, Gate to the *Yuan Qi* Ren 5 *Shi Men*, Stone Gate Ren 6 *Qi Hai*, Sea of *Qi* Ren 8 *Shen Que*, Spirit Palace Gate Ren 15 *Jiu Wei*, Dove Tail Ren 16 *Zhong Ting*, Middle Hall Ren 17 *Tan Zhong*, Middle of the Chest Ren 22 *Tian Tu*, Heavenly Chimney Du 4 *Ming Men*, Gate of Life Du 10 *Ling Tai*, Spirit Tower Du 11 *Shen Dao*, Spirit Path Du 16 *Feng Fu*, Wind Treasury Du 19 *Hou Ding*, Posterior Summit Du 20 *Bai Hui*, One Hundred Meetings Du 24 *Shen Ting*, Spirit Hall *Yin Tang*

indications given in any of these passages, and this has understandably led some writers to question whether they have any particular effect on a person's spirit (see Deadman *et al.*, 1998, p. 50; McDonald, 1992).

It was stated earlier in the chapter that there is a huge variation in the types of names given to different points on the body. For example, some points refer to anatomical features whilst others describe more about the use of the points. The group of points known as the 'Windows of the Sky' are used specifically to enhance the patient's relationship to Heaven. In fact, 'Windows of Heaven' is a more accurate name for them, as *tian* is the word translated as 'sky', whereas 'Heaven' is its more usual translation. (Nevertheless, the authors have chosen to retain the term Windows of the Sky because it is so well known.) Most of the Windows of the Sky points contain the word 'heaven' (*tian*) in their name. The names evoke images of nourishing the part of a person that corresponds to Heaven.

Points that nourish Heaven

The goal of treatment for Daoist practitioners of the Han dynasty was to harmonise the person's *qi* with that of Heaven and Earth. In the Han dynasty, and in many lineages throughout the history of acupuncture, the upper part of the body was regarded as 'resonant' with Heaven.

The names and positions of these Windows in the Sky points (see Table 37.2) indicate that they were considered appropriate for attempting to enhance the connection between the person and Heaven. All Windows are situated upon the neck, with the exception of Lu 3 (upper arm) and PC 1 (chest), where the channels do not ascend as high

Table 37.2 Windows of the Sky points

Element	Windows of the Sky
Wood	None[a]
Fire	SI 16 *Tian Chuang*, Heavenly Window SI 17 *Tian Rong*, Heavenly Appearance PC 1 *Tian Chi*, Heavenly Pond TB 16 *Tian You*, Heavenly Window
Earth	St 9 *Ren Ying*, People Welcome
Metal	Lu 3 *Tian Fu*, Heavenly Treasury LI 18 *Fu Tu*, Support The Prominence
Water	Bl 10 *Tian Zhu*, Heavenly Pillar
Ren mai and *Du mai*	Ren 22 *Tian Tu*, Heavenly Chimney Du 16 *Feng Fu*, Wind Treasury

[a]Unless Gall Bladder 9 is included. See section on Gall Bladder points in Chapter 38.

as the neck. The neck serves as a bridge between the *qi* of the two lower *dan tians* in the torso and the upper *dan tian* in the head.

> What is above the neck is noble and majestic in spirit, which is to manifest the feature of heaven and its kind.
>
> (Tung Chung-Shu; quoted in Chan, 1963, p. 281)

The other reason that practitioners use these points is because they have discovered through their own experience that these points have a heightened ability to affect a person's spirit. That is not to say that these points (and others that predominantly affect the spirit) always produce the effect the practitioner hopes for. This is, of course, true of all the points on the body. There are many reason for a lack of effect. For example, lack of sufficiently deep rapport, unfocused intention (*yi*) on the part of the practitioner or poor point location can all lead to treatment falling short of the practitioner's hopes and expectations. Also, the patient may not yet be in sufficiently harmonious balance to be able to benefit fully from this treatment.

Using the Windows of the Sky

Connecting with Heaven

The Windows of the Sky are indicated when a patient's spirit is diminished and out of touch with the *qi* of Heaven. People who are in touch with Heaven are able to derive happiness from their contact with the outside world. They are open to the wonder of a glorious day, music, beautiful scenery and the splendour of nature and life. As a classic of the Han dynasty put it:

> One able to nourish what Heaven generates and not interfere with it is called 'Son of Heaven'.
>
> (Lushi Chunqiu; quoted in Lo, 2001, p. 25)

It has never been easy to 'nourish what Heaven generates', but city life, materialism and the decline in interest in spiritual matters has made it harder than ever for patients in our culture and time. Everybody knows what it is like to be so tired, preoccupied, upset or low that for short periods of time they seem to lose touch with the beauty of life. Their connection with Heaven is temporarily dimmed.

Practitioners usually only need to intervene when the connection has been weak for some time. In this case the intensity or prolonged nature of the patients' emotional distress has eroded their connection to Heaven. They may have lost clarity, enthusiasm, hope or the ability to generate necessary change in their lives. Their *qi* no longer moves freely and harmoniously. Their sense of purpose and inspiration have become swamped by stagnation, melancholia, anxiety and frustration. As the *Huainanzi* says:

> Thus to attend to affairs while not being in accord with Heaven is to rebel against one's own nature.
>
> (Major, 1993, Chapter 3)

When to use the Windows of the Sky points

These points are most commonly used when acupuncture treatment has already succeeded in bringing about considerable improvement in the patient's health. Ideally patients already have improved vitality and many signs and symptoms have improved. The pulses no longer have major discrepancies in strength or quality. The problem is that the patients are not actually 'enjoying' better health. Their spirits are still depressed, and they tend to see the dark and negative side of life.

The Windows of the Sky can be used effectively in these situations. They can make subtle, or not so subtle, improvements in the person's spirit. Opening the Windows of the Sky has been compared to opening a skylight in a room so that the patient can see some light. The result of this is that the person may see new possibilities in what had seemed hopelessly blocked situations. Their awareness of nature, sense of wonder and love of life are enhanced. They have increased vitality and spontaneity which make it possible to initiate change where before movement had been stifled.

The Windows of the Sky can also be used when the practitioner is unable to bring about any change in the person's health and well-being at all. This is only appropriate if this lack of progress is because the patient's connection to Heaven is weak. If, on the other hand, patients are not progressing because they are very depleted or because there are major imbalances between the Elements, then these points will have less effect. In this case the practitioner should probably consider whether there is some other factor that is impeding progress. This may be an incorrect CF diagnosis, a block to treatment or a severe imbalance in another Element. If the practitioner decides that the diagnosis is fundamentally accurate, the use of one or more of the Windows of the Sky can initiate change that is not otherwise being achieved.

It is important not to force patients to see and hear before they are ready. If they have been in a metaphorical dark prison for a long time, then they will only be able to deal with a small ray of light at first. When the patient has adapted to this, other spirit points or windows can be used so that more inspiration is gradually allowed in.

How to use the Windows in treatment

It is best to use the points on the channels of the patient's CF. In general the best response is achieved when Windows are used with only a few other points. They are often combined with the *yuan* source points or other command points on the same channel.

Some practitioners prefer to use the command points first before using the Window. This gives the *qi* some vitality before the Window is opened. (In practice, the Windows are almost always tonified on the channels of deficient Elements.) Others prefer to treat the Window first. In this case, if a significant pulse change is felt or there is a change in the patient's colour, sound, odour or emotion, then there in no need to treat any other points on the channel. If there is little or no change in these signs, then a command point can be added.

Adverse reactions to treatment

On rare occasions a patient will experience either a sudden lowering of mood or become more manic. This usually occurs if the window is opened before the patient is ready. If a reaction happens, the best way to stabilise the *qi* is usually to treat the *yuan* source point on the channels treated. Treatment to 'ground' the person using points for the lower *dan tian* is also effective. This normally settles the spirit and returns it to a more stable condition. Sometimes this second treatment stabilises the effect of the Window to such an extent that the patient is actually significantly better than before.

Other points with 'tian' in their name

There are nine other points on the body that have *tian* in their name, and all of them are situated on the upper part of the body. The presence of *tian* in the name was intended to convey something of how the point can affect a person's connection with the *qi* of Heaven. These points are:

- LI 17   *Tian Ding*   Heavenly Vessel
- Sp 18   *Tian Xi*   Heavenly Stream
- SI 11   *Tian Zong*   Heavenly Ancestor
- Bl 7   *Tong Tian*   Heavenly Connection
- PC 2   *Tian Quan*   Heavenly Spring
- TB 10   *Tian Jing*   Heavenly Well
- TB 15   *Tian Liao*   Heavenly Foramen
- GB 9   *Tian Chong*   Heavenly Surge

The Kidney chest points

This grouping of points, from Kidney 22 to 27, is situated upon the chest in the intercostal spaces. Kidney 22 (*Bu Lang*, Walking on the Verandah) is the exit point of the Kidney channel. The points higher than Kidney 22 on the channel appear to be more connected to the Organs sited in the Upper Burner than to the Kidneys. *Ling Shu* Chapter 16 describes how the *qi* 'entering the Kidneys and flowing into the Pericardium, it scatters in the chest...'(Sunu, 1985).

Three of the Kidney chest points refer specifically to the spirit (see Table 37.3). The name of each point relates to the two different spirits of the Heart, the *shen* and the *ling*. Kidney 26 (*Yu Zhong*, Elegant Centre) and Kidney 27 (*Shu Fu*, Empty Treasury) are used less often, but can still generate significant changes in the pulses and the person's spirit.

Whereas the main effect of the Windows of the Sky is in their ability to improve a person's connection to Heaven, this area in the chest, the middle *dan tian*, governs our connection to other people and the world of the '10,000 things'.

Use of the Kidney chest points

The Kidney chest points are normally used to supplement treatment that is being carried out on other Organs. They are especially useful when the *qi* of

Table 37.3 Kidney chest points

Name	Number
Shen Feng, Spirit Seal	Kid 23
Ling Xu, Spirit Burial Ground	Kid 24
Shen Cang, Spirit Storehouse	Kid 25

the Kidneys, Heart, Pericardium and Lungs has been depleted through sadness, grief, fear and shock. Their main effect is to strengthen. They are often used when the patient's spirit is depleted and they are struggling to cope with the rough and tumble of daily life, relationships, going to work, looking after the children, etc.

These points are particularly indicated when the person's spirit is devastated by feelings of rejection and heartbreak. When bereavement or the ending of a relationship disturbs this area these points can help the person to re-engage with life and people. Whereas the Windows of the Sky can provide a glimmer of light, the Kidney chest points are most effective at fortifying and enlivening the person's spirit. Moxibustion is frequently used on these points. (See Chapter 41 for more details on each point.)

The Kidney chest points are not the only points that have a particularly powerful effect on this area: *Ren* 17, PC 1, Sp 18, Sp 21, Ht 2, PC 2, Lu 3, Bl 43, Bl 44, *Du* 10 and *Du* 11 are all situated at the same level of the chest.

The outer back *shu* points

The points adjacent to the back *shu* points of the five major *yin* organs are all linked to points associated with the spirit of each Organ. Each point refers to parts of a building. These names imply that these points give each spirit a 'residence'. The outer back *shu* points of the *yin* Organs are listed in Table 37.4.

The *yang* Organs of the Gall Bladder, Triple Burner and Stomach also have points lying adjacent to them, but there is none linked to the Large Intestine, Small Intestine or Bladder. There is also a point that lies adjacent to the Pericardium. The outer back *shu* points of these *yang* Organs and the Pericardium are listed in Table 37.5.

Table 37.4 The outer back *shu* points of the *yin* Organs

Name	Number	Adjacent to:
Door of *Po*	Bl 42	Bl 13 (Lung)
Shen Hall	Bl 44	Bl 15 (Heart)
Hun Gate	Bl 47	Bl 18 (Liver)
Yi Dwelling	Bl 49	Bl 20 (Spleen)
Zhi Room	Bl 52	Bl 23 (Kidney)

Table 37.5 The outer back *shu* points of the *yang* Organs and Pericardium

Name	Number	Adjacent to:
Vitals Back *Shu* point	Bl 43	Bl 14 (Pericardium)
Yang Essence	Bl 48	Bl 19 (Gall Bladder)
Stomach Granary	Bl 50	Bl 21 (Stomach)
Vitals Gate	Bl 51	Bl 22 (Triple Burner)

All of these points are powerful spirit points that are frequently used by Five Element Constitutional Acupuncturists. They are especially useful when depletion of the Organ has meant that its 'spirit' has become weakened and/or agitated.

These points are normally used as part of the treatment being carried out on the CF. There is a tendency to use the points on the *yin* organs somewhat more than those on the *yang* organs, but they are often paired together. (In the case of the Heart, Lung and Kidney there is no true counterpart for the paired *yang* Organ, so obviously they are not paired together.)

Other points that treat the spirit

Points with either *shen* or *ling* in their name are frequently used to treat the spirit.

Shen

As described in Chapter 3, *shen* can mean the spirit of the Heart in some contexts and the person's spirit in others. The word *shen* is found in eight points (two of these were also included in the Kidney chest points above).

- GB 13   *Ben Shen*   Root of the Spirit
- Ht 7   *Shen Men*   Spirit Gate
- Bl 44   *Shen Tang*   Spirit Hall
- Kid 23   *Shen Feng*   Spirit Seal
- Kid 25   *Shen Cang*   Spirit Storehouse
- *Ren* 8   *Shen Que*   Spirit Palace Gate
- *Du* 11   *Shen Dao*   Spirit Path
- *Du* 24   *Shen Ting*   Spirit Hall

(Only two of these points directly relate to the Heart – Ht 7 and Bl 44, the outer back *shu* point of the Heart. As discussed in Chapter 41, Kid 23 and 25 can be used to treat the Heart, as can *Du* 11.)

Ling

The *ling* is of crucial importance in acupuncture (see Appendix A for more on the *ling*). It is this character that gives the great classic of acupuncture the *Ling Shu*, usually translated as the 'Spiritual Pivot', its name. *Ling* is also usually translated as 'spirit' when it occurs in the names of five of the acupuncture points (one of these was also included in the Kidney chest points above):

- GB 18   *Cheng Ling*   Receiving Spirit
- Ht 2   *Qing Ling*   Blue-Green Spirit
- Ht 4   *Ling Dao*   Spirit Path
- Kid 24   *Ling Xu*   Spirit Burial Ground
- *Du* 10   *Ling Tai*   Spirit Tower

Conclusion – using points to treat the spirit level

It is not always necessary to use the points discussed in this chapter. If a patient is relatively healthy and strong, treatment on command points may generate all the change that is needed at that time. For other patients, however, it is necessary to treat the spirit. This is one of the greatest challenges for the practitioner of this style of acupuncture.

When the body suffers more than the spirit it may be appropriate to focus much of the treatment on the body. But often it is the weakness and disharmony of the spirit that underlies the physical suffering. When the spirit and mind are struggling then the practitioner should concentrate on treating the CF to nourish the root.

A practitioner harmonises Heaven and Earth in a patient in order to redress their imbalance.

> In general in the life of human beings
> Heaven brings forth the vital essence,
> Earth brings forward the body.
> Unite these two to make a whole person.
> When they are in harmony, there is vitality;
> When they are not in harmony, there is no vitality.

(the pre-Han classic Nei Yeh; quoted in Roth, 1986)

Summary

1 Patients can change and feel better in themselves from needling any point on the body.

2 The rapport between the practitioner and patient and the intention (*yi*) of the practitioner are crucial to the effect of any point or combination of points.

3 The effect of some acupuncture points is primarily on the patient's spirit.

4 The ancient names of some points allude to their individual characteristics and their effects on the spirit.

5 The Windows of the Sky, the Kidney chest points and the outer back *shu* points are groups of points that have their own characteristics and effect on the spirit.

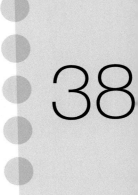

Lung and Large Intestine points

Introduction

In this and the following chapters we describe the points Five Element Constitutional Acupuncturists most frequently use. It must first be stressed, however, that using *any* point on a channel, especially one of the Organs of the person's Constitutional Factor, will create some change. Even if a point is one that is not regarded as specifically affecting the spirit, treatment on the CF usually affects how patients feel in themselves. People who require treatment at the spirit level may not be sufficiently affected by using simple points, however. In this case the art lies in selecting specific points that will more directly affect their spirit.

The characteristics of the points discussed in this chapter come partly from the point names and also the type of point, such as *yuan* source, *luo* junction, back *shu* point, etc. Other known uses of the points are also included and the authors also add much from their personal experience. The actions of the points according to the substances and pathogenic factors are not discussed. (For more on these TCM indications, see Deadman *et al.*, 1998; Ellis *et al.*, 1989; Lade, 1989; Maciocia, 1989.)

Lung points (Table 38.1)

The primary Lung channel

The Lung channel begins at Lu 1 in the third intercostal space. The pathway arches over the axilla and travels down the lateral side of the biceps muscle to the flexure of the elbow. It then runs over the anterior radial side of the forearm to the wrist, over the thenar eminence of the hand, and ends at the radial side of the thumb. It then connects to the Large Intestine channel at LI 4.

Lung 1 *Zhong Fu*, Central Treasury: Entry point, Lung front *mu* point

Needle depth 0.3–0.5 cun; moxa cones 3–5

All points on the Lung channel help a patient to receive *qi* and connect with Heaven, as the Lungs are the 'Receiver of Q*i* from the Heavens'. This Lung point, in particular, has the ability to tonify not just the Lung *qi*, but also the *qi* of the whole chest (*zong qi*).

The Spleen and the Lungs connect at this point and their relationship is particularly close. The Spleen is the 'mother' of the Lungs on the *sheng* cycle. The name *zhong*, which means central, probably refers to this connection, as *zhong qi* is the *qi* of the Stomach and Spleen.

Fu means a treasury. A *fu* can also be a place where riches are stored. Using this point can revitalise

Table 38.1 Commonly used points on the Lung channel

Yuan source point	Lung 9
Luo junction point	Lung 7
Tonification point	Lung 9
Sedation point	Lung 5
Back *shu* point	Bladder 13
Outer Back *shu* point	Bladder 42
Horary point	Lung 8
Xi cleft point	Lung 6
Entry point	Lung 1
Exit point	Lung 7
Window of the Sky	Lung 3

deficient Lung *qi* and reinvigorate the mind and spirit. When the Lung *qi* becomes depleted people can have difficulty receiving inspiration from Heaven. People whose Lungs have become deficient often feel grief and sadness and easily become melancholy or lifeless or lose a sense of purpose. Enhancing the Lung *qi* and the *qi* of the chest enables the person to reconnect with inspiration from Heaven and experience greater meaning in their life.

This is the Entry point. Entry–Exit blocks between the Liver and Lung are frequently found, so this point is commonly used in this context.

Patient Example

An elderly woman who was a Wood CF was not thriving when being treated on the channels of the Wood Element. Although Liv 14 had been treated, Lu 1 had not been used. Only after clearing an Entry–Exit block using both Liv 14 and Lu 1 did she start to improve. Over time the connection between these channels twice more became obstructed and tonifying Lu 1 on each occasion produced substantial improvement.

Lung 2 *Yun Men*, Cloud Gate

Needle depth 0.3–0.5 cun; *moxa cones 3–5*

The reference to clouds in the name of this point probably refers to the importance of the Lungs and a person's contact with Heaven. It implies that this is a gateway through the clouds. Clouds can be associated with grief, sadness and depression. As on a grey overcast day, people need a gate through the clouds to find inspiration and light. The cloud referred to in the point's name could also be a reference to the fluids that are present in the Upper Burner, which are said to be like a 'mist' (*Ling Shu* Chapter 30). The point is used in similar ways as Lu 1 in assisting patients to reconnect with Heaven. It is, however, slightly less powerful.

Lung 3 *Tian Fu*, Heavenly Treasury Window of the Sky

Needle depth 0.5–1.0 cun; *no moxa*

Like Lu 1, this point is a treasury or *fu*. A treasury is a place where a person can go to receive richness and quality or to increase reserves if they are low. Whereas Lu 1 is a Central Treasury, situated on the torso, this is a Heavenly Treasury. It is a Window of the Sky and often used with LI 18, the Window of the Sky on its paired channel. This point can lift the spirit and help people who have become cut off from the inspiration that Heaven gives them as their birthright. It is especially helpful if people have been unable to participate in life or have become locked inside themselves due to grief and sadness.

Lung 4 *Xia Bai*, Guarding White

Needle depth 0.5–1.0 cun; *moxa cones 3–5*

White is the colour resonant with the Metal Element. This point is sometimes used as an adjunct to Lu 1, 2 and 3. It is not, however, generally regarded as being as powerful as these other points.

Lung 5 *Chi Ze*, Foot Marsh: Water point, sedation point

Needle depth 0.5–1.0 cun; *moxa cones 3–5*

This is the sedation point and Water point. It dries up fluid if the Lungs are too wet. This is especially useful if there is phlegm in the Lungs. In this case it is usually sedated. As a sedation point it can also send *qi* down to the Kidneys along the *sheng* cycle and can affect the Lower Burner if it is retaining fluids. This point can also bring fluidity to the Lungs if they are dry. Physically this may manifest as a dry cough but it can also show as a lack of fluidity in the mind and spirit. This commonly leads to mental or spiritual rigidity. It is often paired with LI 2, the Water and sedation point of the Large Intestine.

Lung 6 *Kong Zui*, Greatest Hole: *xi* cleft point

Needle depth 0.5–1.0 cun; moxa cones 3–5

The *xi* cleft point is tonified when the Lungs are depleted and reduced when full. It is often used in acute conditions. Physically this may be an acute lung infection. Mentally and spiritually this may be acute sorrow and sadness that is arising from the Lungs. This may be due to grief experienced when a person is bereaved or the acute sense of pain due to losing someone or something.

Lung 7 *Lie Que*, Broken Sequence: Exit point, *luo* junction point, opening point of *Ren mai*

Needle depth 0.3–0.5 cun; moxa cones 3–5

This point is predominantly used as the *luo* junction point to balance the two Organs in the Element. It is therefore commonly paired with LI 6 (*luo* junction) or 4 (*yuan* source). It is also used for its powerful effect on the Organ and its special effect on the lungs, throat, nose and head. It calms and settles the spirit, allowing a person with tight or shallow breathing to breathe more deeply. It also enables tension to be released if the throat is tight. By opening the throat it can encourage a person to weep, especially if grief and sadness have been repressed for a long period of time.

Lung 8 *Jing Qu*, Channel (or Meridian) Ditch: Metal point, horary point

Needle depth 0.1–0.3 cun; moxa cones 3–5

This is the Metal point and therefore the horary point between 3.00 and 5.00 a.m. Even if not used at the appropriate time of day, this is a powerful point to tonify the Lungs. Some practitioners use it in the autumn as the 'seasonal' horary point. The Metal point within the Metal Element clears stagnation or negativity from a person's mind and spirit by bringing clear, clean and vital *qi* to the Lungs. It is interesting to note that the word *jing* means 'to pass through' or 'things running lengthways' (Hicks, 1999, p. 6). This point name suggests that it assists in cleansing the Element.

Lung 9 *Tai Yuan*, Very Great Abyss: *yuan* source point, tonification point, Earth point, special point for Arteries and Blood Vessels

Needle depth 0.2–0.3 cun; moxa cones 3–5

This is the source point and is often used with LI 4 when the practitioner is 'testing' whether a patient is a Metal CF. The name of this point refers to its ability to raise a person's *qi* from a deep source. The word *yuan*, which translates as abyss, also portrays a spring bubbling from the depths (Allan, 1997, p. 76). It can strengthen and restore people who are depleted or who have low reserves. It can also help a person whose mind and spirit are metaphorically stuck in an abyss. In this case it can help to raise people out of the depths of despair and enable them to have greater stability and control.

This point is so dynamic and reliable that it is easily the most commonly used point on the channel. It is also the Earth point and tonification point and is therefore used when the pulse of the Spleen is stronger than that of the Lung. In this case the mother Element, Earth, nurtures and stabilises its child, the Metal Element.

Lung 10 *Yu Ji*, Fish Border: Fire point

Needle depth 0.3–0.7 cun; no moxa

This is the Fire point and is most commonly used to warm up deficient and cold Lung *qi*. It may be used to warm a person who is detached and inert and has difficulty making contact with other people. Caution is needed when using moxibustion on this point. It is important not to heat up the Metal to such a degree that it becomes 'molten'.

This point can be stimulated to transfer *qi* from the *yin* Organs of the Fire Element into the Lungs.

Patient Example

A very withdrawn Metal CF man in his thirties was spending colossal amounts of time on his own, mainly either at his computer or running. Warming his Lungs by using this point was the most effective treatment he received, both in terms of quality of pulse change and change in his behaviour and attitudes.

Lung 11 *Shao Shang*, Lesser *Shang*: Wood point

Needle depth 0.1 cun; *no moxa*

Shang is the musical note resonant with Metal. Except for occasional use as the Wood point on the Lung channel this point is not commonly used.

Bladder 13 *Fei Shu*: Lung back *shu* point

Needle depth 0.3–0.5 cun; *moxa cones 7–15*

This point is frequently used to enhance the Lung *qi*. It can be used in many situations, for example, when the Lung is full or deficient and in both chronic and acute conditions. It is especially strengthening and nourishing when a person has weak Lungs due to long-term grief or depletion of the Lung Organ. This is often the point of choice for acute problems in the lungs.

Bladder 42 *Po Hu*, Door of *Po*

Needle depth 0.3–0.5 cun; *moxa cones 7–15*

This point is commonly used to treat the spirit by opening the door to the *po*. (For more on the *po*, see Chapters 3 and 18, this volume.) It helps people to reconnect with deeper aspects of the spirit of the Metal Element and to receive *qi* from the Heavens. Using this point can enable people to let go of grief and sadness that has depleted their spirits. It can also be used to strengthen people who feel over-sensitive to others or vulnerable to 'psychic' attack. This point is situated adjacent to the Lung back *shu* point and on top of the Lung Organ and is sometimes used with Bl 13 for a stronger and deeper effect.

Other points used to treat the Lungs

Other points used to treat the Lungs are *Ren* 17, *Ren* 18–22, Bl 43 and Kid 27.

Large Intestine points

(Table 38.2)

The primary Large Intestine channel

The Large Intestine channel starts on the radial side of the index finger, runs up the radial side of the forearm to the elbow, then on to the lateral side of the upper arm. The pathway continues up to the

Table 38.2 Commonly used points on the Large Intestine channel

Yuan source point	Large Intestine 4
Luo junction point	Large Intestine 6
Tonification point	Large Intestine 11
Sedation point	Large Intestine 2
Back *shu* point	Bladder 25
Outer Back *shu* point	None
Horary point	Large Intestine 1
Xi cleft point	Large Intestine 7
Entry point	Large Intestine 4
Exit point	Large Intestine 20
Window of the Sky	Large Intestine 18

shoulder and the large muscle of the neck to the mandible and upper jaw, where it crosses the upper lip before ending at LI 20 at the far side of the nose. Here it joins with the Stomach channel at St 1.

Large Intestine 1 *Shang Yang*, Metal *Yang*: Metal point, horary point

Needle depth 0.1 cun; *moxa cones 3–5*

As in Lu 11, the character *shang* is the musical note resonant with Metal. *Yang* refers to the fact that the Large Intestine is the *yang* Organ of the Metal Element. This is the horary point and is therefore commonly paired with Lu 8. If used between 7 and 9 a.m. it is a powerful point to tonify the Large Intestine. It can still have a powerful effect even if it is not used during horary time. Some practitioners also use it in the autumn as the 'seasonal' horary point. The Metal point within the Metal Element encourages the Large Intestine to clear stagnation from the mind and spirit so that a person can let go of emotional negativity.

Large Intestine 2 *Er Jian*, Second Interval: Water point, sedation point

Needle depth 0.2–0.3 cun; *moxa cones 3–5*

This point is the sedation point and can be used with Lung 5 if the pulses of the Metal Element are full. It can also be used to bring moisture and fluidity to cool the Large Intestine if it is too hot.

Large Intestine 3 *San Jian*, Third Interval: Wood point

Needle depth 0.3–0.7 cun; moxa cones 3–5

This point is seldom used except when the practitioner wishes to treat the Wood within the Metal.

Large Intestine 4 *He Gu*, Joining Valley: *yuan* source point, Entry point

Needle depth 0.5–0.8 cun; moxa cones 5–7

The source point of the Large Intestine is a frequently used point with a large variety of applications. Like all source points, it is used to 'test' whether the person is a Metal CF. In this case it is often used with Lu 9, the Lung source point.

It is also used to augment the use of other points on the channel, especially body points such as LI 15, 17, 18 or 20 or Bl 25, the back *shu* point or St 25, the front *mu* point. Like all source points, it is also used generally to stimulate or sedate the Large Intestine *qi*.

The Large Intestine is responsible for disposing of waste in the body, mind and spirit. If it is incapable of eliminating rubbish then the Lungs cannot receive *qi* from Heaven and the patient does not thrive. This point can play an important role in assisting in the process of letting go on all levels. If sadness and grief have caused the *qi* to become deficient, many people find that they cannot let go of their sense of loss and melancholy. Only by 'letting go' at the source of their suffering can the person begin to re-experience inspiration and a true zest for life.

This is the point of entry for the Large Intestine channel and can be used with Lu 7 if a block is suspected between these two Organs. Coupled with Bl 59 it is used to detoxify the body from the effects of medication, recreational drugs, alcohol, etc. This combination is known as the Great Eliminator.

Sedated in conjunction with Liv 3 (and known as the Four Gates), this point has a very relaxing effect on the body and can clear spasms and tension. It can also calm a patient's spirit, enabling a person who is agitated to settle inside. It is an important point for patients who have problems in the face such as the ears, eyes, mouth and nose.

LI 4 can be massaged or moxa can be used in the event of a patient fainting during treatment, especially if the patient has needles in the lower part of the body. (See Chapter 34 on needle technique for more on the points for treating needle shock.) This point is forbidden in pregnancy.

Large Intestine 5 *Yang Xi*, *Yang* Stream: Fire point

Needle depth 0.3–0.5 cun; moxa cones 3–5

This is the Fire point. This point can be sedated if the patient is in a manic state. The Organs of the Metal Element are particularly prone to becoming cold and inert, and this point is more commonly used to warm and nourish.

Large Intestine 6 *Pian Li*, Slanting Passage: *luo* junction point

Needle depth 0.5–0.8 cun; moxa cones 3–5

This is the *luo* junction point and is commonly used in conjunction with Lu 7 or 9. When used together these points create greater equilibrium between the Lung and Large Intestine. This enables a person to achieve greater harmony and balance mentally and spiritually. It is particularly used to assist the person 'transmit along the road' (*chuan dao*) thoughts and feelings that are no longer relevant to the time (Larre and Rochat de la Vallée, 1992b, p. 103).

Large Intestine 7 *Wen Liu*, Warm Flow: *xi* cleft point

Needle depth 0.5–1.0 cun; moxa cones 5–30

This is the *xi* cleft point and is therefore sometimes paired with Lu 6 to assist these two Organs in their functions. Because of the implications of the name, moxibustion and stimulation with a needle are often used in order to warm and soften the Metal Element. Metal CFs who have become cold and inert are thus enabled to 'go with the flow' in their lives (Hicks, 1999, p. 7).

Large Intestine 8 *Xia Lian*, Lower Ridge

Needle depth 0.5–1.0 cun; moxa cones 3–5

This point is not frequently used although, in a similar way to LI 5, it is effective in calming a patient with manic behaviour (Deadman *et al.*, 1998, p. 118).

Large Intestine 9 *Shan Lian*, Upper Ridge

Needle depth 0.5–1.0 cun; moxa cones 5–10

This point becomes spontaneously tender at the first sign of 'brain fatigue' from mentally overworking.

Large Intestine 11 *Qu Chi*, Crooked Pond: Earth point, tonification point, *He* sea point

Needle depth 0.8–1.2 cun*; moxa cones 5–10*

As the tonification point, this is stimulated in order to strengthen the *qi* of the Large Intestine. This is particularly beneficial when the pulse of the Stomach is stronger than that of the Large Intestine when it joins the mother, the Stomach, to its child the Large Intestine. Because of its connection with the Earth Element, this point is beneficial when stability is needed in the Large Intestine. This point is extremely invigorating and can strongly tonify a patient's *qi*. Along with LI 4, it is an important point for patients who have problems in the face such as the ears, eyes, mouth and nose (Ellis *et al.*, 1988, p. 99).

Large Intestine 15 *Jian Yu*, Shoulder Joint

Needle depth 0.7–1.5 cun*; moxa cones 5–7*

This point is the most commonly used point to treat chronic and acute problems of the shoulder.

Large Intestine 17 *Tian Ding*, Heavenly Vessel

Needle depth 0.3–0.5 cun*; moxa cones 3–5*

This point is situated on the neck, and has the word *tian* in its name, so it is used to treat the spirit. The neck is a person's bridge with their heavenly *qi* and this point can particularly be used when the patient is suffering from a lack of clarity. In this case it can clear the mind and encourage people to let go of any emotions they are holding on to, especially grief and sadness.

Large Intestine 18 *Fu Tu*, Support the Prominence: Window of the Sky point

Needle depth 0.3–0.5 cun*; moxa cones 3–5*

This is the Window of the Sky point on the channel and as such it is a very important point to treat a patient's mind and spirit. It brings light and clarity to the person. It is primarily used to give a lift to a person whose spirit has become diminished and weighed down under the influence of sadness and grief. This is especially indicated when the *qi* has become weakened and the person has become cut off from their spirit. This point can be used to summon the *qi* so that the person can start to reconnect with the *qi* of Heaven again.

> ### Patient Example
>
> A patient had been unable to form a new relationship since the break-up of a relationship some years previously. After this point and Lu 3 had been used he said that he felt ready to try again to achieve intimacy with someone. Within two months he started a new relationship.

Large Intestine 20 *Ying Xiang*, Welcome Fragrance: Exit point, meeting point of St and LI

Needle depth 0.3–0.5 cun*; no moxa*

This point is located at the entrance of the nose. It is the Exit point and links to the Stomach channel at St 1. These two channels comprise the two channels of the *yang ming*, which is described as 'rich in *qi* and blood'. If the connection between these channels is blocked, the person may experience problems in the nose, sinuses or eye. They may also suffer from a wide range of digestive symptoms or dysfunction in the mind and spirit. The name of this point may also refer to the connection between the Large Intestine and Stomach. If rubbish has accumulated in the Large Intestine, this is dispersed when it is joined with the Stomach where there is fragrance (Hicks, 1999, p. 9).

Bladder 25: Large Intestine back *shu* point

Needle depth 0.7–1.2 cun*; moxa cones 7–15*

This point is often used in combination with Bl 13 in order to stimulate the *qi* of the Metal Element. As the back *shu* point of the Large Intestine it has a strong fortifying effect on the Large Intestine Organ. Although not specifically a spirit point, by strengthening the Organ, it can invigorate and revitalise a person on every level. It is also frequently used to treat problems of the lower *jiao*, such as constipation, diarrhoea and lumbar pain.

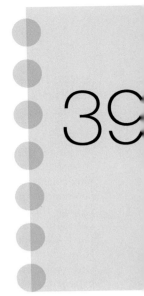

Stomach and Spleen points

Stomach points (Table 39.1)

The primary pathway of the Stomach channel

The Stomach channel begins below the eye, travels down the cheek, loops backwards along the angle of the jaw and ascends in front of the ear to the upper corner of the forehead. From the jaw a pathway runs down the side of the throat to travel transversely out along the superior edge of the collarbone, and then to descend down the nipple line, passing through the breast and to the side of the umbilicus, to the groin. Here the channel moves out transversely to continue down the front of the thigh, the lateral border of the patella and tibia, and then over the top of the foot to end at the lateral side of the second toe. It then joins the Spleen channel at Sp 1.

Stomach 1 *Cheng Qi*, Receive Tears: Entry point

Needle depth 0.3–0.5 cun; *no moxa*

This is the Entry point that receives *qi* from LI 20, the Exit point of the Large Intestine. It is most commonly used to clear Entry–Exit blocks between these two channels.

The Large Intestine and Stomach channels together constitute the *yang ming* channel.

Stomach 4 *Di Cang*, Earth Granary: meeting point of St and LI

Needle depth 0.3–0.5 cun; *no moxa*

The name of this point alludes to both the Earth Element and a granary, the place where reserves of food are stored. *Su Wen* Chapter 8 says that the Stomach and Spleen are responsible for 'storehouses and granaries'. This point is situated at the corner of the mouth and is used when people are having problems with digestion. More rarely it can be used if people have difficulties with their attitude to food.

Stomach 8 *Tou Wei*, Corner of the Head: meeting point of St and GB

Needle depth 0.5–0.8 cun; *no moxa*

This point is used to clear the head if it feels stuffy or congested. It is also used when overthinking (*si*) has 'knotted' (*jie*) the *qi* and people are 'tying themselves up in knots' (see Chapter 5, this volume). In this case they may be preoccupied or continually worrying about their problems. Another translation of the name of this point is Head Tied.

Stomach 9 *Ren Ying*, People Welcome: Window of the Sky, point of sea of *qi*

Needle depth 0.3–0.5 cun; *no moxa*

This is an extremely powerful point. Chapter 33 of the *Ling Shu* designates it as one of the 'seas of *qi*' and it can be used to strengthen a person's *qi*.

It is the only Window of the Sky on the channels of the Earth Element. One tendency of Earth CFs, or people whose Earth Elements have become

Table 39.1 Commonly used points on the Stomach channel	
Yuan source point	Stomach 42
Luo junction point	Stomach 40
Tonification point	Stomach 41
Sedation point	Stomach 45
Back *shu* point	Bladder 21
Outer Back *shu* point	Bladder 50
Horary point	Stomach 36
Xi cleft point	Stomach 34
Entry point	Stomach 1
Exit point	Stomach 42
Window of the Sky	Stomach 9

distressed, is to find it difficult to experience intimate contact. However much they like the idea of letting people show empathetic concern towards them, in practice they find it hard to allow themselves to soften sufficiently to let it in. 'People Welcome' can be used to help people establish more satisfying relationships with those who care for them.

Stomach 12 *Qu Pen*, Broken Bowl

Needle depth 0.3–0.5 cun; *moxa cones 3–5*

This point is located in the supraclavicular fossa, which is shaped like a bowl. The name of this point also evokes the Chinese saying, 'My rice bowl is broken', which is used when people say that they are no longer able to support or feed themselves. This point can be used when a patient is unable to nourish and sustain themselves physically or spiritually.

An alternative name for this point is *Tian Gai*, Heaven Cover. This evokes a further image. In ancient times Heaven was visualised as an inverted bowl. This was supported by the four main mountains of China. It was said that if this bowl was broken, then Heaven would be sundered and contact would be broken. The implication is that this point connects people to the heavens and subsequently to their spirit (Hicks, 1999, p.11).

Stomach 14 *Ku Fang*, Storehouse

Needle depth 0.3–0.5 cun; *moxa cones 3–5*

This point draws on the reserves of *qi* that are held in the 'storehouses and granaries'.

Stomach 19 *Bu Rong*, Not Contained

Needle depth 0.5–0.8 cun; *moxa cones 3–5*

This point has also been named 'not at ease'. It is situated in the stomach region and can be used when the Stomach *qi* rebels so patients are unable to digest their food. The result may be vomiting, belching or nausea. This may be from a physical cause such as overeating or for emotional reasons such as anxiety or worry.

Stomach 20 *Cheng Man*, Receiving Fullness

Needle depth 0.5–1.0 cun; *moxa cones 3–5*

The name of this point has implications concerning the tendency of people whose Earth Element is distressed to feel dissatisfied and deprived. Using this point may help to fill the void they feel in their centre.

Stomach 21 *Liang Men*, Beam Gate

Needle depth 0.5–1.0 cun; *moxa cones 5–15*

This point is at the level of *Ren* 12 and is an important point for digestion. Opening this gate can enable people to digest and assimilate thoughts as well as food, especially if their thoughts are stuck or obsessive.

Stomach 22 *Guan Men*, Border Gate

Needle depth 0.8–1.0 cun; *moxa cones 5–15*

This point is similar to the previous point and encourages physical, mental and spiritual digestion.

Stomach 23 *Tai Yi*, Supreme Unity

Needle depth 0.7–1.0 cun; *moxa cones 5–15*

The name *Tai Yi* refers to the state of undifferentiated unity that existed before the arising of *yin* and *yang* and the division of Heaven and Earth. Located in the middle of the torso, the name refers to the age-old division of the body between the upper part, resonant with Heaven, and the lower, resonant with Earth.[1]

It has a long recorded history of being used to treat problems that arise in a person's spirit

---

[1]It is typical of the syncretic nature of Chinese medicine that the body can be divided into two (Heaven and Earth) or into three (Heaven–Man–Earth).

(Chan, 1963, p. 281). This point is especially useful for Earth CFs who are either excessively 'grounded' in the material world or 'ungrounded' and internally unstable, making it hard for them to cope effectively with day-to-day life. This point can balance these aspects and bring people stability and harmony within.

Stomach 25 *Tian Shu*, Heavenly Pivot: Large Intestine front *mu* point, point to release Internal Dragons

Needle depth 0.7–1.2 cun*; moxa cones 5–15*

Tian Shu is the name of the central star in the Northern Dipper, around which the other six stars revolve. This point lies at the intersection of Heaven and Earth in the body:

> As the body resembles heaven and earth, the waist serves as a sash ... What is above the sash is all *yang* and what is below the sash is all *yin*, each with its own function.
>
> The *yang* is the material force of heaven, and the *yin* is the material force of earth.
>
> (Tung Chung-Shu; Chan, 1963, p. 281)

Certainly the name implies that it is a point of special importance, and few points have so many alternative names. It is situated on the lower *dan tian* and can enable a person to have both stability and a connection to the earth as well as an ability to contact the heavens and reconnect the spirit. It is especially useful when people are mentally unstable and prone to emotional swings.

This point is particularly useful for Earth CFs who feel insecure and unstable. This point is often paired with Spleen 15, Great Horizontal, the Spleen point alongside it. This implies that the vertical connection between Heaven and Earth is complemented by the horizontal movement generated by Spleen 15.

This point is one of those used when releasing the 'Internal Dragons'.

Patient Example

A woman in her late fifties had an extremely worried disposition and she found it difficult to feel internally secure and stable. At the root of this characteristic was her extremely depleted Earth Element. Treatment on 'command points' and the back *shu* points brought some improvement to her symptoms, pulses and colour, but she did not seem to be changing in herself. Tonifying St 25 and Sp 15 together initiated a more profound change in her state of mind and mood than any of the other point combinations.

Stomach 27 *Da Ju*, Great Fullness

Needle depth 0.7–1.2 cun*; moxa cones 5–10*

This point is mainly used for its local effect, especially when the Stomach Organ causes symptoms lower down in the digestive tract. It is also sometimes used to fill an internal void in a similar way to St 20.

Stomach 28 *Shui Dao*, Water Way

Needle depth 0.7–1.2 cun*; moxa cones 5–10*

This point is used for problems with fluids in the lower burner. It is often combined with *Ren* 4 and sometimes with Spleen 13.

Stomach 29 *Gui Lai*, The Return

Needle depth 0.7–1.2 cun*; moxa cones 5–10*

The name of this point probably refers to the menstrual cycle. Regulating the menstrual cycle is one of the main uses for this point.

Stomach 30 *Qi Chong*, Surging *Qi*

Needle depth 0.5–1.0 cun*; moxa cones 7*

This is an extremely powerful point, as the name implies. It can be used to treat both the *jing* via the *Chong mai* (one of the Eight Extraordinary Channels) and the Earth *qi* via its connection to the Stomach and the Sea of Nourishment (*Ling Shu*, Chapter 33). Using this point can therefore strongly invigorate a person's *qi* and enhance the Stomach and Spleen. This point is underused owing to its location in the groin.

Stomach 32 *Fu Tu*, Prostrate Hare: point to release Internal Dragons

Needle depth 1.0–1.5 cun*; moxa cones 3–5*

This point is one of the points used when releasing the 'Internal Dragons'.

Stomach 36 *Zu San Li*, Leg Three: *Li* Earth point, horary point, point of Sea of Nourishment

Needle depth 0.5–1.0 cun*; moxa cones 7–20*

The name of this point suggests that if this point is treated people will be able to walk another three *li*, about 1 mile or 1.6 kilometres.

This is a major point to nourish the Stomach. Metaphorically it is similar to giving chicken soup, one of the most nourishing dishes in the Chinese cuisine. It is such a strengthening point that it has a very potent effect, especially if it is used between 7 and 9 a.m., the horary time. Some practitioners also use this point as a 'seasonal' horary point in the late summer between August and October. (In countries that move the clock in order to have a 'Summer Time', in summer this point can be used to maximum effect an hour later than during 'Winter Time'.)

As the Earth point within the Earth Element it can benefit patients who have any kind of imbalance in the Earth Element, enabling them to assimilate at all levels. At a physical level it can enhance the immune system and strengthen resistance to disease. Mentally and spiritually it can bring great stability to people who are feeling emotionally unstable or insecure. It helps to calm the mind and spirit if patients are worried, anxious or obsessive. It can also clear the mind if people have been intensively working by studying or over-thinking.

St 36 can be used in the event of a patient fainting during treatment, especially if the patient has needles in the upper part of the body. (See Chapter 34 for more on the points for treating needle shock.)

Stomach 37 *Shang Ju Xu*, Upper Great Void

Needle depth 0.3–0.5 cun; *moxa cones 3–5*

This point is sometimes used as the upper *He* sea point of the Large Intestine for acute problems in the Organ, such as constipation or diarrhoea. It is rarely used to treat the Stomach.

Stomach 39 *Xia Ju Xu*, Lower Great Void

Needle depth 0.5–1.0 cun; *moxa cones 3–5*

This point is sometimes used as the lower *He* sea point of the Small Intestine for acute problems in this Organ. Like St 37, it is rarely used for treating the Stomach.

Stomach 40 *Feng Long*, Abundant Prosperity: *luo* junction point

Needle depth 0.5–1.0 cun; *moxa cones 3–5*

The point name gives some idea of the richness, abundance and prosperity that can be accessed from its use. This point is the *luo* junction point and is very

commonly used to treat symptoms of both the body and spirit. It is often combined with Sp 4 or 3. The stabilising effects of the junction point can help to bring a person greater balance and harmony and reconnection to the Earth.

Stomach 41 *Jie Xi*, Released Stream: Fire point, tonification point, point to release Internal Dragons

Needle depth 0.5–0.7 cun; *moxa cones 3–5*

This is the Fire point and tonification point. It is therefore commonly used if the pulses of the Small Intestine and Triple Burner are stronger than those of the Stomach. In this case it will reconnect the mother Element, Fire, to the Earth. Even if there is not an obvious discrepancy in the strength of the pulses, tonification points are often used to assist the natural working of the *sheng* cycle and create a clear passageway between the Elements.

This point is one of those used when releasing the 'Internal Dragons'.

Patient Example

A patient who was a young professional woman in her early thirties had a long history of eating disorders and anorexia. She was a Fire CF. Her pulses were very deficient and for many years her Fire Element had not been nourishing her Earth Element, the next Element on the *sheng* cycle. The tonification points of Earth, St 41 and Sp 2, evoked a better response on her Earth pulses than other command points such as St 42, 36, 40 and Sp 3, 4 and 6.

Stomach 42 *Chong Yang*, Surging *Yang*: Exit point, *yuan* source point

Needle depth 0.3–0.5 cun; *moxa cones 3–5*

This is the *yuan* source point and is therefore a very frequently used point. It is often sedated if the person is agitated and disturbed and the Stomach pulse is full (Surging *Yang*). It is a frequently used point when a patient fluctuates between mania and depression. More commonly it is tonified in order to strengthen and revitalise the *qi* of the Stomach.

St 42 is also the Exit point of the Stomach channel and joins to Sp 1, the Entry point of the Spleen.

Stomach 43 *Xian Gu*, Sinking Valley: *shu* stream point, Wood point

Needle depth 0.3–0.5 cun; *moxa cones 3–5*
This is the Wood point and it is rarely used. It is occasionally used with Sp 1, although being on a *yang* channel it cannot transfer *qi* from the Wood Element. (See Chapters 34 and 36, this volume, for explanation of transfers of *qi* across the *ke* cycle.)

Stomach 44 *Nei Ting*, Inner Courtyard: Water point

Needle depth 0.3–0.5 cun; *moxa cones 3–5*
This is the Water point and can therefore be used with Sp 9 to affect the balance of the Water in the Earth. It is especially useful when the Stomach is too hot, causing the patient to feel agitated and restless.

Using a sedating needle action can help to calm the patient.

Stomach 45 *Li Du*, Harsh Exchange/Strict Mouth: Metal point, sedation point

Needle depth 0.1 cun; *moxa cones 3–5*
This name is very hard to translate and may even mean 'Rapid Raising of Spirits' (see Hicks, 1999, p. 15). It is the Metal point and is therefore used as the sedation point. If used in this way it can transmit *qi* to the Large Intestine when the pulse of the Stomach is full.

Bladder 21 *Wei Shu*: Stomach back *shu* point

Needle depth 0.5–0.7 cun; *moxa cones 7–15*
This point is commonly used to tonify the Stomach and connects directly to the Organ itself. It has a strongly enhancing effect on the Organ and is often used to improve the 'rotting and ripening' function of the Stomach. Like other back *shu* points, it also has the effect of strengthening the patient's mind and spirit by increasing the *qi* of the Stomach Organ.

This point can help to revitalise people who are tired and lethargic and enable them to assimilate and digest food, thoughts and information. It may also help people who feel they lack a centre to feel more stable and grounded. It is usually used in combination with the Spleen back *shu* point.

Bladder 50 *Wei Cang*, Stomach Granary

Needle depth 0.3–0.5 cun; *moxa cones 5–10*
This outer back *shu* point is probably underused, largely because the names of the outer back *shu* points of the *yang* Organs are not as evocative as those of the *yin* Organs. This point is a powerful point in assisting the Stomach in its role of being responsible for 'storehouses and granaries'. It can enable a person to digest thoughts and ideas. It can be used on its own or with Bl 51, the outer back *shu* point of the Spleen, or with Bl 20, the Stomach back *shu* point.

Other points used to treat the Stomach

One other point used to treat the Stomach is *Ren 12*.

Spleen points (Table 39.2)

The primary pathway of the Spleen channel

The Spleen channel begins on the medial side of the big toe, travels along the medial edge of the foot, passes anterior to the malleolus at the ankle bone and up the inside of the leg on the posterior border of the tibia. From here it continues upwards over the medial aspect of the knee and thigh and then up to

Table 39.2 Commonly used points on the Spleen channel	
Yuan source point	Spleen 3
Luo junction point	Spleen 4
Tonification point	Spleen 2
Sedation point	Spleen 5
Back *shu* point	Bladder 20
Outer Back *shu* point	Bladder 49
Horary point	Spleen 3
Xi cleft point	Spleen 8
Entry point	Spleen 1
Exit point	Spleen 21
Window of the Sky	None

the abdomen, passing through the stomach and spleen organs. From the spleen and stomach it then travels through the diaphragm to join Sp 17, 18, 19, 20 and 21. It then connects to the Heart channel at Ht 1.

Spleen 1 *Yin Bai*, Hidden White: Wood point, Entry point

Needle depth 0.3–0.5 cun*; moxa cones 3–5*

The presence of white in this point name probably refers to the close connection between the Spleen and the Lungs of the Metal Element. The Spleen constitutes the foot *tai yin*, the Lungs the hand *tai yin*. (For a list of the channel's connections such as *tai yang*, etc., see Cheng, 1987, p. 19.)

This is the Entry point and Wood point on the channel. It can therefore be used to transfer *qi* from the Liver across the *ke* cycle. This point is also used when patients have symptoms of mania or mental agitation. In this case sedating the point can calm the person.

Patient Example

A patient in his forties had a long history of irritable bowel syndrome. His symptoms included alternating constipation and loose stools, flatulence, discomfort in the lower abdomen and a general feeling of malaise and fatigue. He was an Earth CF, with very deficient Earth pulses and full Wood pulses. (Liver *qi* stagnation invades the Spleen was the TCM diagnosis.) Tonifying the Earth Element yielded some improvement and reducing the Wood as well was moderately successful. Transferring *qi* from the Liver to the Spleen by tonifying Sp 1 brought about a breakthrough in his treatment.

Spleen 2 *Da Du*, Great Capital: Fire point, tonification point

Needle depth 0.1–0.3 cun*; moxa cones 3–5*

As the Fire point and tonification point, this point is commonly used, often in combination with St 41. It can be used to transfer *qi* from the Heart and Pericardium, to improve the connection between these Organs along the *sheng* cycle, and to join the mother to her child. This point can also be used to warm up a person with a cold and deficient Spleen. Its use can bring back warmth and vitality to the spirit.

Spleen 3 *Tai Bai*, Supreme White: Earth point, horary point, *yuan* source point

Needle depth 0.3–0.5 cun*; moxa cones 3–5*

Tai Bai is the name of the planet Venus, which is associated with the Metal Element. Like Sp 1, this is probably either a reference to the connection with the Lungs through the *tai yin* or through the mother–child connection.

This point is extremely important for bringing vitality and stability to the Spleen. This is the Earth point, the horary point between 9 and 11 a.m., and also the *yuan* source point. This combination of uses means that it is the most frequently used point on the Spleen channel. It is often paired with St 42 (*yuan* source) or St 36 (horary).

When used as a horary point between 9 and 11 a.m., this point strongly enhances the *qi* of the Spleen. Unlike some other horary points, it can be used during sociable hours, enabling practitioners to use it on many of their Earth CF patients. As the Earth point within the Earth Element, Sp 3 will also invigorate the Spleen at other times of day and it can bring stability and equilibrium to patients with imbalanced Earth. This point is also used as a seasonal horary point by some practitioners in the late summer between late August and October. If a patient feels muzzy-headed due to poor Spleen transformation function, this point can move the *qi*, creating greater mental clarity.

Spleen 4 *Gong Sun*, Grandfather and Grandson: *luo* junction point, opening point of *Chong* (penetrating) *Mai*

Needle depth 0.3–0.5 cun*; moxa cones 3–5*

Gong Sun is the family name of Huang Di, the Yellow Emperor. He was a legendary emperor during a dynasty associated with the Earth Element (Hicks, 1999, p. 16).

This point is the *luo* junction point and is commonly used along with St 40 or 42. Creating equilibrium between these two Organs can be especially beneficial to patients who have instability in the Earth Element. Sp 4 is also the Opening Point of the *Chong mai* (one of the Eight Extraordinary Channels; for more on this see Maciocia, 1989, pp. 360–361). This makes it an outstandingly powerful point that is especially beneficial when people have lassitude due to depleted *qi*. It is also useful for digestive complaints, especially nausea or poor appetite.

Spleen 5 *Shang Qiu, Shang* Mound: Metal point, sedation point

Needle depth 0.3–0.5 cun; moxa cones 3–5

Shang is the musical note resonant with Metal and this is the Metal point on the channel. It can be stimulated to tonify the Metal within the Earth. This is the sedation point and it is normally reduced when the Spleen is full. It then transmits *qi* along the *sheng* cycle to the Lungs, its child.

Spleen 6 *San Yin Jiao*, Three *Yin* Crossing: meeting point of three *yin* of leg

Needle depth 0.5–1.0 cun; moxa cones 3–5

This is an extremely powerful point that can be used to treat the Spleen, Kidney and Liver. It should not be used if practitioners are still 'testing' the CF as they will not get clear feedback as to which Organ is generating the pulse changes. Practitioners should take care that all three Organs have approximately the same level of *qi* if they wish to stimulate or reduce using this point. If indicated, this point can have a profound effect on a person's psyche with a strong 'calm the spirit' action. It is often helpful for insomnia and anxiety as well as enabling a person to have greater mental clarity and calmness.

This point directly affects the uterus and can stimulate labour. It is therefore forbidden in pregnancy.

Spleen 8 *Di Ji*, Earth's Pivot: *xi* cleft point

Needle depth 0.5–1.0 cun; moxa cones 3–5

This is the *xi* cleft point. In the *Ode to Elucidate Mysteries* it says:

> Man consists of top, middle and bottom. The major points for these three areas are Great Enveloping (Sp 21), Heavenly Pivot (St 25) and Earth's Pivot (Sp 8).
>
> (Deadman *et al.*, 1998, p. 194)

Here 'top, middle and bottom' is a way of describing Heaven, Man and Earth.

Earth's Pivot is a crucial point for enhancing the *qi* of the Spleen, particularly for its effect on the functions of the Middle and Lower Burner. As a *xi* cleft point, it is also used for acute problems, especially acute period pains. It can also be used when a patient is sluggish, tired and worn out, and it improves the Spleen's ability to transform and transport on all levels.

Spleen 9 *Yin Ling Quan, Yin* Mound Spring: Water point

Needle depth 0.5–1.2 cun; moxa cones 3–5

This is the Water point on the channel. It can be used if the practitioner wishes to regulate the balance of the Water in the Earth and can especially be used when the Earth is waterlogged, in which case it will be sedated. (The use of this point by TCM practitioners to clear Damp is based upon its Five Element usage.)

Spleen 10 *Xue Hai*, Sea of Blood

Needle depth 0.5–1.2 cun; moxa cones 3–5

As the name suggests, this point is most commonly used to affect a patient's Blood.

Spleen 12 *Chong Men*, Surging Gate: meeting point of Spleen and Liver

Needle depth 0.5–1.0 cun; moxa cones 3–5

This point has a connection to the Liver channel and is sometimes used to treat problems in the Lower Burner caused by the Spleen and Liver.

Spleen 13 *Fu She*, Treasury Dwelling

Needle depth 0.5–1.0 cun; moxa cones 5–10

This is sometimes used with other lower abdominal points, such as *Ren* 3, 4 or 5, Kid 12 or 13, or St 27, 28 or 29, to treat symptoms in the Lower Burner. This point can also be used to good effect for enhancing Spleen *qi* in general.

Spleen 15 *Da Heng*, Great Horizontal

Needle depth 0.7–1.2 cun; moxa cones 5–10

This point is often combined with St 25, which lies next to it. Physically it has an effect on the lower abdomen, especially the bowels. It also centres the mind and spirit, especially if a patient feels internally unstable and insecure. It is indicated if a person has a propensity to sadness, weeping and sighing (Deadman *et al.*, 1998, p. 200). Its main effect is to stabilise the *qi* of the Spleen.

Spleen 16 *Fu Ai*, Abdomen Sorrow

Needle depth 0.5–1.0 cun; moxa cones 5–10

This point can be used to lift the spirit of patients whose emotional life has become unstable due to imbalance in the Earth Element, especially if it is causing symptoms in the abdomen.

Spleen 18 *Tian Xi*, Heavenly Stream

Needle depth 0.3–0.5 cun; moxa cones 3–5

Tian in the name of this point refers both to its location on the upper part of the body, and also to the point's ability to help the patient to reconnect with the *qi* of Heaven. Sited over the middle *dan tian*, this point is capable of bringing great vitality and nourishment to the patient. It is possibly underrated for its ability to treat Earth CFs at the level of the spirit.

Spleen 20 *Zhou Rong*, Encircling Glory

Needle depth 0.3–0.5 cun; moxa cones 3–5

This point is often used to treat the spirit on Earth CFs. The name suggests nurturing and supporting a patient. It is especially useful for stimulating *qi* that has become 'knotted' and led to the patient becoming worried, preoccupied and depressed. This point is situated close to Lu 1 and can be used to help the Spleen assist the Lungs for problems in the lungs.

This point has an alternative name of *zhou ying*. This refers to ying qi or 'nutritive *qi*', which is a component of '*zhen qi*' or 'true *qi*', that originates in the Lungs. This also alludes to the close relationship between this point and the Lungs.

Spleen 21 *Da Bao*, Great Enveloping: Exit point, general *luo* junction point

Needle depth 0.3–0.5 cun; moxa cones 5–10

This point is the Exit point, connecting to the Heart channel at Ht 1. It is commonly used in this respect and more generally to regulate the *qi* and Blood in the chest.

Worry, excessive intellectual activity, instability and uncertainty in the circumstances of a person's life and a lack of supportive and caring relationships can all lead to a person becoming increasingly troubled in their mind and spirit. This is a powerful point for raising the spirit of someone whose spirit has become diminished and oppressed due to dysfunction of the Spleen.

Patient Example

A patient in her late forties was failing to adjust well to changing circumstances in her life. She was an Earth CF whose children had been an excessive focus in her life. They were now adolescent and she worried about them a great deal. Her husband had left her, leaving her isolated in terms of companionship, and anxious about her future. She reported that she was unable to concentrate, and was constantly tired and low in spirits. Treatment on Earth was only moderately successful until Sp 21 was tonified. After this there was a marked improvement in her spirit and she initiated several positive changes in her life. These included re-training as a nurse and finding other interests and friendships that helped her to focus less on her children.

Bladder 20 *Pi Shu*: Spleen back *shu* point

Needle depth 0.5–0.7 cun; moxa cones 7–15

Like all the back *shu* points, this point is used frequently and can have a powerful effect on a patient's general well-being. Through strengthening the Spleen Organ, a patient can be strengthened at all levels. This point is particularly indicated when the Spleen *qi* is severely depleted and sluggish.

Bladder 49 *Yi She*, Yi Dwelling

Needle depth 0.3–0.5 cun; moxa cones 5–10

This point lies next to the Spleen back *shu* point and can be combined with it. It is especially used to treat the *yi*, the faculty for the cognitive, reflective and organisational processes of the mind. *Si*, worry or 'over-thinking', 'knots' the *qi*, leading to the *yi* losing its 'dwelling'. When the *yi* is affected patients may ruminate and worry about problems and be unable to think clearly. They may also feel confused and muzzy-headed. This point can have a profound effect and can calm the patient, allowing the *yi* to settle. A healthy *yi* allows patients to access their intention and maintain focused awareness.

Other points used to treat the Spleen

Other points used to treat the Spleen are *Ren* 4 and 10.

Heart and Small Intestine points

Heart points (Table 40.1)

The primary pathway of the Heart channel

The deep pathway of the Heart originates in the heart organ and ascends along the aorta through the lungs to the axilla, where it becomes superficial. It then runs along the medial aspect of the arm from the axilla to the little finger. Here it connects with the Small Intestine channel at St 1.

Heart 1 *Ji Quan*, Supreme Spring: Entry point

Needle depth 0.5–1.0 cun; moxa cones 3–5

The word 'supreme' in the name refers to the importance placed on the Heart amongst the Organs. 'The Heart holds the office of lord and sovereign. The radiance of the *shen* stems from it' (Larre and Rochat de la Vallée, 1992b, p. 33). This point is like a spring of *qi* that can be drawn on to nourish the Heart on all levels, especially when a patient is upset, anxious or distressed. It may be used early on in treatment if command points have not affected the patient's spirit. When used it can have a direct and immediate effect on the Heart, enabling a patient to regain equilibrium and calmness. It can also be used when

sadness has weakened the *qi* and can help to summon the *qi* back to its normal movement. It enables a patient to open the heart and connect to the spirit. This is a very reliable and effective point to strengthen and nourish the Heart.

This point is also commonly used as the Entry point and is linked to the Exit point of the Spleen, Sp 21. It is interesting to note that *qi gong* and meditation practitioners keep this area relaxed and open while practising. They thereby allow the *qi* to flow freely from the heart to the arms and hands. This allows the hands to stay warm and the heart to become relaxed and settled.

Patient Example

A male patient in his forties had started getting severe palpitations. He attributed the onset of symptoms to his inner conflict over whether to stay in his marriage. He was a Fire CF and treatment on all four of the Fire Organs helped settle the Heart somewhat. Ht 1 was used at the third treatment and produced a very substantial pulse change. His symptoms were very much better after the treatment. For better or for worse, he left his wife a couple of months later.

Heart 2 *Qing Ling*, Blue-Green Spirit

Needle depth 0.3–0.5 cun; moxa cones 3–5

Qing (inadequately translated as blue-green) is the colour of living vegetation and is closely related to the word *sheng* or creation (as in the *sheng* cycle). Following on from the Supreme Spring, this point gives life and vitality to the Heart, specifically the *ling*.

Table 40.1 Commonly used points on the Heart channel

Yuan source point	Heart 7
Luo junction point	Heart 5
Tonification point	Heart 9
Sedation point	Heart 7
Back *shu* point	Bladder 15
Outer Back *shu* point	Bladder 44
Horary point	Heart 8
Xi cleft point	Heart 6
Entry point	Heart 1
Exit point	Heart 9
Window of the Sky	None

Regrettably it is not a very reliable point, often yielding little change. It is situated on a level with the other points that affect the middle *dan tian* and is sometimes said to be forbidden to needle.

Heart 3 *Shao Hai*, Lesser Sea: Water point

Needle depth 0.5–1.0 cun; moxa cones 3–5

This is the Water point on the Heart. Water controls Fire and this point will cool and calm the Heart if a patient is agitated, restless or has too much heat. This point can also be used to transfer *qi* from the Kidneys to the Heart across the *ke* cycle.

Heart 4 *Ling Dao*, Spirit Path: Metal point

Needle depth 0.3–0.5 cun; moxa cones 3–5

This is another point on the Heart channel with *ling* in its name. The *dao* means the way. In this context *dao* can either be translated as 'the pathway of the Heart channel' or, more profoundly, as 'the way of the *dao*'. It is especially indicated when the spirit is agitated from deficiency or if the patient feels miserable and sad and needs to be reconnected to their path.

It is also indicated if people suddenly lose their voices or are struck dumb – especially if there is an emotional cause such as a sudden shock, fright or agitation. This point is sometimes used in combination with Heart 7.

Heart 5 *Tong Li*, Penetrating the Interior: *luo* junction point

Needle depth 0.3–0.5 cun; moxa cones 3–5

This point is the *luo* connecting point and this may partially account for the name, as *tong* can also mean connecting. This point has a long history of being used to treat the spirit. The *Ode to the Jade Dragon* says of this point: '*Tong Li* treats a frightenable Heart' (Deadman *et al.*, 1998, p. 214). It is especially used when the Heart has been unsettled by shock and trauma and it can bring stability and strength to the *shen*. It can also be used when a patient is easily startled and disturbed emotionally. Using this point enables the *qi* to penetrate deeper inside to affect the patient's spirit.

This point can also balance the Heart and Small Intestine Organs when used as the *luo* connecting point. In this case it is often used with SI 4 or SI 7. Combining this point with the Small Intestine points brings stability to the Element, especially when the two paired Organs are out of harmony.

The point is also powerful physically, with a particular effect on the tongue and speech. It can be used for stuttering and many other speech disorders arising from the Heart.

Heart 6 *Yin Xi Yin*, Cleft: *xi* cleft (accumulation) point

Needle depth 0.3–0.5 cun; moxa cones 3–5

The name partly refers to the fact that is the *xi* cleft point. It is commonly used for more acute conditions affecting the Heart, especially when the patient is restless, anxious or agitated due to the *qi* floating on the surface. Using this point helps the *qi* to settle and calm. This point also has an alternative name of *shi gong* – stone palace. The Chinese use the term 'stone house' to indicate something firm and enduring. This can also indicate that the point is where something firm and enduring can be found (Hicks, 1999, p. 21).

Heart 7 *Shen Men*, Spirit Gate: *shu* stream point, Earth point, *yuan* source point, sedation point

Needle depth 0.3–0.5 cun; moxa cones 5–7

This is the most frequently used point on the Heart channel. It is a very flexible point with a wide variety of uses for any condition of the Heart. Its name, Spirit Gate, serves to give some insight into its ability to strongly affect the Heart spirit. *Shen Men* was also a name given by many Daoists to the eyes (Hicks, 1999, p. 21) and it is through the eyes that the practitioner can notice the vitality and brightness of a person's spirit.

This point is the *yuan* source point and also the sedation point. It is an excellent point to sedate when the patient's Heart pulse is either full or very agitated. Its main use, however, is to strengthen the Heart and for this use it is extraordinary, often having an immediate effect during the treatment. As the *yuan* source point it is often used with SI 4 when the practitioner is 'testing' whether a patient is a Fire CF.

The power of this point can often be seen most dramatically when treating a person who is suffering from shock. As *Su Wen* says:

> When there is starting with *jing* the Heart no longer has a place to rely on. The *shen* no longer has a place to refer to, planned thought no longer has a place to settle. This is how the *qi* is in disorder (*luan*).

(Larre and Rochat de la Vallée, 1996, p. 61)

Patient Example

A patient who was a nurse in her late twenties rang a practitioner for an emergency appointment. Questioning eventually elicited that she had been involved in a moderately serious car accident the previous day, but she was almost incapable of speech. After tonification of *shen men* she spoke perfectly normally and afterwards reported that she felt completely back to her usual self. The only point used was Ht 7.

Heart 8 *Shao Fu*, Lesser Treasury: Fire point, horary point

Needle depth 0.3–0.5 cun; *moxa cones 3–5*

Like Heart 3 and Heart 9, this point has *shao* in its name. This is because the Heart channel is also the channel of the hand *shao yin*. This is the horary point (11 a.m.–1 p.m.) and is often used in this context, especially when the Heart *qi* is deficient. It is also the Fire point within the Fire and is indicated when a patient is sad, worried and fearful, especially fearful of other people (Deadman *et al.*, 1998, p. 221). It is a very warming point, so care must be taken if the patient is already inclined to be too hot.

Heart 9 *Shao Chong*, Lesser Rushing: Wood point, tonification point, Exit point

Needle depth 0.1 cun; *moxa cones 3–5*

This is the Wood point and tonification point. Given the propensity of the Wood pulses to be more full than those of Fire, this point is very commonly tonified and it connects the mother Element, Wood, to the child, Fire. As its name implies, its use produces a surge of vitality and strength to the Heart. It is the point of exit, linking to SI 1.

Bladder 15 *Xin Shu*: Heart back *shu* point

Needle depth 0.5–0.7 cun; *moxa cones 3–5*

This point is commonly used, although some care should be taken with people whose Heart is very fragile. The practitioner should ensure that tonifying the Heart is an effective treatment principle by using Heart command points before using this point. Used in the right context, it will have a direct effect on the Heart Organ itself and can thus strengthen the Heart physically or at the level of the spirit. It can be used in many contexts, for example, if a patient is emotionally disturbed, anxious, sad and miserable, and also for a patient who is broken-hearted from a relationship ending.

Bladder 44 *Shen Tang*, Spirit Hall

Needle depth 0.3–0.5 cun; *moxa cones 3–5*

The outer back *shu* point of the Heart can be used to affect the *shen* and give it a place of 'residence'. The point has a powerful action and primarily strengthens and stabilises the Heart spirit.

Other points used to treat the Heart

Other points to treat the Heart include Kid 23, Kid 24, Kid 25, *Ren* 14, *Ren* 16, *Ren* 17, *Du* 10, *Du* 11 and *Du* 14.

Small Intestine points

(Table 40.2)

The primary pathway of the Small Intestine channel

The Small Intestine channel runs from the ulnar side of the little finger up the ulnar side of the forearm, then along the posterior aspect of the upper arm and

Table 40.2 Commonly used points on the Small Intestine channel

Yuan source point	Small Intestine 4
Luo junction point	Small Intestine 7
Tonification point	Small Intestine 3
Sedation point	Small Intestine 8
Back *shu* point	Bladder 27
Outer Back *shu* point	None
Horary point	Small Intestine 5
Xi cleft point	Small Intestine 6
Entry point	Small Intestine 1
Exit point	Small Intestine 19
Window of the Sky	Small Intestine 16 & 17

shoulder. It then zigzags over the shoulder-blade before reaching the base of the neck. From here it travels across the side of the neck to the jaw and the cheek and then turns sharply back to the ear, where it ends at SI 19. Here it joins the Bl channel at Bl 1.

Small Intestine 1 *Shou Ze*, Lesser Marsh: Metal point, Entry point

Needle depth 0.1 cun; moxa cones 3–5

This is the Entry point and Metal point. It is only occasionally used to regulate the Metal within the Small Intestine. It is more frequently used as the point of entry.

Small Intestine 2 *Qian Qu*; Forward Valley: Water point

Needle depth 0.3–0.5 cun; moxa cones 3–7

This is the Water point and can be used to moisten the Small Intestine.

Patient Example

A teenage patient had severe red eczema on his hands. He was a Fire CF who was mainly treated on the Small Intestine. Treatment on different Small Intestine points was helpful but, somewhat at wit's end, the practitioner stimulated SI 2 and Ht 3 in order to moisten and cool the two Organs. The patient's skin markedly improved and repeated treatment on these points (and others) produced an almost complete disappearance of symptoms. Over time the patient also became considerably more confident in himself.

Small Intestine 3 *Hou Xi*, Back Stream: Wood point, tonification point, opening point of *Du* channel

Needle depth 0.3–0.7 cun; moxa cones 3–7

This is the Wood point and tonification point and it is often paired with Ht 9. Using it will create balance between the Wood and Fire along the *sheng* cycle. It is used if the Wood Element is fuller than its child, the Fire. As this is a common situation it is a frequently used point. This point is also known for its effect on the mind and spirit and can be used to steady emotional swings.

As the Wood point within the Small Intestine it can also enable people to make decisions when they have difficulty sorting out their future direction in life. The above function may also be because of the point's connection to the *Du mai*, which affects the brain and therefore helps to clarify a person's thinking.

Small Intestine 4 *Wang Gu*, Wrist Bone: *yuan* source point

Needle depth 0.3–0.5 cun; moxa cones 3–7

As the *yuan* source point of the Small Intestine, this point is excellent for strengthening or calming the Small Intestine. Like all *yuan* source points, it is the preferred point to use when a practitioner is assessing whether a patient is a Small Intestine CF. This point is frequently used by practitioners of Five Element Constitutional Acupuncture and can have a profound effect on a patient's well-being and ability to separate pure from impure on all levels.

Small Intestine 5 *Yang Gu*, Yang Valley: Fire point, horary point

Needle depth 0.3–0.5 cun; moxa cones 3–7

This is the Fire point and the horary point between 1 p.m. and 3 p.m. It is often used as the horary point as its timing is in the middle of the day. It is a powerful point and can be used to shake up and invigorate the Small Intestine and enable people to acquire greater mental clarity and calmness. The point promotes mental clarity and appropriate decision making, assisting the Small Intestine to separate the pure from the impure (Deadman *et al.*, 1998, p. 405).

Small Intestine 6 *Yang Lao*, Nourishing the Old: *xi* cleft (accumulation) point

Needle depth 0.3–0.5 cun; *moxa cones 3–5*

This is the *xi* cleft point. The name of this point has meant that it has been used throughout history to treat people who are suffering from problems associated with old age.

Small Intestine 7 *Zhi Zheng*: branch to the Heart channel, *luo* junction point

Needle depth 0.3–0.7 cun; *moxa cones 3–7*

The scholars seem to be sure that in this context *zheng*, which can be translated as 'correct', 'to put right' or 'to regulate', pertains to the Heart channel. They may well be correct because, as the *luo* point, it connects to the Heart channel via either Ht 7 or Ht 5. The name might also be referring to the Small Intestine's role of 'separating the pure from the impure', however, and therefore correcting and regulating. Either way, this point's use in assisting the Small Intestine in this role is often underrated. This is a powerful point for the mind and spirit, particularly in regard to helping the person resolve ambivalences and confusions. The 'Methods of acupuncture and moxibustion' from the *Golden Mirror of Medicine* recommends it for 'depression and knotting of all seven emotions' (Deadman *et al.*, 1998, p. 238).

Small Intestine 8 *Xiao Hai*, Small Sea: Earth point, sedation point

Needle depth 0.3–0.5 cun; *moxa cones 3–5*

This is the Earth point and therefore the sedation point. It is occasionally used to regulate the Earth within the Small Intestine, but it is mainly used for its local effect on the elbow.

Small Intestine 11 *Tian Zong*, Heavenly Ancestor

Needle depth 0.3–0.8 cun; *moxa cones 3–7*

This point is situated on the upper part of the body, like all the points with *tian* in their name. It is one of the most important spirit points on the Small Intestine channel. A Chinese story tells of a mythical Heavenly Ancestor who had the task of separating *yin* (earth) and *yang* (heaven) from its primeval state of chaos (Hicks, 1999, p. 23). This point is used to help clear the internal mental and spiritual chaos of someone who has lost clarity and certainty.

Small Intestine 16 *Tian Chuang*, Heavenly Window: Window of the Sky

Needle depth 0.3–0.7 cun; *moxa cones 5–10*

This is one of the two Windows of the Sky points that has 'window' in its name. *Chuang* is a small window designed to allow smoke and steam (and by extension, *qi*) to circulate and escape. This point is excellent for giving people a lift when they have become unable to find a resolution for their difficulties. When their ability to separate the 'pure from the impure' has become seriously impaired and they cannot see their way ahead clearly, this point can often be of enormous benefit.

Small Intestine 17 *Tian Rong*, Heavenly Appearance: Window of the Sky

Needle depth 0.3–0.7 cun; *moxa cones 3–5*

Whether this is a Window of the Sky or not, its effect is primarily upon the spirit (see the section on Windows of the Sky in Chapter 37, this volume). It does not seem to be as powerful as the previous point but still has the effect of lifting the spirit and clarifying the mind. It is also effective for problems of hearing.

Small Intestine 19 *Ting Gong*, Listening Palace: Exit point

Needle depth 0.5–0.8 cun; *no moxa*

This is the Exit point of the channel, linking to the Bladder channel at Bl 1. A block between the Small

Intestine and Bladder channels is a quite common Exit–Entry block. Its application in treating many hearing problems has been well documented. Less well known is its use for people who can't discriminate or make sense of what they hear due to imbalance of the Small Intestine.

Patient Example

A patient in his fifties was a Fire CF. His general lack of clarity indicated that one of the Organs affected was the Small Intestine. One of his problems was poor hearing. The practitioner wondered about the cause of it when the patient mentioned that his wife was incessantly talking and this got on his nerves. An important point used during his treatment was SI 19. His health improved overall from treatment and his relationship with his wife also became easier. Although his hearing never substantially improved, his ability to take things in did. During one treatment he mentioned that he found it easier to listen to his wife because he felt so much better in himself.

Bladder 27 *Xiao Chang Shu*: Small Intestine back *shu* point

Needle depth 0.7–1.2 cun; moxa cones 7–15

Situated on the sacrum this point is used for problems of the lower back, but its main use is to strengthen the Small Intestine. Although not a spirit point, it can strengthen a patient on all levels by benefiting the Small Intestine Organ. It is often combined with Bl 15.

Other points used to treat the Small Intestine

Ren 4 can also be used to treat the Small Intestine.

Bladder and Kidney points

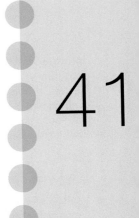

41

CHAPTER CONTENTS

The use of the back *shu* and outer back *shu* points on the Bladder channel that affect the various Organs are discussed in the section of the respective Organ.

Bladder points (Table 41.1)

The primary pathway of the Bladder channel

The Bladder channel begins at the inner corner of the eye. It ascends the forehead and travels over the head to the nape of the neck. From here it divides into two pathways. The first pathway is the inner Bladder line. This travels down the back at 1.5 *cun* from the medial line. It then passes over the buttock and travels down the back of the thigh to the knee crease. While travelling down the back it enters the kidneys then the bladder. The second pathway is the outer bladder line. This travels down the back at 3 *cun* from the medial line and passes over the buttock and down the back of the calf. The two lines join at the knee crease at Bl 40. From here the pathway travels over the gastrocnemius muscle, posterior to the external malleolus, over the calcaneus and along the external edge of the 5th metatarsal to the exit point Bl 67. Here it connects with the Kidney channel at Kid 1.

Bladder 1 *Jing Ming*, Bright Eyes: Meeting point of Bl, SI, St; Entry point

Needle depth 0.3–0.5 cun; no moxa

Ming is the same word that in the phrase *shen ming* is translated as the 'radiance of the spirits'. The eyes are often regarded as the best indicator of the state of a person's spirit. When the eyes shine the spirit is flourishing. This point is the first point on the Bladder channel and is used with SI 19 if a patient has an Entry–Exit block between the two channels.

It is also an important point to bring dynamism and vitality to patients who are deficient and depleted in the *qi* of their Water Element. It also can have a profound effect on a person's spirit and can bring lubrication to a person who is lacking in fluidity and flexibility at this level. This point may be beneficial to patients who cling to old habits because they are fearful of making changes. It also can have an important local effect on the eyes and is used for many eye problems.

Bladder 10 *Tian Zhu*, Heavenly Pillar: Window of the Sky, point of sea of *qi*

Needle depth 0.5–0.8 cun; moxa cones 3–5

The pillar referred to in the name is probably the trapezius muscle, but *tian zhu* is also the name of a star. Its location at the top of the spine might also indicate its importance in helping people to stand erect and to 'face up to' what is happening to them (Hicks, 1999, p. 25).

This point is extremely powerful, being both a Window of the Sky and a sea of *qi*. In the absence of many other points that treat the person's spirit on the Bladder channel, there is a tendency to use

Table 41.1 Commonly used points on the Bladder channel

Yuan source point	Bladder 64
Luo junction point	Bladder 58
Tonification point	Bladder 67
Sedation point	Bladder 65
Back *shu* point	Bladder 28
Outer Back *shu* point	None
Horary point	Bladder 66
Xi cleft point	Bladder 63
Entry point	Bladder 1
Exit point	Bladder 67
Window of the Sky	Bladder 10

this point often. It can also help people to gain new perspectives on areas of their lives.

Bladder 11 *Da Zhu*, Great Shuttle

Needle depth 0.5–0.7 cun; moxa cones 3–7
This is one of the points used in the External Dragons combination.

Bladder 12 *Feng Men*, Wind Gate

Needle depth 0.5–0.7 cun; moxa cones 5–10
This point can be reduced or tonified for problems in the Lungs.

Bladder 17 *Ge Shu*, Diaphragm *shu* point

Needle depth 0.5–0.7 cun; moxa cones 7–15
Although no emphasis is placed in Five Element Constitutional Acupuncture on the Blood (*xue*), this point is sometimes used if the person is suffering from disorders of the Blood.

Bladder 28 *Pang Guang Shu*: Bladder back *shu* point

Needle depth 0.7–1.2 cun; moxa cones 7–15
A very valuable point for treating problems of the bladder, painful conditions in the sacrum and for strengthening the Bladder in general. Like other back *shu* points, it can strengthen the Organ directly.

By doing this it can strengthen a person at any level of the body, mind and spirit. This is one of the points of choice when the Water Element or lower *jiao* has been affected by cold. Moxibustion would be used in this case.

Bladder 40 *Wei Zhong*, Supporting the Middle:[1] Earth point

Needle depth 0.5–1.0 cun; moxa cones 3–5
This point has also been called 'equilibrium middle'. This is the Earth point and, as the name implies, it also has the ability to stabilise and bring equilibrium to the Organ. Although it is very useful for local problems and for problems in the lower back, it is not commonly used by practitioners of Five Element Constitutional Acupuncture.

Bladder 45 *Yi Xi*, Cry of Pain

Needle depth 0.3–0.5 cun; moxa cones 5–10
Yi and *Xi* are both said to denote the kinds of sighing sounds that the patient utters when this point is palpated. This is presumably due to a releasing of *qi* in the area of the diaphragm. Some practitioners use this point to support people's spirits when they need internal strength. Its strengthening effect is probably due to it effectively being the outer back *shu* point of the Governor Vessel.

Bladder 58 *Fei Yang*, Fly and Scatter: *luo* junction point

Needle depth 0.7–1.0 cun; moxa cones 3–7
Tonifying this point can bringing vitality and energy to a patient who feels sluggish and depleted. It is the *luo* junction point, so it is often paired with Kid 4 and Kid 3. Using these Bladder and Kidney points in combination can bring stability to the Element, especially if the two paired Organs are out of harmony.

Bladder 59 *Fu Yang*, Instep *Yang*

Needle depth 0.5–1.0 cun; moxa cones 3–7
This point is sometimes paired with LI 4 in order to eliminate toxins from the body, in a combination known as the Great Eliminator.

---

[1] J. R. Worsley used Wu Wei-ping's numbering system for the Bladder channel. This accounts for different numbers being allocated for Bladder 40–54. Bladder 40 in the Chinese numbering system accords with Bladder 54 in Wu Wei-ping's (see Worsley, 1982, for the numbering system he used).

Bladder 60 *Kun Lun*, Mountain: Fire point

Needle depth 0.3–0.7 cun; moxa cones 3–7

In a well-known legend in Chinese mythology, the *Kun Lun* mountain is a mythical mountain in the far west of China (found in the *Huainanzi*, Chapter 4, and other texts). Believed to be unattainable, it is surrounded by a vermilion lake (this is the Fire point) and is the source of the Yellow River. This mountain is thought to possess powerful *qi* and offer spiritual and physical renewal (Lade, 1989, p. 171).

Although the name may partly refer to the external malleolus, which is situated close by, this story indicates that this is a powerful point on the channel. It is often used in the treatment of chronic back pain anywhere along the spine, especially if this is associated with deficiency in the Bladder and Kidney channels. Much of this point's strength comes from its ability to warm the Bladder and to keep the Water from becoming too cold. Cold Water will cause people to become stiff and contracted in their movements and in their spirits. It can also cause pain. Warming the Water will free the person up so that they can move with greater flexibility. Moxa should be used with care if a patient has signs of Heat, but if indicated then moxa can be used to great effect. This point should not be used in pregnancy.

Patient Example

A female patient in her fifties was a Water CF. Her main complaint was tiredness and increasing anxiety, which she realised was often completely inappropriate. Tonifying her Water had good results and the pulse changes from moxibustion were better than from needling. On three occasions Bl 60 was used along with Kid 2, the Fire point on the Kidneys. The use of this point made a clear improvement in the tiredness and anxiety.

Bladder 61 *Pu Can*, Servant's Respect: point to release External Dragons

Needle depth 0.3–0.5 cun; moxa cones 3–7

This point is used in the External Dragons combination.

Bladder 62 S*hen Mai*, Extended Vessel

Needle depth 0.3–0.5 cun; moxa cones 3–5

This powerful point is the opening point of the *Yang Heel Vessel*. It can create dynamic changes when people have low energy due to a deficient Water Element. It can also have an effect of sending the *qi* down from the head and calming the spirit if someone has extreme fear and fright, insomnia, mania or hyperactivity.

Bladder 63 *Jin Men*, Golden Gate: *xi* cleft point

Needle depth 0.3–0.5 cun; moxa cones 3–5

Gold is almost pure *yang* in its nature and is a Daoist symbol for incorruptibility (Lade, 1989, p. 175). Like other *xi* cleft points, it can be used in acute situations and especially in acute fear or anxiety arising from an imbalance in the Water Element. It can also be used to warm up a deficient and cold Bladder.

Bladder 64 *Jing Gu*, Capital Bone: *yuan* source point

Needle depth 0.3–0.5 cun; moxa cones 3–7

As the *yuan* source point this is a very reliable point for strengthening the Bladder. Like other *yuan* source points it is commonly used when testing for the CF. In this case it is often used in conjunction with Kid 3, the *yuan* source point of the Kidney. It also has a general strengthening effect and can bring calmness to patients who are fearful. It is an excellent distal point when other points higher on the channel are used.

Bladder 65 *Shu Gu*, Bone Binder: *shu* stream point, Wood point, sedation point

Needle depth 0.3–0.5 cun; moxa cones 3–5

This point is the sedation point but it is rarely used as the pulse of this Organ is seldom full. It is the Wood point.

Bladder 66 *Zu Tong Gu*, Passing Valley: Water point, horary point

Needle depth 0.2–0.3 cun; moxa cones 3–5

This is the Water and horary point between 3 p.m. and 5 p.m. It is often paired with Kid 10 and can be used to shake up and invigorate the Bladder, especially in the late afternoon. Because it is the Water point within the Water Element it can also have a powerful effect at other times of day and can bring moisture and lubrication to the Bladder. Some practitioners use it as a 'seasonal' horary point during the winter.

Bladder 67 *Zhi Yin*, Extremity of *Yin*: Metal point, tonification point, Exit point

Needle depth 0.1 cun; *moxa cones 3–5*

This is the Metal and tonification point. As the tonification point it can reconnect the mother Element, Metal, to the child, Water, along the *sheng* cycle. It is common for the Metal pulses to be significantly stronger than the Water pulses so it is a frequently used point.

This point is also used in the treatment of Husband–Wife imbalances.

Other points used to treat the Bladder

Several points on the lower abdomen are sometimes used to treat particular problems of the bladder, for example, *Ren 2*, *Ren 3*, *Ren 6*, Bl 31 and 32, but no other points on the Bladder channel are commonly used as part of the long-term treatment of a Water CF.

Kidney points (Table 41.2)

The primary pathway of the Kidney channel

The primary pathway of the Kidney channel starts on the sole of the foot at Kid 1. It then runs up the navicular bone and behind the medial malleolus

Table 41.2 Commonly used points on the Kidney channel

Yuan source point	Kidney 1
Luo junction point	Kidney 4
Tonification point	Kidney 7
Sedation point	Kidney 1
Back *shu* point	Bladder 23
Outer Back *shu* point	Bladder 52
Horary point	Kidney 10
Xi cleft point	Kidney 5
Entry point	Kidney 1
Exit point	Kidney 22
Window of the Sky	None

before travelling up the medial side of the leg and moving up to the groin. On the leg it intersects the Spleen meridian at Sp 6. The channel then ascends the abdomen and travels over the chest before proceeding along the throat and ending at the root of the tongue. The channel exits at Kid 22 where it joins the Pericardium channel at PC 1.

Kidney 1 *Yong Quan*, Bubbling Spring: Wood point, sedation point, Entry point

Needle depth 0.3–0.5 cun; *moxa cones 3–5*

This is the only point on the sole of the foot. As the first point and Entry point on the Kidney channel, it is compared to a spring where the *qi* 'bubbles' up from the Earth. The name gives an image of pure, fresh, revitalising water replenishing a person, so understandably this point can powerfully enliven a person's Kidney *qi* when tonified. It is often paired with Bladder 1, the Entry point of the Bladder, which can also have an invigorating effect.

This point can also descend *qi* that has risen to the upper part of the body. For example, if a person has heat rising to the head or feels agitated due to imbalance in the Kidney *qi*, this point can bring the *qi* downwards to the feet. Because of this action this point has a very calming effect.

It is the Wood point and sedation point, but it is rarely used in this respect because patients' Water is rarely fuller than their Wood.

Practitioners of *qi gong* make contact with the Earth *qi* at this point. Contact with this point while standing allows practitioners to root and descend their *qi* or absorb the invigorating *qi* of the Earth up through the feet and into the *dan tian*.

Kidney 2 *Run Gu*, Blazing Valley: Fire point

Needle depth 0.3–0.5 cun; *moxa cones 3–5*

At this point the spring has turned into a valley. The word 'blazing' is referring to the fact that this is the Fire point. This point can warm people who are chilly and lethargic because their Water is too cold. Care should be taken with moxa as this point has an extremely powerful warming effect. Kid 2 can also cool people who easily flush up and become restless because the Water is too warm. If used in this context this point is usually sedated.

Kidney 3 *Tai Xi*, Greater Mountain Stream: *yuan* source point, Earth point

Needle depth 0.3–0.5 cun; moxa cones 3–5

This is the *yuan* source point and Earth point. As the *yuan* source point of the Kidneys it has special significance, due to the *yuan qi* being stored between the two Kidneys and the Kidneys' role in storing the *jing*. *Yuan qi* is '*jing* in *qi* form'.

This point is commonly used for any problem arising from the Kidneys and it has a powerful effect. Like other *yuan* source points it is commonly used when testing for the CF. In this case it is often used in conjunction with Bl 64, the *yuan* source point of the Bladder. It is also one of the points used in the treatment of Husband–Wife imbalances, as it can transfer *qi* across the *ke* cycle from the Spleen.

Kidney 4 *Da Zhong*, Great Cup: *luo* junction point

Needle depth 0.3–0.5 cun; moxa cones 3–5

A cup is a receptacle to store fluid and this may refer to the key role of the Kidneys and Bladder in the control and storage of fluids in the body. This point links the Kidneys and Bladder as it is the *luo* junction point and it is often used in combination with Bl 58 or Bl 64. If these two Organs are out of balance, this combination of points can have an extremely stabilising effect on the Element.

This point also has a strong effect on a person's emotions and is particularly noted for its powerful effect in calming a patient's fear, especially when the Kidneys are depleted, causing a person's will to be deficient (Deadman *et al.*, 1998, p. 342). This may result in symptoms such as a lack of confidence or withdrawal and an inability to leave the safety of the home.

Kidney 5 *Shui Quan*, Water Spring: *xi* cleft point

Needle depth 0.3–0.5 cun; moxa cones 3–5

This point is called Water Spring, a place where water is always available. This is the *xi* cleft point and can be used for general support of the Kidneys and also when treating acute conditions.

Kidney 6 *Zhao Hai*, Shining Sea: opening point of *Yin Qiao Mai*

Needle depth 0.3–0.5 cun; moxa cones 3–5

The image of the 'Shining Sea' is provided by the fire of the 'Blazing Valley', which lies close by, shining on the water (Ellis *et al.*, 1989, p. 201). As a sea it can also be seen as a huge reservoir of water. This is a very moistening point and can be used if a person's Water Element has become too dry or hot. This is generally a very dynamic and invigorating point. It is especially powerful due its role as the opening point on the *Yin* Heel Vessel, one of the Eight Extra channels (for more on the *Yin* Heel Vessel, see Maciocia, 1989, p. 362).

Kidney 7 *Fu Liu*, Returning Current: *jing* river point, Metal point, tonification point

Needle depth 0.3–0.5 cun; moxa cones 3–5

The name of this point still maintains the imagery of water that is found in Kidney points 1 to 6. It has an alternative name of *Fui Bai*, Bearing White, which alludes to this point's function as the Metal point on the channel. As the Metal point it is therefore the tonification point and is very commonly used to strengthen the Kidneys by connecting the mother, Metal, to her child, Water. It is one of the four points used to treat Husband–Wife imbalances.

Kidney 9 *Zhu Bin*, Building up the River Bank

Needle depth 0.5–0.7 cun; moxa cones 3–5

Zhu Bin can be translated in several different ways; for example, as well as the name above, it can also be called 'Guest House'. Consequently it is difficult to be clear about the meaning intended for the name of this point (Hicks, 1999, p. 33). The name 'Building up the River Bank' brings to mind the fact that uncontrolled water arising from flooding was a major concern in many parts of China. In the building of canals in England, the internal bank is often 'puddled' or patted, a process that makes the bank less porous. There are many historical references to the treatment of psychological disorders, such as madness, mania, raging fury and cursing, through the use of this point (Deadman *et al.*, 1998, p. 349).

This point is often used at the 3rd, 6th and 9th months of pregnancy to strengthen the Kidneys and enhance the subsequent health of the child.

Kidney 10 *Yin Gu Yin*, Valley: Water point, horary point

Needle depth 0.7–1.0 cun; *moxa cones 3–5*

The point name gives another reference to the passage of water. This is the Water point and horary point between 5 p.m. and 7 p.m. It is a commonly used point that can have a powerful effect during horary time, when it can shake up and revitalise the Kidney *qi*. It can also invigorate a patient's *qi* if it is used as the Water point within the Water Element. Some practitioners also use this point as the 'seasonal horary' during the winter.

Kidney 12 *Da He*, Great Brightness

Needle depth 0.5–1.0 cun; *moxa cones 5–10*

Situated next to *Ren 3*, this point affects the centre of *qi*, that is located in this area. It can be used to great effect for problems in this area and also to re-invigorate a person whose Water Element is depleted.

Kidney 13 *Qi Xue*, *Qi* Cave

Needle depth 0.5–1.0 cun; *moxa cones 5–10*

This point has two alternative names, *Bao Men*, Gate of the Womb, and *Zi Hu*, Door of Infants. These names indicate this point, sited next to the important point *Ren 4*, is mainly used to treat the womb and issues of fertility. There is much anecdotal evidence of this point being used successfully to help women conceive.

Kidney 16 *Huang Shu*, Vitals: *shu* point

Needle depth 0.5–1.0 cun; *moxa cones 7–10*

This point is one of the band of points that encircles the lower *dan tian* and can be used to enhance the *qi* that is stored in this area. The word *huang* here alludes to the *dan tian*. It is particularly used to help restore depleted vitality, in body or spirit. It is especially useful to calm the spirit if the Heart and Kidney *qi* have lost their connection and the spirit has become unsettled.

Kidney 21 *You Men*, Dark Gate

Needle depth 0.3–0.7 cun; *moxa cones 3–5*

This point can be used to good effect when a patient is suffering from phobias or is being overwhelmed by fearfulness.

Kidney 22 *Bu Lang*, Walking on the Verandah: Exit point

Needle depth 0.3–0.7 cun; *moxa cones 3–5*

This is the first of the Kidney chest points (see Chapter 36, this volume, 'Using Points to Treat the Spirit'). It is also the Exit point of the Kidney channel, linking to PC 1, the Entry point of the Pericardium. Verandahs are the first places people walk to beyond the interiors of their homes. They can be safe places for fearful people to go when first venturing out into the world or for asthmatics who wake in the night to sit (Hicks, 1999, p. 35). This point can also be translated as Corridor Walk, referring to the points of the Kidney channel travelling by steps up the ribcage (Ellis *et al.*, 1989, p. 218).

Kidney 23 *Shen Feng*, *Shen* Seal

Needle depth 0.3–0.5 cun; *moxa cones 3–5*

A seal is the traditional way that people assert their identity on a document. Like the other Kidney chest points, it is used not only to treat Water CFs but also to support Fire or Metal CFs. This is partly because of its location on the chest. It has the effect of strengthening and nourishing the spirit and giving a person a better sense of their own identity. It is especially helpful when people's sense of self is weak as a result of their Heart and Pericardium being disturbed by intense emotions, such as sadness and shock.

Kidney 24 *Ling Xu Ling*, Burial Ground

Needle depth 0.3–0.5 cun; *moxa cones 3–5*

The *ling* is the *yin* aspect of the Heart spirit and the word *xu* also has *yin* connotations, i.e. meaning hidden, dark or obscure. This is an important point to resurrect the spirit. It is used when a person has become resigned and depleted by the vicissitudes of life. It can help to reach into some of the darker recesses of the spirit in order to help people to re-engage more fully with life, especially if they have lost purpose and direction.

Kidney 25 *Shen Cang*, Spirit Storehouse

Needle depth 0.3–0.5 cun; *moxa cones 3–5*

Storing, *cang*, is one of the roles of the Water Element, as winter is the time for storing. This point refers to the storehouse of the *shen*. It is used when a person needs to call on reserves at the level of the spirit. It is the last of the three Kidney chest points that refer to the spirit specifically. All these points are sited over the middle *dan tian*. It can be used in similar situations to Kid 23 and 24 and is very commonly used in association with treatment on the Heart and Pericardium. It is perhaps the point of choice in situations when the intensity of feelings of rejection and loneliness have devastated the stability and strength of a person's *shen*.

Kidney 26 *Yu Zhong*, Elegant Centre

Needle depth 0.3–0.5 cun; moxa cones 3–5

Zhong refers to the old name for the centre of *qi* that resides in the chest (see *Ren* 17). As this point and the next are slightly further away from the middle *dan tian*, they are not quite as powerful for the spirit as the preceding points. This point is quite commonly used, however, to strengthen a person's spirit in conjunction with treatment on the Kidneys.

Kidney 27 *Shu Fu*, *Shu* Treasury

Needle depth 0.3–0.5 cun; moxa cones 3–5

This is the last point on the Kidney channel and it is the least powerful Kidney chest point for treating the spirit level. It is a *fu*, or treasury, which is a place where reserves of *qi* can be accessed and drawn on.

Bladder 23 *Shen Shu*: Kidney back *shu* point, point to release the External Dragons

Needle depth 0.5–1.2 cun; moxa cones 3–15

One of a ring of points around the area of the lower *dan tian*, this point is commonly used to bolster, strengthen and warm the Kidneys. By treating the Organ directly, the Kidney can be strengthened at all levels.

Bladder 52 *Zhi Shi*, *Zhi* Dwelling

Needle depth 0.5–1.0 cun; moxa cones 7–15

As the *zhi* or Will Dwelling, this point is used to strengthen the spirit of the Kidneys. When the spirit of a Water CF has become imbalanced, it can manifest either as overwhelming ambition and willpower or conversely as the lack of the requisite driving force to motivate or generate change or embrace life. This point will bring either of these extremes into a better balance.

The state of the *zhi* is also important in relation to the *shen*, as in many ways the Water/Fire relationship is central to the person's *yin/yang* balance. The *Huainanzi* expresses the close relationship of these two aspects of the human spirit.

> The *shen* is the inexhaustible reservoir of *zhi*; when this inexhaustible reservoir is clear and pure, *zhi* shines forth. *Zhi* is the storehouse of the Heart. Through perfect *zhi*, the Heart is in balance.
>
> (quoted in Larre and Rochat de la Vallée, 1995, p. 66)

Other points used to treat the Kidneys

The points *Ren* 1, *Ren* 4, *Ren* 8, *Du* 1 and *Du* 4 can also be used to supplement treatment on the Kidneys.

Pericardium and Triple Burner points

42

CHAPTER CONTENTS

Pericardium points (Table 42.1)

The primary pathway of the Pericardium channel

The primary pathway of the Pericardium begins just lateral to the nipple at PC 1. It then arches over the axilla to travel down the medial surface of the arm and forearm, across the middle of the wrist and palm, to end at the tip of the middle finger. Here it joins the Triple Burner channel at TB 1.

Pericardium 1 *Tian Chi*, Heavenly Pond: Window of the Sky, Entry point

Needle depth 0.2–0.4 cun; moxa cones 3–5. No moxa or needle on women

An early name for the Pericardium was *Dan Zhong*, which is hard to translate but means the chest as a centre of *qi* in the body (Larre and Rochat de la Vallée, 1992b, pp. 81–97). The deep channel of the Pericardium starts in the middle of the chest, in the middle *dan tian*, and comes to the surface at the Heavenly Pond. The word *tian* in the name denotes this point's ability to affect the spirit. *Chi*, a pond, is a place where the *qi* collects before it flows into the Pericardium channel (Ellis *et al.*, 1989, p. 223). This point is a powerful point to affect the spirit level of the Pericardium.

Although this point is a Window of the Sky, it (like Lu 3) is not situated on the neck. When sadness or heartbreak has depleted a person's spirit, the effect of this point is unmatched by any other point on the Pericardium. Sadness affects the *qi* of the heart and sends the *qi* downwards. This point can lift the *qi* again, enabling the person to regain strength and vitality in their Heart-Protector. This in turn means that a person is more able to let people in or keep them out appropriately and without feeling too vulnerable. Regrettably, due to the location, it is not usually possible to use this point on a woman.

This is also the point of entry on the channel. If the connection between Kid 22 and PC 1 is blocked it can cause a person to feel shut off in their ability to relate to others.

Pericardium 2 *Tian Quan*, Heavenly Spring

Needle depth 0.5–0.7 cun; moxa cones 3–5

Although this point is on the arm, it forms part of the band of points that rings the middle *dan tian* at the level of the heart. Like Ht 1, which lies nearby, this point has *quan* or spring in its name. Both points have the effect of enlivening the *qi* in the channel and can be depended upon to give the patient vitality and strength as well as the ability to connect with their spirit.

PC 2 is the best alternative to PC 1 for a woman: that is, as a window or as an entry point.

Tian quan is not as effective for treating physical symptoms as emotional ones. If a patient is experiencing heart problems such as palpitations or arrhythmias due to problems in the Pericardium, command points or the back *shu* point often have a better

DOI: 10.1016/B978-0-7020-3175-5.00042-5

Table 42.1 Commonly used points on the Pericardium channel

Yuan source point	Pericardium 7
Luo junction point	Pericardium 6
Tonification point	Pericardium 9
Sedation point	Pericardium 7
Back shu point	Bladder 14
Outer Back shu point	Bladder 43
Horary point	Pericardium 8
Xi cleft point	Pericardium 4
Entry point	Pericardium 1
Exit point	Pericardium 8
Window of the Sky	Pericardium 1

effect. On the other hand, if patients are having difficulties in their emotional life then PC 1 and 2 are more clearly indicated.

Pericardium 3 *Qu Ze*, Crooked Marsh: Water point

Needle depth 0.5–0.7 cun; moxa cones 3–5

The water referred to in PC 1 is a pool, where its power is contained. In PC 2 it is surging and active. At this point the flow has slowed and has combined with the earth to form a marsh which the Chinese consider is a fertile place.

As the Water point, this point can be used to transfer *qi* across the *ke* cycle from the Kidneys or to regulate Water within the Pericardium. Putting Water on the Fire will calm and cool a patient who is restless, agitated and anxious due to too much Heat in the Pericardium.

Pericardium 4 *Xi Men*, Cleft Gate: *xi* cleft point

Needle depth 0.5–0.7 cun; moxa cones 3–5

This is the *xi* cleft point and it is commonly used to strengthen the *qi* of the Pericardium. It is especially useful in acute situations. Physically it can soothe the Pericardium if a patient has chest pains. It also has a strong emotional effect and can be used to calm a person who feels anxious, fearful or frightened

(Deadman *et al.*, 1998, p. 374) or who has had a sudden emotional upset affecting the Pericardium. It can be paired with TB 7.

Pericardium 5 *Jian Shi*, The Intermediary: Metal point, meeting of three *yin* of arm

Needle depth 0.5–0.7 cun; moxa cones 3–5

The name of this point alludes to the Pericardium's function of assisting the Heart and being responsible for the Heart's communications with the other Organs. This is the Metal point, although it is rarely used in this context.

Pericardium 6 *Nei Guan*, Inner Gate: *luo* junction point

Needle depth 0.5–0.7 cun; moxa cones 3–5

This potent and frequently used point is the *luo* connecting point of the Pericardium. It lies on the opposite side of the arm from the *luo* connecting point of the Triple Burner, the Outer Gate. Using PC 6 and TB 5 together can bring harmony and stability to the Fire Element when these two Organs are out of balance.

The name Inner Gate describes the point's ability to reach the inner aspect of a person. This point has the ability to enhance the *qi* of the Pericardium and subsequently the *qi* of all the Organs of the Upper Burner, especially when a person becomes oppressed by sadness or lack of joy. Opening this gate can ease a constricted chest and strengthen the *qi* of the Upper Burner if it has become depleted. This allows patients to brighten and settle in their mind and spirit.

This point has a potent effect on symptoms of nausea and sickness and has been much researched in this respect over recent years.

Pericardium 7 *Da Ling*, Great Mound: *yuan* source point, Earth point, sedation point

Needle depth 0.3–0.5 cun; moxa cones 3–5

This is the *yuan* source point and the Earth point. It lies alongside the *yuan* source point of the Lungs, which also has 'great' in its name.[1] This point, like Pericardium 6, is invaluable for the treatment of

---

[1] The *yuan* source points of the *yin* Organs all have names denoting great power. All three of the *yuan* source points on the foot *yin* channels have *tai*, which usually translates as 'greatest' or 'great', in their names.

the Pericardium when the spirit of the person is suffused with sadness, feelings of rejection, loneliness and lack of joy. Like other *yuan* source points, it is commonly used when testing for the CF. In this case it is often used in conjunction with TB 4, the *yuan* source point of the Triple Burner.

Pericardium 8 *Lao Gong*, Palace of Weariness: Fire point, horary point, Exit point

Needle depth 0.3–0.5 cun; *moxa cones 3–5*

This is the Fire point and horary point between 7 p.m. and 9 p.m. when it can be used to shake up and enhance the *qi* of the Pericardium. It is also used by some practitioners as the 'seasonal' horary point in the summer. It is also the Exit point and joins the Triple Burner channel at TB 1.

As the Fire point within the Fire Element, this is a very potent point. When the Pericardium lacks warmth it is unable to fulfil its role of being the source of 'elation and joy' (*Su Wen* Chapter 8; Larre and Rochat de la Vallée, 1992b, p. 81). Lack of joy (*bu le*) is the consequence of a Pericardium that has become cold and lifeless. As long as there is no risk of overheating the Organ, moxibustion can be very effective at enlivening the Protector of the Heart.

Patient Example

A patient in his forties had a seemingly extremely robust constitution. He had musculo-skeletal pain but also said in the initial consultation that he had been impotent for some years. He was obsessed with sexual fantasies and had not been in a sexual relationship for some years. He also felt the cold severely. He was a Fire CF and acupuncture and moxibustion on the PC and TB led to his sexuality becoming better balanced. The Palace of Weariness, especially, made a difference to his physical impotence.

Pericardium 9 *Zhong Chong*, Rushing into the Middle: Wood point, tonification point

Needle depth 0.3–0.5 cun; *moxa cones 3–5*

This is the last point on the Pericardium channel. Its name is similar to *dan zhong*, the area at the other end of the channel, in the middle of the chest. This

is the tonification point and Wood point. Using this point joins the Wood, the mother, with the Fire, its child, along the *sheng* cycle. It is common for the Wood to have more abundant *qi* than the Fire, so this point is used frequently. It can enhance and invigorate the Pericardium and is often paired with TB 3.

Bladder 14 *Jue Yin Shu*: Pericardium back *shu* point

Needle depth 0.5–0.7 cun; *moxa cones 3–7*

The Pericardium is here referred to by its name as the hand *jue yin*. The *jue yin* (Liver and Pericardium) is responsible for Blood (*xue*) and the vessels (*mai*), which are the 'pathways of animation' (Larre and Rochat de la Vallée, 1995, p. 5). This point particularly stabilises and strengthens the Pericardium. It can have a direct effect on the Pericardium Organ/function itself and can thus strengthen a person at any level.

Bladder 43 *Gao Huang Shu*, Gao Huang back *shu* point

Needle depth 0.3–0.5 cun; *moxa cones 7–50*

The *Gao Huang* is an area of the body that forms the border between the Upper and Middle Burner, between the middle *dan tian* and the abdomen. When a person is extremely depleted and has chronic and almost incurable diseases, the illness may have lodged in this space. This region is said to be very hard to influence with acupuncture. One of the best ways to affect it is by using moxibustion on this point which is said to tonify the *qi* of the whole body. Sun Si-miao in *The Thousand Ducat Formulas* says of this point: 'there is no illness it cannot treat' (Deadman *et al.*, 1998, p. 304).

This point is also used as an adjunct to treatment on the Pericardium. It will warm, strengthen and nourish the *qi* of the chest especially on patients whose CF is in the Pericardium or Heart. This point can have a large number of moxa cones used on it. Sometimes up to 50 are used. This can be a useful point to warm a Fire CF who is internally cold. Moxa on this point can also normalise the blood count of a patients with anaemia.

Other points used to treat the Pericardium

Other points to treat the Pericardium include Kid 23, Kid 24, Kid 25, *Ren* 15, *Ren* 16 and *Ren* 17.

Triple Burner points (Table 42.2)

The primary pathway of the Triple Burner channel

The Triple Burner channel begins at the ulnar nail point of the ring finger and runs over the back of the hand and posterior surface of the forearm to the back of the elbow. From here it ascends the upper arm to the shoulder and then the neck, winds round the ear and then crosses over the temple to end at the outer extremity of the eyebrow. Here it joins the Gall Bladder channel at GB 1.

Triple Burner 1 *Guan Chong*, Rushing the Frontier Gate: Metal point, Entry point

Needle depth 0.1 cun; moxa cones 3–5

This is the Metal point and the point of Entry of the Triple Burner, following on from the Exit point of the Pericardium, PC 8.

Triple Burner 2 *Ye Men*, Fluid Gate: Water point

Needle depth 0.3–0.5 cun; moxa cones 3–5

Like the previous point, this point is also a gate. This time it is the Fluid Gate. One of the key functions of the Triple Burner is the 'regulation of fluids'. This

point is the Water point and when stimulated it can increase fluid secretions. The fluids referred to are *ye*, which are fluids that are found deep in the organs and structures of the body, such as the joints, spinal column, bone marrow and brain. These fluids are viscous and do not move rapidly.

Triple Burner 3 *Zhong Zhu*, Middle Islet: Wood point, tonification point

Needle depth 0.3–0.5 cun; moxa cones 3–5

Here is another reference to *zhong*, but this time it is on the Triple Burner channel (see PC 9 and Ht 9 for other points with *zhong* in the name). An old name for *yuan* was *zhong* and this point probably refers to the Triple Burner's function of distributing the *yuan qi* around the body. It is interesting to note that the *Ling Shu* refers to the Triple Burner as *zhong du*, the 'central river' (Ellis *et al.*, 1989, p. 238).

This point is the Wood point and tonification point. By using this point the mother Element, Wood, is connected to the child, Fire. This is a commonly used point because the Wood Element is often fuller than the Fire. This point can strongly tonify the Triple Burner and can also have the effect of raising a person's spirits (Maciocia, 1989, p. 439).

Table 42.2 Commonly used points on the Triple Burner channel

Yuan source point	Triple Burner 4
Luo junction point	Triple Burner 5
Tonification point	Triple Burner 3
Sedation point	Triple Burner 10
Back *shu* point	Bladder 22
Outer Back *shu* point	Bladder 51
Horary point	Triple Burner 6
Xi cleft point	Triple Burner 7
Entry point	Triple Burner 1
Exit point	Triple Burner 22
Window of the Sky	Triple Burner 16

Patient Example

A patient in her fifties complained of depression and migraines. She was a Wood CF with very full Wood pulses but she was lacking in joy and smelt scorched. She also had very deficient Pericardium and Triple Burner pulses. Sedating various points on the Liver and Gall Bladder channels, including the sedation points, enabled her to feel substantially better. The use of the tonification points on Pericardium and Triple Burner (PC 9 and TB 3), however, to transfer *qi* from Wood created a greater level of balance between these Elements. This had not been attained by treating the Wood Element alone.

Triple Burner 4 *Yang Chi, Yang* Pond: *yuan* source point

Needle depth 0.3–0.5 cun; moxa cones 3–5

This is an important strengthening point. It is the *yuan* source point on the Triple Burner channel and one function of the Triple Burner is to distribute *yuan qi*. As the *yuan* source point it is most commonly used to test if a person is a Fire CF. In this case it is used with PC 7, the *yuan* source point of the Pericardium.

Practitioners in some Japanese lineages tonify this point at each treatment to tonify the *yang* (College of Traditional Acupuncture, 2000). This is partly because, in general, Japanese practitioners are inclined to focus on the Triple Burner's role in assisting the *ming men* in the creation of the body's warmth and temperature regulation (see Mole, 1994).

Triple Burner 5 *Wai Guan*, Outer Gate: *luo* junction point, opening point of *Yang Wei* (linking) *Mai*

Needle depth 0.5–0.8 cun; *moxa cones 3–5*
This is the *luo* junction point and it is frequently used. It is often combined with PC 6 or PC 7. The combination of these points can create great stability in the Fire Element if the Pericardium and Triple Burner are out of balance.

The Inner Gate (PC 6) and the Outer Gate are often used together and are complementary. As the names imply, they can enable people to find a balance between opening up and closing down to the outside world, other people and themselves.

Fevers place a particular strain on the Pericardium and Triple Burner. The Pericardium has to protect the Heart from the heat and the Triple Burner has to harmonise the temperature and fluids in the body. After a person has had a fever it is very common for the Pericardium and Triple Burner pulses to be depleted and a person to be pale and lacking joy, vitality and stamina. This point is especially effective in this situation.

Triple Burner 6 *Zhi Gou*, Branching Ditch: Fire point, horary point

Needle depth 0.5–0.8 cun; *moxa cones 5–7*
This is the Fire point and horary point between 9 p.m. and 11 p.m. Due to it being active as a horary point during unsocial hours, it is rarely used in this context. As the Fire point within the Fire Element it is also often used with PC 8 to warm up a cold and sluggish Pericardium and Triple Burner. Too much moxa on this point could overheat the Triple Burner and dry up fluids, so moxa should only be used if it has proved to have been effective on other Triple Burner points.

Triple Burner 7 *Hui Zong*, Assembly of Ancestors: *xi* cleft point

Needle depth 0.5–0.8 cun; *moxa cones 5–7*
This is the *xi* cleft point. There is some disagreement concerning the translation of the name, but the word *zong* is the same as the word used for the *qi* that activates the chest. Like other *xi* cleft points, this point acts as a reservoir of *qi*. It can be used when extra *qi* is required in treatment, for instance when acute conditions affect the Triple Burner.

Triple Burner 10 *Tian Jing*, Heavenly Well: Earth point, sedation point

Needle depth 0.3–0.5 cun; *moxa cones 3–5*
The word *jing* or 'well' is likely to refer to the enormous hollow in which this point is found. The word *tian* indicates that this point can influence a person's relationship to Heaven. It may seem unusual to name a point so relatively low in the body with the word *tian*, but when the arm hangs down this point is at the same level as Stomach 25, *Tian Shu*. It marks the border of the lower half of the body, which is resonant with Earth, and the upper part of the body, which is resonant with Heaven. The name *tian* indicates that this point can affect a person's spirit. It is not, however, a commonly used point.

This point is the Earth point and sedation point. It is rarely used as the sedation point as the pulse of the Triple Burner is seldom full. It is sometimes used to regulate the Earth within the Triple Burner.

Triple Burner 11 *Qing Leng Yuan*, Clear Cold Abyss

Needle depth 0.3–0.5 cun; *moxa cones 3–5*
The main use of this point is either to warm the Triple Burner if it has become cold and lifeless or to cool and calm it if it is too hot.

Triple Burner 15 *Tian Liao*, Heavenly Foramen

Needle depth 0.3–0.5 cun; *moxa cones 5–7*
This point is the uppermost point of the Triple Burner on the torso, hence it has *tian* in its name. This is a powerful point for treating people who feel oppressed in the chest, heart or Upper Burner, especially if this is caused by depletion of the Triple Burner.

Triple Burner 16 *Tian You*, Heavenly Window: Window of the Sky

Needle depth 0.3–0.5 cun; no moxa

This Window of the Sky point can have a dramatic effect. The word *you* or window can also be translated as 'enlightenment', and windows are also the 'ears' and 'eyes' of the head. This point has an unparalleled ability to bring in lightness and to uplift a person whose spirit has become bowed down by sadness and lack of joy.

Triple Burner 22 *He Liao*, Harmony Foramen: Exit point

Needle depth 0.1–0.3 cun; moxa cones 3–5

This is the Exit point joining to the Gall Bladder channel at GB 1. This Exit–Entry block should always be considered if there are local problems in one temple.

Triple Burner 23 *Si Zhu Kong*, Silk Bamboo Hollow

Needle depth 0.3–0.5 cun; no moxa

The eyebrow is often compared to a bamboo leaf (Ellis *et al.*, 1989, p. 250). Bamboo is renowned for forming its flower inside the hollow stem. This name implies that a hidden quality resides at this point. It can be used to regulate the Triple Burner when there is instability, for example, if a person is struggling to maintain a stable temperature or mood.

Bladder 22 *San Jiao Shu*, Triple Burner *shu*

Needle depth 0.5–1.0 cun; moxa cones 7–15

Whether the Triple Burner truly has a 'form' or not has been much debated. There is no doubt, however, that its energetic centre is in the 'space between the two Kidneys' or the *ming men* (see Chapter 12). The back *shu* point is located near this area. Stimulating this point with a needle or moxibustion is effective at boosting the vitality and internal warmth of a person whose Ministerial Fire has become deficient. Although not a spirit point it can be used to strengthen the Triple Burner Organ/function. This can benefit a patient at all levels.

Patient Example

A patient in her sixties had been extremely ill with influenza followed by bronchitis. A lengthy period of convalescence had failed to restore her to her previous level of vitality. She was a Fire CF and treatment using the back *shu* points of the Pericardium and Triple Burner along with Bladder 43 and Governor Vessel 4 had an extremely beneficial effect.

Bladder 51 *Huang Men*, Vitals Gate

Needle depth 0.3–0.5 cun; moxa cones 7–15

This is not the *gao huang* referred to in Bladder 43, the outer back *shu* point of the Pericardium. The word *huang* is connected to the lower *dan tian*. Situated above the 'space between the two Kidneys', this point fortifies the Triple Burner in particular and the lower *dan tian* in general.

Other points used to treat the Triple Burner

Other points used to treat the Triple Burner are *Ren* 5, 7, 12 and 17.

Gall Bladder and Liver points

43

Gall Bladder points (Table 43.1)

The primary pathway of the Gall Bladder channel

The Gall Bladder channel begins at the outer canthus at the corner of the eye. It then travels across the temple and ascends in front of the ear to the corner of the forehead. Next it doubles back and descends behind the ear, only to zigzag once more over the side of the head to the forehead and back to the rear of the head. From here it travels down the neck to cross to the front of the shoulder and then on to the axilla. It then zigzags forwards and down across the side of the chest and then backwards and down to the person's side at the level of the waist. From here it moves forwards and down again to the front of the anterior iliac crest of the hip bone and backwards and down to the hip. It then continues down the lateral side of the thigh, knee and lower leg, in front of the lateral malleolus of the ankle and over the top of the foot. It ends at the lateral side of the fourth toe at GB 41 where it connects to Liv 1.

Gall Bladder 1 *Tong Zi Liao*, Pupil Foramen: Entry point

Needle depth 0.3–0.5 cun; moxa cones 3–5

This is the point of Entry, which is linked to the point of Exit of the Triple Burner channel at TB 22. A block between these two channels can cause local problems, such as temporal headaches, neuralgia and eye problems. Releasing this block can transform patients' minds and spirits and give them greater insight or vision as well as calm their anger and irritability.

Gall Bladder 9 *Tian Chong*, Heaven Rushing

Needle depth 0.3–0.5 cun; moxa cones 3–5

Ma Shi, a Ming dynasty physician, thought there was a mistake in *Ling Shu* Chapter 2 which states that Small Intestine 17 is a Window of the Sky. This was because SI 17 was given as a point on the *shao yang* or Gall Bladder channel. As this point has *tian* in its name some people assume that it is really the Window of the Sky described in the *Ling Shu*. Whether this is true or not, the name Heaven Rushing marks this point out as a spirit point. In contrast, neighbouring points on the channel generally have topographical names.

Situated on the head, this point has a powerful effect on the mind and spirit when the Gall Bladder is either full or deficient. It can help patients to have

DOI: 10.1016/B978-0-7020-3175-5.00043-7

Table 43.1 Commonly used points on the Gall Bladder channel

Yuan source point	Gall Bladder 40
Luo junction point	Gall Bladder 37
Tonification point	Gall Bladder 43
Sedation point	Gall Bladder 38
Back shu point	Bladder 19
Outer Back shu point	Bladder 48
Horary point	Gall Bladder 41
Xi cleft point	Gall Bladder 36
Entry point	Gall Bladder 1
Exit point	Gall Bladder 41
Window of the Sky	None

greater clarity of mind and spirit and to improve their ability to make decisions. It is also indicated if a patient is fearful and timid if it is a result of Gall Bladder deficiency.

Gall Bladder 12 Wan Gu, Mastoid Process

Needle depth 0.3–0.5 cun; moxa cones 3–5
This point can be used for insomnia arising from the Gall Bladder and Liver especially if combined with Bl 18 and 19 (Maciocia, 1989, p. 445).

Gall Bladder 13 Ben Shen, Root of the Spirit

Needle depth 0.3–0.5 cun; moxa cones 3–5
Ben Shen is the name of Chapter 8 of the *Ling Shu*, the chapter with the fullest discussion on the spirit in the *Nei Jing*. The *shen* is regarded as the 'root' of the person and it is also essential that the *shen* is properly rooted in a person. This point along with GB 15 and 16 has a powerful effect on the mind and spirit. As it is located over the upper *dan tian*, it can be reduced to calm a person if the *shen* is agitated. This is especially effective when anger has made the *qi* 'rise', creating too much heat or recurring angry thoughts. It is also indicated when a patient has persistent and unreasonable jealousy, anxiety or worry (Maciocia, 1989, p. 446).

Ben Shen can also enable a person to become more assertive, creative or decisive if a person's Gall Bladder is deficient.

Gall Bladder 15 Tou Lin Qi, Head above Tears

Needle depth 0.3–0.5 cun; moxa cones 3–5

This point is used to stabilise the mind and spirit when a patient has emotional swings. It can also be tonified to strengthen the spirit when the Gall Bladder is deficient.

It is sometimes combined with GB 41, *Zu Lin Qi*, Foot above Tears.

Gall Bladder 16 Mu Chuang, Eye Window

Needle depth 0.3–0.5 cun; moxa cones 3–5

As well as treating afflictions of the eyes, this point can also be used to expand a person's insight and vision.

Patient Example

An elderly patient had suffered from severe migraines, which affected his vision, for many years. He was of an irascible temperament and thought that his migraines were largely the result of his intense feelings of frustration. Using this point on two consecutive occasions made an enormous difference to the intensity, duration and frequency of his migraines and he became less bad-tempered over the same period of time.

Gall Bladder 17 Zheng Ying, Upright Living

Needle depth 0.3–0.5 cun; moxa cones 3–5
Zheng Ying can mean fear or solitude and this may be an indication for the use of this point for calming the spirit (Ellis *et al.*, 1989, p. 267).

Gall Bladder 18 Cheng Ling, Receiving Spirit

Needle depth 0.3–0.5 cun; moxa cones 3–5

This point affects the person's *ling*, the *yin* counterpart to the *shen*. It is one of the best points to use to treat people's spirits, especially if they are troubled by obsessional thoughts or dementia. This point is also said to connect a person's spirit to the universal *qi* (College of Traditional Acupuncture, 2000). It is located lateral to *Du 20*, which is at the highest point on top of the head.

Gall Bladder 20 *Feng Chi*, Wind Pond

Needle depth 0.5–0.8 cun; *moxa cones 7–10*

This is a powerful point that can be used for its local effect, as well as for problems in the head and eyes.

Gall Bladder 24 *Ri Yu*, Sun and Moon: front *mu* point of Gall Bladder

Needle depth 0.3–0.5 cun; *moxa cones 5–7*

The name refers to the expression 'clear as the sun and moon', which indicates a clear and decisive mind. The combined characters for 'sun' and 'moon' form the word *ming*, which means 'intelligent', 'clear' or 'understand'. These are the qualities that people strive to achieve when their Gall Bladder is deficient.

This point is mentioned in *Su Wen* (along with the back *shu* point) for the treatment of indecisiveness resulting from Gall Bladder deficiency. As the sun represents *yang* and the moon *yin*, the name of the point implies a balancing of *yin* and *yang* in the Gall Bladder. It is probably the most important point for people who are struggling with indecision, confusion or excessive rigidity due to an imbalanced Gall Bladder.

There may also be a link in the name to the eyes, the sense organ associated with the Wood Element, as the left eye is known as the sun and the right eye is known as the moon. It is also the front *mu* point.

Gall Bladder 25 *Jing Men*, Capital Gate: front *mu* point of Kidneys

Needle depth 0.3–0.5 cun; *moxa cones 7–10*

This is the front *mu* point of the Kidneys but it is often used to treat the Gall Bladder. This point is situated on the side of the body in the region of the Gall Bladder and it can strongly move *qi* that is stuck in or around the Gall Bladder Organ.

Gall Bladder 30 *Huan Tiao*, Jumping Circle

Needle depth 1.5–2.5 cun; *moxa cones 7–20*

This point has a strong local effect on the hip and lower back.

Gall Bladder 34 *Yang Ling Quan*, Yang Mound Spring: Earth point, special point for tendons

Needle depth 0.5–1.0 cun; *moxa cones 7–10*

This is the Earth point, so it is often combined with Liv 3. It is a powerful point and is normally used to regulate the Earth within the Wood and can generally stabilise the Element.

It is also the *hui* gathering point for the tendons. It is commonly used when the muscles and/or tendons are inflexible or rigid or to encourage the body to heal injured tendons.

This point is also used if people are timid and fearful of people 'as if about to be apprehended' (Deadman *et al.*, 1998, p. 452).

Gall Bladder 36 *Wai Qiu*, Outer Mound

Needle depth 0.5–0.8 cun; *moxa cones 3–5*

This is the *xi* cleft point and can be used to treat acute Gall Bladder problems.

Gall Bladder 37 *Guang Ming*, Bright and Clear: *luo* junction point

Needle depth 0.7–1.0 cun; *moxa cones 5–7*

The name 'bright and clear' undoubtedly refers in part to this point's potent effect upon the eyes and vision. A lack of brightness and clarity, however, are also common symptoms when a person's Gall Bladder is dysfunctional. This point is commonly used to assist the patient to become more decisive and clear thinking.

GB 37 is also the *luo* junction point. It is often paired with Liv 5, although it can be combined with Liv 3. Using these points together can bring stability to the two Organs within the Element if they are out of balance.

Gall Bladder 38 *Yang Fu*, Yang Support: Fire point, sedation point

Needle depth 0.5–0.7 cun; *moxa cones 5–7*

This is the Fire point and the sedation point. Using this point joins Wood to Fire, along the *sheng* cycle. It is often combined with Liv 2 when the Wood Element is full and the Fire deficient. As this is a common situation, this point is frequently used.

Gall Bladder 39 *Xuan Zhong*, Hanging Cup: Special point for bone marrow

Needle depth 0.3–0.5 cun; moxa cones 5–7

This point is mainly used to strengthen the bones and the marrow, especially when people also have weak Kidneys.

Gall Bladder 40 *Qiu Xu*, Wilderness Mound: *yuan* source point

Needle depth 0.3–0.7 cun; moxa cones 3–5

This is the *yuan* source point and is usually combined with Liv 3. Whereas Liv 3 is often paired with GB 34 for more physical symptoms, GB 40 is preferred when the priority is to bring about a change in the person's spirit. Because they are the *yuan* source points, the combination of GB 40 and Liv 3 are often the first points used to test whether a person is a Wood CF.

Gall Bladder 41 *Zu Lin Qi*, Foot above Tears: Wood point, horary point, Exit point, opening point of *Dai mai*

Needle depth 0.3–0.5 cun; moxa cones 3–5

This is the Wood point and horary point between 11 p.m. and 1 a.m. It is therefore usually combined with Liv 1. Because Gall Bladder horary time is at night, this point is rarely, if ever, used as a horary point. It can, however, be used to calm a hyperactive Gall Bladder during the day, between 11 a.m. and 1 p.m., the Gall Bladder low time. Some practitioners use this point as a 'seasonal horary' during the spring, especially if the Wood Element is deficient.

This is also the Wood point within the Wood Element and it can treat the essence of the Element, enabling people to grow and develop when they have difficulty moving forward. It can be used to calm a person's anger and impatience or enable a person to have more courage and decisiveness. It is a very powerful point and is equally effective, whether sedated or tonified. It is particularly effective for treating Gall Bladder problems in the upper part of the body including eye, breast or neck conditions.

It is also the Exit point and connects to Liv 1 both as Wood points and as Entry–Exit points. GB 41 is also the opening point of the *Dai mai*, one of the Eight Extra channels. (For more on the Extraordinary Channels, see Maciocia, 1989, p. 361.)

Gall Bladder 43 *Xia Xi*, Pinched Ravine: Water point, tonification point

Needle depth 0.3–0.5 cun; moxa cones 3–5

This is an essential point for tonifying the Gall Bladder. It is the tonification and Water point and is therefore often paired with Liv 8. As the Water Element is rarely fuller than the Wood Element it is seldom used as a tonification point. It is used to bring moisture to the Wood Element, however. The tendency of some Wood CFs to become brittle and rigid in their body or spirit can be counteracted by enhancing the Water within the Wood.

If the Gall Bladder is too hot, causing anger, frustration and emotional volatility, this point can be sedated to cool the person.

Gall Bladder 44 *Zu Qiao Yin*, Foot Hole: *yin* Metal point

Needle depth 0.1 cun; moxa cones 3–5

This is the Metal point and is only used if the practitioner wishes to affect the balance of the Metal within the Wood.

Bladder 19 *Dan Shu*: Gall Bladder back *shu* point

Needle depth 0.5–0.7 cun; moxa cones 3–7

This is an essential and commonly used point to either tonify or sedate the Gall Bladder. By affecting the Organ directly, this point can affect a person on all levels of body, mind and spirit. Moxibustion is commonly used if the Gall Bladder is deficient.

Bladder 48 *Yang Gang*, *Yang* Net

Needle depth 0.3–0.5 cun; moxa cones 3–5

This is an effective point for treating the mental and spiritual aspects of the Gall Bladder, especially to enable a person to make clear decisions and judgements.

Liver points (Table 43.2)

The primary pathway of the Liver channel

The Liver channel begins on the lateral side of the big toe and travels over the top of the foot to the medial side of the lower leg where it meets the Spleen

Table 43.2 Commonly used points on the Liver channel

Yuan source point	Liver 3
Luo junction point	Liver 5
Tonification point	Liver 8
Sedation point	Liver 2
Back *shu* point	Bladder 18
Outer Back *shu* point	Bladder 47
Horary point	Liver 1
Xi cleft point	Liver 6
Entry point	Liver 1
Exit point	Liver 14
Window of the Sky	None

channel at Sp 6. About halfway up the shin bone it crosses the Spleen channel to go to the back of the medial surface of the lower leg.

It continues up the medial surface of the thigh to the groin, curves around the genitals and moves upwards to the tip of the eleventh rib. From here it skirts around the stomach and enters the Liver and Gall Bladder organs. The pathway then moves out over the abdomen to the bottom of the ribcage and ends in the ribs, below the breast at Liv 14. Here it joins the Lung channel at Lu 1.

Liver 1 *Da Dun*, Great Mound: Wood point, horary point, Entry point

Needle depth 0.1–0.2 cun; *moxa cones 3–7*

This is the Entry point, Wood point and the horary point between 1 a.m. and 3 a.m. It is used in a similar way to the Gall Bladder horary point, however, during the Liver low time (between 1 and 3 in the afternoon) to calm a hyperactive Liver. It is also sometimes used as a 'seasonal horary' in the spring, especially if the Wood Element is deficient.

As the Wood point in the Wood Element, this point provides a powerful surge of vitality to the Liver when tonified. It can also have a strong calming effect when reduced. Moxibustion is commonly used.

Liver 2 *Xing Jian*, Moving Between: Fire point, sedation point

Needle depth 0.3–0.5 cun; *moxa cones 3–7*

This is the Fire point and sedation point. As the pulses of the Wood Element are commonly full, the sedation points are frequently used. Using this point improves the connection between the Wood Element and the Fire Element along the *sheng* cycle.

The Liver can easily become agitated and over-heated due to frustration or toxic substances, such as some foods, recreational drugs or some prescribed medicines. There may, therefore, be too much Fire within the Wood. Patients may feel rage, hot inside or have a red face. As anger makes the *qi* 'rise', they may also literally become 'hot headed' and have a tendency to have headaches and migraines. This point can be very effective at cooling and calming down the Liver in this situation.

Liver 3 *Tai Chong*, Great Surging: *yuan* source point, Earth point

Needle depth 0.3–0.5 cun; *moxa cones 3–7*

This is the most frequently used point on the Liver channel. It is extremely effective when tonified or sedated and can literally provide the Liver with a great surge of *qi*. It is the *yuan* source point and, like other *yuan* source points, it is commonly used when testing the CF. In this case it is used in conjunction with GB 40, the *yuan* source point of the Gall Bladder.

This point is an extremely calming point. It is also very effective if the Liver *qi* fails to move in a relaxed and smooth way due to suppressed anger. This can cause depression or mood swings and can manifest in a multitude of physical symptoms such as a tight chest, digestive problems, sighing, pre-menstrual tension, eye problems or headaches. It can also be sedated with LI 4 to create a more strongly calming and relaxing action and to also clear spasms and tension.

This point is also the Earth point and it helps to generate increased stability in the Liver.

Liver 4 *Zhong Feng*, Middle Seal: Metal point

Needle depth 0.3–0.5 cun; *moxa cones 3–7*

The main use of this point is to transfer *qi* across the *ke* cycle, when a patient has a Husband–Wife imbalance. Tonifying this point moves *qi* from the Lung to the Liver.

Liver 5 *Li Gou*, Wormwood Canal: *luo* junction point

Needle depth 0.3–0.5 cun; *moxa cones 3–7*

As the *luo* junction point of the channel this is often combined with GB 37, although it can be paired with GB 40. Using these Liver and Gall Bladder points in combination can bring stability to the Element, especially if the two paired Organs are out of harmony. Its name may be a reference to its ability to connect the two Organs of the Wood Element.

This point can calm a person who is depressed or oppressed due to imbalance in the Liver *qi*. It may be especially useful if a person feels constricted in the throat due to emotional difficulties and tension. It also connects to the genitals. Moxibustion is commonly used if the Liver is deficient.

Liver 6 *Zhong Du*, Middle Capital: *xi* cleft point

Needle depth 0.3–0.8 cun; *moxa cones 3–5*

This is the *xi* cleft point and it is especially indicated when the Liver *qi* is not moving smoothly. It has a particular effect on the genital area.

Liver 8 *Qu Quan*, Crooked Spring: Water point, tonification point

Needle depth 0.5–0.8 cun; *moxa cones 3–5*

This is the tonification point and Water point. Using it will connect the Kidney, the child, to the Liver, the mother. Although the pulse of the Kidney is seldom fuller than the Liver pulse, this point can very effectively join these two Organs along the *sheng* cycle and it is frequently used to tonify the Liver. It can also bring flexibility to a person if their Wood has become brittle, dry and inflexible, causing them to have difficulty responding to changes happening in their lives.

Liver 13 *Zhang Men*, Chapter Gate: Spleen front *mu* point, special point for five *yin* Organs

Needle depth 0.5–0.8 cun; *moxa cones 3–7*

The word *zhang* was originally used to denote the camphor laurel tree and therefore, by extension, any valuable wood (Ellis *et al.*, 1989, p. 301).

All points on the body with *men* in the name are powerful. A 'gate' has the ability to open and close and serves as a transition between two different places. This gate has a powerful effect on the middle *jiao* and is also situated close to the Liver Organ itself. It can powerfully affect the body as well as the spirit. Physically it can be used for many digestive disorders arising from the Liver. As a spirit point it can be used to support people who are having difficulties moving through transition phases in their lives or who have difficulties planning for the future.

This point is the front *mu* point of the Spleen and can be used to harmonise the relationship between the Spleen and Liver.

Liver 14 *Qi Men*, Gate of Hope: Liver front *mu* point, Exit point, meeting point of Spleen and Liver

Needle depth 0.3–0.5 cun; *moxa cones 3–7*

Qi Men was a title for the commander of the Royal Guard (Hicks, 1999, p. 49). This is a reference to the Liver's role as the holder of 'general of the armed forces' in *Su Wen* Chapter 8 (Larre and Rochat de la Vallée, 1992b, p. 151). The Liver's responsibility for the 'conception of plans' in the same passage is also indicated in the name of this point.

This is an important point on the Liver channel for treating both the mind and spirit. Like Liv 13, it is located close to the Liver Organ itself. It can be used if people's Liver *qi* is not moving freely, causing them to have difficulty asserting themselves or attempting to initiate change. This can lead to a lack of creativity and a tendency for people to lack a clear vision of their future. People need hope in order to face the future and this is often what they lack when the Liver is suffering. This lack of any enthusiasm for the future is a hallmark of depression that originates in the Liver. There are no Windows of the Sky on the Liver channel but this point has the ability to bring light and hope to a person who is gloomy and depressed and whose horizons have become limited.

It is the Exit point on the Liver channel, linking the channel to the Lung channel at Lu 1.

Bladder 18 *Gan Shu*: Liver back *shu* point

Needle depth 0.5–0.7 cun; *moxa cones 7–15*

Like all the other back *shu* points, this point is frequently used, especially to tonify the Liver. Its direct effect on the Liver Organ can help a person physically, mentally and spiritually.

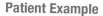

Patient Example

A patient in her late thirties had a long history of heroin, methadone and cannabis abuse, although she held an important post in a publishing company. She was very successful in her work but her personal life and view of her future were bleak. She was assertive at work and in contrast almost completely unassertive in her personal relationships. Treatment took place over a considerable period of time and there were no startling breakthroughs at any stage. She was a Fire CF but treatment on her Wood was crucial to her recovery. 'Gate of Hope' was used several times, after which she always reported a lifting in spirits and on two occasions expressed a greater determination and motivation to change.

Bladder 47 *Hun Men*, Gate of the *Hun*

Needle depth 0.3–0.5 cun; *moxa cones 3–7*
The *hun* are said to come and go when a person sleeps. The *men*, which indicates a large gate, helps govern this aspect of the *hun*. This point has a profound effect on a person's spirit and especially on the *hun*, the spiritual aspect of the Liver.

It can bring about a lifting of the spirits, increased clarity of mind and relief from oppression and constraint caused by unresolved feelings of anger. It will also 'root' the *hun* if a person is having difficulty making plans, cannot find a direction or purpose in life or is generally unsettled due to an imbalance in the Liver. This point can also enable a person to sleep soundly at night if an unrooted *hun* has caused a person to have vague feelings of fear at night or to sleep walk (Maciocia, 1989, p. 421).

Other points used to treat the Liver

Other points used to treat the Liver are *Ren* 4, *Du* 8, *Du* 20 and Sp 6.

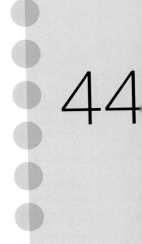

Ren and *Du* channel points

CHAPTER CONTENTS

Introduction

Practitioners of Five Element Constitutional Acupuncture use the *Ren* and *Du* channels for three main reasons:

- for their effect on the deep pathways of the channels through the *jiaohui*, which can be translated as 're-union' or 'intersection' points
- for their 'segmental' correspondence, for example, *Du* 8 is on the same level as the back *shu* point of the Liver and affects the Liver
- for their use in treating local problems in the channels

(These channels are sometimes translated as the Conception vessel (CV) and Governor vessel (GV). 'Conception' vessel is not, however, an accurate translation and Directing vessel is more accurate. Because of this mistranslation we have decided to use the Chinese names of *Ren* and *Du*.)

Ren points

The primary pathway of the *Ren* channel

The *Ren* channel begins on the perineum, rises up the midline over the abdomen, chest and throat and ends at the centre of the chin.

Ren 1 *Hui Yin*, Meeting of *Yin*: Entry point of *Ren mai*, *Du mai* and *Chong mai*, luo junction point of *Ren mai*

Needle depth 0.8–1.2 cun; no moxa

This point is an important focus in some Daoist meditation techniques. It is the *yin* extremity of the circuit of *qi* sometimes known as the 'small circulation' or the 'micro-cosmic' orbit. This circuit travels up the *Du* channel through *Du* 20 and down the *Ren* channel. *Ren* 1 is the most *yin* point on the body, lying in a dark and hidden location. *Du* 20, which lies opposite it on the head, at its uppermost pole, is the most *yang*. Because of its location, this point is underused. It is the meeting point of *yin qi* in the body. One of its alternative names is 'Seabed', which both alludes to its position at the bottom of the torso and also to its extreme *yin* nature (Hicks, 1999, p. 50).

This is a powerful point to invoke change when treatment on the 12 channels is failing to strengthen the patient. This point calms and anchors the spirit. It can be used to treat the spirit when people are struggling to cope or they have reached breaking point.

This is the Entry point for the *Ren mai* and is used when the practitioner is treating a *Ren/Du* block (see Chapter 33 for discussion of this treatment).

Ren 3 *Zhong Ji*, Utmost Middle: Bladder front *mu* point, meeting point of *Ren*, Spleen, Liver and Kidney

Needle depth 0.5–1.0 cun; moxa cones 5–15

In ancient texts about sexual cultivation, with which there is a good deal of overlap with Chinese medicine, the *zhong ji* is the name given to the centre of *qi* in this area. It is also an old name for the uterus (Lo, 2001, p. 45). This point is mainly used to treat both chronic and acute problems of the bladder. It is also a re-union point that connects to the Liver, Spleen and Kidney channels. It can be used to treat problems in the Lower Burner, especially when any of these three Organs are implicated.

Ren 4 *Guan Yuan*, Gate to the *Yuan Qi*: Small Intestine front *mu* point, meeting point of *Ren*, Spleen, Liver and Kidney

Needle depth 0.5–1.0 cun; *moxa cones 5–15*

This point is a gate to the *yuan qi*. It can therefore be used to enhance this fundamental form of *qi*. It affects the *qi* of the Kidneys (see Chapter 12, this volume, for discussion about the *qi* between the two Kidneys) and enhances the lower *dan tian*, which is also referred to as the cinnabar field. Cinnabar is a mineral thought to have a near perfect balance of *yin* and *yang*. It was highly prized by Daoist alchemists. *Ren* 4, 5 and 6 are all points in the 'cinnabar field'. By focusing on this area practitioners of *qi gong* transform, root and store *yuan qi*. (For more about the cinnabar field, see Lade, 1989, p. 255.)

Moxibustion is often used on this point if the uterus is cold and a woman is experiencing menstrual or fertility problems. It is sometimes used for male impotence or problems with the sperm. It can also be tonified to 'anchor' the spirit if a patient is anxious or restless. It is also a re-union point of the Liver, Spleen and Kidney channels, so it is used to affect these Organs, especially when they are causing symptoms in the Lower Burner.

Ren 5 *Shi Men*, Stone Gate: Triple Burner front *mu* point

Needle depth 0.5–1.0 cun; *moxa cones 5–15*
The name *Shi Men* translates as a 'stone woman', which is a barren woman. Some texts warn practitioners that needling this point can make a woman infertile.

This is the front *mu* or alarm point of the Triple Burner and it is used to affect the *qi* of the Triple Burner. Like *Ren* 4, it is also a part of the cinnabar field. Because of its location and its link with the Triple Burner, it particularly affects the *yuan qi*. Like *Ren* 4, this is a 'gate' of *qi* and it is a powerful point for reviving a person who has become depleted in vitality of body and/or spirit. Moxibustion is commonly used if this area is cold.

Ren 6 *Qi Hai*, Sea of *Qi*

Needle depth 0.5–1.0 cun; *moxa cones 5–15*

This point is a major energy centre and like *Ren* 4 and 5 it affects the lower *dan tian* and the cinnabar field. This is one of the most powerful points for affecting the Kidney *qi* and thereby a person's deepest vitality. Moxibustion is commonly used if this area is cold.

Ren 7 *Yin Jiao*, *Yin* Crossing

Needle depth 0.5–1.0 cun; *moxa cones 5–15*

This is a re-union point for the Triple Burner, Pericardium and Kidney. It is occasionally used to treat problems due to imbalances in temperature or fluid in the Lower Burner. It is a less commonly used point for treating the lower *dan tian* than the above points.

Ren 8 *Shen Que*, Spirit Palace Gate

Needle forbidden; moxa cones 3–30

This point lies on the navel and it is here that *qi* enters an embryo. This point was consequently regarded as a vital gate into the body. Some early Daoists considered the navel to be the seat of the *Tai yi*, the Supreme Unity; thus, this point has a strong connection to the spirit. This is a powerful point for building up a patient who is exhausted and worn out at a deep level and lacks vitality in the spirit. Only moxibustion can be used on this point and the moxa is placed on a bed of salt.

Ren 9 *Shui Fen*, Water Division

Needle depth 0.5–1.0 cun; *moxa cones 5–15*

As the name suggests, this point is used to regulate fluids in the Lower and Middle Burners.

Ren 10 *Xia Wan*, Lower Epigastrium: meeting point of *Ren* and Spleen

Needle depth 0.5–1.0 cun; *moxa cones 5–15*

Through its meeting with the Spleen channel this point is sometimes used to help the Spleen, especially if the person is experiencing problems in the Middle Burner.

Ren 12 *Zhong Wan*, Middle of the Epigastrium: Stomach front *mu* point, special point for *yang* Organs, Middle Burner front *mu* point

Needle depth 0.5–1.2 cun*; moxa cones 5–15*

An alternative name for this point is *Tai Cang*, Supreme Granary, which refers to its prime role of affecting the Stomach. This point is commonly used in addition to command points when treating the Stomach channel. It can have a profound effect on the stomach if a person feels nauseous.

Ren 14 *Ju Que*, Greatest Palace Gate: Heart front *mu* point

Needle depth 0.3–0.8 cun*; moxa cones 5–15*

This is the palace of the emperor, which is the Heart. It is the front *mu* or alarm point of the Heart and it affects the Heart directly, as it is on its deep pathway. It is one of the most commonly used points to treat the Heart spirit or *shen*. It is often tonified when a person is depleted and lacking in spirit. Using this point can sometimes have an immediate effect on raising people's spirits when they are feeling miserable or joyless. It can also be sedated to calm people who feel out of control and agitated in their spirits.

Ren 15 *Jiu Wei*, Dove Tail: *luo* junction point of *Ren mai*, *yuan* source point of five *yin* Organs, point to release Internal Dragons

Needle depth 0.3–0.5 cun*; moxa cones 3–5*

The name obviously refers to its physical location. It is located at the end of the xiphoid process of the sternum, which apparently looks like a turtle dove. An alternative name is *Shen Fu*, Spirit Storehouse. This is the front *mu* point for the Pericardium and it is frequently tender on palpation. It is commonly used to treat the Pericardium, and is used in much the same way as *Ren* 14 is used to treat the Heart. These two points can sometimes be used in combination when the spirit of both the Heart and the Heart-Protector are in need of support.

This point (or to be precise, an extra point lying very slightly below it) is one of the points used when releasing the Internal Dragons.

Ren 16 *Zhong Ting*, Middle Hall

Needle depth 0.3–0.5 cun*; moxa cones 3–5*

Although not commonly used, this point can be used to treat the Heart and Pericardium, particularly when they are severely depleted.

Ren 17 *Tan Zhong*, Middle of the Chest: Pericardium and Upper Burner front *mu* point, special point for *qi*, point of sea of *qi*

Needle depth 0.3–0.5 cun*; moxa cones 3–5*

Tan Zhong was an early name for the Pericardium and this point can be used to treat the Pericardium as well as the other Organs of the Upper Burner. Another name for this point is *Shang Qi Hai*, the Upper Sea of *qi*. It is the front *mu* point of the Upper Burner and this name reflects its importance in regulating the *qi* of this area. This point is commonly used with moxibustion to warm the Organs of the Upper Burner when they are deficient and cold.

Ren 20 *Hua Gai*, Flower Covering

Needle depth 0.3–0.5 cun*; moxa cones 3–5*

Hua Gai was the name of the canopy over the Emperor's carriage. The Lungs can be compared to a canopy over the Heart, which is the emperor of the body. This point is seldom used but can be effective in treating disorders affecting the upper part of the Lungs.

Ren 22 *Tian Tu*, Heavenly Chimney: Window of the Sky

Needle depth 0.5–1.0 cun*; moxa cones 3–7*

This is a Window of the Sky. This point is less commonly used than the Windows of the Sky situated on the main channels. It can be used to augment treatment on the CF or other Elements, especially when the throat or speech is affected causing a person to have difficulty communicating with others. It is sometimes treated in combination with *Du* 16, the Window of the Sky on the *Du* channel.

Ren 24 *Cheng Jian*, Receiving Fluid: Exit point

Needle depth 0.2–0.3 cun*; moxa cones 3–7*

This is the Exit point of the *Ren* channel and it can be used to clear an Entry–Exit block between the *Ren* and *Du* channels.

Du points

The primary pathway of the *Du* channel

The *Du* channel begins at the base of the spine, travels up the midline of the back to the nape of the neck, over the top of the head, down the forehead and nose, over the upper lip and ends on the upper gum.

Du 1 *Chang Qiang*, Long Strength: Entry point, *luo* junction point of *Du*

Needle depth 0.5–1.0 cun; moxa cones 5–15

This point is underused point owing to its location. It is the Entry point of the *Du mai* and is used when there is an Entry–Exit block between the *Ren* and *Du* channels. It can be used to strengthen the *Du* channel and the spine. Zhou Mei-sheng said of this point that, 'This channel together with the backbone forms a strong pillar of the human body and manifests stoutness of the Kidney *qi*' (quoted in Hicks, 1999, p. 54).

Du 4 *Ming Men*, Gate of Life

Needle depth 0.3–0.8 cun; moxa cones 5–15

This is a very important point due to its location directly over the *ming men* or 'space between the two Kidneys'. This is where the Kidney essence or *jing* is stored and it is also the centre of the vital warmth of the body. It is located on the same level as the inner and outer back *shu* points of the Kidneys.

The name *ming men* can be translated as the 'gate of life' or 'gate of destiny'. If this gate is closed, people can have difficulty fulfilling their destiny as they will not have access to their *jing* or essence. This point is especially indicated to warm, tonify and revitalise the Kidney *qi* if it is cold and depleted. It can be used if people are severely lacking in physical vitality and/or vitality in their spirit. An alternative name is *Jing Gong*, or Palace of the *Jing*. Moxibustion is commonly used when a person is cold but care should be taken not to moxa this point if a person is hot as they can become overheated. It is also used for local problems in the back.

Du 8 *Jin Suo*, Contracted Tendon

Needle depth 0.3–0.8 cun; moxa cones 3–5

This point is located in the area of the back *shu* point of the Liver. It is used to assist the Liver and Gall Bladder in their role of regulating the tendons and muscles of the body. As the name indicates, the point is most commonly sedated rather than tonified in order to relax contraction and spasm of the musculature, especially when the muscles of the back are tense.

Du 10 *Ling Tai*, Spirit Tower

Needle depth 0.3–0.8 cun; moxa cones 3–5

Ling Tai was a name used for the Heart in some early Daoist texts. The emperor Wen Wang had a tall tower built, which he called *ling tai*, from which he could survey his realm and subjects (Hicks, 1999, p. 55). This point is situated just below the back *shu* point of the Heart. It strengthens people's spirit at a deep level. It can be used after patients have already made some progress with treatment and it can awaken the spirit when a patient needs to take stock and prepare for the next stage of their growth and development.

Du 11 *Shen Dao*, Spirit Path

Needle depth 0.3–0.8 cun; moxa cones 3–5

This point is situated on the same level as the back *shu* points of the Heart. It is often used to strengthen the person's spirit. It can be used with *Du* 10 because, once the spirit has been awakened, it then needs to move forward along its path. These points can together have a profound effect on a person's spiritual development. It is interesting to note that like the Kidney points at the same level on the front of the body (Kid 24 and 25), a point that primarily affects the *ling* is followed by a point that nourishes the *shen*.

Du 12 *Shen Zhu*, Body Pillar

Needle depth 0.3–0.8 cun; moxa cones 5–30

This point is situated between the back *shu* points of the Lungs. It is mainly used to support treatment on the Lungs. The name refers to the spine and the *Du mai* and the point is also used to benefit the upper spine and back. Some practitioners also use this point to support a patient who has 'collapsed' either in their body or spirit.

Du 13 *Tao Dao*, Kiln Path

Needle depth 0.3–0.8 cun; *moxa cones 3–7*

This point is mainly used for local problems although Zhou Mei-sheng wrote, 'The point can give comfort, make one happy and contented' (quoted in Hicks, 1999, p. 56).

Du 14 *Da Zhui*, Great Hammer

Needle depth 0.3–0.8 cun; *moxa cones 5–15*

This powerful point is used to shake up and re-invigorate a person's *qi*, especially if other points are failing to generate change in a person. Being the 'influential point of *yang*', with connections to all the *yang* channels, it tonifies the *yang qi* and therefore the warmth and vitality of the person.

Du 16 *Feng Fu*, Wind Treasury: Window of the Sky, point of Sea of Marrow

Needle depth 0.3–0.7 cun; *moxa cones 5–30*

This point is less commonly used than the Windows situated on the main channels. It can, however, be an important point because this area is easily blocked or closed off by tense neck muscles and poor posture caused by stress. Using this point can clear the head, allowing a person to see and hear more clearly and have greater perspective on possibilities for their future. It can also encourage a better connection and integration of the body with the mind and spirit.

Du 19 *Hou Ding*, Posterior Summit: point of Sea of Marrow

Needle depth 0.3–0.5 cun; *moxa cones 3–7*

This point is commonly sedated in conjunction with *Du* 20. It calms the mind and spirit and is especially used in acute situations such as when a patient is severely agitated and disturbed. In this case it soothes and settles the mind. It is sometimes used to calm a patient who is agitated, before the practitioner tonifies the underlying deficiency.

Du 20 *Bai Hui*, One Hundred Meetings: meeting point of all *yang* channels, point of Sea of Marrow, point to release External Dragons

Needle depth 0.3–0.5 cun; *moxa cones 3–7*

The Daoist text, 'Daoist Storehouse', says that the head is the meeting place of the hundred spirits (College of Traditional Acupuncture, 2000). This point sits at the very top of the head, in a large soft fontanelle. It was therefore perceived as the point where the influences of Heaven most easily entered the body. It is commonly used with *Du* 19 (see above).

This point also connects with the deep pathway of the Liver. It can be used to treat the spirit, especially when the Liver is affected. In this case the patient may be agitated due to anger or frustration or lacking vitality of the spirit due to deficiency. It can also be used to lift the spirits when a patient is depressed or dejected.

This point is used to release the External Dragons.

Du 24 *Shen Ting*, Spirit Courtyard

Needle depth 0.3–0.5 cun; *moxa cones 3–5*

Ting or courtyard refers to the upper *dan tian* (Bertschinger, 1991, p. 142). This point is used to calm the mind and spirit, in much the same way as *Du* 19 and 20. It is sometimes used in conjunction with these points and also with *Yin Tang* or Seal Hall, which is situated between the eyebrows. (*Yin tang* is on the line of the *Du* channel but is not one of its points. It is a very calming and relaxing point.)

Du 26 *Ren Zhong*, Middle of the Man: Exit point

Needle depth 0.3–0.5 cun; *no moxa*

This point lies in the groove below the nose. The name of this point arises because the nose receives 'the five *qi* from the Heaven' and the mouth 'receives the five *qi* from the earth' (Hicks, 1999, p. 57). Man stands between Heaven and earth and hence this point is 'the middle of the man'. This point is effective when used to calm a patient whose mind and spirit are agitated. It can also restore consciousness. The unconsciousness can arise either from a physical cause such as concussion, seizure or fainting or in the mind and spirit if the *shen* is disturbed or obstructed. In the *Ode of Xi-hong* it says, 'The ability of *Ren Zhong* to treat mania disorder is supreme' (quoted in Deadman *et al.*, 1998, p. 560).

Du 28 *Yin Jiao*, Mouth Crossing

Needle depth 0.1–0.2 cun; *no moxa*

This is the exit point on the *Du mai* and is used when clearing an Entry–Exit block between the *Ren* and *Du* channels.

Section 7

Treatment

Treatment planning

CHAPTER CONTENTS

Introduction

Having taken the patient's case history and made a diagnosis, the practitioner is now ready to plan the treatment. The first section describes the three main stages of treatment planning. The second section takes this to a greater depth and describes some guidelines for treatment planning. The third section then describes how to deal with patients who are not progressing sufficiently.

The three main stages of treatment planning

These are:

1 summarising the diagnosis
2 forming an overall treatment strategy
3 planning the individual treatments

Summarising the diagnosis

When making the diagnosis the practitioner picks out the significant findings from the case history and answers some basic questions such as:

- What is the patient's CF?
- Which other Elements are in distress?
- Are there any important blocks to treatment?
- What is the primary level of body, mind or spirit?

The case history should be detailed and if possible written in the patient's own words. It should give the specifics of the patient's complaint(s) and also information about the main systems such as sleep, appetite, bowels, etc. It should additionally contain details of the patient's health, personal and family history, relationships and present situation as well as a physical examination (see Chapter 24; see also checklist for a traditional diagnosis in Appendix F).

At this stage of treatment planning it is useful to have a summary of the answers to the questions listed above. An example of this appears below. Variations in the headings may occur, but most of these headings are essential. The example below is written in some depth and many practitioners will write this in a more shorthand form.

Diagnosis Sheet

Name: Josephine Bloggs, Age 46

Patient's main complaint: Poor sleep, anxiety, lack of confidence.

Secondary complaints: Headaches prior to periods. Occasional backache.

CF: Fire. Josephine looks lack of red beside her eyes. Although she appeared to enjoy interacting with me she only stayed animated if I kept contact with her. The rest of the time she seemed to drop into a flat and sad state with a joyless voice tone. Occasionally a brilliant smile would fleetingly light up her whole face, but it would quickly fade and the rest of the time she found it hard to raise a smile. When carrying out the physical examination I smelt a scorched odour.

Pulses: Her third position and her Ht and SI pulses were very deficient.

Left		Right	
SI −2	Ht −2	Lu −1	LI −1
GB +½	Liv +½	Sp −1	St −1
Bl −2	Kid −2	PC −2	TB −2

Next most likely CF: Wood. She has a green colour around her mouth. At times she can seem overly assertive. At other times her ability to assert herself seems normal. She expresses a lot of frustration about her personal life. Wood may need additional help later on in treatment. Her Liv and GB pulses felt slightly full.

Other Elements: Earth. She took sympathy well and I could not see any yellow colour or hear any singing. Water. She gets anxious but this seems more to do with her Heart. She showed appropriate fear when asked about the future. No blue colour. Metal. She seemed to take in respect well. Could go back and do more tests on Metal.

Blocks:

H–W: No reason to suspect.

AE: Possible, need to test.

Possession: *Internal:* Possible, eyes glazed over and has many 'spooky dreams' *External:* Unlikely

Entry–Exit: Possibly between Wood and Metal, re-evaluate after first few treatments.

Level

Body: No apparent reason to think so. Problems seem to arise from internal rather than external or miscellaneous causes.

Mind: Josephine often does not think clearly, but there are many times in her work and when chatting in the treatment room where her mind works well.

Spirit: Josephine has a worn, hurt look, deep in her eyes. It is not always there, but shows when she is unattended and I look back. Primary level is spirit.

Physical examination: Upper and Lower Burners are cold. Front *mu* point for Heart – *Ren* 14 – is tender. Akabane: Heart 15/7; Spleen 5/10.

Any uncertainty about the diagnosis should be expressed on this sheet. For example, if practitioners can't decide between two CFs, then they may state which one it is *more* likely to be and give a case for both. Indeed, in the full text of the case history, any information gained from each Element should be noted. This may include colour, sound, emotion, odour, 'golden keys' or any other secondary diagnostic information.

Forming an overall treatment strategy

When the summary of the diagnosis is complete, the practitioner can plan the treatment strategy. The diagnosis indicates the general direction of treatment. The treatment strategy then specifies the overall way that the treatments might be carried out.

Planning a treatment strategy

Planning an effective treatment strategy involves discussion of these questions:

1 Which treatment principles to use and order of priority?

2 What are the appropriate points to use?

3 What is the appropriate number of points to use?

4 Is moxa appropriate? If so, how much, and on which points?

5 Might there be any patient variations? For example, the patient may be particularly irritable and have other pre-menstrual signs prior to her period.

6 Are there lifestyle changes that the patient needs to make?

7 What change might the practitioner expect to see when the patient gets better?

Treatment principles

Treatment principles describe the treatment that will be carried out and help the practitioner to choose which points to use. The practitioner formulates the treatment principles from the areas listed on the diagnosis sheet and the case history. Each treatment principle will be different according to the patients' diagnoses. Here are some examples:

1 strengthen and warm the Earth CF

2 balance Husband–Wife imbalance

3 remove Aggressive Energy

4 strengthen Metal CF at the level of the Spirit

Below is an example of a treatment strategy made by Josephine's practitioner before her treatment began. Once the main treatment principles have been formed, they should also be prioritised and listed in the order that the treatment might be carried out.

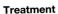

Treatment Strategy for Josephine
Treatment principles and order of priority

- Release the Internal Dragons.
- Check for Aggressive Energy.
- Balance Akabane.
- Strengthen and warm Fire CF at the spirit level.
- Treat Wood Element if necessary.

Examples of appropriate points to use

1. **Release Internal Dragons:** Point below *Ren* 15, St 25, St 32, St 41
2. **Clear Aggressive Energy:** Bl 13, 14, 18, 20 and 23
3. **Balance Akabane:** Ht 5 Right side
4. **Warm Fire CF:** Examples could be TB 4 and PC 7, TB 3 and PC 9, TB 5 and PC 6, Bl 14 and 22 with moxa and needle. If need to treat Heart and Small Intestine side of Fire use SI 4 and Ht 7, SI 3 and Ht 9, SI 5 and Ht 8, Bl 27 and 15, etc. Later spirit points such as Bl 43, *Ren* 15, PC 2, etc. or Ht 1, SI 11, *Ren* 14, etc., might be included.
5. **Treat Wood:** Liv 3, GB 40 and other points on the Wood channels.

Appropriate number of points to use

Small number of points as treatment is directed to spirit level.

Moxa, if appropriate how much, and on which points?

Patient feels the cold and upper and lower *jiao* are cold so moxa is appropriate. Use on points of Fire Element.

Patient variations

May need to treat her Wood Element prior to her period.

Lifestyle changes that the patient may need to make

Suggest she finishes working and has some quiet time before going to bed in order to help sleep. Suggest she eats a nourishing diet and not on the run.

How to assess if the patient is improving

The deep look of hurt in her eyes will be lessened. She will be able to laugh more. She will be able to consider entering a relationship. Her sleep will be better. Her periods will be heavier. She will be calmer and less anxious. Her pulses will become stronger and more settled.

Planning the individual treatments

Having created a treatment strategy, practitioners can then plan what they will do on the actual day of treatment.

Planning the first treatment

The first treatment is different from subsequent treatments. This is because the practitioner is not yet certain about the diagnosis and is still at the stage of testing the CF. Some blocks may also need to be cleared before treatment can progress.

Planning subsequent treatments

At the start of all subsequent treatments practitioners obtain feedback from patients about their progress. Based on this feedback, the practitioner then plans the next treatment. According to the patient's progress the treatment principles may be reassessed and changed. Alternatively they may be kept the same. The skill of taking feedback and assessing the patient's response to an individual treatment is a crucial part of the planning process. Failure to do this can result in irrelevant and ineffective treatments. The more carefully the options are considered, the quicker the practitioner's experience accumulates. This process also enables practitioners to take a fresh approach to every treatment and ensures that they don't become stale or routine after seeing a patient over a period of time. Once the CF has been established the Five Element Constitutional Acupuncturist may change the points used at the treatment. These will vary according to the state of the patient.

Some guidelines for treatment planning

When deciding which treatment to carry out, the practitioner follows various guidelines. Some of these may be irrelevant for a particular treatment, but the practitioner should consider them all and be guided by them in the right circumstances. Some different areas that are considered are:

1. clearing blocks first
2. treating the CF
3. correcting left/right imbalances (Akabane)
4. how many points to use in one treatment
5. the frequency of treatment
6. if treatment is not sufficiently effective, what are the possibilities?
7. responding to a patient's lack of progress
8. prognosis

Clearing blocks first

The process of clearing and strengthening

If any of the four blocks to treatment discussed in Chapters 29–33 are present, they must be cleared first. Without clearing one or more of the four blocks first, the normal strengthening or balancing treatments are less likely to be effective. The 'blocks' are:

- Possession
- Aggressive Energy
- Husband–Wife imbalance
- Entry–Exit blocks

The process for clearing a block is given in the chapters on blocks to treatment (Chapters 29–33, this volume).

If more than one block is present, then they should be cleared in the order listed above. The order of priority implies that some blocks are more pervasive than others. For example, it may be difficult to clear Aggressive Energy if the patient is possessed.

Do the blocks get cleared in one treatment?

A block is frequently cleared in a single treatment. On the other hand some blocks such as a Husband–Wife imbalance can take more than one treatment to resolve completely.

Sometimes blocks can return after they have been cleared and the practitioner should then be prepared to repeat the treatment. At the same time, the practitioner needs to attempt to understand why the block has recurred. For example, a block between Liv 14 and Lu 1 may reappear for a number of different reasons. One reason may be a serious condition, such as a tumour, existing in the lungs. Alternatively it may be because a person frequently becomes overwhelmed by resentment because of an ongoing life situation.

The reappearance of a block may raise further questions about the patient's state of health. In the case of possession, one treatment is often sufficient, but there are cases where the treatment is repeated to very good effect. Patients whose spirit is weak and who are still in the situation that caused the possession can become possessed again. If this occurs, the treatment is repeated. When the patient is clear again, there is a new urgency to begin the strengthening process to avoid a further regression.

Clearing blocks during ongoing treatment

Normally practitioners clear any blocks they think are present before moving on to treating the patient's

CF. There are two situations, however, when a block may need to be treated at a later stage in the patient's treatment.

Firstly, the block may have been present when treatment commenced, but was not apparent to the practitioner. It may only emerge later that this block is preventing the treatment from progressing at its normal rate. Clearing the block then allows treatment to progress normally.

Secondly, but less commonly, a block may arise after treatment has begun. In this case it is usually because the patient's physical or psychological health has deteriorated significantly. For example, if the patient contracts a major illness it may be worth re-testing for Aggressive Energy. If the patient becomes extremely psychologically traumatised, possession should at least be considered. A Husband–Wife imbalance may arise if the patient becomes very distressed, especially if it is concerning an intimate relationship. Husband–Wife imbalances may also arise if the patient's health deteriorates to such an extent that their grip on life itself is starting to loosen.

Entry–Exit blocks are the exception to this rule. They are often not apparent at the beginning of treatment and become evident as treatment progresses. This sometimes occurs when a patient has previously been making good progress. As extra *qi* is generated from treatment an Entry or Exit connection that was previously partially blocked can become seriously blocked because a greater amount of *qi* is travelling through it. In this case the treatment may stop working until the block has been cleared.

Correcting left/right imbalances

If a patient has an imbalance between the channel on the left and right sides (an Akabane imbalance), this can be corrected by treating the side of the patient that is the weakest. This imbalance is found by heating the nail points of the channels. Its presence is indicated when there is a disparity between the time it takes to warm the nail point on one side as opposed to the other. For example, if the number of passes on the Spleen nail points is 10 on the left and 5 on the right, then the left side is weaker. This is notated as 10/5. To treat the above imbalance, the Spleen *luo* junction point (Sp 4) is tonified on the left side. The test is then carried out again and the practitioner usually finds that the Akabane has become balanced. If it is still imbalanced then the *yuan* source point of the affected side can also be treated. (See Chapter 28, this volume, for more about the Akabane test.)

If the patient has a number of Akabane imbalances, then the first one to be treated should be the one associated with the CF if it is imbalanced. This will often balance the other left/right imbalances. If the other channels remain imbalanced then the practitioner should treat the first channel along the *sheng* cycle.

This may then balance the following channels. It is not always necessary to treat these left/right imbalances as they will often automatically balance when the CF is treated.

Treating the CF

The main priority

Once blocks are cleared, the practitioner's main priority is to treat the CF (see Chapters 29–33 for the needle techniques used). Because of the extremely chronic and fundamental nature of the CF, it is inevitably out of harmony with the other Elements. By treating it the practitioner is attempting to bring it into greater harmony with the other Elements.

Most frequently the CF Element is tonified. The pulses determine the practitioner's choice of needle technique. Sometimes the Wood Element and occasionally the Earth Element require sedation. The choice of points is somewhat different whether tonifying and sedating, so they will be dealt with separately.[1]

First, however, the notion of 'testing the CF' will be considered.

Testing and verifying the CF

When treating the CF, the first few treatments are primarily concerned with testing the accuracy of the diagnosis. It is important for the practitioner to find and treat the CF, as it is the backbone of treatment and it nourishes the root cause of the patient's condition. Whatever the diagnosis, based on colour, sound, emotion and odour, it is the response of the

patient that provides the ultimate verification. The key evidence for a correct CF is whether:

1 The patient changes in mind and spirit. This is usually manifested by patients expressing that they feel 'better in themselves'.

2 The pulses become more harmonious and the overall strength and quality of all pulse positions improves.

3 The practitioner perceives improvement in the person's signs such as colour, sound, emotion and odour or the sparkle in the eyes.

4 The patient's complaints improve.

The CF pulse change

Often the confirmation of the CF comes during the treatment when the pulses change and come into greater harmony. Harmony means that the pulses become more similar and even. This kind of overall improvement in the pulses, from treating one Element, is sometimes known as a 'CF pulse change'. It is interpreted as 'all the Officials or Organs working together' and is a good indication that what has been treated is the CF. It is unnecessary for the practitioner to feel an increase in the strength of the Organ that has been treated.

Five Element Constitutional Acupuncturists learn to assess the effectiveness of the treatment during the session. They will evaluate the change to the overall balance and harmony amongst the pulses. If the first needle achieves a striking balance, it might be wise to stop, as balance is often more important than strengthening.

How much the pulses change during a treatment is dependent on a number of issues including the nature of the patient's complaint and how ill the patient is to begin with. Some patients have more obvious pulse changes than others. With experience the practitioner becomes more adept at knowing what is a reasonable expectation of change for a particular patient, although even with experience this can still be a difficult issue.

Tonifying

When tonifying the patient's *qi*, the practitioner uses the needle technique described in Chapter 34, this volume. Most tonification takes a few seconds to carry out as the needles are not retained. When a patient is agitated the needles may be retained for longer, however, as retention is likely to have a more calming effect.

---

[1] This is one area where the shortage of Five Element theory leads to confusion. TCM theory helps to explain the difference between fullness and deficiency. This is explained further in the final chapter in this book (Chapter 48) on integration of TCM and Five Element theory. For example, the main reason the Wood and Earth Elements are sedated is that Liver *qi* stagnation and Damp (a pathogenic factor not discussed in Five Element theory) are present. This creates a full condition that requires elimination.

When the CF is being tested the best points to use first are the source points. In the example above, the practitioner thinks that the CF is Fire but knows it could be Wood. The points the Five Element Constitutional Acupuncturist uses at the first treatment will probably be the source points of Fire. In this case a 'CF treatment' would consist of needling, in sequence, TB 4 and PC 7 or SI 4 and Ht 7 or possibly all of these points (see the section 'The two sides of Fire' below).

Once the source points have been used, there are a number of other points on the channel of the CF Element that might be considered. These could be:

- tonification points
- junction points
- horary points
- Element points
- back *shu* points
- points appropriate to the level, for example, Windows of the Sky, outer back *shu* points or spirit points

Sedating

When sedating the patient's *qi*, the principle is much the same as when tonifying. Sedation needle technique is described in Chapter 34.

The practitioner needs to be aware that at some stage later in treatment it may become appropriate to change to tonifying rather than sedating the patient's CF. The key for the practitioner lies in knowing when to change. The reverse, changing from tonifying to sedating, is not something that occurs in longer-term treatment. It could, however, happen as a one-off situation in a treatment, or there may be a period during the switch from sedating to tonifying where the practitioner is unsure about the appropriate needle technique.

Although most patients with full pulses have underlying deficiency, there are a few patients who always need to have their *qi* sedated. These are frequently Wood CFs. Although some Wood CFs start treatment with a full Liver, its underlying deficiency may only become apparent later on. For other patients the Liver always remains full.

As with tonification technique, source points are often the first points the practitioner uses when sedating the patient's *qi*. Other points that might be used could be:

- sedation points
- junction points
- back *shu* points
- Element points
- points appropriate to the level, such as spirit level points

Using body and command points together

Often body points and command points are used in the same treatment. In this case the same needle technique is employed for both sets of points. For example, if the Wood pulse is full and the *yuan* source points, Liv 3 and GB 40, are being sedated, then the body points Liv 14 and GB 24 would also be sedated if used in that treatment. If, on the other hand, the Metal pulses are deficient and LI 11 and Lu 9 are used as tonification points, then if the back *shu* points, Bl 25 and Bl 13, were also used they would also be tonified.

The two sides of Fire

The Wood, Earth, Metal and Water Elements each have two Organs connected with them – a *yin* Organ and a *yang* Organ. The Fire Element has four – two *yin* and two *yang* Organs. Five Element Constitutional Acupuncturists usually consider that there are 'two sides of Fire'. Some patients have their CF on the Pericardium and Triple Burner side of Fire, while others have their CF on the Small Intestine and Heart side. When testing for the CF, the practitioner assumes that the patient's CF lies in one pair or the other. The testing process is therefore slightly more complex than for the other four Elements.

When testing the CF on a patient diagnosed as a Fire CF, the Five Element Constitutional Acupuncturist usually starts by testing the Pericardium and Triple Burner side of Fire. If the treatment creates changes similar to those described in the section above, 'Testing and verifying the CF', the practitioner will carry out no further treatment. If, however, this creates little or no change in the patient or the pulses, then the practitioner may decide to also treat the Heart and Small Intestine. She or he will then assess which side of Fire creates the best change and continue treating these Organs during further treatments.

Having treated many Fire CFs, practitioners become more able to determine which side of Fire they should focus treatment on before treating the patient. They often do this by paying attention to the patient's characteristics or from the pulses. If the pulses of one pairing in the Fire Element are significantly weaker than the other, then it is a good, but not conclusive, indication that the key Organs are in that pair. The issue remains, however, that colour, sound, emotion and odour may lead practitioners to Fire, but it does not tell them which Organs. (See Chapter 12, this volume, on the Organs of the Fire Element.)

Occasionally a patient responds well to treatment on two of the Organs of Fire other than the paired Organs. This is most frequently the Heart and the Pericardium, but it can be other combinations. If this is the case the practitioner should continue treatment on these two Organs but bear in mind that this may change. In the case of, for instance, the Heart and Pericardium, the Heart may have been traumatised and only need temporary help until it is strong enough to allow the Pericardium to keep it well protected.

Moving from 'testing the CF' to 'treating the CF'

There is no set rule as to how long it takes practitioners to confirm the diagnosis of their patient's CF. Sometimes the practitioner knows that the correct CF has been treated after only one treatment. For example, greater harmony between the pulses may be felt at the time of treatment. The patient may also change in other ways, such as in the facial colour, emotional state or sparkle in the eyes. The patient may then return for the next treatment feeling better in her or himself and saying that some symptoms have improved. This feedback is simple and straightforward. The practitioner will now continue and move from testing to treating the CF.

Often treatment is not so straightforward, however. For example, the practitioner may notice some *slight* improvement in the pulses or patient, and think it *may* be the CF but not be sure. In this case more than one treatment needs to be carried out before the practitioner can say with absolute certainty that treatment is being given on the patient's CF.

In the first few treatments it is best for practitioners to only treat points connected to what they think is the CF and to avoid treating other Elements. This ensures that the patient's feedback is clear, and has only come about from changes to the CF Element.

How long should the practitioner remain 'testing' the CF

It is usually best to treat an Element at least three times before deciding to abandon it. Usually after this time practitioners are either sure that the treatment is being carried out on the CF or not. They can then move from 'testing' to 'treating the CF' or move to testing another CF.

Occasionally, good results arise from treating an Element and it *appears* to be the patient's CF. Later, however, this 'runs out' and no longer has its initial beneficial effect. This may either be due to a block such as an Entry–Exit block arising or because that Element is significantly imbalanced but it is not the CF. In this situation the practitioner needs to go back and reassess which Element needs to be treated. As Entry–Exit blocks are most commonly found preceding the CF it is sometimes best for the practitioner to treat this before giving up on the diagnosis. If this doesn't have a beneficial effect, the practitioner may move on to testing another Element.

Some practitioners tend to switch their CF diagnosis too early. Some tend to persist stubbornly with an Element when it is patently not yielding sufficient change. The art lies in finding a middle way between these extremes.

How many points to use in one treatment?

Treatments should be kept simple

In general Five Element Constitutional Acupuncturists keep treatments simple and use only a small number of points. For example, when testing the CF in the first few treatments, it is wise to stay with treating only the *yuan* source points or the other points listed in the sections on tonification or sedation.

When the patient is progressing and the CF is established, the back *shu* points might be used in conjunction with the source points. This is a stronger treatment, but it is still simple. If, on the other hand, the practitioner decides to focus treatment on the patient's spirit, then possibly the Windows of the Sky, for example, PC 1 (Heavenly Pond) and TB 16 (Heavenly Window), might be used, again perhaps in conjunction with the source points or other command points.

It is not possible to specify the number of points to use per treatment, but one or two on each channel is normal. Each point is usually treated bilaterally. It is also usual practice for the practitioner to treat each pair of Organs in an Element unless the practitioner detects a marked difference in the pulse response to the Organs. For example, a Water CF will usually respond well to both the Kidneys and Bladder being treated. If, however, treatment using points on the Kidney channel has a beneficial effect on the pulses whereas points on the Bladder have little or no effect, then the practitioner might decide to only treat the Kidneys.

Pulse changes

The practitioner must monitor the pulse changes achieved during a treatment. Although there is no scale to measure the degree of harmonisation, if a good degree of change is achieved, then it is wise to stop. Even if further points had been planned, it is often best to finish if the pulses have significantly improved overall. Thus the real criterion for a good treatment is not the number of points used, but the quality of change on the pulses. With experience the practitioner becomes better at knowing when to stop. This is a core skill for the practitioner to develop.

Minimum intervention

In practice, new practitioners are often tempted to do too much. It is easy for them to think that if there has only been a small pulse change, adding more points will be the solution. The key to successful treatments predominantly lies in the accuracy of the diagnosis, not in believing that more points will generate more change. If practitioners are really unsure of the diagnosis, then it is better for them to limit themselves to two points only. The emphasis is then on going back to basics and really finding out if the treatment principles are correct rather than using more points.

Using the pulses to assess the treatment

The notion of using the pulse changes to test whether a treatment is effective has another application other than testing and verifying the CF. The 'CF pulse change', although not the final arbiter, can indicate that an Element is the CF. In a similar way it can be used in each treatment to test out various options.

For example, at the end of a treatment, the practitioner may notice that although almost all of the

pulses respond well to the CF treatment, the Water Element consistently does not. There may be other reasons (for example an Entry–Exit block), but the practitioner may suspect that treatment of the Water Element would be a good supplement to the CF treatment.

In this situation, it is best to treat the Water Element at some later stage. When treating another Element it is best to treat it before the CF. This gives the practitioner an opportunity to compare the resulting pulse change with previous pulse changes from treating the CF. If the Water Element points create an overall pulse change (a matter of degree), it can be assumed that further inclusion of points on these channels may be effective.

Treatments are also tests in that the practitioner can use them to gain information concerning whether the patient responds well to:

- mainly 'command' points
- 'spirit' level points
- body and command points combined
- tonification or sedation treatments
- treatment on Elements other than the CF
- particular points or combinations of points
- moxibustion

The frequency of treatment

One of the most difficult issues for practitioners is how often to treat their patients. Is it better to treat a particular patient every day, every week or every month? Are more frequent treatments better? Is there an optimum time between one treatment and the next?

Chinese medicine has some general guidelines about the frequency of treatment. The more acute the problem, the more frequent the treatment should be. The treatments should be less frequent if the problem is more chronic. 'Frequent' means daily or even twice a day. 'Less frequent', as for the chronic condition, means approximately weekly at the start of the patient's treatment.

Because Five Element Constitutional Acupuncture is usually used with chronic conditions, the view taken is that treatment should usually begin on a weekly basis. Ideally, however, it would be best if the practitioner could monitor changes to the patient's pulses more frequently. For example, if practitioners could take their patients' pulses every day, they would discover that the initial change on the pulses often gradually diminishes in the days following a treatment. When the patient returns, the pulses are possibly better than before the previous visit, but less good than immediately after the previous treatment.

This is often reflected in what patients say. For example, at first patients may commonly say things like, 'I was much better for four or five days and then I started to slip back.' If it was possible the best option would be for the practitioner to monitor the patient's pulses and carry out the next treatment just as the patient began to drop back.

Practitioners sometimes can follow this ideal condition. Patients with severe chronic and empty conditions can be treated two or even three times a week initially and then move on to weekly treatments. It is important to remember, however, that some of the best changes may occur in the 24 to 48 hours following a treatment, so the practitioner must take great care if treating again before this time period has elapsed.

Weekly treatment is usual at first. After some treatments when patients return on a weekly basis and say they are still well, the practitioner will often extend this to fortnightly treatments. As the patient gets better this is gradually extended from fortnightly to three-weekly, monthly, two-monthly and finally, seasonal treatments.

Some patients continue having weekly treatments for a long period of time whilst others move to fortnightly treatments quickly. This depends on the patient's initial state of health and also on their rate of progress. Sometimes patients may return for their weekly treatment and say they feel well. They may also have pulses that have remained the same as they were at the end of the previous treatment. In this situation the correct option may be to not treat the patient during that session.

Dealing with patients who are not progressing sufficiently

If treatment is not sufficiently effective, what are the possibilities?

(Table 45.1)

Practitioners expect the treatment that follows their diagnosis to produce good results. Sometimes, however, this is not the case. There may have been no progress at all, some progress, or sometimes spectacular progress, followed by a levelling off or even a relapse. At whatever stage this occurs, it is necessary to consider other options. Even experienced practitioners find a list of possible options useful.

Firstly, the practitioner reviews the patient's file which lists the treatments given and the feedback received at the subsequent treatment. This may give the practitioner clues about which treatments have been effective and which have not. The main reasons why treatment is not progressing are discussed below.

Wrong CF

There are many reasons why practitioners diagnose the wrong CF, but it is usually because they have misread or been unable to discern the correct colour, sound, emotion and odour. Sometimes these indicators are not consistent. For example, a patient who has taken drugs can have damaged the Liver sufficiently for green to appear on the face. It may also be difficult for the practitioner to gain a clear picture of patients' usual emotional predispositions when they have recently had an experience, such as a bereavement, which has created an intense emotional upheaval.

Missed block

Any one or more of the four blocks may not have been cleared or has been cleared and returned. The practitioner needs to re-evaluate whether the patient could have any of these blocks. Pulse diagnosis is crucial to the diagnosis of Entry–Exit blocks and Husband–Wife imbalances. Understanding the patient's internal world enables the practitioner to diagnose possession. If Aggressive Energy is suspected, it is best to carry out the treatment, as it is not invasive.

Incorrect level

The patient may have progressed in some ways, but treatment has not sufficiently reached them on the level of body, mind or spirit. In this case the patient may have progressed reasonably well at first, but is no longer benefiting significantly from subsequent treatments. Practitioners may recognise the situation when patients seem to be getting everything (or almost everything) they originally came for, but are curiously unmoved. For example, a Water CF had a severe back problem. In spite of

Table 45.1 Is treatment on the correct CF?

	Signs of treating on the CF	Signs of not treating on the CF
Pulse changes	There is an overall change on the pulses	Only the pulse of the Element treated changes
	The pulses of the CF Organs change less than the other pulses or not at all	There is no harmonisation of the pulses as a whole
	If there has been fullness this gets stronger before settling to a more harmonised pulse	If there has been a fullness on the pulse this just disappears and the pulse becomes weak
Patient changes	The patient looks livelier – colour, sound, emotion, odour change	There is no change in colour, sound, emotion or odour
	The patient feels 'better in self'	The patient does not feel better in her/himself
	The patient feels better about the future	There is no sense of the patient moving forward and making progress
	There may be an exacerbation after the treatment. This settles and then the patient feels better	There may be an aggravation (rather than exacerbation) after treatment. After this settles the patient does not feel better
	The patient copes better with life	Treatment doesn't hold. The patient may feel better for a while then it runs out
	There is a change in her/his relationship to health in a fundamental way	The patient sometimes feels better but sometimes doesn't
	The patient is more able to make lifestyle changes in her/his life	The patient finds it difficult to make lifestyle changes
	The patient no longer notices symptoms or a large number of symptoms just go away	The patient's symptoms change but each symptom seems to have to be dealt with individually
	The eyes look more shiny	There is no change in the patient's eyes
	The patient switches in her/his consciousness from symptom to self	The patient only notices changes to her/his symptoms
	The patient seems more robust	There is no change in the patient's overall robustness

being once again fully functional, the patient said to the practitioner, 'When am I going to be *really* better?'

Sometimes the body benefits more than the mind and spirit. Sometimes it is the other way around. In these situations the practitioner needs to vary some of the points used in order to initiate change at the appropriate level.

Another Element is too imbalanced

In some situations treatment centred on the CF is not successful because another Element is so imbalanced that it obstructs improvement. For example,

a patient may be a Water CF but the Heart or Pericardium has been affected by a recent relationship break-up, or a patient who is a Wood CF may have depleted Water due to overworking. Pulse diagnosis, colour, sound, emotion, odour or secondary indications are the tools that may reveal to the practitioner which Element needs to be treated directly.

Inconsistent and irregular treatment

A patient may have started to get better and the practitioner and the patient have high hopes. Then after some time the patient realises that progress is not really continuing. Often in this case, the problem is that treatment has not been consistent. A week has been missed for holidays, another because of a funeral. Sometimes the patient and practitioner have agreed to reduce the number of treatments and the frequency is no longer enough. Although improvement has occurred, the patient's treatment has not been consistent enough for it to hold and for the patient to progress. The time will come, however, when the patient will be able to come less frequently.

Treatment is not strong enough

Many patients benefit enormously from very simple treatments using just one point on each of the channels of the CF. It is best to start treating a new patient with very few points, as minimum intervention is always an ideal. Some patients, however, may need stronger points or more points in each treatment. For example, they may need the back *shu* points and more moxa if they are to benefit sufficiently.

Incorrect needle technique or inaccurate point location

Inaccurate needle technique is most common on the Wood Element. The practitioner is sedating when she or he should be tonifying, or vice versa. Inaccurate point location is also, of course, a reason for many ineffective treatments.

Lifestyle issues

A patient may have a lifestyle issue that is interfering with treatment. For example, a Fire CF patient who is easily disturbed and gets into extreme emotional states, regularly has arguments with her partner. This causes the patient's Heart to become agitated. The patient requires several weeks of tranquillity for her *shen* to stabilise, but this seems impossible. Another patient who is an Earth CF, has eating patterns that consistently work against the progress achieved by treatment.

When the patient's lifestyle is a problem, the practitioner needs to discuss the issue with the patient and support the patient in finding a way to make a change. Some practitioners are tempted to blame the patient's lifestyle for the failure of treatment. Although this may sometimes be so, it can also be a way of ignoring other issues, such as the accuracy of the diagnosis.

Patient Example

A Fire CF would feel better immediately after treatment, but when she went home she would invariably row with her husband and the effect of the treatment would be lost. Finally, the practitioner asked if she could manage not to row after treatment and she decided to visit her sister in another part of the country for six weeks. The practitioner arranged for another practitioner to treat her and she stabilised. When she returned she was strong enough to tell husband that they needed not to row and begin to sort out their relationship. After this had happened, progress was made.

Rapport

Some patients fail to thrive owing to a lack of rapport between patient and practitioner. There are obviously no easy solutions to this, but the practitioner must strive to break through the barriers that are present.

Responding to a patient's lack of progress

If a patient is making poor or no progress, practitioners might reflect on which two or three of the above options are the most likely explanation. They may then decide on which course of action to take, for instance they may decide to:

1 make further investigations, for example, about the patient's lifestyle;
2 return to the diagnosis and thoroughly revisit colour, sound, emotion and odour;
3 look at the frequency of treatment and selection of points.

As they become more experienced, practitioners consider the above options almost constantly. All of the above suggestions presuppose, however, that the practitioner is getting correct feedback and knows whether the patient is getting better. Practitioners need to consider how they make this judgement and how they take in the patient's feedback.

Prognosis

Prognosis is the art of forecasting the course of a disease and how it might respond if addressed by a specific form of treatment. When patients ask, 'How long will it take for me to get better?', they are asking the practitioner to assess their prognosis. It is a natural question to ask and impossible for practitioners to answer with any certainty as there are many variations as to how each individual reacts. There are, however, generalisations that practitioners can make which can be helpful:

The longer the patient has had a problem, the longer it will take to clear it

A back problem that has come on in the last three months will generally respond better than one that has been present for 15 years.

The more complicated the patient's problems, the longer they will take to improve

Obviously some patients are very ill at some level and their passage back to health will be difficult. 'Complicated' can have various meanings, however. A patient may, for example, have had a problem for which she or he has taken medication. This may have led to a side effect that is being treated by yet another medication. This can take time to unravel in treatment. When patients are taking many medications, they may also take longer to improve, especially if the medication has been taken for a long period of time or is having a profound effect on the patient's body, mind and spirit.

The more the person's life situation exacerbates the problem, the longer it takes to improve

Some people are in situations that improve their physical, mental and spiritual health and others are not. For example, Fire CFs who are in relationships that enhance their ability to give and receive warmth and love generally progress better than those who are in less nourishing relationships. People's needs are different and their deep needs are shaped to a large extent by their underlying Elemental imbalances. If patients are in situations that nourish their Elements in daily life, they are likely to achieve better health than those who don't. Having said this, many patients who are in difficult circumstances find that treatment enables them to make changes to enhance their lives. Many become more satisfied with their 'lot' after having treatment. In these circumstances patients may progress rapidly.

The deeper the source of the illness, the longer the treatment will take

Someone whose spirit has been deeply affected by grief for 40 years cannot be expected to heal as quickly as someone who has been affected by grief for only a year. This guideline can be easy to apply with some patients and be more difficult with others. When taking a patient's case history, the practitioner should aim to understand how deeply the spirit has been affected and for how long.

The effect of lifestyle habits

Those with lifestyle habits antagonistic to their health take longer to get well. Poor dietary habits, not getting enough sleep, working too hard, over-exercising, not exercising at all, living in an abusive relationship, taking recreational drugs and many other factors will mitigate against treatment and prolong the process of getting better.

Putting these together

The above list describes some of the main circumstances that affect a patient's prognosis. Through experience practitioners gain a better understanding of how long various people take to get better. Then they can apply the above considerations in individual cases. 'How long will it take?' is never an easy question. Experienced practitioners get better at estimating this, but most also have experiences of apparently easy patients who took a long time to improve and the apparently difficult patients who got better in two or three treatments.

Making an assessment of the patient's prognosis allows practitioners to become clearer about the rate at which patients might progress during their first few treatments, and also later on when the diagnosis is confirmed. For some patients slow but small changes can be counted as good progress. For others more rapid changes might be expected.

Taking feedback

Two types of feedback

Taking feedback is essential in order for the practitioner to plan the next treatment. The practitioner will get detailed information at each treatment as to how the patient is progressing following the last visit. This has two aspects to it. There is, on the one hand, what the patient tells the practitioner and, on the other, what the practitioner can observe about the patient. Both are important.

It is important for the practitioner to have a clear and detailed description of the patient's complaints. Some of this will derive from the patient's answer to the question, 'How will you know you are getting better?' Another part will come from the questioning of systems and monitoring improvement in areas such as sleep, appetite, bowels, etc. Yet more will derive from areas that the patient did not complain about, but the practitioner observed about the patient. For example, the patient may have breathing problems or very dry skin, but never complained about them. Monitoring these changes will be additional confirmation for the practitioner that the patient is making progress.

The non-verbal signs could be the patient's:

- pulses
- general appearance
- colour
- sound
- emotion
- odour
- posture
- gestures and movements
- facial expression
- brightness of eyes
- other areas noticed

The practitioner often first looks at the patient's general appearance and then looks in detail at the other components. The pulses are a significant sign and practitioners often ask themselves if the change that took place in the pulses at the previous treatment is still holding or have the pulses slipped back to their original character.

To test whether the treatment plan is working, it is essential to have accurate and objective feedback.

Remembering what has changed

Because Five Element Constitutional Acupuncturists rely heavily on sensory feedback, it is essential for them to monitor how the patient's non-verbal signs are changing over the course of treatment. For example, in relation to the colour, the patient may be less green beside the eyes or the pulses may be more harmonious. These judgements presuppose that the practitioner can remember what she or he saw and compare this to how the patient is now presenting.

To compare the look of the patient's face or the brightness in the eye before and after treatment can be essential to knowing whether the treatment was successful.

Patients are not necessarily immediately aware of how they are changing from treatment and practitioners cannot always rely on the patient's verbal report. Patients can sometimes have improvements in their general well-being or vitality but not be aware of this until their specific symptoms improve. The practitioner may have, however, noticed that the patient's improved appearance, colour and pulses indicate that they are getting better.

Practitioners are not equal in their ability to observe and record feedback. Some practitioners find this difficult and some find it easy. This skill is rarely pointed out or taught. Recording sensory impressions can help the learning process. Practice is important.

Summary

1 The three main stages of treatment planning are:
   - summarising the diagnosis
   - forming an overall treatment strategy
   - planning individual treatments.
2 When deciding on which treatment to carry out:
   - Blocks are cleared first.
   - The main priority is to then treat the CF.
3 The CF is confirmed by:
   - Whether the patient changes in her or his spirit. This is usually manifested by the patient expressing in some way that he or she 'feels better in her/himself'.
   - The pulses become more harmonious and the strength of all pulse positions improves.
   - The practitioner perceives improvement in the person's signs or how she or he is in her/himself.
   - The person's complaints improve.
4 The choice of needle technique is determined by the pulses.
5 The frequency of treatment is important.
6 Pulse changes are significant when evaluating treatment.
7 When treatment is not working, the possibilities should be investigated systematically.

Treatment – pulling it all together

46

Introduction

The goal of a diagnosis is to understand the nature of a patient's physical, mental and spiritual imbalances as clearly as possible. Diagnosis should answer four questions:

* What is the person's CF?
* Which other Elements/Organs are in distress?
* Are there any 'blocks' to successful treatment?
* What is the primary level of treatment – body, mind or spirit?

The previous chapter described various methods practitioners can use to answer these questions in order to form a diagnosis. Once these questions have been answered, practitioners move on to the first stage of treatment which is based on 'testing' the diagnosis. When practitioners are certain of the CF, and are sure that any blocks have been cleared, they then need to discover how best to treat each individual patient. Some useful question to ask are:

* Does the patient primarily need treatment using command points?
* Does the patient need to be treated using points that focus on the spirit?
* Does the patient need to be treated on any other Elements besides the CF?
* Does the patient flourish with a small number of points or is a large number preferable?
* Will the patient benefit from moxa?

In the rest of this chapter are two longer case histories followed by another six shorter ones. These illustrate some of the various kinds of diagnoses and treatments practitioners might carry out. The names of patients and some aspects of the case history have been changed for confidentiality.

Patient 1 – Andrew

Andrew was 45 and single. He seemed friendly but rather distant when he first met his practitioner. He told her that he worked as a computer programmer and had been in the job for 4 years.

Main complaint

Andrew had been suffering from insomnia for the last 3 years. He said 'I toss and turn and feel fidgety and too cold and it sometimes takes me two hours to get off to sleep. It's bad even if I feel tired when I go to bed'. He didn't know why it had come on, 'just

DOI: 10.1016/B978-0-7020-3175-5.00046-2

one of those things', but it was now bad about 80% of the time. (*His practitioner tested Earth at this point and gave him sympathy which he accepted and moved through easily.*) He said he didn't usually wake once he'd gone off to sleep although he'd occasionally wake in the early hours around 3 a.m. The insomnia was worse if he was stressed or feeling upset.

Secondary complaint

His secondary complaint was asthma. He'd had this since he was 10 years old. It had come on gradually and did not cause him much trouble these days although it was worse when he exerted himself. The asthma had been bad when he was a teenager but now caused him very little problem as long as he took his daily inhaler.

Present situation

Andrew worked very hard as a computer programmer and indicated that he loved the status and good financial rewards he gained from it. The job was now 'too easy'. In the past he had changed jobs frequently and he thought he might look for another job soon. He also had difficulty with his boss at times, 'the boss can be overbearing and pushy and doesn't always understand things as well as I do. Like yesterday he was putting pressure on me to finish my current job without knowing what exactly I needed to do' (*the practitioner tested Wood here and suggested that this must be frustrating. Andrew agreed and got slightly angry – the practitioner judged this to be appropriate*).

Andrew had very little social life although he had a sporadic sexual relationship with a colleague. He had had a few relationships in the past but all were fairly short lived. He had had a major relationship for two years when he was in his thirties but she'd gone off with someone else. He admitted that it had left a big hole in his life. (*He choked up as he talked about this – indicating that he was still feeling some loss.*)

Questioning the systems

Andrew's appetite was good. He loved food and cooking and he talked about some cookery classes he had enjoyed. (*The practitioner thought his joy came and went smoothly but he still seemed a little flat.*) About twice a week he had indigestion and this could be quite painful, especially after a big meal. Antacid tablets helped this. Andrew also mentioned that his energy levels were down on what they used to be and had been worse for three years, since not sleeping well. He said his bowels were normal and he might go twice a day and they would be slightly loose. He had had a rumbling appendix several years ago. This was no problem now. The practitioner wondered if it might come back but Andrew said he didn't think it would. (*The practitioner thought this was an appropriate response and he could reassure himself.*) He had a tendency to feel the cold rather than the heat. Urination, perspiration and other systems were all normal.

The pulses

Left		Right	
SI −1	Ht −1	Lu −2	LI −2
GB − ½	Liv − ½	Sp −1	St −1
Bl −2	Kid −2	PC −2	TB −2

Andrew's pulses were all very deficient and the Liver and Gall Bladder were the strongest pulses.

Family history

His relationship with his father had been very poor. His father had been a very successful entrepreneur who had little time for his son and his approval had been inextricably linked to his son's level of academic and sporting achievement. He had been closer to his mother and she had died a few years ago. He showed little emotion about this and said he had not had difficulty accepting her death. He now saw his father 'sporadically'.

The diagnosis

Andrew appeared to be a Metal CF. The practitioner thought his colour was white, voice tone weeping and the odour rotten. His grief seemed to be his most inappropriate emotion. At times he seemed to be extremely inert with little sense of loss when it might have been expected. At other times he would choke up and appeared to be feeling a lot of grief. When the practitioner showed him respect and appreciation for his achievements he had been unable to take this in.

Supporting evidence for the diagnosis was also present in his relationship with his father and the way he was driven to find ways of feeling better about himself in relation to his financial and career status. The practitioner also noted that although Andrew said that he had been unaffected by the death of his mother, the commencement of his insomnia had coincided with this. He also sometimes woke at 3 a.m., which is the horary time for the Lung.

He was also slightly irritable at times and had some green around the eyes. These both indicated that his Wood Element was imbalanced. The practitioner considered that there was a possibility of an Entry–Exit block between the Liver and Lung, especially as the pulse of the Liver was considerably fuller than that of the Lung.

The practitioner was also concerned to see an improvement in his Fire Element as he was also quite lacking in joy.

The practitioner's diagnosis sheet looked like this:

Diagnosis Sheet

Name: Andrew, Age 45

Patient's main complaint: Insomnia – tosses and turns and can't get off to sleep.

Secondary complaints: Asthma

CF: Metal. Andrew looks white, has a weeping voice tone and has a rotten odour. His grief seems to be his most inappropriate emotion and he swings between grief and a lack of grief.

Next most likely CF: Fire. He seems to find it difficult to raise much joy.

Other Elements: Wood. He seems to be somewhat irritable and be green around the eyes. Earth. He accepts sympathy smoothly and does not appear to sing or be yellow. Water. Appears to be able to reassure himself. He shows appropriate fear when asked about the future. No blue colour. Metal.

Blocks:

  H–W: Don't think so.

  AE: Possible, need to test.

  Possession: Internal or external: Unlikely.

  Entry–Exit: Pulses, colour and emotion indicate this is possible between Wood and Metal.

Level

  Body: No apparent reason to think so.

  Mind: Andrew seems to be able to think very clearly.

  Spirit: I think this is the primary level, as he seems inert and unable to respond.

Physical Examination: Upper Burner is cold.

Akabane: Sp 5/16

The treatment strategy was as follows:

Treatment Strategy for Andrew

Treatment principles and order of priority

* Check for Aggressive Energy.
* Strengthen and warm Metal CF at the spirit level.
* Treat Fire Element if necessary.
* Clear Liver/Lung block.

Examples of appropriate points to use

1. **Clear Aggressive Energy:** Bl 13, 14, 18, 20 and 23
2. **Balance Akabane:** Sp 4
3. **Treat Metal CF:** Examples could be Lu 9, LI 4, Lu 8, LI 1, LI 11, Bl 13, Bl 25
4. **Treat Fire CF:** TB 4, PC 7, SI 4, Ht 7 and other points.

Appropriate number of points to use

Suspect will need only a small number of points as treatment is directed to spirit level.

Moxa, if appropriate how much, and on which points?

Moxa will be appropriate as patient feels the cold and the upper *jiao* is cold.

Lifestyle changes that the patient may need to make

Ensure spends some time relaxing before going to bed as can work late on his computer. May need to consider eating earlier as currently eats late at night.

How to assess if the patient is improving

May become less inert and able to express emotions. He may wish to have more interaction with others at work and create a more social life. Expect his sleep, asthma and indigestion to improve. Expect his pulses to become stronger and more harmonious.

Treatment 1

At the first treatment the practitioner tested for Aggressive Energy on Bl 13, 14, 18, 20 and 23. There was no redness around the needles and the pulses didn't change, so the result was negative

The practitioner then decided to correct the Akabane imbalance on the Spleen and treated the *luo* junction point Sp 4 on the right side. This corrected the imbalance and brought up the Spleen pulse but no other pulses.

The practitioner then went on to 'test' the CF and treated the *yuan* source points of the Metal Element, Lu 9 and LI 4. These were tonified without retention. This produced an excellent pulse change. The Lungs and Large Intestine barely changed but all the other pulses came up and harmonised to a similar quantity.

The rear positions remained more deficient. Moxibustion was then added to the same points. This had the effect of making all the pulses feel slightly stronger. Usually moxa cones are used *before* needling. In this case it was added *after* the needles to support the effect of the needle.

Treatment 2

Andrew reported that he felt more energetic for a couple of days but otherwise was much the same as ever. The pulses had gone back to how they were at the commencement of treatment. The practitioner decided to test for the presence of an Entry–Exit block between the Liver and Lung. This was based on the discrepancy between the pulses of these two Organs, the green colour, irritability and the presence of asthma – a symptom situated between the Exit point of the Liver and the Entry point of the Lung.

Liv 14 and Lu 1 were both tonified as both Organs were deficient. The change on the pulses was striking.

Left		Right	
SI −1	Ht −1	Lu −1	LI −1
GB −1	Liv −1	Sp −1	St −1
Bl −1	Kid −1	PC −1	TB −1

All the pulses had changed and were now harmonious in terms of strength and quality. Despite being tonified, the Wood pulses were now more deficient, so they were more in harmony with the other pulses.

The *yuan* source points of Metal were then tonified again. This created a slight strengthening in all of the pulses.

Treatment 3

Andrew reported substantial improvement in his sleep and he was now getting off to sleep more easily most nights. His asthma and indigestion had also improved and he said that he had felt 'on very good form all week. Really cheerful and better energy.' There was no longer any green on the face. The pulses were slightly weaker than at the end of the previous treatment but the increase in harmony had been maintained.

The practitioner used moxibustion and tonification on the tonification points of Metal – Lu 9 and LI 11. All the pulses felt stronger at the end of treatment.

Treatment 4

Andrew said that progress had been maintained. He was sleeping better and had also reduced using his inhaler. He said he had been surprised to find that he needed to use it only once a day instead of the previous twice. He had also dramatically reduced his antacid consumption. He said that he felt 'really well'. The practitioner did not treat the patient that week.

Treatment 5

Andrew had had an upsetting appraisal at work. His supervisor obviously did not hold him in anything like as much regard as he had thought he deserved. His sleeping and chest had been worse, as had his mood. His indigestion was fine. On examination his pulses were as follows:

Left		Right	
SI −1	Ht −1	Lu −2	LI −2
GB −1	Liv −1	Sp −1	St −1
Bl −1	Kid −1	PC −1	TB −1

The practitioner thought that strengthening of the pulses was needed. The back *shu* points of the Lungs and Large Intestine – BL 13 and 25 – were tonified and moxa was used. The pulses felt stronger after this treatment. The practitioner had intended to also use the *yuan* source points if the change had been moderate, but did not need to use them.

Treatment 6

Two weeks elapsed, as the practitioner was on holiday, but the patient said he felt much better after the previous treatment. He commented that he had been very low for about 24 hours and then felt much better in himself (see Appendix E on treatment reactions). His sleeping and general energy had also improved. He had also on the practitioner's advice been eating earlier in the day.

The practitioner tonified the *luo* junction points Lu 7 and LI 6 with moxa. All the pulses felt better.

Further treatments

The patient continued to benefit from treatment. Nearly all of the treatment was focused on the Metal

Element. Other point combinations used were the Windows of the Sky, Lu 3 and LI 18, Bl 42 with the tonification points, and *Du* 12 with the *yuan* source points.

After treatment 6, Andrew's treatment was spaced to fortnightly and rapidly moved onto monthly visits. He continued to come for treatment even though his physical symptoms had improved. This was because he had noticed that treatment had a positive effect on his well-being. He felt able to consolidate the previously casual relationship with his work colleague and they were even talking of moving in together. On one occasion the practitioner sedated his Wood as he was furious with his girlfriend and the pulse was very full. In general his Wood remained much better than before the Entry–Exit treatment. His indigestion never returned and he was less irritable. He also had fewer problems with his asthma, only needing to use his inhaler occasionally. He still had occasional bouts of insomnia but these were less prolonged. He also felt generally warmer in temperature.

On a couple of occasions the practitioner tonified his Pericardium and Triple Burner. Although he was obviously jollier than before, the pulses were inclined to remain low and the practitioner thought there was scope for improvement in this area. Treatment yielded only very slight pulse change and the practitioner did not persist.

Patient 2 – Bernice

Bernice was 56 and married. She had one child, aged 28, from a previous marriage. She looked young for her age and was well dressed but also pale and drawn.

Main complaint

Bernice said she had been very anxious and depressed since she had split up from her husband nine months previously. 'We're still seeing each other and are trying to make a go of it, but the fact he wanted to break up was a complete shock.' Although somewhat anxious before, she had completely lost her emotional stability since the break-up. She was getting mood swings and had not felt herself at all. She admitted that he had always been a philanderer but she loved him. She now thought about him obsessively. She had been offered antidepressants but had refused to take them. (*Bernice related this in a flat and joyless voice*

tone and she also cried. She accepted and appeared to enjoy the sympathy the practitioner offered. The practitioner noticed that her eyes looked very dull and lifeless.)

Secondary complaints

She had low energy and no vitality since her husband left. She also found it hard to sleep at night and would wake intermittently thinking about her husband and their situation and finding it hard to get off again. She also complained of some pain in her left shoulder that had been there for the last six months. This caused her no restriction in movements and tended to be worse when she was tired.

Present situation

Bernice ran the administration department of a large company in her home town. She said she loved her job and enjoyed both the organisation and overseeing her staff of six. She brightened up and became more animated when talking about it. She had been off work a lot recently because of the break-up and although the company had been sympathetic they were now putting her under pressure to work more regularly again. She said she felt frustrated by this but understood why they were doing it. (*Her practitioner thought that her response was appropriate.*) When questioned about any possibility of losing her job she looked a bit hesitant but said she didn't think this would be a problem. (*The practitioner didn't think this was really enough to check her response to fear and decided to test again later.*)

Bernice said she lived on her own but her husband occasionally visited at weekends. The house was on the market as she couldn't afford to pay the mortgage.

Family and personal history

She had been a 'war baby'. Bernice's mother had been mentally ill and her father in the US army. The father had abandoned the family when she was a few months old and she had been taken from her mother when she was 7 years old and sent to boarding school. 'I loved the school because it gave me stability and I had one very close friend.' She said she was still in contact with her mother. She described herself as 'an introverted child' and said she didn't really come out of herself until her teens. 'I now have issues to do with abandonment.' (*She related this sometimes laughing and at other times sounding very flat. When her practitioner gave her respect for how she'd survived this ordeal she agreed and said she thought she'd survived it well. Her practitioner also told her how young she looked – at this Bernice completely brightened up and her whole face lit up.)*

The systems

Her appetite had been poor since the break-up, although previously it had been good. She had lost a stone in weight and had to force herself to eat. Her bowels and urination were normal. She had had a hysterectomy when she was in her late forties. Before this her periods had been heavy with clots. She would often feel cold. She loved the summer and hated the winter and dull damp weather. Sometimes she would feel hot and sweaty when she woke in the night.

The pulses

Left		Right	
SI −2	Ht −2	Lu − ½	LI − ½
GB −1	Liv −1	Sp − ½	St − ½
Bl −2	Kid −2	PC −1	TB −1

The diagnosis

The practitioner thought Bernice was a Fire CF. Her colour was lack of red and voice tone was usually lacking in laughter although with some inappropriate laughter too. Her emotions seemed to swing between joy and a lack of joy and she would either be flat and joyless or brighten up and be quite animated. She was unsure of the odour but thought it might be scorched. Bernice had also seemed to enjoy the sympathy she received from her practitioner. Rapport between the patient and the practitioner had been good. The practitioner thought that this was important as Bernice needed to open up and talk about her feelings.

Secondary diagnostic information also indicated Fire as her CF. Her vulnerability and lack of 'heart protection' had always been a striking aspect of her personality. Relationships were extremely important to her and, due to her childhood experiences, she was terrified of being abandoned. Some other symptoms such as her poor sleep and anxiety also pointed to Fire. The practitioner wondered

if her shoulder pain on the left side might be arising from a weakness in her Heart and Heart-Protector.

Other symptoms indicated Earth as a possibility, for example, her poor appetite, some secondary diagnostic factors, such as extreme tenderness on the Spleen front *mu* point and a cold middle *jiao*. The practitioner also considered whether she had a Husband–Wife imbalance. This was based on the difference in the pulses between the left and right wrists and also her confusion, obsessive thoughts and not feeling 'herself' since her husband had left. The practitioner was, however, not sure of this diagnosis. Below is the practitioner's diagnosis sheet.

Diagnosis Sheet

Name: Bernice, Age 56

Patient's main complaint: Anxiety and depression since break up of marriage nine months ago.

Secondary complaints: Poor sleep, aching left shoulder.

CF: Fire. Bernice looked lack of red, has a voice tone that swings between being flat and excessively joyful. I think she had a scorched odour. Her joy seems to be her most imbalanced emotion.

Next most likely CF: Earth. She likes sympathy and also has obsessive thoughts about her ex-husband. She has a poor appetite and a cold middle *jiao*.

Other Elements: Wood. She says she has 'mood swings', which could be to do with suppressed anger but I think these are to do with her joy and sadness. Water. She is quite fearful especially to do with being abandoned but again think this is more to do with the Fire Element. Need to test this again. Metal. A lot of issues in her past that she might have grief about but she seems to have dealt with these well.

Blocks:

H–W: This is a possibility but not sure.

AE: A possibility too; need to test.

Possession: Internal or external: Possible but I don't think so.

Entry–Exit: Could be a block between Spleen and Heart.

Level

Body: Not a lot of physical symptoms.

Mind: Has obsessive thoughts but think comes from her spirit level.

Spirit: Think problems stem from this level. Her eyes look dull and lacking in spirit and her posture is slumped. She feels unable to move forward in her life and needs internal strength to give her emotional stability.

Physical examination: Middle Burner is cold. Left shoulder is also cold. Front *mu* point Spleen tender

The treatment strategy was as follows:

Treatment Strategy for Bernice

Treatment principles and order of priority

- Check for Aggressive Energy.
- Strengthen and warm Fire CF at the spirit level.
- Balance Husband–Wife imbalance if necessary.
- Treat Earth Element if necessary.

Examples of appropriate points to use

1. **Clear Aggressive Energy:** Bl 13, 14, 18, 20 and 23
2. **Treat Fire CF:** Examples could be TB 4, PC 7, TB 3, PC 9, TB 5, PC 6, Bl 14, Bl 22, Bl 43, *Ren* 15, TB 16, PC 2 or SI 4, Ht 7, SI 3, Ht 9, Bl 15, Bl 44, Bl 28, *Ren* 14, etc.

Appropriate number of points to use

Small number of points as treatment is directed to spirit level
If treat Husband-Wife more points may be needed.

Moxa, if appropriate how much, and on which points?

Moxa may be appropriate. Patient feels the cold and the middle *jiao* is cold. She does, however, sometimes wake feeling hot so this should be used with care.

Lifestyle changes that the patient may need to make

Bernice's major issue is dealing with the situation with her husband. Expect to see some change in how she deals with this. Expect her to be able to eat more as she becomes more balanced.

How to assess if the patient is improving

Her eyes may become brighter and her posture more erect. She may become strong enough to take control of her life and have greater emotional stability. She may have improvements in sleep, obsessive thoughts and anxiety levels and be able to work more regularly.

Treatment 1

The practitioner tapped for Aggressive Energy first. This was negative. She then went on to 'test' for the CF and tonified the *yuan* source points of the Fire Element TB 4 and PC 7. There was some change in the pulses. Although it was small, it was enough for the practitioner to think that the PC and TB might be the side of Fire that was the CF, so she decided to stop treatment at this point.

Pulses before treatment				Pulses after treatment			
Left		Right		Left		Right	
SI −2	Ht −2	Lu − ½	LI − ½	SI −1	Ht −1	Lu − ½	LI − ½
GB −1	Liv −1	Sp − ½	St − ½	GB −1	Liv −1	Sp ✓	St ✓
Bl −2	Kid −2	PC −1	TB −1	Bl −1	Kid −1	PC −1	TB −1

Treatment 2

The practitioner arranged for Bernice to return in four days' time. Bernice reported that she had felt very emotional after treatment and was very tearful. She said, 'it was very scary as I felt even more vulnerable.' The patient said she was still 'not quite right'. The practitioner was very surprised by this strong reaction as she had expected a more positive change in Bernice's symptoms.

The practitioner considered two choices for treatment. One was to treat the Small Intestine and Heart side of Fire and the other to assume she had a Husband–Wife imbalance and to set about re-balancing this. She suspected that Bernice's unexpectedly bad reaction pointed to a Husband–Wife imbalance. The previous treatment had affected the pulses on the right wrist and the pulse picture still revealed substantially more strength on the 'wife' side than the 'husband' side on the left. The practitioner decided to move the *qi* from the right side to the left in order to create balance between the two sides.

The combination of points for Husband–Wife was used. These were Bl 67, Kid 7, Kid 3 and Liv 4 and they were all tonified (see Chapter 32). She then treated the *yuan* source points of Heart and Small Intestine. This is commonly done to help the Heart regain control of a chaotic situation but in this case it was also used because the practitioner suspected that Bernice would benefit from treatment on this side of the Fire Element. At the end of the treatment the pulses on both sides were approximately equal in strength.

Treatment 3

The practitioner asked Bernice to return only three days after the treatment to ensure that the imbalance did not reassert itself. Bernice reported that her mood had lightened for a couple of days and that she had felt more stable. Now, however, she felt back to 'square one'. The pulses felt much the same as at the beginning of treatment.

The practitioner repeated the Husband–Wife treatment, knowing that it can be difficult to shift. Owing to feeling better in herself for a time after the previous treatment, the patient was more trusting of the practitioner and she felt more hopeful that a change could be brought about.

At the end of the treatment the practitioner felt that the patient looked different, especially in her eyes, which were brighter, and she was obviously in better spirits. The pulses now had more balance and harmony between the left and right sides.

Left		Right	
SI −1½	Ht −1½	Lu −1	LI −1
GB −1	Liv −1	Sp −1	St −1
Bl −1	Kid −1	PC −1	TB −1

Treatment 4

Bernice came back stating that she felt very different. Although still somewhat low and anxious, she was hardly thinking about her ex-husband. When she did, she no longer had the intense physical or emotional sensations that she had been experiencing. She also reported that she no longer had obsessive thoughts about him.

At this treatment the practitioner decided to go back to testing the Fire Element as the CF and this time treated the *yuan* source points Ht 7 and SI 4. The pulse change was excellent and all of the pulses felt in greater harmony at the end of treatment. They were much less thin, as well as being more relaxed and smooth. The change appeared to confirm that the CF was Fire and that Heart and Small Intestine were likely to be the key Organs. The practitioner was aware that she needed to keep an eye on the pulses to ensure that the Husband–Wife imbalance didn't recur.

Treatment 5

Bernice returned saying that she had felt much better in herself and she felt strong enough to take control of her situation. She talked with her husband and he admitted he had found someone else and had only now felt able to tell her. Although she was devastated when she heard this, she also felt able to move on and leave the relationship behind. She said she wanted to achieve a more satisfying life in terms of her relationships, than the one she had created for herself. 'I know I have a long way to go.'

The practitioner decided to focus treatment on Bernice's *shen*, particularly using spirit points on the Heart and Small Intestine and around the chest. The challenge was to lift her spirit, steady her emotions and settle her anxiety. At this treatment the pulses were edgy, thin and straining. They were significantly lower than when she left the previous time. The practitioner tonified Kid 25 (Spirit Storehouse) followed by Ht 7 and SI 4 again. This yielded a better pulse change than the previous treatment and the pulses felt more settled.

Further treatments

Bernice continued to improve although she had a slight relapse on the eighth treatment after seeing her husband again. Her pulses did not appear to regress, however, and her practitioner was pleased that the Husband–Wife imbalance did not reappear. Over time she felt able to return to work on a more regular basis. Her appetite also improved, and her other symptoms such as her shoulder pain, waking feeling hot and difficulties sleeping went as she felt increasingly independent from her husband and better in herself.

The practitioner often used points which were directed towards the spirit level such as Ht 1, *Ren* 14, Bl 44, SI 11, SI 16 and SI 17 (see Chapter 40 for more on these points). She combined this with command points and other points such as Bl 15 and Bl 27, the back *shu* points. The practitioner cautiously used some moxa as Bernice's heat symptoms subsided and this proved to be beneficial. Her pulses grew less thin and 'edgy' and Bernice gradually became more stable in herself. The Kidney chest points were also used extensively, as were *Du* 10, 11 and 12. The practitioner also did some treatment on the command points of PC and TB with some good effect but never as beneficial as treatment on the Heart and Small Intestines.

Command points on the Stomach and Spleen such as the *yuan* source points, Element points, and tonification points were also used with some good effect later on in treatment and these seemed to give her added stability.

Clearing the Husband–Wife imbalance had moved her *qi* back to a state of internal balance. Strengthening her Fire Element was also very beneficial to her, especially treatment at the spirit level. She grew stronger in herself and reinforced by an encouraging attitude from her practitioner, she became much more sociable and within a year had started a new relationship.

Patient 3 – Caroline

Caroline reported that she had not recovered her usual sense of well-being following a severe respiratory infection two months previously. She relished describing her symptoms and told the practitioner the circumstances of her personal history with great gusto. Her emotion was sympathy, odour fragrant, facial colour yellow with some green. The practitioner was uncertain about her voice tone.

Secondary information also largely supported a diagnosis of an Earth CF. She was a compulsive comfort eater and was extremely unhappy to be away from home for any period of time. She was also quite insecure, easily becoming very emotional and getting 'upset over small things'.

The green colour and other signs indicated that her Wood Element was under strain. The pulses were full, she planned her life to an excessive degree, and she had a marked tendency to be unable to sleep at the most active time of the Liver, 1–3 a.m. She said, 'I just lie there thinking about all the things I have to do.' She found that if she wrote a list, it would often settle her mind and she could get back to sleep. The problems in her Wood Element were exacerbated by drinking at least half a bottle of wine each evening. The pulses were as follows:

Left		Right	
SI ½	Ht ½	Lu −2	LI −2
GB +1	Liv +1	Sp −2	St −2
BI −1	Kid −1	PC −1½	TB −1½

All of Caroline's pulses felt thin. The Metal pulses were very soft and empty. One of the most noticeable aspects of her pulses was their lack of harmony. The Wood pulses were full and the other pulses showed marked discrepancies between them in terms of strength. It is more common to use transfers of *qi* with these kinds of pulse pictures than with pulses that are reasonably uniform in the different positions.

Treatment 1

The practitioner first tapped for Aggressive Energy. This was negative. Next he tonified the *yuan* source points of Earth – St 42 and Sp 3. The pulses after treatment were as follows:

Left		Right	
SI − ½	Ht − ½	Lu −2	LI −2
GB +1	Liv +1	Sp −1½	St −1½
BI −1	Kid −1	PC −1	TB −1

This was a disappointing pulse change, as it only really initiated change on a few of the pulses including the Earth Element which was worked on. This kind of change cast doubt in the practitioner's mind about the CF diagnosis.

Because of the full pulses on the Liver and the weak Lungs, the practitioner then tried clearing an Entry–Exit block between the Liver and Lung – Liv 14 and Lu 1. This might have accounted for the poor pulse change but it did not create any further change in the pulses. The practitioner decided to stop the treatment at this stage, go over the case history again and reassess the diagnosis.

Treatment 2

Much to the practitioner's surprise, the patient reported having felt better over the week. What improvement there had been on the pulses had held well. As it was 10 a.m. the practitioner decided to use the horary points of Earth, St 36 and Sp 3. She also used moxibustion as the patient was cold.

This produced a better pulse change than in the first treatment and the practitioner decided no more treatment was needed that day.

Treatment 3

The patient described feeling more energetic and commented that she was eating less than usual. There was no change in her insomnia, however.

The practitioner was now reassured that the CF probably was correct, based upon the pulse change obtained in the previous treatment and the patient's change in herself. The points used were:

1 Sp 1. This point was tonified to transfer *qi* across the *ke* cycle from the Liver to the Spleen.
2 St 40 (Abundant Splendour) and Sp 4 (Prince's Grandson), the *luo* junction points. These were used to enhance the condition of the Earth. Moxibustion was used.

Caroline's pulses were now starting to become stronger and more vital. The change in the Metal Element from treating the Earth was particularly marked.

Metal follows Earth on the *sheng* cycle, so this indicated that the Earth Element was feeding its 'child'. The fullness in the Wood pulses was still a cause for concern as they were so out of harmony with all the other pulses.

Treatment 4

Caroline was again feeling better and said that she had surprised herself by not getting as upset in a situation as she would have expected. She reported only a slight change in her irritability and insomnia. The practitioner decided to treat her Wood Element as well as her Earth and choose these points:

1 Liv 3 and GB 40, the *yuan* source points of Wood. These were sedated in order to establish more harmony between all of the pulses. The practitioner also had a conversation with her about the Wood Element, how it was causing her problems and how her alcohol consumption was making matters worse. After 20 minutes the Wood pulses no longer felt full.

2 St 41 and Sp 2, the tonification points, were tonified. Moxibustion was also used.

The pulses after treatment are shown below.

Left		Right	
SI − ½	Ht − ½	Lu −1	LI −1
GB ✓	Liv ✓	Sp −1½	St −1½
Bl −1	Kid −1	PC −1	TB −1

Treatment 5

The patient said that she continued to feel energetic and well and she reported a substantial improvement in her insomnia and irritability. She reported that she had been quite upset at times during the week and had been struggling to drink less alcohol. The practitioner was pleased to note that the pulses on the Wood Element had improved and decided that the time was right to focus treatment on the spirit. The treatment principles were to sedate Wood and tonify the Earth Element at the spirit level. The points were:

1 Liv 2 and GB 38, the sedation points, which had the effect of calming the Wood Element and gently transferring *qi* along the *sheng* cycle to the Fire Element.

2 St 25 and Sp 15, Heavenly Pivot and the Great Horizontal. These points had the effect of enhancing the stability of the spirit in the Earth Element.

3 St 42 and Sp 3, the *yuan* source points, were tonified to support the effect of St 25 and Sp 15.

Further treatments

The practitioner carried on treating her weekly for two more treatments, then dropped the frequency of treatments to every two weeks. Treatment was centred on two treatment principles. The first was focused on sedating the Wood Element. This had a good effect and was continued. Points such as the *yuan* source points, sedation, *luo* junction, back *shu* and various points based upon their names, e.g. GB 9, 16 and 24, Liv 13 and 14, were all used.

The second treatment principle was to tonify the Earth Element. Tonification of the Earth Element was the dominant focus of Caroline's treatment. Following treatment 5, the patient was more secure in herself and she also gradually cut down on alcohol. Although points on the body to affect her mind and spirit were used occasionally, most treatments were on the command points or back *shu* points.

The patient was an example of someone who benefited from treatment far more than she had originally envisaged.

Patient 4 – David

David was possessed. His eye contact was almost non-existent and his views on all sorts of subjects, including, for example, his parents, women, black people and his colleagues at work, were chaotic and negative. The practitioner was convinced about this part of the diagnosis but was extremely uncertain about his CF. The other diagnostic indicators, especially the emotion, were difficult to read. This was because she found it hard to understand or have empathy with his internal world. David's facial colour was either green or yellow and his emotion was probably anger.

After the possession treatment had been carried out using the Internal Dragons, David became much easier to relate to and the practitioner decided to start treatment on the Earth Element. This was because she decided that the odour, which had been uncertain, was fragrant, and that the emotion was probably a rejection of sympathy rather than anger. The colour was still unclear and the practitioner did not know the voice tone.

The extent of the transformation on the pulses from treating the *yuan* source points of Earth dispelled any lingering doubts over the CF diagnosis.

Patient 5 – Elisabeth

Elisabeth was either a Metal or Wood CF. Her main complaint was headaches, which came from an imbalance of her Liver. They were brought on by alcohol or bright light and were better on lying down. Her emotion was either grief or lack of anger, her colour both white and green, her voice tone was lack of shouting and her odour was rotten.

Secondary indications were also unclear. For example, she planned a lot and seemed to enjoy the process. Her relationship with her father had been good and she did not seem to be especially concerned about her feelings of inner worth.

When the practitioner commenced treatment by testing for Aggressive Energy, the patient had marked erythema on both Metal and Wood. This implied that Metal was probably primary, as the progression of Aggressive Energy is across the *ke* cycle.

After the Aggressive Energy had been cleared, the colour, sound, emotion and odour became clearer. The lack of anger and green became less marked. The lack of shouting was still somewhat evident but the balance had definitely swung towards the Metal Element being the CF and treatment confirmed this.

Patient 6 – Felicity

Felicity's main complaint was fatigue and low-grade depression. Her CF was Fire and the colour, sound, emotion and odour all pointed to this Element, although she was also often irritable and 'fed up', especially pre-menstrually. She suffered from moderately severe period pains.

Based on secondary indications, her practitioner decided to commence treatment on the Heart and Small Intestine pairing of Fire rather than the Pericardium and Triple Burner. This was based partly on the way that she was so vague and fuzzy when replying to questions. Her practitioner thought that she had difficulty separating pure from impure on a mental and spiritual level. Her relationships had not been much of a problem for her, indicating that the

Pericardium was not the primary Organ involved. There was little difference in quantity between the pulses of the Heart and Small Intestine and those of the Pericardium and Triple Burner.

Treatment 1

The practitioner recorded Felicity's pulses.

Left		Right	
SI −2	Ht −2	Lu −1½	LI −1½
GB ✓	Liv ✓	Sp −1	St −1
Bl −1½	Kid −1½	PC −2	TB −2

Felicity's practitioner decided on the following treatment principles and points on the first treatment:

- tap for AE – negative
- treat Fire Element, Ht 7 and SI 4, *yuan* source points

The pulses changed in this way:

Left		Right	
SI −2	Ht −2	Lu − ½	LI − ½
GB ✓	Liv ✓	Sp − ½	St − ½
Bl −2	Kid −2	PC −1	TB −1

The change on the pulses of the Fire Element indicated that the Heart and Small Intestine was the CF. This was because the pulses of the Heart and Small Intestine did not change, whereas those of the other Organs did. The lack of change on the Wood pulses was noteworthy, however. Although notated as ✓, which would imply that the Organs were in good health, this was not actually the case. Felicity's irritability indicated that the Wood Element was imbalanced. This was supported by the fact that, in regard to strength and quality, the Wood pulses were not in harmony with the other pulses.

Treatment 2

The pulses had only slipped back a little from the end of the previous treatment and Felicity reported that she had felt better over the week. The practitioner used Ht 9 and SI 3 as the tonification points. The tonification points were chosen in an attempt to harmonise the large differential between the Wood pulses and the pulses of the CF, as they transfer *qi* from the Wood Element.

After treatment the pulses were:

Left		Right	
SI −1½	Ht −1½	Lu − ½	LI − ½
GB ✓	Liv ✓	Sp − ½	St − ½
Bl −1	Kid −1	PC −1	TB −1

A good pulse change was achieved. By using these points the practitioner had used minimum intervention at the same time as giving Felicity the opportunity to improve. No further treatment was carried out in that session.

Treatment 3

Felicity had had a good week but was now pre-menstrual and she reported feeling grumpy and irritable. Overall her pulses were stronger than when she first came for treatment. The Wood pulses were very hard again, however, and relatively fuller than the other pulses.

The practitioner sedated GB 40 and Liv 3, the *yuan* source points. The practitioner could have used the sedation points of the Liver and Gall Bladder instead, as they would have created greater harmony between the pulses of the Wood Element and those of the Heart and Small Intestine. As it was the first time the practitioner had treated the Wood, the *yuan* source points were chosen. This was because the response to *yuan* source points gives a clearer picture of the kind of change that can be initiated by treating an Element. The Liver and Gall Bladder were treated first so that the practitioner could end the treatment on the CF. To treat the CF the practitioner tonified Bl 15 and 27, the back *shu* points of the Heart and Small Intestine.

At the end of the treatment all the pulses felt in greater harmony. Most of the pulses felt stronger, with the exception of the Wood pulses, which felt softer and less strong.

Treatment 4

Felicity said that she had been well and had had no period pains at all. The discrepancy in strength and quality between the pulses was now much less

marked than before, particularly between Wood and the other pulses. The practitioner's main concern was to reinvigorate her Fire and enhance her spirit. Her pulses were as follows:

Left		Right	
SI −1½	Ht −1½	Lu − ½	LI − ½
GB − ½	Liv − ½	Sp −1	St −1
Bl −1	Kid −1	PC −1	TB −1

The practitioner tonified two points to treat Felicity's spirit, Ht 1 (Supreme Spring) and SI 11 (Heavenly Ancestor). She then tonified Ht 7 and SI 4 to support the spirit points. After treatment the pulses were as follows:

Left		Right	
SI −1	Ht −1	Lu − ½	LI − ½
GB − ½	Liv − ½	Sp ✓	St ✓
Bl −1	Kid −1	PC − ½	TB − ½

Further treatments

The practitioner's main focus was on tonifying the Heart and Small Intestine, particularly using points to strengthen the spirit. Over the course of the next six months the following points were used on different occasions: Ht 2, 4, 5, 6, 7, 8, 9; SI 3, 4, 5, 6, 7, 12, 16, 17; Bl 15, 27, 44; *Ren* 14; *Du* 10, 11; Kid 24, 25 and 26. Felicity reported progressive improvement in her energy and general well-being and continued treatment because it made her feel 'better than I've ever felt in my whole life'.

The practitioner continued to sedate Felicity's Wood Element when she was pre-menstrual and also once when she was under a lot of stress at work. Over time, Felicity had fewer pre-menstrual symptoms. The practitioner noted that although the pulses could be somewhat fuller pre-menstrually, they were never as full as they had been prior to starting treatment.

The practitioner treated Felicity's Pericardium and Triple Burner on a couple of occasions. These treatments did not generate a significant pulse change, so the practitioner did not continue with these treatments.

Patient 7 – Gordon

Gordon was 7 years old. His main complaint was eczema and bed-wetting was a secondary issue. The practitioner found it difficult to diagnose his predominant emotion. This is sometimes the case with young children because there is little personal history to discuss and it is this area that often evokes most emotion in adults. Gordon's colour was blue, the odour was putrid and the voice tone either groaning or lack of laughter.

The bed-wetting, his craving for salty foods and his love of exciting, dangerous activities gave secondary, but poor-quality, support for a diagnosis of Water as CF. Treatment confirmed that Water was his CF. Both his bed-wetting and the eczema improved with treatment. Further dietary changes also helped the eczema to change substantially.

Patient 8 – Holly

Holly said that she thought she was having a 'nervous breakdown'. She was extremely agitated and was having trouble sleeping. She had recently broken up with an abusive partner and was fearful that he would come to where she was staying and be aggressive. She had a history of unhappy relationships: 'I always seem to fall for the wrong kind of guys.' Her father had been a heavy drinker and during her childhood he had swung between being very loving and violent towards her. She seemed to have very little ability to protect her Heart and her joy was very erratic. Her colour was lack of red and she also showed some blue, her voice tone varied between a lack of laughter and excess laughter. The practitioner did not know the odour. The practitioner diagnosed that her CF was Fire but that there was also some weakness in her Kidneys.

Treatment 1

The practitioner recorded Holly's pulses.

Left		Right	
SI −1½	Ht −1½	Lu −2	LI −2
GB −1	Liv −1	Sp −2	St −2
Bl −2½	Kid −2½	PC −3	TB −3

The practitioner first tested for Aggressive Energy. There was some erythema around the Kidney and Pericardium points. Because of this, the practitioner also tested the back *shu* points of the Heart. There was, however, no pulse change apart from a slight calming of the pulses, so the practitioner concluded that no Aggressive Energy was present.

Next the practitioner tonified PC 7 and TB 4 in order to 'test' if this side of Fire was the CF. This produced no significant change so the practitioner went on to tonify Ht 7 and SI 4. This produced a very slight pulse change. The practitioner was far from happy with the response, but decided to leave it in order to monitor the patient's response.

Treatment 2

The patient reported no change; in fact she had possibly been even more panicky. This could have been due to her former partner increasing his phone calls to her. Because of these circumstances it was difficult for the practitioner to be certain of the feedback. The pulses were much the same as before.

The next points the practitioner used were Ht 9 and SI 3. Because points on the Heart and Small Intestine had produced a better change on the pulses than the Pericardium and Triple Burner, the practitioner chose to focus on these Organs. Little change was felt on the pulses, so the practitioner went on to tonify the Pericardium and Triple Burner again using PC 6 and TB 5 – the *luo* junction points. Once more there was little response.

The practitioner decided to stop there and review the case history again. The practitioner asked himself why treatment was not initiating any significant change. Wrong CF was possible. At one stage the practitioner wondered if he had detected a putrid odour. The practitioner did not think that the patient was possessed or had a Husband–Wife imbalance, but realised that he should not rule them out. Holly was, after all, in great distress in her spirit. The practitioner resolved to test for an Entry–Exit block at the next treatment, and to test either the Heart or the Pericardium.

Treatment 3

Holly reported no change in her condition. The practitioner treated the Entry–Exit points of Heart and Spleen, Ht 1 and Sp 21. No appreciable pulse change was felt, so he went on to the Kidneys and Pericardium and tonified Kid 22 and PC 1. There was some improvement in the pulses generally, but not a great deal. Finally the practitioner used the back *shu* points of the Heart and Pericardium, Bl 14 and 15, in order to treat these Organs more powerfully. There was only a slight change on the pulses.

Treatment 4

Holly had had a slightly better week but the former boyfriend was now leaving her alone, which had certainly helped.

The practitioner resolved to test the Water Element to see if it was the CF. If there was no pulse change from treating Water he planned to go back to tonifying points on the Fire Element, as these would help the spirit more directly.

The practitioner tonified the *yuan* source points of the Bladder and Kidneys, Bl 64 and Kid 3. This produced a very good pulse change.

Left		Right	
SI −1	Ht −1	Lu − ½	LI − ½
GB − ½	Liv − ½	Sp −1½	St −1½
Bl −2	Kid −2	PC −2	TB −2

The patient said that she felt different immediately after the points were treated and she seemed more settled. The practitioner decided not to do any more treatment in order to assess the effect of treating the Water Element as the CF.

Treatment 5

Holly returned saying she felt somewhat better. She was sleeping better and although she still felt anxious said that the 'feelings are no longer so overwhelming'.

The practitioner decided to persist with treating Water as the CF and tonified Kid 24 – Spirit Burial Ground – to strengthen and calm the spirit. He backed this up with the tonification points, Bl 67 and Kid 7.

Further treatments

Holly slowly but surely improved from treatment on the Water Element. Ideally the practitioner always makes a correct CF diagnosis but this, obviously, does not always happen. The key to finding the CF is to use simple treatments that test the diagnosis. In this case the practitioner realised fairly quickly

that Fire was not the CF. Using only simple treatments enabled him to detect this. If he had added more treatment principles and points in an attempt to generate some kind of change in Holly, then the feedback he received would have been less informative. By the time he changed the diagnosis to Water CF the practitioner had persisted with his original diagnosis of Fire for a sufficient amount of time to be fairly certain that it was not the CF.

The practitioner focused treatment almost exclusively on the Water Element. Some of the points he used were Bl 67, 66, 64, 63, 60, 58,10, 1; Kid 1, 2, 3, 4, 5, 6, 7, 9, 10, 16, 23, 24, 25, 27; the back *shu* points and Bl 52; *Ren* 4, 6, 8; and *Du* 4 and 16.

Conclusion

When practising acupuncture, the diagnosis always comes first and the treatment follows. The question the practitioner has to ascertain, however, is whether the diagnosis is correct. Minimal treatments have the advantage of giving the best feedback as to whether the diagnosis is correct. They also give the patient the opportunity to thrive based on the minimum intervention. Minimum intervention allows the patient's *qi* to come into greater harmony, allowing the patient to heal her or himself. It is the experience of many practitioners of Five Element Constitutional Acupuncture that the most profound changes usually happen when treatment is based on one or maybe two treatment principles.

The practitioner needs to discover what makes each individual patient thrive. For example, does this patient thrive with:

- simple command points treatments?
- treatments using points that primarily affect the spirit?
- treatments using spirit points supported with command points?
- moxibustion?
- other Elements also being treated along with the CF?
- treatments based on harmonising the Elements by using *qi* transfers?

Once the diagnosis is confirmed, the practitioner needs to discover the best way to treat each individual patient as this has a huge impact on the efficacy of treatment.

Most importantly perhaps, diagnosis does not end with the case history. At each treatment the practitioner must remain aware of the balance of the Elements and whether any blocks are present. The practitioner also needs to have a long-term strategy about how to address the chronic imbalances. She or he must also be prepared to respond to any immediate needs of the patient should they arise. For example, an Element or Organ may require treatment because of an acute physical or emotional problem.

The depth of the diagnosis is always based on the quality of the diagnostic information the practitioner has identified. Ideally the patient's colour, sound, emotion and odour are all detected at the early stages of diagnosis and all indicate the same Element as the CF. It is even better if the secondary diagnostic indications also support the diagnosis. Obviously this is not always the case, as can be seen in some of the above examples.

The practitioner must base the diagnosis on whatever information she or he has and during the following treatments must strive to plug any holes in the diagnosis. For example, if an odour has not been detected, the practitioner can concentrate on trying to discern this at subsequent treatments.

The practitioner also needs to understand that a diagnosis is only a working hypothesis. Even when the practitioner is confident of a CF, it still needs to be confirmed by the patient's response to treatment. Only when patients are feeling better in themselves and there are overall improvements in the pulses, as well as the symptoms, can the practitioner be sure that the CF diagnosis is correct. As Francis Bacon wrote:

> If a man will begin with certainties, he shall end in doubts; but if he will be content to begin with doubts, he shall end in certainties.
>
> (The Advancement of Learning, 1605)

Section 8

Integration

Integration with TCM – a brief introduction to how a practitioner can integrate the two styles

47

Introduction

This chapter is primarily written for practitioners and students who have a background in TCM and who wish to integrate TCM with Five Element Constitutional Acupuncture. It is also for practitioners who have studied both styles of treatment and who are not currently integrating them.

Some practitioners choose to treat patients using only Five Element Constitutional Acupuncture. For these practitioners there is no need to read this chapter – unless of course they are a little curious! As practitioners we have spent many years using this style of treatment exclusively, so we know the strengths it possesses. Subsequently we have used TCM and Five Element treatment together and believe that there are significant benefits to be gained from using them together.

Integrating different styles of treatment is far from being without precedent. Practitioners of Chinese medicine have always integrated or brought together different lineages. *In the Footsteps of the Yellow Emperor* describes how Five Element Constitutional Acupuncture evolved from many styles of acupuncture treatment from both the Orient and the West (Eckman, 1996). What is currently called

'TCM' was created from the classics of Chinese medicine and thousands of years of clinical practice. It was largely re-formulated during the 1950s and is still changing today (Fruehauf, 1999; Scheid, 2002). All medicine has to adapt to the environment, culture and needs of the people it serves.

Why integrate?

The main benefits of combining the two styles of treatment are as follows:

- Practitioners have a greater variety of diagnostic methods and paradigms to use. This sheds more light on the nature of the patient's suffering and ultimately allows practitioners to treat a wider range of patients.
- The two styles together form a whole. They use the same underlying theory and do not overlap in any inconsistent way.
- The patterns when used in combination are relevant to typical patients in the West.

An integration of the two approaches allows the practitioner to treat a wide range of patients who have conditions stemming from any of the causes of disease. These conditions may vary between acute and chronic problems, problems affecting the channels and/or the Organs, and also between conditions affecting people physically as well as psychologically.

Because practitioners of Five Element Constitutional Acupuncture focus their treatments at the root of the patients' problems, they can help people who have no symptoms but want to improve how they feel. They are also adept at treating patients with a cacophony of symptoms that don't easily fit into any pattern. Both styles of treatment provide something very special to the well-being of the patients they treat.

This chapter will take a practitioner through some important aspects of integrating the two styles of treatment. The following chapter (Chapter 48) will then use case histories to illustrate how an integrated diagnosis and treatment can be carried out.

The similarities and differences between Five Element and TCM styles of treatment

These two systems have the same umbrella term of 'acupuncture' and of course have large areas of theory and practice in common. Where they overlap may seem obvious to many acupuncturists, but it is important to specify them. Following this the differences in each style are clarified. This will provide a foundation for discussion about the benefits of each style and how the two styles can be integrated.

What do the two styles have in common?

Table 47.1 summarises the similarities in emphasis between Five Element and TCM diagnosis and treatment.

How are the two styles different?

Table 47.2 summarises the different emphasis placed on diagnosis and treatment by practitioners of the two traditions.

Integrating the strengths of both styles

The benefits of integration

The well-being of the patient is at the heart of all treatment. The integration of Five Element Constitutional Acupuncture and TCM allows the practitioner to have a wider choice when deciding on which

Table 47.1 Similarities in emphasis between Five Element and TCM diagnosis and treatment

Main area of emphasis	Areas where the two styles overlap
Traditional diagnosis	The structure of the diagnosis carried out by practitioners of both styles of treatment is based around 'to see', 'to feel', 'to ask' and 'to hear'.[a] Practitioners from both traditions ask their patients similar questions from the 'ten questions'. The questions cover areas such as 'food and drink', 'stools and urination' and 'sleep' – all areas that are as important to a patient today as they were 400 years ago.
Observation	Practitioners from both traditions observe signs such as the posture, gestures, facial colour and voice tone. The degree of emphasis varies according to the tradition.
Theory of the Organs/ Officials	TCM describes 'the functions of the *Organs*' and Five Element Constitutional Acupuncture describes 'the functions of the *Officials*'. By using these terms both systems are clarifying that the 'Organs' of Chinese medicine are different from the organs described by a practitioner using a Western medicine diagnosis.
Pulse taking	Both Five Element and TCM practitioners use the pulses as part of their diagnosis. All practitioners feel for pulses at six different positions and at more than one depth on the wrist and all use the first three fingers of the hands when feeling pulses. Pulses have been designated slightly different positions in different lineages of Chinese medicine but there is a consensus over most of the positions.[b]
Point locations	The basic positions of the points and channels are the same for practitioners of both styles.

[a]These four ancient methods of diagnosis were first described in the 'Annals' of Su Ma Qian in the Han dynasty 206–220 BCE (Eckman, 1996, p. 144).
[b]Maciocia, 2005, p. 355.

Table 47.2 Differences in emphasis between Five Element and TCM diagnosis and treatment

Main area of emphasis	Five Element	TCM
Organising theory	Five Element theory	*Yin/yang* theory
Substances	Five Element practice refers mainly to '*qi*' and to the spirit (*shen*), but does not include *jing*, body fluids or blood.	In TCM practice and diagnosis, the full range of Substances is used – *jing*, body fluids, *qi*, blood and *shen*. They are used in diagnosis and point functions.
Aetiology	Internal or emotional causes are emphasised.	External, climatic causes and miscellaneous lifestyle causes are emphasised.
External causes	Emphasis is on the effect of seasons.	Emphasis is on the effect of climate.
Relationship to nature	The observation of nature is regarded as being a major path to understanding people and illness.	There is no emphasis on observing *yin/yang* and the Five Elements in nature.
Ben (root) or *biao* (manifestation)	More emphasis on the *ben* (root) via treatment of the CF or constitution and the Officials. The CF is regarded as the most fundamental imbalance.	Emphasis on both the *ben* (root) and the *biao* (manifestation). Treatment of Pathogenic Factors and *yin/yang*, Substances and Organs, 'syndromes' or 'patterns' cover both *ben* and *biao* according to their context.
Treatment of chronic versus acute	Emphasis on treating chronic conditions especially those resulting from constitutional predispositions and the emotions. Preventive treatment is also carried out.	Emphasis on both chronic and acute illnesses. 'Channel problems' and joint problems commonly treated but many other problems also treated.
Level of treatment	Emphasis on mind and spirit.	Emphasis is on the patterns with no reference to level. 'Nourishing Blood', for example, can affect the mind or spirit.
Diagnosis using signs or symptoms	As the CF patterns are mainly diagnosed via signs (colour, sound, emotion and odour), there is a strong emphasis on signs and sensory acuity of the practitioner.	TCM places a mixed emphasis on signs and symptoms, with often a greater reliance on symptoms.
Pulse diagnosis	Emphasis is on the strength and harmony of the pulses and the changes throughout the process of treatment.	Emphasis is on 28 pulse qualities and combinations of depth, width, strength, shape, rhythm, rate and length. Pulse often not taken after treatment.
Method of questioning	Rapport and assessing the emotions is emphasised. Emphasis is on the patients and *how* they describe their experience. Information about systems is used to assess the progress of treatment.	Emphasis is on factual gathering of information. This information is used to make a diagnosis of the patient's overall patterns of disharmony.
Relationships	Emphasis on the relationship between the Elements through the *sheng* and *ke* cycles.	Emphasis on relationships between the syndromes and how they lead to each other.
Balancing *qi*	Emphasis on harmonising the Five Elements.	Focus on nourishing *yin* and warming *yang*.
Blocks to treatment	Aggressive Energy, Husband–Wife imbalance, possession, Entry–Exit block.	Pathogenic Factors – Wind, Cold, Damp, Dryness, Heat, Fire, Phlegm, Blood Stagnation and *qi* Stagnation.

Table 47.2 Differences in emphasis between Five Element and TCM diagnosis and treatment—cont'd

Main area of emphasis	Five Element	TCM
Number of points used per treatment	Smaller number, 2–6 per treatment.	Larger number, 4–12 per treatment.
Needle technique	Gentle needle techniques. Immediate withdrawal of needle when tonifying (reinforcing). Gentle technique when sedating. (Sedation is most similar to 'even' technique.)	Stronger needle techniques are used when clearing Pathogenic Factors. Needle is retained when reinforcing (tonifying). Even technique is used when reducing but underlying *qi* is deficient.
Width of needles	Finer needles are used because of emphasis on spirit.	Thicker needles are used especially when emphasis is on clearing pathogens.
Moxibustion	Moxa often employed using small cones directly on the skin.	Moxa often used indirectly with moxa stick or on a needle.
Use of points	Emphasis on the category of the point, the 'spirit' and/or the name of the point. Also emphasis on 'command points'.	Emphasis on the 'function' or action of points.
Outcome of treatment	Most emphasis on enhancing the patient's underlying *qi* in order to deal with the main complaints and prevent further potential disease.	Most emphasis on dealing with the patient's presenting condition.
Other areas of diagnosis and treatment specific to the tradition	1. The use of horary points and the Midday–Midnight law. 2. The use of *qi* transfers to move *qi* between Organs.	1. The use of the eight extra channels in order to treat deep levels of imbalance. 2. The use of lifestyle advice, e.g. diet, protection from climatic factors, for patients to use in order to become healthy. 3. The use of tongue diagnosis. 4. The use of the 'Eight Principles' to classify illness.

treatment to choose. Just as Chinese medicine complements the weaknesses of Western medicine, so these two styles of acupuncture complement each other superbly. Integration creates a breadth and depth to the patient's treatment. An integration of these two styles of treatment expands a practitioner's range of treatment possibilities and creates a style which is both flexible and pragmatic. Some of the strengths of each style are specified below. These help the practitioner to determine the desirable qualities that can be used in an integration of both styles of treatment.

The main strengths of Five Element Constitutional Acupuncture and TCM treatments

The main strengths of Five Element Constitutional Acupuncture

- The focus of treatment on the CF or Constitutional Factor which is the underlying weakness of the patient.
- The attention to rapport-making skills. This leads to both trust and commitment from the patient

and to a more internal approach when diagnosing and understanding the patient.

- The notion of 'Officials' rather than Organs and the fact that the understanding of the Organ function is applied to the body, mind and spirit. For example, the Small Intestine 'separates the pure from impure' mentally and spiritually as well as physically. Inability to 'sort things out' mentally can lead to patients feeling unfocused and muzzy-headed and having a lack of discrimination in many areas of their lives including their relationships, work and friendships.
- The notion that treatment can be focused more on one particular level of the person through point selection and intention.
- The recognition of the emotion as an important indicator of and cause of disease. The ability to emotion 'test' in order to find which emotion is the least fluent and most inappropriate.
- The ability to strengthen a person's underlying imbalance in order to relieve symptoms and to prevent illness.
- The understanding of the major blocks (Aggressive Energy, Husband–Wife, possession and Exit–Entry) and how to correct them.
- The importance of using pulse taking to assess the change in the patient during and after a treatment. The importance of the overall balance and harmony of the pulses.
- Minimum intervention, relying on the *sheng* and *ke* cycles to create change in Elements not treated directly.

The main strengths of TCM

- The understanding of the importance of diagnosing and treating a patient's *yin/yang* balance.
- The use of the theory of the Substances (*qi*, blood, *jing*, body fluids and *shen*) in diagnosis. Use of these Substances enables the practitioner to identify signs and symptoms that are grouped together to form patterns of disharmony. For example, patients may be diagnosed as being Heart Blood deficient if they have a number of signs and symptoms including being anxious, easily startled, have poor sleep, poor concentration and postural dizziness.

- The understanding of Pathogenic Factors and their importance as blocks to treatment and also how to clear them and understand their causes. This leads to the understanding of how to treat acute illnesses and the associated process of diagnosis, needling and frequency of treatment.
- The awareness of how the pathology of *yin/yang*, the Organs, Substances and Pathogenic Factors form together as syndromes. This leads to a greater understanding of why a patient's pathology can lead to the manifestation of certain signs and symptoms.
- The recognition of lifestyle and diet as a cause of disease (and linked to syndromes), thus providing a basis for advice to patients.
- The recognition that a problem can sometimes originate in a channel rather than an Organ. 'Channel problems' often cause joint conditions and also acute infections.
- The importance of pulse taking using the 28 qualities. This is geared to the recognition of the disharmony of *yin/yang*, the functions of the Organs, the Substances and the Pathogenic Factors.
- Understanding tongue diagnosis and that this is also linked to the recognition of the disharmony of *yin/yang*, the functions of the Organs, the Substances and the Pathogenic Factors.

Patterns of integration

In an integrated approach to diagnosing and treating, the patterns of the CF and the TCM syndromes form a hierarchy of four levels.

At the deepest level are the five CF patterns, which are mainly diagnosed by the signs of colour, sound, emotion and odour. The CF affects people's core values and beliefs, which in turn influences their emotions and behaviour.

The next level is the basic deficiencies and stagnations associated with the various Organs. These often arise directly from the underlying constitutional imbalance or CF, although they can also arise from other Organs that are under strain. Some examples of these are Spleen *yang* deficiency, Kidney *yin* deficiency, Heart Blood deficiency and Liver *qi* stagnation. The diagnosis of the basic syndromes involves colour, pulse, tongue and various physical symptoms.

Table 47.3 Comparison of patterns within the integrated style

Pattern	Theoretical basis	Recognition: signs and symptoms	Level
CF (Wood, Fire, Earth, Metal or Water)	Element and Officials	Colour Sound Emotion Odour	Affects person at level of identity, core values and beliefs, which in turn affects spirit, mind, emotions and behaviour and leads to syndromes
Basic syndromes (*qi*, blood, *yin* or *yang* deficiency or *qi* stagnation)	Function of the Organs in terms of Substances and *yin/yang*	Pulse Tongue Colour Symptoms	Affects person and bodily functions
Secondary syndromes (Wind, Cold, Damp, Heat or Dryness or Phlegm or Blood stagnation)	Function of the Organs and Pathogenic Factors	Symptoms Pulse Colour Tongue	Affects bodily functions
Channel problems (Acute or chronic problems that have entered the channel but not the Organ)	Knowledge of channels and possible symptomatology	Varying symptoms	Body/channels

The third level, which we call secondary syndromes, involves Pathogenic Factors. Some examples of these are Damp–Heat in the Large Intestine or Cold invading the Stomach. The diagnosis of these is mainly based on symptoms and, to some degree, tongue and pulse signs.

The last level is a channel problem where there is a blockage at a superficial level within a channel and which does not affect the Organ itself. The main symptoms arising from channel problems are musculo-skeletal problems and some acute infections that have not penetrated further into the body.

Table 47.3 illustrates this hierarchy of the patterns of the CF and syndromes. The next chapter (Chapter 48) describes how the two styles are integrated with examples of case histories.

Summary

1 Five Element Constitutional Acupuncture can be used effectively as a style on its own.

2 There are many similarities between TCM and Five Element Constitutional Acupuncture, as they both stem from a common root and tradition. There are also fundamental differences.

3 Integration of two styles allows the two profound paradigms, *yin/yang* and the Five Elements, to be used together.

4 Integration gives the practitioner a wide range of therapeutic possibilities for treating both acute and chronic conditions, as well as enhancing the patient's general well-being.

Case histories illustrating integrated diagnosis and treatment

48

Introduction

The previous chapter described the similarities and differences between Five Element Constitutional Acupuncture and TCM and the strengths and weaknesses of each. This chapter will now take the practitioner through the main stages of an integrated diagnosis and treatment. The purpose of integrated treatment is to give patients a chance to thrive with minimum intervention from treatment. Some general principles for the practitioner to follow when integrating the two styles of treatment are as follows.

- Use the first treatments to confirm the CF. Diagnosis is only a working hypothesis until confirmed by the patient's response to treatment. Because treatment on the CF will affect many other treatment principles, the practitioner often concentrates on using the first few treatments to resolve any areas of uncertainty about it. At this stage the practitioner is therefore less likely to treat other obvious pathologies, such as Blood, *yin* or *qi* deficiency.
- Clear any blocks to treatment if they are severe enough to hold back progress. Aggressive Energy, Possession, Husband–Wife and Entry–Exit blocks should always be cleared first.
- Clear full conditions caused by Pathogenic Factors, Phlegm and Blood Stagnation if they are severe enough to stop treatment on the CF from being successful. If the condition is overwhelmingly full, for example an acute infection, the CF should not be treated at all. The practitioner needs to find a balance between clearing and tonifying when a patient has a mixed condition, i.e. full conditions with marked underlying deficiencies. Because the presence of Pathogenic Factors is often diagnosed more easily than the CF and other deficiencies, there is a tendency for some practitioners to concentrate on clearing pathogens to the detriment of tonifying.
- If treatment on the CF is not generating sufficient improvement in certain signs and symptoms, more treatment principles can be added. Minimum intervention remains a guiding principle.
- If necessary, consider treatment principles that differentiate whether the CF is more *yin* or *yang* deficient or has any substance pathologies such as *qi* or Blood deficient or stagnant.

These principles of integration will be demonstrated using case histories of some patients who have benefited from treatment.

The stages of making an integrated diagnosis and treatment are as follows:

- take the case history – make rapport, ask specific questions and assess the emotions
- make a diagnosis
- draw a diagram of the diagnosis

- formulate treatment principles
- simplify and prioritise the treatment principles
- form a treatment strategy
- decide on points
- carry out the treatment

Case history 1 – Howard

Introduction and making rapport

The case history

Howard was 58 years old and married with two grown-up children. The elder was from a previous marriage. The practitioner's first impression of him was of a friendly and amicable person. He was of medium height and slightly overweight. Howard was out of breath climbing the flight of stairs to the treatment room. He commented as he sat down that he could feel his heart beating from the climb. His main complaint was asthma.

The practitioner first asked Howard to say something about himself – this was in order to get to know him and gain rapport. Howard responded by telling her that he was a school caretaker and that he had been in his job for 25 years and loved it.

Howard was chatty and warm and laughed a lot. He was often making jokes – sometimes at his own expense. (*The practitioner noticed that when given respect or when talking about some poor treatment he had received for his asthma, he would laugh rather than express grief, anger or other emotions. At other times his joy would drop, especially when the practitioner stopped chatting and wrote some notes. At these times he seemed momentarily sad and vulnerable. His joy would then come up again when the conversation recommenced.*)

Main complaint

The diagnosis continued with the practitioner asking him for more specific details about his main complaint. The asthma began over 20 years ago. He had had a bout of bronchitis with frequent coughing so had decided to give up smoking. A couple of days later he developed bronchial asthma and had had it ever since. 'Maybe I should start smoking again!' he quipped.

He described feeling as if a 'brick' was sitting across his chest. He felt as if couldn't get any more air into his lungs as they felt so full and congested. Occasionally he would bring up some thick white phlegm. He also said that his chest was much worse when lying down and he slept with at least three pillows most of the time.

The asthma was controlled by inhalers but as soon as he had a cold or flu it would go to his chest and he would often have a full-blown asthma attack. The last one had been two months ago and he had been taken into hospital and 'pumped full of steroids'. He admitted that he was scared of this happening again and that was why he had come for treatment. (*The practitioner judged that considering the seriousness of the situation that the way he expressed his fear was appropriate.*)

Questioning the systems

Howard said that his sleep was 'dreadful'. It was light and the smallest thing would wake him, even the birds singing. He got off to sleep easily but would then wake at 2–3 a.m. and couldn't get off again. He would then go to sleep after what seemed like a long time and would wake with a muzzy head. (*When the practitioner offered him sympathy about his poor sleep Howard accepted it.*)

Howard said his appetite was 'too good' and he loved to eat. He would often consume dairy products and had a hot milky drink before bed, 'to help him sleep'. He would often bloat after eating and would have loose stools which didn't have a strong odour.

Howard also said he had poor energy and said he felt 'totally worn out'. He loved his job but whereas once it had been easy, it now exhausted him and he was wondering whether it was time to retire.

The practitioner continued to ask Howard specific questions about his health such as thirst, urination and perspiration, and wrote down all of Howard's answers. At the same time she assessed how Howard responded emotionally to her questions.

Personal history

She also asked Howard about his health history, his family health and his personal history. This included questions about areas such as his childhood, emotional stresses, difficult phases in his life and relationships, as well as which areas of his life were most problematic for him. These were all important to get to know Howard as a person. The questions are also important to get a sense of the balance of a patient's emotions. This is easier when they are talking about difficult issues in their life than when describing less problematical topics like perspiration, urination, etc.

Howard described having a happy childhood: 'I always had lots of friends and I could always make them laugh.' He also said that he was generally happy with his life at present but that he thought he suffered from Seasonal Affective Disorder (SAD) and got quite depressed in the winter: 'We're going to move to Italy in the winter months.' He said he thought it had got worse as he became older. When questioned more about this he said things were generally fine and that he didn't wish to dwell on his difficulties. He did, however, mention in passing that his elder daughter from his first marriage was dependent on heroin and this caused him much pain and sadness. He had tried to help her but she didn't seem to want to help herself. (*He looked very sad when talking about this issue. The practitioner noted that she might talk with him some more about this later.*) When asked about his current wife, he laughed and said everything was 'fine', but his eyes and facial expression belied this.

Howard's pulses

Howard's pulses all felt deficient and the practitioner wrote down this pulse picture:

Left		Right	
SI –1	Ht –1 (Floating)	Lu – ½ (Floating)	LI – ½ (Floating)
GB – ½	Liv – ½	Sp – 1½ (Slippery)	St – ½ (Slippery)
Bl – ½	Kid – 1½ (Deep)	PC – 1½	TB –1½ (Deep)

Tongue diagnosis

Howard had a pale, swollen tongue with a midline crack going to the tip. At the rear of the tongue he had a sticky white tongue coating. The tip was redder than the main tongue body.

Physical examination

Having taken Howard's pulses and looked at his tongue, the practitioner carried out other parts of the physical diagnosis such as feeling his three *jiao*, palpating the front *mu* and back *shu* points, testing the Akabane and observing his colour, sound and odour. After the diagnosis was completed and Howard had left, the practitioner went over all the information she had written down. She then wrote up the diagnosis, including drawing a diagnostic diagram.

Diagnosis

Forming a diagnosis

The practitioner knew that she needed to diagnose Howard's whole condition in order for both the root and the manifestation of his problem to improve. This meant that she should identify all of the patterns present. This included his CF as well as any syndromes that were present.

She put these together and drew a diagram. The purpose of the diagram was to give the practitioner an overview of the diagnosis. The diagram could connect Howard's 'patterns' aetiologically and bring in specific internal, external and miscellaneous causes of various patterns. The practitioner also included the signs and symptoms supporting each pattern. This allowed for easier monitoring of Howard's progress.

Howard's CF

The practitioner opted for Howard being a Fire CF. This is because he laughed inappropriately and showed excess joy even when he might have become angry, or suffused with grief. He also showed appropriate fear and accepted sympathy appropriately. At the same time he would drop into sadness and seemed vulnerable and uncertain when the practitioner stopped chatting.

Howard did not want to dwell on his difficulties when questioned. Although he admitted to having SAD in the winter months he did not wish to talk about this and he mentioned but didn't talk in any depth about his daughter's dependency on heroin. He preferred to laugh, chat and joke. Keeping his cup 'half full' was probably a positive way for him to deal with his difficulties – but this was to the detriment of looking at his whole situation and was probably contributing to his underlying depressed condition. To back up the diagnosis of Fire, the practitioner saw a lack of red colour by the side of Howard's eyes and smelt a scorched odour.

The practitioner thought that some of Howard's treatment would need to be directed towards the level of his spirit. She hoped that when Howard felt stronger and trusted her he would probably be able to open up and talk more about himself.

The practitioner also considered whether Howard was suffering from possession, had a Husband–Wife imbalance or had an Entry–Exit block. She did not think that any of these were present.

Making a diagram

Figure 48.1 shows the diagram drawn up by the practitioner. The oblong boxes indicate the main patterns. The oval boxes indicate aetiology and the main signs or symptoms are written next to the boxes. The boxes are joined up by arrows that indicate in which direction the patterns probably affect each other – sometimes the arrow travels in two

directions, indicating that the patterns are both affecting each other.

The diagram shows all of Howard's patterns including the CF. Because the CF underlies all of the other patterns, it is placed at the top of the diagram. Usually (but not always) the CF and the other patterns will involve some of the same Organs. In this case Howard's constitutional imbalance in Fire has led to Heart *qi* and Heart *yin* deficiency. The diagram also describes how the Phlegm–Damp has probably been formed. The cause is likely to be from a combination of a number of factors which are:

1. the constitutional Fire imbalance, which has led to a weak chest and *zong qi*
2. a poor diet with too many Phlegm-forming foods
3. colds (invasions of Wind–Cold) which easily go to the chest

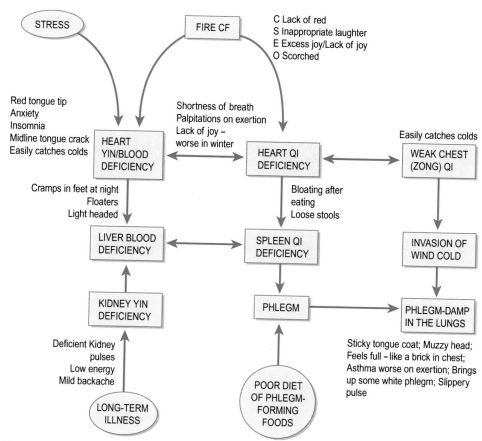

Figure 48.1 • Diagnosis diagram for Howard

Treatment planning

Forming treatment principles

The next stage in the diagnosis is for the practitioner to form treatment principles. These inform the practitioner in the choice of points. The main treatment principles involved in a Five Element diagnosis would be to 'Treat the CF' or to deal with a block such as Aggressive Energy, Possession, Husband–Wife imbalance or Entry–Exit block.

A TCM practitioner would use treatment principles to decide whether to tonify the deficient patterns and to clear full ones.

Putting these together into an integrated diagnosis allows the practitioner to have an overview of all of the treatment priorities – so the first stage of planning treatment is to list all possible treatment principles:

* treat Fire CF
* tonify Heart *qi*
* nourish Heart *yin*
* tonify *zong qi*
* clear Wind–Cold when present
* nourish Liver Blood
* tonify Spleen *qi*
* clear Phlegm
* clear Phlegm–Damp from the Lungs

If the practitioner used all of the patterns listed in the boxes above the result would be confusing. There would be far too many treatment principles. The next stages are to simplify and then prioritise the treatment principles.

Simplifying the treatment principles

In order to simplify the treatment principles, the practitioner eliminated all treatment principles that she believed to be unnecessary. Most of these were ones she expected to be resolved when dealing with other treatment principles.

Some of the treatment principles could easily be simplified. For example, on reflection 'nourish Liver Blood' could be taken out as the Blood deficiency had probably come from the Heart Blood deficiency (more likely as Fire is her CF) combined with Spleen *qi* deficiency. The Wind–Cold was only present occasionally so need not be listed as a main treatment principle. Treating the Fire CF and the treatment principles to do with Heart syndromes could also be merged together. A patient often has syndromes

that are on the same Organ as the CF and the practitioner can often find one or more points that can deal with both of these at the same time.

The practitioner was now left with a smaller number of treatment principles. This was less awkward and made it easier to plan a treatment and choose points. The Treatment principles are now listed as:

* treat Fire CF by tonifying Heart *qi* and Heart *yin*
* tonify Spleen *qi*
* clear Phlegm–Damp from the Lungs
* tonify *zong qi*

Prioritising the treatment principles

The next stage was for the practitioner to prioritise the treatment principles. In order to prioritise the practitioner considered which of the remaining treatment principles she should concentrate on and in which order to use them. To do this, the practitioner listed the treatment principles and put the first and second treatment principles at the top as she thought they were the main priorities. The other three treatment principles were put in brackets as they would not be used immediately but might be brought in later. The list now looks like this:

* treat Fire CF (by tonifying Heart *qi* and nourishing Heart *yin*)
* clear Phlegm–Damp
* (tonify *zong qi*)
* (tonify Spleen *qi*)

She also added:

* (clear Wind–Cold when necessary)

Treatment strategy

The practitioner has now formed a treatment strategy. From the final five treatment principles she decided that her main treatment priorities were to tonify the Fire CF and to clear the Phlegm–Damp from the Lungs. The Phlegm–Damp is causing so much congestion that she thought it needed to be cleared early on in treatment. She recognised that when treating Howard's Fire Element she is likely to need to treat at the spirit level.

She doesn't yet know which of the four Fire 'Officials' are the main ones associated with what she considers to be Howard's CF. It could either be Howard's Pericardium and Triple Burner or his Heart and Small Intestine. She decided to find this out by treating the Pericardium and Triple Burner first and monitoring the response. If the response was not good she would then go on and treat the Heart and Small Intestine. Although the syndromes connected to the Fire CF were Heart syndromes, this did not mean that the Heart was the Organ of the CF as the Heart syndromes also cover the Pericardium.

The practitioner had one more treatment principle she wished to add. This was to test for Aggressive Energy before embarking on any further treatment. This is routinely carried out at the start of the first treatment. Aggressive Energy could have been present because the patient had taken quite a few medicinal drugs for his asthma. He also has some heat signs such as a red tongue tip – so heat could have become trapped in the Organs (see Chapter 30, this volume, for more on this). The practitioner decided not to use moxa as the patient had too many signs of heat.

If Howard had any signs of Wind–Cold invading he was told to ring and arrange treatment immediately so that the practitioner could clear the pathogen before it affected the chest and caused more problems with his asthma.

Treatment

Stages of treatment

For the first treatment the practitioner had three main treatment principles which were:

* test for Aggressive Energy
* treat Fire CF
* clear Phlegm–Damp

If there was no Aggressive Energy the practitioner had decided to test the Fire to see if it was the CF. She decided not to bring in the treatment principle of Clearing Phlegm–Damp on the first treatment. Keeping the treatment simple would not cloud the picture and the practitioner would be clear about how the points affect the patient.

Choosing points

Points for testing for Aggressive Energy

The points for testing Aggressive Energy are Bl 13 (Lung), 14 (Pericardium), 18 (Liver), 20 (Spleen) and 23 (Kidney) + check needles on non points in each of the *jiaos*. The needles are left in at a very superficial level and the practitioner waits to see if an erythema forms around the needle.

Points for testing the CF

The points for testing the CF would be TB 4 and PC 7, and they are tonified without retention. If the pulse response to these is poor, then the practitioner may choose to move on to treat the Heart and Small Intestine. In this case she would tonify Ht 7 and SI 4. Other points on the channels of the CF will be used in later treatments.

Points for clearing the Phlegm–Damp

Points for clearing the Phlegm–Damp could be Lu 5 and St 40 and the needle technique would be 'even'. The practitioner did not use reduction as Howard had an underlying deficiency.

Treatment 1

At the first treatment there was no Aggressive Energy present. The practitioner then used TB 4 and tonified without retention. There was a small pulse change and the pulses felt marginally less deficient.

The second point tonified was PC 7. After this both of the first positions became less floating. There was still a slightly slippery pulse on the Stomach/ Spleen but overall the pulses felt more harmonious and stronger. The practitioner was pleased with this change and decided that this was enough treatment.

Left		Right	
SI –1	Ht –1	Lu –1	LI –1
GB – ½	Liv – ½	Sp – ½	St – ½ (Slippery)
Bl –1	Kid –1 (Deep)	PC –1	TB –1 (Deep)

Treatment 2

Howard reported that he felt much better after treatment. He had more energy, especially at the end of the day. He had also slept better for the first three nights and his recovery rate was much better after exercise. His chest, however, didn't feel much better and it still felt like there was a weight on it. He was still bringing up some phlegm.

Because his chest had not responded the practitioner decided to add one treatment principle and to:

* resolve Phlegm–Damp in the chest
* continue to test the CF.

The first points the practitioner used were Lu 5 and St 40 'even'. After this the pulses all felt slightly more settled and the slippery quality on the Stomach and Spleen diminished. Next she tonified PC 9 and TB 3. These are the tonification points which pull the slightly fuller energy from the Wood Element into the Fire. Howard's pulses felt much more harmonious after treatment.

Left		Right	
SI – ½	Ht – ½	Lu – ½	LI – ½
GB – ½	Liv – ½	Sp – ½	St – ½
Bl –1	Kid –1 (Deep)	PC –1	TB –1 (Deep)

Further treatments

Over the next few months Howard's treatment progressed well. During this time the practitioner cleared Phlegm–Damp for a further five treatments. She used Lu 5 and St 40 and also points such as *Ren* 17 and Lu 1, all with 'even' technique. Howard gradually cut down on his inhalers and also kept his doctor informed of his progress. After 11 treatments he had reduced his Becloforte and Atrovent from 3 to 1 puffs a day. He also hadn't taken Ventolin for 'weeks'. Howard also cut down on 'Phlegm-forming' foods, specifically eating less dairy products and fatty foods. This also helped his chest to become clearer. Howard was treated weekly at first but as he progressed the practitioner spread out the treatments to two-weekly and then on to three- and four-weekly.

On the sixth treatment Howard came in with the beginnings of a cold with a swollen throat, a runny nose and a slight headache. The practitioner 'released the exterior' and 'cleared Wind–Cold' by placing cups on Howard's back over Bl 12 and 13 and using Lu 7 and LI 4 with a mild reducing technique. Howard's cold did not go to his chest, indicating that Howard was probably stronger than before.

As well as Howard's asthma improving, he also had other changes which were profound. By the eighth treatment he was sleeping much better and only occasionally having a bad night's sleep. He also had more energy and reported finding it easier to climb stairs. He still felt somewhat bloated after eating but his loose stools were much better. Although these were symptoms of Spleen *qi* deficiency, the practitioner had not needed to tonify his Spleen as by treating the mother (the Pericardium), the child (the Spleen) had responded.

After 10 treatments Howard told his practitioner he was feeling much happier than before. He said that he hadn't realised how depressed and anxious he had been. It was his nature to be positive, but beneath that positive exterior he had been very unhappy. Now he could be positive without having to force it. The practitioner noticed that Howard did not seem to be so 'high' for much of the time but seemed more balanced and calm in his temperament.

As time went on and Howard's Heart-Protector improved he felt more able to talk about personal issues and was encouraged to talk openly with his wife about his sadness about his daughter from his first marriage. He told his practitioner that 'a problem shared is a problem halved'. Although he could not change the situation he found that she wanted to listen to his worries. 'I've always felt that I shouldn't talk about my difficulties. Now I know I'm liked for who I am, not whether I'm happy or not.'

Later on in treatment the practitioner tested points on the Heart and Small Intestine, but the best change came from treating Pericardium and Triple Burner, so treatment was predominantly focused on this side of Fire.

One of the treatment principles listed was to strengthen the *zong qi*. The practitioner did not find any need to use points on Howard's Lungs as he progressed so well from treatment on the Pericardium and Triple Burner and this in itself strengthened the *zong qi*.

Some of the points the practitioner used to treat Howard's CF were:

- PC 7 and TB 4 (source points)
- PC 9 and TB 3 (tonification points)
- Bl 14 and Bl 22 (back *shu* points)
- PC 6 and TB 5 (Inner and Outer Frontier Gate)
- *Ren* 15 (to treat the spirit)
- PC 2 (Heavenly Pond to treat the spirit)
- Bl 43 (to strengthen deficiency and treat the spirit)

Below are some of the combinations of points used in Howard's treatments:

- Lu 5, *Ren* 17, St 40 (even); PC 6 and TB 5 (tonify)
- Lu 5, St 40, Lu 1 (even); *Ren* 15 and *Ren* 4, PC 7 and TB 4 (tonify)
- *Ren* 17 and Lu 1 (even); Bl 43 and Bl 22 (tonify)
- St 40, Lu 5 (even); PC 9, TB 3 and PC 2 (tonify)

The integrated treatment

The integrated practitioner treats both the CF and the syndromes. If Howard had had his CF treated but not the Phlegm–Damp, he may have felt better in himself but his chest may not have improved as it would have been difficult to shift the pathogen without direct treatment. On the other hand, if the Phlegm–Damp had been treated as well as the underlying Spleen or Lung deficiency, but not the CF, this would have helped Howard's asthma but he would probably have experienced less change in how he 'felt in himself' as a result.

Further examples of integrated diagnosis

The following two case histories with diagrams are shorter than the one above and are designed to provide further examples of integrated diagnosis and treatment.

Case history 2 – Patricia

The case history

Patricia came for treatment having been recommended by a friend. She was 43 years old and had two grown-up children. She worked part-time as a teacher. The practitioner checked that the address she had written down for Patricia was correct. It was wrong. When Patricia realised this she blurted out, 'Well if you can get that wrong you might get my treatment wrong.' The practitioner did not take offence at this but used this piece of information diagnostically – she realised that Patricia was terrified. She could have mistaken her response as anger as it was said forcefully but her eyes and agitated body movements indicated that fear was the emotion. She also realised that she would need to win Patricia's trust before Patricia could comfortably be treated by her. Throughout the diagnosis the practitioner noticed that Patricia looked wary. Over time they seemed to have got over the initial problem about the address but it was difficult for Patricia to settle. Sometimes when asked a personal question Patricia's eyes darted from side to side. At other times she just looked tense and uncomfortable. The practitioner also observed that Patricia's voice had a groaning quality and she had a blue/black colour to the side of her eye.

Main complaint

Patricia told her that her main complaints were migraines and panic attacks. The panic attacks had started three years previously. When one was coming on she noticed that she became dizzy, almost faint, and hot. Her heart would start pounding and voices would sound muffled. She felt a need to go outside and get some fresh air. The panic attacks started when she was going through a divorce and they continued after this was settled. She didn't know what brought them on: 'I can think I'm fine and then suddenly I'll have a panic and I don't know why.' When she had an attack she would take Indovel and this would help it to go away.

Patricia also described having both migraines and headaches. The headaches centred around the eyes and the front of the brow and were 'not very intense'. She had these nearly all of the time. Migraines were brought on by tiredness or were stress related. When she had a migraine her eyes became light sensitive, her vision blurred and her whole head throbbed. She also became irritable and sometimes felt sick. She would feel hotter at these times and would put a cold flannel across her eyes.

Pulse diagnosis

Below is Patricia's pulse picture when she first came for treatment.

Left		Right	
SI –1	Ht –1	LI –1	Lu –1 (All right side thin and floating)
GB –1	Liv –1 (Wiry)	Sp –1	St –1
Bl –2	Kid –2	PC –2	TB –2

Tongue diagnosis

The tongue was pale and slightly swollen. It had a thin white coating and red spots at the tip.

The diagnosis

By the end of the diagnosis Patricia's practitioner had concluded that she was probably a Water CF. This would need to be central to the treatment if it was to get to the root of Patricia's problem. The practitioner had noted the way Patricia responded to joy, sympathy, anger and grief and had concluded that these responses were not significantly inappropriate. None of them induced changes in her voice, eyes, body language, etc. The fear was there all the time, however. It was almost palpable. When she was particularly frightened the practitioner could see the disharmonious movements of *qi* affecting her facial expression, eyes and posture. The practitioner realised that she needed to be reassuring and firm when treating Patricia to ensure that she felt safe when having treatment.

Figure 48.2 shows Patricia's integrated diagnosis and includes other symptoms.

From the diagnosis the practitioner prioritised the treatment principles trying to keep treatment as simple as possible (see previous case history). Minimum intervention is always the goal. The main treatment principles she decided to use were:

- treat Water CF by nourishing Kidney *yin*
- subdue Liver *yang*

Treatment 1

At the start of treatment the practitioner decided to concentrate treatment entirely on the Water CF. This was backed up by the fact that both of Patricia's main complaints had also originated from the Water Element, even though other Elements were involved. The panic attacks were due to Kidney and Heart *yin* deficiency and the migraines to Kidney *yin*

deficiency causing Liver *yin* deficiency and Liver *yang* rising.

Having tapped for Aggressive Energy, which wasn't present, the next stage of treatment was to treat the Water CF. The points the practitioner tonified were the *yuan* source points, Bl 64 and Kid 3. The pulses changed after this and became less floating and also the wiriness on the Liver lessened.

Left		Right	
SI –1	Ht –1	LI –1	Lu –1 (More settled)
GB –1	Liv –1 (Less wiry)	Sp –1	St –1
Bl –2	Kid –2	PC –1½	TB –1½

Treatment 2

Patricia came into the next treatment with a huge smile on her face. She seemed more relaxed and less edgy. She hadn't had a headache since her last period. She also had had only slight signs of panic attacks but they had been much less severe. She had more energy generally even though she didn't realise that she was previously tired. The practitioner treated the Water CF by tonifying Water with Bl 23 and 28 – the back *shu* points – and then used the tonification points Bl 67 and Kid 7.

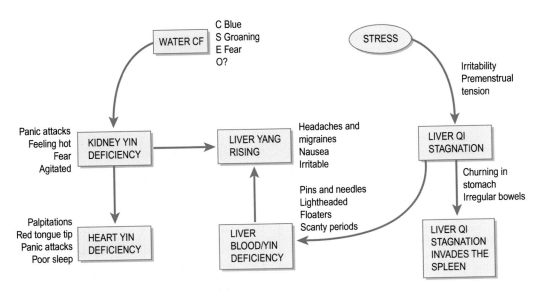

Figure 48.2 • Diagnosis diagram for Patricia

Treatment 3

Patricia continued to improve. The practitioner continued to treat Water and at this point decided to use points to influence the spirit more directly. For this treatment she used Kid 25, Spirit Storehouse. Although Patricia was better in herself she still needed her spirit and reserves supported on a deep level. Without this support the treatment was less likely to hold. As it was the late afternoon the practitioner also added Bl 66 and Kid 10, the horary points, for the Kidney *yin* deficiency.

Treatment 4

Patricia's period was due and she had woken at 6 a.m. with a migraine. She was nauseous and retching. The practitioner decided to treat Patricia's Liver and Gall Bladder directly and subdued Liver *yang* with Liv 2 and GB 38. She then treated the CF tonifying Bl 23 and 52 and Bl 64 and Kid 3.

Further treatments

Patricia continued to make good progress, seeming less wary as she felt the benefits of treatment. Treatment continued to be centred on her Water CF and treating her spirit. The practitioner still subdued the Liver when her period was due. She did not have her Liver Blood nourished as treating the Kidney fed the Liver via the *sheng* cycle.

By the fifth treatment Patricia had come off her Indoval and had had no major panic attacks – although she had a slight dizziness occasionally which disappeared of its own accord. She was much more relaxed and on one occasion even spoke laughingly of her extreme reaction at the start of treatment. She told her practitioner that she felt much stronger and more relaxed in her life generally and that her relationship with her husband had improved as a result.

By the tenth treatment she had had no headaches during the week and had only had slight headaches rather than migraines before her period. Treatment continued and was gradually spread out from two-weekly to monthly. She continues to come on a monthly basis. Her symptoms are much better and she feels considerably more at ease and less stressed.

Case history 3 – Ellena

The case history

Ellena was 60 years old and single. She lived by herself but close to her nephew and sister. When the practitioner met her he had the impression of a person who was gentle and soft, but a bit strange. She talked to herself in the reception, and later when she went to the toilet she left the door slightly open. It emerged during the interview that she had been training as a nurse at the age of 19 and had then been diagnosed as suffering from schizophrenia. She was taking no drugs for this condition and she seemed to be able to speak with some clarity, although without making any real contact with the practitioner.

Main complaint

Her main complaint was a frontal headache which had been caused by a car accident 30 years ago. It injured her head on the left side and she pointed to the Gall Bladder channel. The pain had gradually moved from the side to the front of the head. She now had headaches every two to three weeks; they were an 'irritable ache and discomfort'. She said that hot weather and raw cheese made them worse. It was not clear to her if movement made them better or worse. Later she said, 'I can't concentrate and don't seem to think right. I can't watch TV for a long time – after about half an hour I feel drowsy. It stops me being interested in anything.'

Pulse diagnosis

Left		Right	
SI –1	Ht –1	Lu –1	LI–1 (Generally wiry quality)
GB +1	Liv +1 (Wiry)	St –1	Sp –1 (Wiry/slippery)
Bl –1½	Kid –1½	PC –1	TB –1

The pulses were weak apart from the left-hand side middle position, which was full. The right-hand middle position was slippery. There was a general wiry quality on the pulses.

Tongue diagnosis

The tongue was red-purple at the front and pale red at the back. It had a thickish white coating at the middle and back and it was swollen on the edges with tooth marks.

The diagnosis

The practitioner diagnosed Ellena as being an Earth CF. She had a yellow hue on her face and a fragrant odour. Her voice, however, was quite clipped. Ellena talked incessantly about food throughout the interview and worried a lot about her health – as well as her father's, sister's and brother's health. She complained a lot and often repeated problems over and over again as if continually seeking sympathy and support. She loved it when she was given sympathy and this would often lead to her telling her practitioner in great detail about other problems she had. Ellena, however, also had a somewhat clipped voice and also experienced a lot of frustration in her life.

The practitioner considered whether Ellena was a Wood CF. Her Wood pulses were full and wiry

and she was angry, especially that her sister kept an eye on her and tried to stop her from doing what she wanted to do. The diagram in Figure 48.3 shows Ellena's integrated diagnosis and includes the other symptoms she discussed during the diagnosis.

From the integrated diagnosis the practitioner simplified and then prioritised the treatment principles. The main treatment principles he decided to use were:

- clear Internal Dragons
- clear Phlegm
- treat Earth CF
- move Liver *qi*

Treatment 1

At the first treatment the practitioner decided to clear possession using the Internal Dragons treatment. The patient's symptoms of talking to herself and her lack of awareness of her environment indicated that this treatment was appropriate. The practitioner was unable to make contact with her spirit through her eyes. The 'lights were on but nobody was at home'.

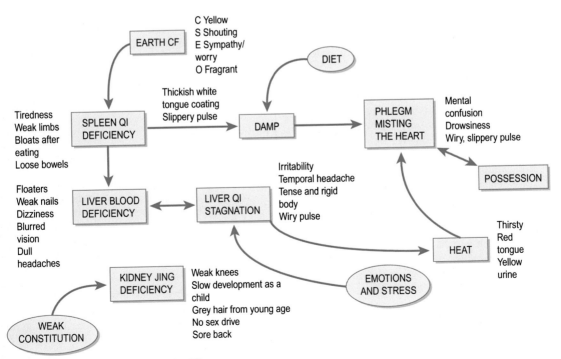

Figure 48.3 • Diagnosis diagram for Ellena

Treatment 2

Following the first treatment she said she felt a little bit better and that her energy was better the following morning. She also commented that several people said she seemed a lot better. The treatment principles for the next treatment were to:

* tap for Aggressive Energy
* clear Phlegm
* test the Earth CF

The test for Aggressive Energy was negative. The practitioner then cleared Phlegm using PC 5 and St 40 (even). The third part of the treatment was to test if she was an Earth CF by tonifying the source points St 42 and Sp 3. After treatment the pulses felt softer and less wiry. The most dramatic pulse change was after treating the CF. As treating Earth had a very positive response on the Wood pulses, it strongly indicated that Earth was the primary imbalance rather than the other way around.

Left		Right	
SI –1	Ht–1	Lu –1	LI –1 (All pulses softer and more harmonious)
GB ✓	Liv ✓	St –1	Sp –1
Bl –1	Kid –1	PC –1	TB –1

Treatment 3

On returning from the treatment Ellena told her practitioner that she had slept really well and that her energy was a bit better. Her stomach had been a bit upset in the morning. She had had a headache which lasted a day with the pain coming and going. The pain, however, was not as strong as before.

The treatment principles for the third treatment were to continue to:

* clear Phlegm
* treat Earth CF

For this treatment the practitioner used the points PC 5 and St 40 again. He then treated the CF with St 36 and Sp 6 (tonify).

After this treatment Ellena reported that her appetite was better and she was enjoying more foods than before. Her energy had also been better. She also had had no headache at all during the week. The practitioner also noted that the patient called

him by his name for the first time and seemed to be more aware of him as a person.

Further treatments

The three treatment principles below were the main ones used for the following five treatments:

* clear Phlegm
* move Liver *qi*
* treat Earth CF

The practitioner decided to add the treatment principle to move Liver *qi* as she had a lot of frustration about her current situation. Moving the Liver *qi* also helped to move the Phlegm. During this time Ellena continued to feel better and even started looking for a job. Her sister, finding that she was so much better, did not keep such a close eye on her all of the time. She consequently felt more relaxed. The biggest changes came about whenever the CF was treated. Some spirit points were used later on in treatment. These included:

* St 25 Heavenly Pivot
* Bl 49 *Yi* Dwelling – the outer back *shu* point of the Spleen
* Sp 20 Encircling Glory
* Sp 18 Heavenly Stream
* St 9 People Welcome – The Window of the Sky

Ellena stopped treatment after 12 treatments when she moved to another part of the country. By this time she felt she was well enough to do without any more treatment. Her practitioner thought she could benefit from further treatments and suggested she go to a practitioner near to where she was moving. As yet it is unclear whether she has taken this up.

Conclusion

The reason for integrating these two styles of treatment is that they complement each other in many ways. Integration allows a practitioner to have an increased range in both the depth and breadth of treatment. This includes an expansion in practical areas such as needle technique, pulse taking and observation or in theoretical areas such as blocks to treatment or the functions of points taught by each style. Using these two styles together allows the practitioner to treat all levels of the patient's body, mind and spirit, as well as acute and chronic problems or problems arising from external, internal or miscellaneous causes.

TCM predominantly focuses on pathologies as they affect the *qi* of body. In this way it offers much to the practitioner of Five Element Constitutional Acupuncture. Howard, for example, had severe Phlegm, which was diagnosed by pulse, tongue and the nature of the asthma. Treatment on the CF alone, nourishing the root, may have cleared it over time, but the TCM treatment protocol of clearing Phlegm yielded rapid improvement. At the same time diagnosis of the constitutional imbalance, the CF, and simple treatments can affect patients at a deep level and profoundly influence how they feel in themselves. Simple treatments on the CF can also eliminate the need for a larger number of treatment principles and thus reduce the number of points used.

TCM offers a more analytical approach to understanding pathology than does the Five Element approach and this is a great strength. Five Element Constitutional Acupuncture is a more intuitive style that focuses on the nature of the person rather than the nature of the illness. An integration of the two styles allows the practitioner to combine the two disciplines that should always form the basis of medical practice, science and art. As the great physician Xu Dachun said:

> Illnesses may be identical, but the persons suffering from them are different.
>
> (Unschuld, 1990, p. 17)

Summary

1 The purpose of integrated treatment is to give patients a chance to thrive with minimum intervention from treatment.

2 Use the first treatments to confirm the CF.

3 Clear any blocks to treatment if they are severe enough to hold back progress.

4 Clear full conditions caused by Pathogenic Factors, Phlegm and Blood stagnation if they are severe enough to stop treatment on the CF from being successful.

5 If treatment on the CF is not generating sufficient improvement in certain signs and symptoms, more treatment principles can be added.

6 Using these two styles together allows the practitioner to treat all levels of the patient's body, mind and spirit, as well as acute and chronic problems or problems arising from external, internal or miscellaneous causes.

Appendix A: Different terms used to describe the spirit

It is useful to consider some terms used to describe the spirit in Chinese medicine. *Shen* is the most commonly used and, depending on the context, means either the spirit of the Heart or the person's spirit in a more generalised sense. The *shen, po, hun, yi* and *zhi* are the spirits of the five major *yin* Organs. They are described in the chapters on the Organs with which they are associated. Two other terms are also used – *jing-shen* and *ling*.

Jing-shen

Jing-shen is the term in Chinese medicine that most closely accords with the use of the word 'spirit', in the way it is used by practitioners of Five Element Constitutional Acupuncture. The following description from an early text describes *jing-shen* thus:

> The *jing-shen* lives in the body like the flame blazing in the candle.
>
> (Loewe, 1993, pp. 154–155)

Like *shen, jing-shen* means different things in different contexts. All the modern Chinese terms that are used to translate English words that start with the prefix 'psycho-' start with *jing-shen*. For example, mental illness is *jing-shen bing* and psychiatry is *jing-shen bing xue*. It can also mean the 'vigour' or 'vitality' that a person exhibits when their body and spirit are both healthy.

In earlier times *jing-shen* meant that combination of inherited temperament and human individuality which constitutes the human spirit.

> The combination of blood and *qi*, the association of essences and spirits (*jing-shen*), this is what makes life, perfectly fulfilling the natural destiny (*xing ming*) of each.
>
> (*Ling Shu* Chapter 47; Lu, 1972)

In an important article on early Daoist concepts of the spirit, the *jing-shen* is defined as 'a rarefied form of *jing* and the manifestation of the transcendent *shen* within the physiological system' (Roth, 1986).

Darwinists attribute significant amounts of human behaviour to man's inherent drive to ensure the survival of the species (for example *The Selfish Gene*, by Richard Dawkins). What many consider to be the strongest driving force in an animal or human, the drive to survive when threatened, is carried in the *jing* and the Kidneys. Fear, the most underlying emotion of all, is the emotion that resonates with the Kidneys.

The concept of *jing-shen* conveys man's dual nature, part animal, part spirit. Animals possess *jing* but they do not possess *shen*. It is the *shen* that gives people their glory, the miracle of human consciousness. Only humans, standing between Heaven and Earth, possess *jing-shen* (see Jarret, 1998, p. 83).

> *Jing* represents any substance full of life, while *shen* represents the heavenly inspiration in each person. *Jing shen* expresses the origin and unfoldment of Heaven and Earth in man.
>
> (Unschuld, 1989, p. 70)

Ling

The *ling* is of crucial importance in acupuncture. It is this character that gives the great classic of acupuncture the *Ling Shu*, usually translated as the 'Spiritual Pivot', its name. *Ling* is also usually translated as 'spirit' when it occurs in the names of five of the acupuncture points (Ht 2, Ht 4, Kid 24, GB 18, and *Du* 10; *shen* also appears in six point names – Ht 7, *Du* 11, *Ren* 8, Bl 44, and Kid 23 and 25).

The character shows rain falling from Heaven onto three mouths and below that, two female shamans dancing. The role of the shaman was to cultivate her or his *ling* in order to draw down the benefits of Heaven on the community.

Ling refers to a calm internal receptive capacity. This is necessary for a person to be able to live in harmony with Heaven. The *ling* was perceived as the *yin* counterpart to the more *yang shen*. The *shen* 'radiates' from the person's eyes whereas the *ling*, which is more *yin*, cannot be discerned so easily from the outside. The radiance of the *shen* is dependent upon the state of the person's *ling*, just as their *yang* is always dependent upon their *yin*. (See Jarret, 1998, pp. 51–56. More on the *ling* can be found in Yang, 1997, p. 28.) In approximately −200 in the *Ta Tai Li* it says:

> The *jing qi* of the *yang* is called *shen*. The *jing qi* of the *yin* is called *ling*. The *shen* and the *ling* are the root of all living creatures.
>
> (Needham, 1956, p. 269)

Like the *shen*, the *ling* only exists in humans and does not exist in lower animals.

No mention is made of *ling* in contemporary Chinese medical books and it can be assumed that this is because the concept is tainted by its shamanistic connotations.

Appendix B: The external and miscellaneous causes of disease

The external causes of disease

The external causes of disease are climatic conditions. They are Wind, Cold, Damp, Dryness, Summer Heat and Fire. They can affect the body either singly or in a combination of two or more pathogens. Under normal circumstances most people can easily 'brave the elements' without being adversely affected by them. There are two common situations when climatic factors can have a detrimental effect. The first is when a person's qi is not strong. This makes them susceptible to certain climatic conditions. The second is if the climatic influence is extreme or prolonged and therefore people can't resist it. People tend to be affected by the climate to which they are most susceptible. For example, people who feel the cold easily are more susceptible to 'Cold' conditions, whereas those of a hotter constitution will be more easily affected by 'Heat'. Some people are more susceptible to Damp weather whilst others are most affected by Wind or Dryness.

Wind

'Wind' (feng) in the body closely matches what the Chinese observed in the environment. Wind is something that arises suddenly and goes through many rapid changes. It is often located on the outside of the body and moves in an upward direction. Wind can also make the body shake. Any symptom with these qualities is called Wind. For example, the common cold or influenza has many of these qualities, as do joint pains that move from place to place in the body. Wind can include windy weather, draughts, fans or air conditioning as well as sudden change in temperature, such as moving from a warm building into the cold. Prolonged exposure to this climate can cause Wind but it is diagnosed by the presence of the symptoms of Wind rather than by knowing the cause.

Cold

Cold (han) stops normal movement and warmth and causes the tissues to contract. This contraction causes pain. Pain from cold is intense and 'biting' in nature and is relieved by applying warmth. Chilblains or frostbite are two of the most obvious results of cold. Cold can penetrate the tendons and cause the joints to become painful, white and contracted. It can also cause some abdominal pain leading to menstrual cramps, diarrhoea, epigastric pain or an inability to digest food. Cold puts extra stress on the organs of those who are already ill, especially old and frail people. As with Wind, Cold is diagnosed by the presence of the symptoms of Cold rather than by knowing that the patient has been caught in cold conditions.

Damp

Damp is a common cause of disease for many people in Britain and other countries that are wet or humid. Living in a damp house, staying by or on water, remaining in wet clothes or sitting on damp grass can all affect people who are vulnerable to this condition. Damp is heavy in nature and causes people to feel sluggish and stiff. It mainly affects the lower half of the body. Unlike Wind, which comes and goes quickly, Damp is 'sticky and lingering' and is therefore more difficult to clear. Symptoms of Damp include a stuffy chest, a bloated stomach or abdomen, feeling heavy headed or poor concentration. In the lower part of the body it can cause bowel problems, fluid retention, discharges or a heavy feeling in the legs. Damp often creates a desire to lie down. Like the Wind and Cold, Damp is diagnosed by the presence of the symptoms.

Dryness

Dryness is most common in hot, dry areas such as Arizona. Alternatively it can arise from central heating or during aeroplane flights. It is rarely found in damp countries like Britain. Dryness can create any 'dry' symptoms such as a dry nose, throat, lungs or dry skin. The presence of the symptoms of dryness in the body is enough to make a diagnosis and patients may not have been aware of having been in a dry atmosphere.

Summer Heat and Fire

Summer Heat and Fire are similar although not identical. Summer Heat is more likely to arise from the external environment, for example, spending too long in the sun or in places like hot kitchens or laundries. Fire, on the other hand, arises from the inside and is slightly more 'solid' than summer heat. It can be caused if the other pathogenic factors of Wind, Cold, Damp or Dryness are trapped in the body for a time. In this case they can combine together and start generating Heat. For the purposes of this section, Summer Heat and Fire will be referred to jointly as 'Heat'.

Heat moves in an upward direction and can make people restless. It can disturb the mind and spirit, causing anxiety and agitation. It can show itself in one area only, such as a red hot painful joint. It can also arise all over the body causing people to feel hot. Sunstroke is an obvious symptom arising from the heat, but there are many others. For example, Heat can combine with Damp causing inflammation. When people have an infection with a high fever they are affected by a combination of Wind and Heat.

The miscellaneous causes of disease

The miscellaneous causes of disease cover areas such as diet, overwork, exercise and sex. (Constitution and *jing* is also a miscellaneous cause of disease; see Chapter 3, this volume, for more on *jing*.) Most of these are to do with patients' lifestyles. In the twenty-first century people are less in contact with the natural rhythms of nature and the seasons than at any other time in history. They are also working longer and harder, breathing in more polluted air and often have poorer dietary habits. For these reasons the miscellaneous causes are a common cause of disease in most Western societies.

Diet

The Chinese understood that poor dietary habits are a major cause of illness and they especially affect the Stomach and Spleen. In response to this they created many dietary 'rules' that have been passed down through countless generations. These rules are flexible because everyone differs slightly in their dietary needs. In general, eating a well-proportioned diet will help people to maintain an efficiently functioning digestive system. Eating a varied diet, at regular times and without eating too late at night is also important, as is the temperature of food, the speed of eating it and the environment in which it is eaten. It is now common practice for many people to eat on the run during a short lunch break. This does not allow enough time for their food to be digested and nourish them. A poor diet can in turn lower resistance to disease and cause people to feel tired and depressed. A balanced diet consists of approximately 40–45% vegetables and 40–45% grains. More nutritious foods such as meat or dairy produce are richer and should be kept to a maximum of about 10–15%.

Work and rest

Chinese medicine puts great emphasis on the balance of activity and rest. In China most people will have a rest after lunch before they start working again. In the UK and the USA people may work through their lunch breaks and on into the afternoon – often on a diet of sandwiches and other cold foods. Overwork can adversely affect their Kidneys and cold food their Stomach and Spleen. 'Modern' times have dictated that people work harder and for longer periods and people tend not to take the time to replenish their *qi*. Along with this, people who do not take time off to recuperate from an infection risk severely weakening themselves. Their bodies can become too weak to throw off infection and this is a major cause of post-viral diseases. Other issues, such as the fulfilment people gain from their work and the amount of time they spend relaxing, are also extremely important if people wish to maintain their health.

Exercise

The correct balance between too much and too little exercise varies from individual to individual and it is important for people to take notice of their body's needs. Some people have been known to over-stimulate themselves to the point of collapse because they are obsessed by fitness. This generally weakens their *qi* and specifically their Kidneys and Spleen. Too little activity is just as bad. Studies have found that children are taking one-third less exercise than they were in the 1930s. In these days of increased car use, more television and computer games, children easily miss out on exercise.

Sex

The Chinese recognised that too much sex can be a cause of disease. They warned that this is especially important for men rather than women. Men can wear out their Kidney *jing* if they ejaculate too often. This can result in possible back problems, tiredness and premature ageing. The issue of what exactly is too much sex has been much debated in many texts throughout Chinese history. There is a natural balance between too much and too little sex. Too little sex can lead to much frustration and resentment, also possibly causing illness. In general the 'right' amount of sex could be said to be as much as satisfies each couple and is part of a fulfilling relationship for them both.

> Illnesses hover constantly about us, their seeds blown by the wind, but they do not set into the terrain unless the terrain is ready to receive them.
>
> (Claud Bernard)

> Bernard is right; the pathogen is nothing, the terrain is everything.
>
> (Louis Pasteur, the discoverer of bacteria, on his deathbed)

Appendix C: Four Needle Technique

The Four Needle technique is used in Five Element Constitutional Acupuncture for transferring *qi* from one Organ to another. It was first developed by the Korean monk, Sa Am, in the seventeenth century. It (or variants) is commonly used by Korean and Japanese practitioners for treating the root cause of a person's illness. (For example, it is used by the eminent practitioners Kuon Dowon in Korea and Nanagiya in Japan; see Eckman, 1996.)

Four Needle technique is based on Five Element theory that *qi* can be transferred from one Element to another along the *sheng* and *ke* cycles. This is in keeping with the principle expressed in *Su Wen* Chapter 5:

> If there is a *qi* deficiency in a particular location or channel, the *qi* can be conducted or guided from other channels to supplement the weakness.
>
> (Ni, 1995)

The Four Needle technique uses 'command' points to transfer *qi* and supports this by treating the Element that 'controls' the Element that is being primarily treated. In Five Element Constitutional Acupuncture it is only used if the practitioner is unable to harmonise the *qi* of two Elements along the *sheng* cycle. This is particularly the case when treating a Husband–Wife imbalance (see Chapter 32, this volume).

It can be used to tonify an Organ or to sedate it, although tonification is far more common.

Tonification

The principle of tonification is to tonify the horary point on the 'mother' Organ to give it a boost and to tonify the tonification point on the deficient Organ to transfer the *qi* from the 'mother'. At the same time the Element point of the 'controlling' Element is sedated on the deficient Organ as well as the horary/Element point on the Organ that controls the deficient Organ. This lessens the 'control' of the Organ and makes the transfer more effective.

In the case of the Kidneys, therefore, the following points are tonified:

- Lu 8 – the horary/Element point
- Kid 7 – the tonification point

At the same time, the following points are sedated:

- Kid 3 – the Earth point (Earth controls Water)
- Sp 3 – the horary/Element point

In practice, unless practitioners use the Four Needle technique often, they look up the combination of points from the following table (Table C.1).

Sedation

The Four Needle technique can also be used to sedate an Organ, although this is used less than the tonification technique. The principle here is to sedate the sedation point on the affected Organ along with the horary/Element point on the 'child' Organ. The point resonant with the Element that controls the Organ is simultaneously tonified along with the horary point on the controlling Organ.

The points are given in Table C.2.

Table C.1 Four Needle technique – points used to tonify an Organ

Organ	Tonify	Tonify	Sedate	Sedate
Lung	Lu 9	Sp 3	Lu 10	Ht 8
Large Intestine	LI 11	St 36	LI 5	SI 5
Stomach	St 41	SI 5	St 43	GB 41
Spleen	Sp 2	Ht 8	Sp 1	Liv 1
Heart	Ht 9	Liv 1	Ht 3	Kid 10
Small Intestine	SI 3	GB 41	SI 2	Bl 66
Bladder	Bl 67	LI 1	Bl 40	St 36
Kidney	Kid 7	Lu 8	Kid 3	Sp 3
Pericardium	PC 9	Liv 1	PC 3	Kid 10
Triple Burner	TB 3	GB 41	TB 2	Bl 66
Gall Bladder	GB 43	Bl 66	GB 44	LI 1
Liver	Liv 8	Kid 10	Liv 4	Lu 8

Table C.2 Four Needle technique – points used to sedate an Organ

Organ	Sedate	Sedate	Tonify	Tonify
Lung	Lu 5	Kid 10	Lu 10	Ht 8
Large Intestine	LI 2	Bl 66	LI 5	SI 5
Stomach	St 45	LI 1	St 43	GB 41
Spleen	Sp 5	Lu 8	Sp 1	Liv 1
Heart	Ht 7	Sp 3	Ht 3	Kid 10
Small Intestine	SI 8	St 36	SI 2	Bl 66
Bladder	Bl 65	GB 41	Bl 40	St 36
Kidney	Kid 1	Liv 1	Kid 3	Sp 3
Pericardium	PC 7	Sp 3	PC 3	Kid 10
Triple Burner	TB 10	St 36	TB 2	Bl 66
Gall Bladder	GB 38	SI 5	GB 44	LI 1
Liver	Liv 2	Ht 8	Liv 4	Lu 8

Appendix D: Blocks from scars

Occasionally a scar that traverses or lies along a channel can impede a patient's *qi*. The scar may be from an operation or an injury. As normal healing takes place, the *qi* that has been affected will usually rejoin. In this case there will be no after-effects from the initial trauma.

Signs and symptoms of a blockage from a scar

If the scar is causing a blockage, it may cause discomfort or pain around the area even after it has healed on the surface. The patient may also say that the trauma took a long time to heal. Sometimes, although not always, this may have been due to infection on the site of the scar. The blockage from the scar may prevent the treatment from progressing as expected.

Treating a scar

To clear a block from a scar, insert needles into points on the blocked channel on either side of it.

For example, a common site for a scar is along the *Ren* channel after abdominal surgery. In this case choose points above and below the scar – such as *Ren* 2 and *Ren* 7. Tonify the points and retain the needles for at least 5–10 minutes to enable the *qi* to rejoin. When a scar traverses several channels, treat the points above and below the scar on each channel. The treatment may need to be repeated a few times in order that the *qi* is fully connected again.

Appendix E: Treatment reactions

The 'Law of Cure'

Origins

Constantine Hering (1800–1880), who was a student of Samuel Hahnemann (the originator of homeopathy), was the originator of the 'Law of Cure'. Although most of its roots are not found in Chinese medicine, it is still a useful tool to enable a practitioner to understand how the treatment process takes its course.

The Law

The Law of Cure states that during the course of treatment some patients will experience their symptoms:

(i) *Moving from the inside out.* For example, a patient can bring up phlegm as it is cleared from their system. Patients often feel better 'in themselves' before their symptoms start to clear.

(ii) *Moving from above to below.* For example, a pain may travel down a limb as it gets better until it clears from the extremities.

(iii) *Recurring in the reverse order from which they appeared.* For example, a patient may *briefly* experience a recurrence of some emotion or symptom from a past trauma before feeling better. This should only last from 24 to 48 hours after the treatment and after this the patient should feel better than before having the treatment.

A healing crisis

The Law of Cure does not stem from the theory of Chinese medicine. Most practitioners of Chinese medicine do, however, understand that patients may experience a 'healing crisis' after a treatment. A healing crisis is similar to point (iii) above in that patients often feel temporarily worse for 12–48 hours and then feel better than before they had the treatment. A healing crisis may be an important part of a patient's healing process. Some typical characteristics of a healing crisis are as follows:

- It usually has a rapid onset.
- Although the symptoms may be severe, the patient is not brought down by them and she or he retains a sense of well-being throughout the reaction.

It is useful to warn patients that on some rare occasions they may experience this positive reaction to treatment. It is essential to reassure the patient if a reaction occurs.

A treatment aggravation

If a patient has a reaction to treatment but the symptom is *not* cleared from the patient's system, then it is called an 'aggravation' rather than a healing crisis. If a patient has an aggravation they may *not* experience feeling better for up to 48 hours after the treatment and their symptoms may then

DOI: 10.1016/B978-0-7020-3175-5.00058-9

return to how they were prior to the treatment. In this case it may be necessary to reassess the treatment strategy before treating the patient again. It is tempting for some practitioners to hide behind the Law of Cure or a healing crisis when a patient has an aggravation. It is important, however, for the practitioner to recognise the difference between these two reactions in order to assess the true effect treatment is having on the patient.

Appendix F: Checklist for a traditional diagnosis

Name; age; address; telephone; e-mail; status; children; occupation

Main complaint

What is it? When did it start and what was happening around that time? Where is it located? What is its quality and intensity? If continuous or intermittent and if intermittent, its frequency? What makes it worse or better? What can or cannot the person do as a result of the problem? Associated symptoms? What other treatments has the patient tried? Any medication she or he has taken?

Secondary complaint(s)

Same as above.

Health history

• Birth: premature, health at birth • Early childhood: breast-fed or not, rashes, digestion, illnesses (mumps, scarlet fever, rheumatic fever, whooping cough, etc.) • Other past illnesses: accidents, injuries or visits to hospital • Drugs taken: medicinal or recreational, including alcohol • Smoking • Health of parents • Family diseases: siblings and their health.

Personal history

Relationship with parents and siblings and other significant relatives. Friends at school. Significant friends. Significant teachers, mentors or authority figures. Marriages and sexual relationships. Children. Difficult periods in the patient's life. Career. Religion. Hopes for the future.

Present situation

Married or living with partner. Housing (personal living accommodation). Jobs, friendships, children. Religious or spiritual beliefs. Hobbies and interests. Hopes for the future.

To ask: Questioning the systems

1. Sleep
2. Appetite, food and taste
3. Thirst and drink
4. Bowels
5. Urine
6. Temperature preference and sweating
7. Women's issues: (i) menstruation; (ii) discharges; (iii) pregnancy and childbirth; (iv) menopause
8. Head and body
9. Eyes and ears
10. Thorax and abdomen
11. Pain
12. Climate and season

DOI: 10.1016/B978-0-7020-3175-5.00059-0

To feel

Pulse diagnosis. Three *jiao*. Front *mu* and/or back *shu* points. Abdominal diagnosis. Palpating the channels. Palpating musculo-skeletal areas. Structural diagnosis of joints. Skin: temperature, moisture, texture. Nails: strength, ridges. Akabane test. Assessing for moxibustion.

Appendix G: Outcomes for treatment

The judgement as to whether treatment is working or not is often a sensitive one and depends on what criteria are used to judge this. Getting these criteria clear is worth some time and effort, but first the practitioner needs to acknowledge that there are two judges.

Different points of view

When deciding whether the patient is getting better, both the patient and the practitioner have a point of view. The patient brings the problem in the first place and so must, surely, know if they are getting better. The practitioner has treated many patients and has seen patients get better in a variety of ways so she or he also has a point of view.

In addition, Five Element Constitutional Acupuncture is not like taking an aspirin for a headache. The aspirin is successful if it goes straight to the headache and takes it away. It needs to do nothing else. Five Element Constitutional Acupuncture, by contrast, clears blocks and addresses a patient's constitutional imbalance. It specifically does not address the symptom of the headache by taking it away. Rather it treats the underlying *cause* of the headache so that it can get better. These differing points of view are examined below.

The patient's point of view

It seems obvious that patients will judge treatment according to its effect on the symptoms they initially complain about. They frequently want something to be taken away. What they want removed may be some form of pain or some disability, something that hurts or something their bodies now do badly. They do not always want their symptoms taken away, however. What patients ask for is conditioned strongly by what they would usually request of their doctor.

As treatment progresses, and patients feel better, they often understand that it is possible to ask for more than this. For example, they may start to have more vitality and feel more like they used to when they were younger. As a result, patients often change their outcomes for treatment. How they are changing as a person may become a greater priority than how their symptoms are changing. For instance, they may become more focused on their internal growth and development as they find that treatment helps them to feel better in themselves. In this case they are moving more *towards* feeling better than *away from* their symptom. It is important to monitor these changes so that the patient can receive the most benefit from treatment. This process is often labelled 'from symptom to self'.

A negotiated point of view

Towards the end of the case history the practitioner may ask the patient, 'How will you know you are getting better?' or 'How will you know that coming for treatment is worthwhile?' This question is equivalent to the request, 'What are your criteria for getting better and judging how you have benefited from treatment?' The answer to this question will provide the practitioner with milestones along the patient's road to health. If the patient is passing by these milestones, the diagnosis is being confirmed and supports

DOI: 10.1016/B978-0-7020-3175-5.00060-7

both the patient's and the practitioner's confidence in the treatment.

Sometimes the answer to this question is obvious as it relates directly to the patient's complaint. Sometimes, however, the practitioners are surprised. Whatever the answer, this is how the patient is proposing to judge the results of treatment. For this reason, when practitioners know the patient's criteria for getting better, it is useful to ask themselves the following questions.

- *Does the patient have any criteria for getting better?* Occasionally patients say something like, 'I just want to try acupuncture and see what it can do.' At this stage the practitioner would encourage the patient to think more seriously about treatment and come up with some desirable improvements in their health.

- *Is the patient only asking for negative outcomes, that is, what they want to exclude from their life?* If so, the practitioner may try to encourage them to also have some positive ones. For example, switching from, 'I don't want to feel tired and droopy any more' to 'I want to feel more like I did when I was in my twenties and I want to wake up thinking about what I am going to do.' One reason for this is that a conversation about negative outcomes can both dig the patient into a deeper rut and also drain both the practitioner and patient. Conversations about positive outcomes tend to lift people and specify a direction so that the outcomes are more likely to occur.

- *Are any parts of the patient's criteria unrealistic?* If so, it is better to let them know this at the beginning of treatment. For example, a patient may think that treatment can completely cure a degenerative disease. If this is the case the practitioner and patient need to have a discussion and find more realistic outcomes. These may include helping the patient to deal with the illness better, creating some improvement (but not necessarily a 'cure') and if possible stopping further deterioration.

- *Are the patient's criteria high enough?* If patients only ask for more mobility in the shoulder joint and the practitioner thinks that they might also have more energy, be able to breathe better and feel better in themselves, then the practitioner should let the patient know about these possibilities. One reason is that when these areas improve the patient may not realise that it was the acupuncture that helped this. The practitioner is also educating the patient to understand the overall benefits of acupuncture and this is better in the end for both the practitioner and patient.

It is worth making the effort to clarify both the practitioner's and the patient's outcomes for treatment. By doing this the practitioner usually helps the patient to avoid disappointment, makes the treatments more enjoyable and widens the patient's understanding of what acupuncture can do. In turn, the patient is likely to continue having treatment for longer and gain more benefit.

Appendix H: Diagnosing and treating element within element

We mentioned in Chapter 4 that sometimes the CF diagnosis goes one step further; that is, to the Element within the Element. If someone is a Fire CF, for example, a deeper diagnosis is to determine which Element is out of balance within the Fire. Is it Fire, Earth, Metal, Water or Wood? To make this diagnosis, as with all Five Element diagnoses, the basis is colour, sound, emotion and odour. This is a subtle level of diagnosis and is usually only undertaken after many years of practise and thus many years of observing colour, sound, emotion and odour.

The student will be aware that there are many shades of each colour. The same is true for sounds, emotions and odours. So initially the judgement when labelling these indicators is often to say, for example, that this colour look more like green than anything else. This allows the CF diagnosis to proceed.

A common overlap of colours is between yellow and green. The practitioner may ask 'Is this colour more green or more yellow?'. A similar process can occur with sounds, emotions and odours. Without doubt, it is better to concentrate on labelling the predominant colour, sound emotion or odour when first starting to practise. This is a sufficient task in itself.

However, at some point, after working on the CF with positive results, the practitioner may begin to wonder about a patient's Element within Element. When refining the diagnosis in this way, overlaps with respect to colour, sound, emotion and odour become important. The Metal CF who also looks slightly blue within the white, who tends to groan and who frequently responds to difficult situations with fear, may well have the Water Element imbalanced within the Metal.

How can the practitioner respond? In the first place, it is useful to keep in mind the phrase from the Hippocratic oath 'do no harm'. The practitioner may question if there are any points that have an Element within Element that might be harmful? For example, for a Fire CF, evidence may have accumulated that the patient is dry and too hot. In this case strengthening the Fire points of the Fire Element (using Ht 8 or PC 8) may seem to be inappropriate even if Fire within Fire is indicated by the colour, sound, emotion and odour. However, the other indicators may have been pointing to Water within Fire. So a judgement is made that treating the Water within Fire (using Ht 3 or PC 3) would probably be safe. The question then arises about how to proceed.

One first step would be to strengthen Water itself by using the source points of the Kidney and Bladder. If the Element within Element *is* Water within Fire, then simply strengthening Water itself would, in turn, have some impact on the Water within Fire. Determining the effectiveness of a second Element may give some support to a diagnosis primarily based on the colour, sound, emotion and odour. The practitioner may also evaluate the overall effect on the pulses of strengthening Water and notice, for example, if it is similar to a 'normal' CF pulse change (see Chapter 28).

DOI: 10.1016/B978-0-7020-3175-5.00061-9

The next step, and these steps might occur over more than one treatment, would be to treat the proposed Element within the CF. Again, the results would be assessed by the quality of pulse change, the patient's response at the time and the patient's feedback at the next treatment.

Experience suggests that, albeit very subtle, deepening diagnosis and treatment in this way can bring excellent results. (For an extended case history try Shifrin, Shouting for Sympathy, p. 169 in McPherson and Kaptchuk, 1997.)

Bibliography

Academy of Traditional Chinese Medicine: *An outline of Chinese acupuncture*, Beijing, 1975, Foreign Languages Press.

Allan S: *The Way of Water and Sprouts of Virtue*, Albany, 1997, State University of New York Press.

Anonymous: *Discussions of kidney diseases*, Hebei, 1979a, People's Publishing House.

Anonymous: *Chinese medical classics (Nei Ching and Nan Ching)*, Miami, FL, 1979b, Occidental Institute of Chinese Studies Alumni Association.

Anonymous: *The essentials of Chinese acupuncture*, Beijing, 1993, Foreign Languages Press.

Auden WH, Kronenberger L: *The Faber book of aphorisms*, London, 1962, Faber & Faber.

Austin M: *Acupuncture therapy*, New York, 1983, ASI.

Auteroche B, Gervais G, Auteroche M, Navailalh P, Toui-Kan E: *Acupuncture and moxibustion: a guide to clinical practice*, Edinburgh, 1992, Churchill Livingstone.

Becker E: *The denial of death*, New York, 1975, The Free Press.

Beinfield H, Korngold E: *Between Heaven and Earth*, New York, 1991, Ballantine Books.

Bensky D, Barolet R: *Formulas and strategies*, Washington, 2009, Eastland Press.

Bergson H: *Creative evolution*, London, 1988, Dover.

Bertschinger R: *The golden needle*, Edinburgh, 1991, Churchill Livingstone.

Birch S: Naming the unnameable: a historical study of radial pulse six position diagnosis, *Journal of the Traditional Acupuncture Society* 12:2–13, 1992.

Birch S: What is the Sanjiao, Triple Burner? An exploration, *European Journal of Oriental Medicine* 4(2):49–57, 2003.

Birch S, Felt R: *Understanding acupuncture*, Edinburgh, 1998, Churchill Livingstone.

Brooks M: *Instant rapport*, New York, 1989, Warner Books.

Bynner W: *The way of life according to Lao Tzu*, New York, 1962, Capricorn Books.

Carrithers M: *The category of the person*, Cambridge, 1985, Cambridge University Press.

Chan W: *Sources of Chinese tradition*, New York, 1960, Columbia University Press.

Chan W: *A source book in Chinese philosophy*, Princeton, 1963, Princeton University Press.

Chen EM: *Tao te Ching*, New York, 1989, Paragon House.

Cheng X, editor: *Chinese acupuncture and moxibustion*, Beijing, 1999, Foreign Languages Press.

Chia M: *Transform stress into vitality*, Huntington, NY, 1985, Healing Tao Books.

Chuang YM: *The historical development of acupuncture*, Los Angeles, CA, 1991, Oriental Healing Arts Institute.

Chung IK: *Shen Nung Ben Tsao (Shen Nong Ben Cao)*, Beijing, 1982, Chih Chu Ban She.

Cialdini RB: *Influence – science and practice*, Boston, MA, 2001, Allyn & Bacon.

Cleary T: *The human element*, Boston, MA, 1996, Shambhala.

Cleary T: *The essential Confucius*, Edison, NJ, 1998, Castle Books.

Cleary T: *The spirit of Tao*, Boston, MA, 2000, Shambhala.

Cleary T: *The inner teachings of Daoism*, Boston, MA, 2001, Shambhala.

Clearly T, translator: *Sun Tzu: The art of war*, Boston, MA, 2002, Shambhala.

Cleary T: *The Taoist I Ching*, Boston, MA, 2005, Shambhala.

College of Traditional Acupuncture: *Acupuncture point compendium*, Leamington Spa, 2000, College of Traditional Acupuncture.

Connelly D: *Traditional acupuncture: the law of the Five Elements*, Columbia, MD, 1994, The Centre for Traditional Acupuncture.

Dale J: Diversity amidst unity? Responses to a survey of acupuncture practitioners, *European Journal of Oriental Medicine* 2(1):48–54, 1996.

Davis S: The cosmobiological balance of the emotional and spiritual worlds: phenomenological structuralism in traditional Chinese medicine, thought, culture, *Medicine and Psychiatry* 20:83–123, 1996.

Dawkins R: *The selfish gene*, Oxford Paperbacks, 2009, Oxford.

De Bary WT, Watson B, Chan WT: *Sources of Chinese tradition*, New York, 1960, Columbia University Press.

Deadman P, Al-Khafaji M, Baker K: *A manual of acupuncture*, Hove, 2005, Journal of Chinese Medicine Publications.

Denmei S: *Introduction to meridian therapy*, Seattle, WA, 1990, Eastland Press.

Dey T: *Soothing the troubled mind*, Brookline, MA, 2000, Paradigm Publications.

Eckman P: *In the footsteps of the Yellow Emperor*, San Francisco, CA, 1996, Cypress Book Company.

Ekman P: *Emotions revealed*, New York, 2007, Times Books.

Ekman P, Friesen WV: *Unmasking the face*, Englewood Cliffs, NJ, 2003, Prentice-Hall.

Ellis A, Wiseman N, Boss K: *The fundamentals of Chinese acupuncture*, Brookline, MA, 1988, Paradigm Publications.

Ellis A, Wiseman N, Boss K: *Grasping the wind*, Brookline, MA, 1993, Paradigm Publications.

Evans D: *Emotion, the science of sentiment*, Oxford, 2002, Oxford University Press.

Felt R, Zmiewski P: *Acumoxa therapy*, vol 1, Brookline, MA, 1993, Paradigm Publications.

Flaws B: Four LA blocks to treatment, *Traditional Acupuncture Society Journal* 6:5–8, 1989.

Flaws B: Keeping up with the Jones's, *Journal of Chinese Medicine* 35:27–29, 1991.

Flaws B, Lake J: *Chinese medical psychiatry*, Boulder, CO, 2000, Blue Poppy Press.

Frantzis BK: *Opening the energy gates of your body*, Berkeley, CA, 2006, North Atlantic Books.

Fruehauf H: *The Five Organ networks of Chinese medicine*, Portland, OR, 1998, Institute for Traditional Medicine.

Fruehauf H: Chinese medicine in crisis, *Journal of Chinese Medicine* 61:6–14, 1999.

Gascoigne S: *The manual of conventional medicine for alternative practitioners*, Richmond, VA, 1993, Jigme Press.

Gauquelin M: *How atmospheric conditions affect your health*, New York, 1980, ASI.

Goleman D: *Emotional intelligence*, London, 2005, Bloomsbury.

Hammer L: *Chinese pulse diagnosis*, Seattle, WA, 2001, Eastland Press.

Harlow H, Harlow M: Social deprivation in monkeys, *Sci Am* 207(5):136–146, 1962.

Hicks A: *77 Ways to improve your wellbeing*, Oxford, 2009, How To Books.

Hicks A, Hicks J: *Healing your emotions*, London, 1999, Thorsons.

Hicks S: *Acupuncture point names*. Privately published, 1999. Available from info@cicm.org.uk.

Hill S: *Reclaiming the wisdom of the body*, London, 2000, Constable.

Holford P: *Optimum nutrition for the mind*, London, 2003, Piatkus.

Housheng L, Peiyu L: *Three hundred questions on qigong exercises*, Guanzhai China, 1994, Guangdong Science and Technology Press.

Hsu E: *The transmission of Chinese medicine*, Cambridge, 1999, Cambridge University Press.

Hsu E, editor: *Innovation in Chinese medicine*, Cambridge, 2001, Cambridge University Press.

Jarrett L: *Nourishing destiny*, Stockport, MA, 1998, Spirit Path Press.

Kaptchuk T: *The web that has no weaver*, Chicago, 2000, Contemporary Publishing Group.

Kornfield J: *A path with heart*, London, 2002, Rider.

Lade A: *Acupuncture points: images and functions*, Seattle, WA, 2005, Eastland Press.

Larre C: *The way of heaven*, Cambridge, 1996, Monkey Press.

Larre C, Rochat de la Vallée E: *The secret treatise of the spiritual orchid*, Cambridge, 1992, Monkey Press.

Larre C, Rochat de la Vallée E: *Rooted in spirit*, New York, 1995, Station Hill Press.

Larre C, Rochat de la Vallée E: *The seven emotions*, Cambridge, 1996, Monkey Press.

Larre C, Rochat de la Vallée E: *Heart Master and Triple Burner*, Cambridge, 1998, Monkey Press.

Larre C, Rochat de la Vallée E: *The Liver*, Cambridge, 1999, Monkey Press.

Larre C, Rochat de la Vallée E: *The Lung*, Cambridge, 2001, Monkey Press.

Larre C, Rochat de la Vallée E: *Spleen and Stomach*, Cambridge, 2004, Monkey Press.

Larre C, Schatz J, Rochat de la Vallée E: *Survey of traditional Chinese medicine*, Paris, 1986, Institut Ricci.

Lavier J: *Histoire, doctrine et practique de l'acupuncture chinoise*, Paris, 1966, Tchou.

Lawson-Wood D, Lawson-Wood J: *Five Elements of acupuncture and Chinese massage*, Bradford, 1965, Health Science Press.

Liu Y: *The essential book of traditional Chinese medicine*, Beijing and San Francisco, 1988, People's Medical Publishing House and the United States–China Educational Institute.

Lo V: Crossing the *Neiguan*, 'inner pass': a *nei/wai* 'inner/outer' distinction in early Chinese medicine, *International Society for the History of East Asian Science, Technology and Medicine*, 17:15–65, 2000.

Lo V: The influence of nurturing life culture on the devolment of Western Han acumoxa therapy. In Hsu E, editor: *Innovation in Chinese medicine*, Cambridge, 2001, Cambridge University Press, pp 19–51.

Lo V: Translation of *Yinshu* given at a seminar at University College, London, 25 February 2003, 2003.

Loewe M, editor: *Early Chinese texts: a bibliographical guide*, Berkeley, CA, 1993, SSEC and Institute of East Asian Studies, University of California.

Lu GD, Needham J: *Celestial lancets: a history and rationale of acupuncture and moxibustion*, Cambridge, 1980, Cambridge University Press.

Lu H: *A complete translation of the Yellow Emperor's classic of internal medicine (Nei Jing and Nan Jing)*, Vancouver, 1972, Academy of Oriental Heritage.

Maciocia G: The psyche in Chinese medicine, *The European Journal* 1(1):10–18, 1993.

Maciocia G: *The foundations of Chinese medicine*, Edinburgh, 2005, Churchill Livingstone.

Maciocia G: *The practice of Chinese medicine*, Edinburgh, 2008, Churchill Livingstone.

McDonald J: Curtains for the Windows of the Sky, *Pacific Journal of Oriental Medicine* 14:11–18, 1992.

MacPherson H, Kaptchuk T: *Acupuncture in practice*, Edinburgh, 1997, Churchill Livingstone.

Major J: *Heaven and Earth in early Han thought*, New York, 1993, State University of New York.

Manaka Y, Itaya K, Birch S: *Chasing the dragon's tail*, Brookline MA, 1995, Paradigm Publications.

Mann F: *The treatment of disease by acupuncture*, London, 1963, Heinemann.

Mann F: *Acupuncture: The ancient Chinese art of healing*, London, 1971, Heinemann.

Martin P: *The sickening mind*, London, 1997, Harper Collins.

Matsumoto K, Birch S: *Five Elements and ten stems*, Brookline, MA, 1993a, Paradigm Publications.

Matsumoto K, Birch S: *Hara diagnosis, reflections on the sea*, Brookline, MA, 1993b, Paradigm Publications.

Merton T: (trans) *The way of Chuang Tzu*, London, 1970, George Allen & Unwin.

Mole P: The Triple Burner, *European Journal of Oriental Medicine* 1(3):42–46, 1994.

Mole P: Give me that old time religion, *European Journal of Oriental Medicine* 2(5):27–33, 1998.

Moody R: *Life after life*, Covington, GA, 2001, Bantam Books.

Morgan LH: *Ancient society, or researches in the lines of human progress from savagery through barbarism to civilisation*, New York, 1877, Holt.

Needham J: *Science and civilisation in China*, vol 2, Cambridge, 1956, Cambridge University Press.

Ni M: *The Yellow Emperor's classic of medicine*, Boston, MA, 1995, Shambhala.

O'Connor J, Seymour J: *Introducing neuro-linguistic programming*, London, 2003, Thorsons.

Patel A, Knapp M: *The cost of mental health in England. Mental Health Research Review 5*, 1998, Centre for the Economics of Mental Health.

Pert C: *The molecules of emotion. Why we feel what we feel*, New York, 1999, Scribner.

Porkert M: *The theoretical foundations of Chinese medicine*, Cambridge, MA, 1982, MIT Press.

Reber A, Reber E: *The Penguin dictionary of psychology*, London, 1985, Penguin.

Requena Y: *Character and health. The relationship of acupuncture and psychology*, Brookline, MA, 1989, Paradigm Publications.

Richardson J: *The magic of rapport*, Capitola, CA, 2000, Meta Publications.

Ronan C, Needham J: *The shorter science and civilisation in China*, vol 1, Cambridge, 1993, Cambridge University Press.

Rose K, Zhang YH: *A brief history of qi*, Brookline, MA, 2001, Paradigm Publications.

Rossi E: *Shen: Psycho-emotional aspects of Chinese medicine*, Edinburgh, 2007, Elsevier.

Roth H: The Early Taoist concept of *shen*: a ghost in the machine. In *Sagehood and systematizing thought in warring states and Han China*, 1986, Asian Studies Programme, Bowdoin College, pp 47–56.

Scheid V: *Yin/yang and the five phases*, *Traditional Acupuncture Society Journal* 3:14–22, 1988.

Scheid V: *Chinese medicine in contemporary China*, Durham, NC, 2002, Duke University Press.

Scheid V, Bensky D: Medicine as signification – moving towards healing power in the Chinese medical tradition, *European Journal of Oriental Medicine* 2(6):32–41, 1998.

Schipper K: *The Taoist body*, Berkeley, CA, 1993, University of California Press.

Schmidt H: Constitutional acupuncture therapy, *Traditional Acupuncture Society Journal* 8:10–16, 1990.

Scott J: Pulse diagnosis, *Journal of Chinese Medicine* 14:2–14, 1984.

Sivin N: *Traditional medicine in contemporary China*, 1987, University of Michigan: Center for Chinese Studies.

Soulié de Morant G: *Chinese acupuncture*, Brookline, MA, 1994, Paradigm Publications.

Stationery Office : *Department of Health statistics of prescriptions dispensed in FHSA's England 1985–1996*, London, 1996, Stationery Office.

Sun SM: *Supplemental wings to the thousand ducat prescriptions, Qian Jin Fang*, Beijing, 1982, People's Press.

Sunu K: *The canon of acupuncture*, Los Angeles, CA, 1985, Yuin University Press.

Thibodeau G, Patton K: *The human body in health and disease*, London, 1992, Mosby.

Tzu S: *The art of war*, Boston, MA, 1991, Shambhala.

Unschuld P: *Nan Ching*, Berkeley, CA, 1986, University of California Press.

Unschuld P: *Introductory readings in Chinese medicine*, Dordrecht, 1988, Kluwer Academic.

Unschuld P: *Approaches to Chinese medical literature*, Dordrecht, 1989, Kluwer.

Unschuld P: *Forgotten traditions of ancient Chinese medicine*, Brookline, MA, 1990, Paradigm Publications.

Unschuld P: *Medicine in China. A history of ideas*, Berkeley, CA, 1992, University of California Press.

Veith I: *The Yellow Emperor's classic of internal medicine*, Berkeley, CA, 1972, University of California Press.

Waley A: *The way and its power*, London, 1965, George Allen & Unwin.

Wang W, translator: *I Hsien*, Shanghai, 1990, Shanghai san lien shen tien.

Watson B: *Chuang Tzu basic writings*, New York, 1964, Columbia University Press.

Weiger L: *Chinese characters*, New York, 1965, Dover.

Wilhelm R: *I Ching or book of changes*, London, 1951, Routledge & Kegan Paul.

Willmont D: *Energetic physiology of acupuncture point names*, Roslindale, 2001, Will Mountain Press.

Wiseman N: *Glossary of Chinese medical terms and acupuncture points*, Brookline, MA, 1993, Paradigm Publications.

Wiseman N, Ellis A, Zmienski P: *The fundamentals of Chinese medicine*, Brookline, MA, 1995, Paradigm Publications.

Worsley JR: *Traditional Chinese acupuncture*, vol 1, Meridians and points, Tisbury, 1982, Element Books.

Worsley J: Professor J. R. Worsley. A profile, *Traditional Acupuncture Society Journal* 1:1–2, 1987.

Worsley JR: *Traditional acupuncture*, vol II, Traditional diagnosis, Leamington Spa, 1990, College of Traditional Acupuncture.

Worsley JR: *The Five Elements and the Officials*, vol III, 1998, JR & JB Worsley.

Wu JN: *Ling Shu or the spiritual pivot*, Washington, DC, 1993, Taoist Center.

Xinghua B, Baron RB: Flood control and the origins of acupuncture in ancient China, *Journal of Chinese Medicine* no. 67, 2001.

Yang JM: *The root of Chinese Chi Kung*, Roslindale, 1997, Yang's Martial Arts Association Publication Centre.

Yang S, Chace C: *Huang Fu Mi: The systematic classic of acupuncture and moxibustion*, Boulder, CO, 1994, Blue Poppy Press.

Young P: *Understanding NLP*, Carmarthen, 2004, Crown House Publishing.

Zhang YH, Rose K: *Who can ride the dragon?*, Brookline, MA, 2000, Paradigm Publications.

Zhen J: *Da Cheng*, Hong Kong, 1996, Guang Publishing Company.

Zhou Y: *Discussions on the character of medicine by famous physicians of past dynasties*, Changsha, 1983, People's Publishing Company.

Glossary

Aggressive Energy A form of 'perverse' (*xie*) or 'polluted' *qi* that can occur in the *yin* Organs.

Back *shu* points The Back *shu* points lie on the Bladder channel next to the spine. There is one point for each of the Organs and they have a powerful effect by making direct contact with the Organ.

Ben The root of a person's imbalance.

Biao The manifestation of a person's imbalance.

Blood Blood is rarely mentioned in Five Element Constitutional Acupuncture. It moistens and nourishes the body and houses the *shen*.

Channels The pathways or 'meridians' of *qi*. There are 12 main channels that are linked to each Organ as well as the *Ren* and *Du* channels, which traverse the back and front of the body. Other channels, less used in Five Element Constitutional Acupuncture, are the Eight Extraordinary channels, the *luo* channels, the divergent channels, the *luo*-connecting channels and the muscles and cutaneous channels.

CF (Constitutional Factor) A person's constitutionally weakest Element. The main focus of treatment in Five Element Constitutional Acupuncture.

Cun Measurement used for point location. For example, there are 12 *cun* between the wrist and elbow creases.

Dan tian Three centres of *qi* in the body. The lower *dan tian*, situated just below the navel, is usually regarded as the most important.

Dao The 'way' or 'principle' that underlies and organises all creation.

Dong qi 'Stirring' *qi*, virtually synonymous with *yuan qi*.

Dragons The combinations of points used to treat 'possession'.

Du channel The channel of the *Du mai* (one of the extraordinary vessels). It runs up the spine and over the head, ending in the mouth.

Eight Extraordinary Vessels The eight vessels that act as reservoirs of *qi* for the channels. Each vessel has its own functions (see Maciocia, 2005, pp. 819–887).

Five Elements/Phases The five different qualities of *qi* that form once the *Dao* divides. Best exemplified by the cyclical succession of the seasons.

Huang A minor centre of *qi* in the body, often translated as 'vitals'.

Hun The 'ethereal' spirit of the Liver.

Jing One of the 'three treasures' of humanity. Stored in the Kidneys; it is our essence or genetic inheritance.

Jing-shen The human spirit. A union of our genetic inheritance and what heaven bestows on us.

Jingyan Usually translated as 'experience', but it implies a level of excellence that can only come with experience.

Ke cycle The 'controlling' cycle between Elements.

Ling The *yin* aspect of the spirit of the Heart. It is now usually excluded from Chinese medicine.

Ming men Sited between the kidneys, it generates the body's warmth.

Official Description of an Organ as given in *Su Wen* Chapter 8.

Organ A complex system that focuses upon a wide range of functions rather than just the anatomical structure.

Pathogenic factors The 'external' causes of disease, i.e. climatic factors, which can 'invade' a person's *qi*.

Phlegm Phlegm usually arises from the condensation of body fluids. It can mean the same as in the West, but can also have wider meaning. For example, Phlegm can 'obstruct' the Heart, causing psychological problems, as well as muzzy heads, nodules and bony protuberances.

Po The 'corporeal' spirit of the Lungs.

Points The places on the channels of the body where the *qi* can be most easily influenced.

Possession A term used to describe when a person is no longer fully in control of their mind or spirit.

Pulse diagnosis A traditional method of feeling the pulse in different positions on the wrist to diagnose the condition of the Organs, *qi* and Blood.

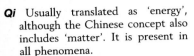

Qi Usually translated as 'energy', although the Chinese concept also includes 'matter'. It is present in all phenomena.

Qi gong Exercises designed to move and harmonise a person's *qi*.

Rapport The bond of trust and intimacy that exists between people.

Ren 'Benevolence' or 'compassion'.

Ren channel The channel of the *Ren mai* (one of the extraordinary vessels). It runs up the front of the body.

Resonances The 'associations' or 'correspondences' between the Elements, seasons, emotions, odours, climates, etc.

Shen In some contexts the 'spirit' of the Heart, in others the person's spirit in its entirety.

Sheng cycle The cycle of 'creation' or 'engendering' between the Elements.

Substances The various manifestations of *qi* in various degrees of density. They are body fluids, Blood, *jing*, *qi* and *shen*.

Syndrome A pattern of disharmony in an Organ which is defined by pathology of *yin/yang*, substances and pathogenic factors.

Tai ji Exercises designed to move and harmonise the *qi* in the body.

Wei qi The body's defensive or protective *qi* which is governed by the Lungs.

Xie qi 'Perverse' or 'polluted' *qi*. Unhealthy *qi*.

Yi Thought and intention. The spirit of the Spleen.

Yin/Yang When the Dao divides into two, *yin*, the passive principle, and *yang*, the active principle, become manifest.

Yuan qi *Jing* in *qi* form.

Zheng qi 'Upright' or healthy *qi*.

Zhi The human will. The spirit of the Kidneys.

Zong qi The *qi* of the chest.

Index

NB: Page numbers followed by *f* indicate figures; *t* indicate tables; *b* indicate boxes

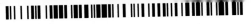

Printed in the United States
By Bookmasters